CLINICAL
OBSTETRICS &
GYNAECOLOGY

This book is dedicated to the millions of women worldwide who will suffer disability, lose their babies or lose their lives through the want of adequate reproductive healthcare.

CLINICAL
OBSTETRICS &
GYNAECOLOGY

FOURTH EDITION

BRIAN A. MAGOWAN MBCHB FRCOG DIPFETMED
Consultant Obstetrician and Gynaecologist
Borders General Hospital
Melrose, UK

PHILIP OWEN MBBCH MD FRCOG
Consultant Obstetrician and Gynaecologist
Princess Royal Maternity Unit
Glasgow, UK

ANDREW THOMSON MBCHB MRCOG MD
Consultant Obstetrician and Gynaecologist
Royal Alexandra Hospital
Paisley, UK

ELSEVIER

ELSEVIER

Notices

ISBN: 978-0-7020-7404-2
International ISBN: 978-0-7020-7405-9
e-ISBN: 978-0-7020-7407-3
Printed in China
Last digit is the print number: 9 8 7 6 5 4 3 2

Content Strategist: Pauline Graham
Content Development Specialist: Nani Clansey
Project Manager: Andrew Riley
Design: Patrick Ferguson
Illustration Manager: Amy Faith Heyden
Marketing Manager: Deborah Watkins

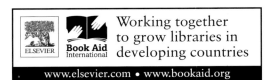

Working together
to grow libraries in
developing countries

www.elsevier.com • www.bookaid.org

Preface

Obstetrics and gynaecology continues to evolve, and we have been keen to reflect this in our new fourth edition. In particular, we have streamlined some areas to allow new practical guidance on how to make the most of your clinical time spent in the speciality, and we have also added online videos to support this.

What remains constant, however, are the many challenges that obstetrics and gynaecology continues to offer: from the ethics of assisted conception treatments through the global importance of contraception, the challenges of gynaecological cancer care and the dilemmas of prenatal diagnosis, there is much with which to become familiar. Although there have been many global advances, hundreds of thousands of women are still dying each year from treatable pregnancy complications, nearly all in under-resourced countries. Many hurdles remain and these are still ours and hopefully now yours to overcome.

Wherever you study or practise obstetrics and gynaecology, a sound knowledge of the clinical aspects will underpin your understanding of this specialty and maximize your ability to learn about and contribute to the care of women. This book is aimed at providing you with that knowledge.

Brian A. Magowan
Philip Owen
Andrew Thomson

List of Contributors

The editors would like to acknowledge and offer grateful thanks for the input of all previous editions' contributors, without whom this new edition would not have been possible.

Charles Ameh MB BS DRH MPH FWACS (OBGYN)
Clinical Lecturer, Maternal and Newborn Health
Liverpool School of Tropical Medicine
Liverpool, UK

Claire Austin MBChB
Specialty Registrar Obstetrics and Gynaecology
South East Scotland, UK

Fraser Barratt BMedSci (Hons)
Obstetrics and Gynaecology Medical Student
Edinburgh University

Susan Brechin FRCOG, MD, FFSRH, FHEA, MIPM
Clinical Lead Sexual Health
Consultant in Sexual & Reproductive Health
NHS Grampian (Honorary Senior Clinical Lecturer, Aberdeen University)
Aberdeen, UK

Janet Brennan MD FRCOG
Consultant in Fetal and Maternal Medicine
Southern General Hospital
Glasgow, UK

Nynke van den Broek PhD FRCOG DTM&H
Professor in Maternal and Newborn Health
Liverpool School of Tropical Medicine
Liverpool, UK

Audrey Brown MRCOG
Consultant in Sexual and Reproductive Healthcare
Sandyford Initiative
Glasgow, UK

Eilidh S. Bruce BSc(Hons)
Obstetrics and Gynaecology Medical Student
Edinburgh University

Kevin Burton MD MRCOG
Consultant Gynaecology Oncologist
Glasgow Royal Infirmary
Glasgow, UK

Sharon Cameron MD
Honorary Professor
University of Edinburgh
Edinburgh, UK

Dan Clutterbuck FRCP MRCGP DFSRH
Consultant in Genitourinary and HIV Medicine
NHS Lothian University Hospitals Division
Edinburgh, UK

Simon Crawford MD MBA FRCS(Ed) MRCOG
Consultant Gynaecological Oncology Surgeon
Southampton University Hospitals NHS Foundation Trust
Southampton, UK

Kate Darlow MRCOG
Consultant Obstetrician and Gynaecologist
Borders General Hospital
Melrose, UK

Angela Davidson MBBS MRCPCH
Registrar in Paediatrics
The Royal Infirmary of Edinburgh
Edinburgh, UK

Mary Ross Davie PhD RM
Country Director, Royal College of Midwives
Scotland, UK

David R. FitzPatrick MD FRCP(Ed)
Professor and Joint Head, Medical and Developmental Genetics
Western General Hospital
Edinburgh, UK

David Gerber MRCPsych MBA
Clinical Lead for Psychosexual and Transgender Services
Sandyford Initiative
Glasgow, UK

Janice Gibson MBChB MD MRCOG
Consultant Obstetrician & Subspecialist in Maternal and Fetal Medicine
The Southern General Hospital
Glasgow, UK

Karen Guerrero FRCOG
NHR Senior Clinical Fellow and Lead Urogynaecologist
NHS Glasgow and Clyde
Queen Elizabeth University Hospital
Glasgow, UK

Kirun Gunganah MBBS, MRCP(UK), MRCP (Diabetes and Endocrinology), PGCME
Consultant in diabetes and Endocrinology
Newham University Hospital
London, UK

Daniel Hufton MBBS MRCPCH
Specialty Registrar in Paediatrics
Neonatal Unit, Simpson Centre for Reproductive Health
Royal Infirmary Edinburgh
Edinburgh, UK

Lorna Hutchison MBChB, MRCOG
Specialist Trainee in Obstetrics and Gynaecology
West of Scotland, UK

Stamatina Iliodromiti PhD, MD, MSc, MRCOG
Department of Obstetrics and Gynaecology
University of Glasgow
Glasgow, UK

Marie Anne Ledingham MBchB, MD, MRCOG, DFFP
Consultant Obstetrician and Fetal Maternal Medicine Specialist
NHS Greater Glasgow and Clyde
Scotland, UK

Mary Ann Lumsden MBBS FRCOG MD
Honorary Consultant Gynaecologist
Glasgow Royal Infirmary
Professor of Gynaecology and Medical Education
Clinical Head of Reproductive and Maternal Medicine
University of Glasgow
Glasgow, UK

Marjory MacLean MRCOG MD
Consultant Obstetrician
Ayrshire Maternity Unit
University Hospital of Crosshouse
Kilmarnock, UK

Brian Magowan MBCHB FRCOG DIPFETMED
Consultant Obstetrician and Gynaecologist
Borders General Hospital
Melrose, UK

Mayank Madhra MBChB MRCOG
Specialty Registrar Obstetrics and Gynaecology
South East Scotland, UK

Kay McAllister MRCOG
Consultant in Sexual and Reproductive Healthcare
Sandyford, Glasgow, UK

Jennifer McKay
FY2 in Obstetrics and Gynaecology, The Borders General Hospital
Melrose UK

Mohamed Mehasseb MBBCh, MSc, MD, MRCOG, PhD
Consultant Gynaecological Surgeon and Oncologist
Glasgow Royal Infirmar
Glasgow, UK

Hannah Mitchell MRCOG Bsc
Teaching Fellow
Imperial College Healthcare Trust
London, UK

Deirdre Murphy MD FRCOG
Professor of Obstetrics and Head of Department
Trinity College Dublin, University Hospital
Dublin, Ireland

Savita Brito-Mutunayagam MBchB (hons), BMedSci, DFSRH
Specialist Registrar in Sexual and Reproductive Health
Aberdeen, UK

Scott Nelson MRCOG PhD
Muirhead Professor of Obstetrics & Gynaecology
University of Glasgow
Glasgow,UK

Catherine Nelson Piercy MA FRCP FRCOG
Professor of Obstetric Medicine
Guy's and St Thomas' Foundation Hospital and Imperial College Healthcare Trust
London, UK

Philip Owen MBBCh MD FRCOG
Consultant Obstetrician and Gynaecologist
Department of Obstetrics
Princess Royal Maternity Unit
Glasgow, UK

Andrew Pearson BSc (MedSci)(Hons), DTM&H, MRCOG
Specialty Registrar Obstetrics and Gynaecology
South East Scotland, UK

Neelam Potdar MBBS, MD, MRCOG
Subspecialist Reproductive Medicine
Consultant Gynaecologist, Honorary Senior Lecturer
University Hospitals of Leicester NHS Trust
Leicester, UK

Jennifer Sassarini MBChB, PhD, MRCOG
Consultant Obstetrician and Gynaecologist
School of Medicine, College of Medical
Veterinary and Life Sciences
University of Glasgow
Glasgow, UK

Philip Savage MRCOG FRCP
Consultant Medical Oncologist
Charing Cross Hospital
London, UK

Andrew H. Shennan MBBS FRCOG MD
Professor of Obstetrics
King's College London and Clinical Director South London CRN
London, UK

Andrew Thomson MBChB MRCOG MD
Consultant Obstetrician and Gynaecologist
Royal Alexandra Hospital
Paisley UK

Derek Tufnell FRCOG
Consultant Obstetrician and Gynaecologist
Bradford Teaching Hospitals Foundation NHS Trust
Bradford, UK

Veenu Tyagi MRCOG
consultant urogynaecologist
NHS Greater Glasgow and Clyde
Queen Elizabeth University Hospital Glasgow

Brooke Vandermolen MBBS BSc
Specialty Registrar Obstetrics and Gynaecology
Women's Health Division
St Thomas Hospital
London, UK

Alex Viner MBChB
Specialty Registrar Obstetrics and Gynaecology
South East Scotland, UK

Cara Williams MRCOG
Consultant Gynaecologist
Liverpool Women's NHS Foundation Trust and Alder Hey Children's NHS Foundation Trust
Liverpool, UK

Video Table of Contents

Video List of Contributors

Claire Austin MBChB
Specialty Registrar Obstetrics and Gynaecology
South East Scotland, UK

Susan Brechin FRCOG, MD, FFSRH, FHEA, MIPM
Clinical Lead Sexual Health,
Consultant in Sexual & Reproductive Health,
NHS Grampian (Honorary Senior Clinical Lecturer, Aberdeen University)
Aberdeen, UK

Savita Brito-Mutunayagam MBchB (hons), BMedSci, DFSRH
Specialist Registrar in Sexual and Reproductive Health
Aberdeen, UK

Dan Clutterbuck FRCP MRCGP DFSRH
Consultant in Genitourinary and HIV Medicine
NHS Lothian University Hospitals Division
Edinburgh UK

Lorna Hutchison MBChB, MRCOG
Specialist Trainee in Obstetrics and Gynaecology
West of Scotland, UK

Mary Ann Lumsden MBBS FRCOG MD
Honorary Consultant Gynaecologist
Glasgow Royal Infirmary
Professor of Gynaecology and Medical Education
Clinical Head of Reproductive and Maternal Medicine
University of Glasgow
Glasgow, UK

Mayank Madhra MB ChB MRCOG
Specialty Registrar Obstetrics and Gynaecology
South East Scotland, UK

Brian Magowan MBCHB FRCOG DIPFETMED
Consultant Obstetrician and Gynaecologist
Borders General Hospital
Melrose, UK

Andrew Pearson BSc (MedSci)(Hons), DTM&H, MRCOG
Specialty Registrar Obstetrics and Gynaecology
South East Scotland, UK

Neelam Potdar MBBS, MD, MRCOG
Consultant Gynaecologist
Subspecialist Reproductive Medicine
Department of Gynaecology
Kensington Building
University Hospitals of Leicester NHS Trust
Leicester, UK

Contents

1

Clinical pelvic anatomy

Introduction

A thorough understanding of pelvic anatomy is essential for clinical practice. Not only does it facilitate an understanding of the process of labour, it also allows an appreciation of the mechanisms of sexual function and reproduction, and establishes a background to the understanding of gynaecological pathology. Congenital abnormalities are discussed in Chapter 3.

Obstetric anatomy

The bony pelvis

The girdle of bones formed by the sacrum and the two innominate bones has several important functions (Fig. 1.1). It supports the weight of the upper body, and transmits the stresses of weight bearing to the lower limbs via the acetabulae. It provides firm attachments for the supporting tissues of the pelvic floor, including the sphincters of the lower bowel and bladder, and it forms the bony margins of the birth canal, accommodating the passage of the fetus during labour.

The birth canal is bounded by the true pelvis, i.e. that part of the bony girdle which lies below the pelvic brim – the lower parts of the two innominate bones and the sacrum. These bones are bound together at the sacroiliac joints, and at the symphysis pubis anteriorly. The brim is outlined by the promontory of the sacrum, the sacral alae, the iliopectineal lines and the symphysis. The pelvic outlet is bounded by bone and ligament including the tip of the sacrum, the sacrotuberous ligaments, the ischial tuberosities and the subpubic arch (of rounded 'Norman' shape) formed by the fused rami of the ischial and pubic bones. In the erect posture the pelvic brim is inclined at an angle of 65–70° to the horizontal. Because of the curvature of the sacrum, the axis of the pelvis (the pathway of descent of the fetal head in labour) is a J-shaped curve (Fig. 1.2).

The change in the cross-sectional shape of the birth canal at different levels is fundamentally important in understanding the mechanics of labour. The canal can be envisaged initially as a sector of a curved cylinder of about 12 cm diameter (Fig. 1.2). The stresses of weight bearing at the brim level in the average woman tend to flatten the inlet a little, reducing the anteroposterior diameter but increasing the transverse diameter. In the lower pelvis, the counterpressure through the necks of the femora tends to compress the pelvis from the sides, reducing the transverse diameters of this part of the pelvis (Fig. 1.1). At an intermediate level, opposite the third segment of the sacrum, the canal retains a circular cross-section. With this picture in mind, the 'average' diameters of the pelvis at brim, cavity, and outlet levels can be readily understood (Table 1.1).

The distortions from a circular cross-section, however, are very modest. If, in circumstances of malnutrition or metabolic bone disease, the consolidation of bone is impaired, more gross distortion of the pelvic shape is liable to occur, and labour is likely to involve mechanical difficulty. This is termed cephalopelvic disproportion. The changing cross-sectional shape of the true pelvis at different levels – transverse oval at the brim and anteroposterior oval at the outlet – usually determines a fundamental feature of labour, i.e. that the ovoid fetal head enters the brim with its longer (anteroposterior) diameter in a transverse or oblique position, but rotates during descent to bring the longer head diameter into the longer anteroposterior diameter of the outlet before the time of birth. This rotation is necessary because of the relatively large size of the human fetal head at term, which reflects the unique size and development of the fetal brain.

In most affluent countries, marked pelvic deformation is rare. Pelvimetry using X-rays, computed tomography or magnetic resonance imaging scans can be used to measure the pelvic diameters but is of limited clinical value in predicting the likelihood of a successful vaginal delivery. Mechanical difficulty in labour is assessed by close observation of the progress of dilatation of the cervix, and of descent, assessed by both abdominal and vaginal examination.

The pelvic organs during pregnancy

The uterus

The uterus is a remarkable organ, composed largely of smooth muscle (the myometrium), which increases in weight during pregnancy from about 40 g to around 1000 g as the myometrial muscle fibres undergo both hyperplasia and hypertrophy (Fig. 1.3). It provides a 'protected' implantation site for the genetically 'foreign' fertilized ovum, accommodates the developing fetus as it grows and, finally, expels it into the outside world during labour.

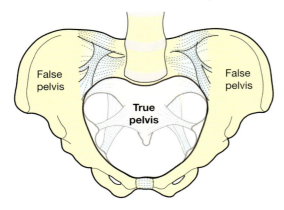

Fig. 1.1 The 'true' and 'false' pelvis.

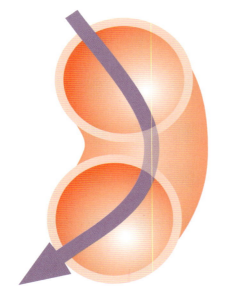

Fig. 1.2 The birth canal resembles a curved cylinder.

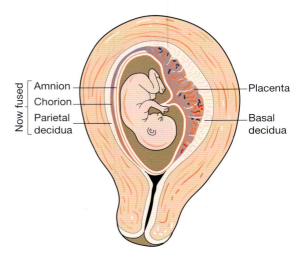

Fig. 1.3 The uterus and developing fetus at 12 weeks' gestation.

Table 1.1	Average pelvic diameters		
	Diameter		
Level	**Direction**		**Size (cm)**
Inlet	Anteroposterior		11.5
	Transverse		13
Cavity	All diameters		12
Outlet	Anteroposterior		12.5
	Transverse intertuberous		11
	Interspinous		10.5

Whereas the body of the uterus is formed from a thick layer of plain muscle, the cervix, which communicates with the upper vagina, is largely composed of denser collagenous tissue. This forms a rigid collar, retaining the fetus in utero as the myometrium hypertrophies and stretches. The junctional area between the body and cervix is known as the isthmus, which, in late pregnancy and labour, undergoes dilatation and thinning, forming the lower segment of the uterus. It is through this thinned area that the uterine wall is incised during caesarean section.

The uterine arteries, branches of the anterior division of the internal iliac arteries, become tortuous and coiled within the uterine wall (Fig. 1.4). Innervation of the uterus is derived from both sympathetic and parasympathetic systems, and the functional significance of the motor pathways is incompletely understood. Drugs that stimulate alpha-adrenergic receptors activate the myometrium, whereas beta-adrenergic drugs have an inhibitory effect, and both beta-agonists and alpha-antagonists have been used in attempts to inhibit premature labour. Afferent fibres from the cervix enter the spinal cord via the pelvic splanchnic (parasympathetic) nerves (S2,3,4). Pain stimuli during labour from the fundus and body of the uterus travel via the hypogastric (sympathetic) plexus, and enter the spinal cord at the level of the lower thoracic segments.

The cervix

This becomes more vascular and softens in early pregnancy. The mucous secretion from the endocervical glands becomes thick and tenacious, forming a mechanical barrier to ascending infection. In late pregnancy the cervix 'ripens' – the dense mesh of collagen fibres loosens, as fluid is taken up by the hydrophilic mucopolysaccharides that occupy the interstices between the collagen bundles. This allows the cervix to become shorter as its upper part expands.

Additional changes

The ligaments of the sacroiliac and symphyseal joints become more extensible under the influence of pregnancy hormones. As a result, the pelvic girdle has more 'give' during labour. The increased mobility of the joints may result in backache or symphyseal pain.

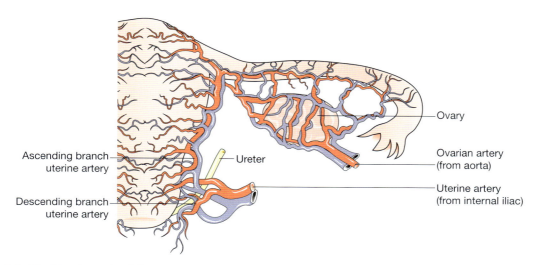

Fig. 1.4   **The blood supply of the uterus, fallopian tube and ovary (posterior view).**

The urinary tract in pregnancy

Frequency of micturition is often noticed in early pregnancy. As pregnancy advances, the ureters become dilated, probably due to the relaxing effect of progesterone on the smooth muscle wall, but also in part due to the mechanical effects of the gravid uterus. The urinary tract is therefore more vulnerable to ascending infection (acute pyelonephritis) in comparison to non-pregnancy.

The perineum

This term usually refers to the area of skin between the vaginal orifice and the anus. The underlying musculature at the outlet of the pelvis, surrounding the lower vagina and the anal canal, is important in the maintenance of bowel and urinary continence, and in sexual response. The muscles intermesh to form a firm pyramidal support, the perineal body, between the lower third of the posterior vaginal wall and the anal canal (Fig. 1.5). The tissues of the perineal body are often markedly stretched during the expulsive second stage of labour and may be torn as the head is delivered. Injury to the anal sphincters may lead to impaired anal continence of faeces and/or flatus. Poor healing of an episiotomy or tear is liable to result in scarring, which may cause dyspareunia (pain during intercourse).

Anatomical points for obstetric analgesia

Pudendal nerve block

Knowledge of the pudendal nerves is important in obstetrics because they may be blocked to minimize pain during instrumental delivery, and because their integrity is vital for visceral muscular support and for sphincter function. These nerves, which innervate the vulva and perineum, are derived from the second, third and fourth sacral roots (see Fig. 1.2). On each side the nerve passes behind the sacrospinous ligament close to the tip of the ischial spine and re-enters the pelvis, along with the pudendal blood vessels, in the pudendal canal. After giving off an inferior rectal branch, they divide into the perineal nerves and the dorsal nerves of the clitoris. Motor fibres of the pudendal nerve supply the levator ani, the superficial and deep perineal muscles, and the voluntary urethral sphincter. Sensory fibres innervate the central areas of the vulva and perineum. The peripheral skin areas are supplied by branches of the ilioinguinal nerve, the genitofemoral nerve and the posterior femoral cutaneous nerve (Fig. 1.6). The pudendal nerve can be blocked by an injection of local anaesthetic just below the tip of the ischial spine, as described in Fig. 30.13.

Spinal block

The spinal cord ends at the level of L1–2. A spinal injection at the level of the L3–4 space will produce excellent analgesia up to around the level of the T10 nerve root or above, depending on the position of the patient and the volume of local anaesthetic used.

Epidural block

The epidural space, between the dura and the periosteum and ligaments of the spinal canal, is about 4 mm deep. Epidural injection of local anaesthetic blocks the spinal nerve roots as they traverse the space.

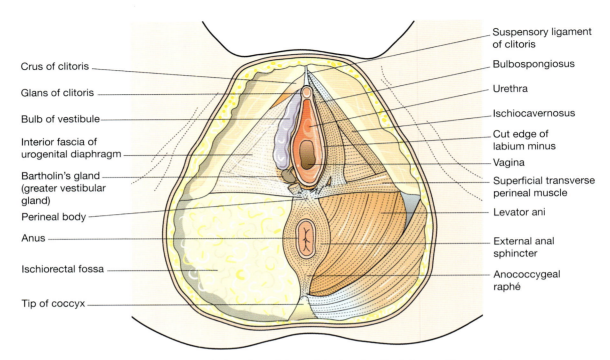

Crus of clitoris

Glans of clitoris

Bulb of vestibule

Interior fascia of
urogenital diaphragm

Bartholin's gland
(greater vestibular
gland)

Perineal body

Anus

Ischiorectal fossa

Tip of coccyx

Suspensory ligament
of clitoris

Bulbospongiosus

Urethra

Ischiocavernosus

Cut edge of
labium minus

Vagina

Superficial transverse
perineal muscle

Levator ani

External anal
sphincter

Anococcygeal
raphé

Fig. 1.5 The perineum: a view from below the pelvic outlet, showing the intermeshing muscles.

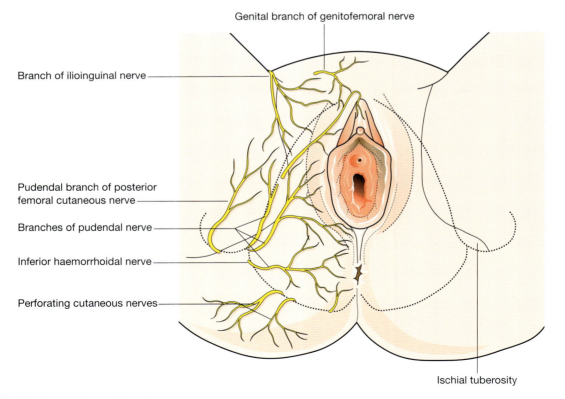

Genital branch of genitofemoral nerve

Branch of ilioinguinal nerve

Pudendal branch of posterior
femoral cutaneous nerve

Branches of pudendal nerve

Inferior haemorrhoidal nerve

Perforating cutaneous nerves

Ischial tuberosity

Fig. 1.6 Innervation of the vulva.

Gynaecological anatomy

The uterus

The uterus has the shape of a slightly flattened pear, and measures 7.5 × 5.0 × 2.5 cm. Its principal named parts are the fundus, the cornua, the body and the cervix (Fig. 1.7).

It forms part of the genital tract, lying in close proximity to the urinary tract anteriorly and the lower bowel behind. All three tracts traverse the pelvic floor in the hiatus between the two bellies of the levator ani muscle. Clinically this means that a problem in one tract can readily affect another (Fig. 1.8).

The uterine cavity is around 6 or 7 cm in length and forms a flattened slit, with the anterior and posterior walls in virtual contact. The wall has three layers: the endometrium (innermost), the myometrium and the peritoneum (outermost).

Endometrium

The endometrium is the epithelial lining of the cavity. The surface consists of a single layer of columnar ciliated cells, with invaginations forming uterine mucus-secreting glands within a cellular stroma. It undergoes cyclical changes in both the glands and stroma, leading to shedding and renewal about every 28 days.

There are two layers: a superficial functional layer which is shed monthly, and a basal layer which is not shed, and from which the new functional layer is regenerated. The epithelium of the functional layer shows active proliferative changes after a menstrual period until ovulation occurs, when the endometrial glands undergo secretory changes. Permanent destruction of the basal layer will result in amenorrhoea. This fact forms the basis for ablative techniques for the treatment of menorrhagia.

The normal changes in endometrial histology during the menstrual cycle are determined by changing secretion of ovarian steroid hormones. If the endometrium is exposed to sustained oestrogenic stimulation, whether endogenous or exogenous, it may become hyperplastic. Benign hyperplasia may precede malignant change.

Myometrium

The smooth muscle fibres of the uterine wall do not form distinct layers. While the outermost fibres are predominantly longitudinal, continuous with the musculature of the uterine tubes above and the vaginal wall below, the main thickness of the uterine wall is formed from a mesh of criss-crossing spiral strands. The individual muscle cells contain filaments of actin and myosin, which interact to generate contractions. During labour, the propagation of contractile excitation throughout the uterine wall is facilitated by the formation of 'gap junctions' between adjacent muscle cells. As a result, the spread of excitation resembles that in a syncytium.

Peritoneum

The posterior surface of the uterus is completely covered by peritoneum, which passes down over the posterior fornix of the vagina into the pouch of Douglas. Anteriorly, the

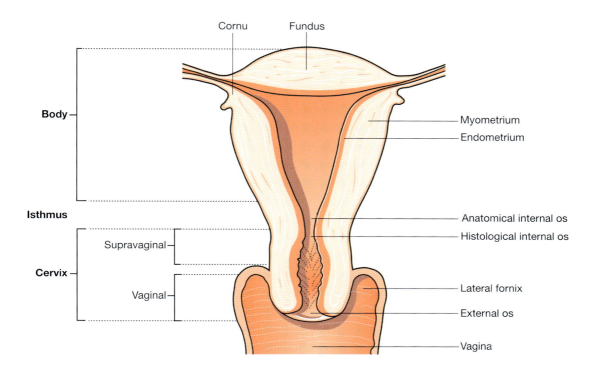

Fig. 1.7 Coronal section of the uterus.

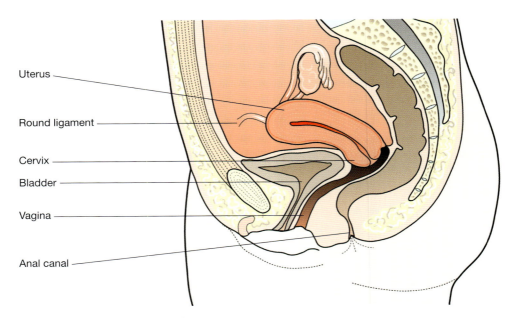

Uterus

Round ligament

Cervix

Bladder

Vagina

Anal canal

Fig. 1.8 **Female pelvic organs: sagittal view.**

peritoneum is reflected off the uterus at a much higher level onto the superior surface of the bladder.

The cervix

The cervix connects the uterus and vagina, and projects into the upper vagina. The 'gutter' surrounding this projection comprises the vaginal fornices – lateral, anterior and posterior. The cervix is about 2.5 cm long; the shorter part of it, which lies above the fornices, is termed the 'supravaginal part'. The endocervical canal is fusiform in shape between the external and internal os. After childbirth, the external os loses its circular shape and resembles a transverse slit. The epithelial lining of the canal is a columnar mucous membrane with an anterior and posterior longitudinal ridge, from which shallow palmate folds extend; hence the name 'arbor vitae'.

There are numerous glands secreting mucus that becomes more abundant and less viscous at the time of ovulation in mid-cycle. The vaginal surface of the cervix is covered with stratified squamous epithelium, similar to that lining the vagina. The squamocolumnar junction (histological external os) commonly does not correspond to the anatomical os, but may lie either above or external to the anatomical os. This 'tidal zone', within which the epithelial junction migrates at different stages of life, is termed the transformation zone. The ebb and flow of the squamocolumnar junction is influenced by oestrogenic stimulation. In the newborn female, and in pregnancy particularly, outgrowth of the columnar epithelium is very common, forming a bright pink 'rosette' around the external os. This appearance has been misnamed an 'erosion', but the epithelial covering, though delicate, is intact. In cases where the cervix has undergone deep bilateral laceration during childbirth, the resulting anterior and posterior lips tend to evert, exposing the glandular epithelium of the canal widely. This appearance is termed 'ectropion'.

Clinical aspects

The transformation zone is typically the area where precancerous change occurs. This can be detected by microscopic assessment of a cervical cytological smear. If the duct of a cervical gland becomes occluded, the gland distends with mucus to form a retention cyst (or Nabothian follicle). Multiple follicles are not uncommon, giving the cervix an irregular nodular feel and appearance. The body of the uterus is usually angled forward in relation to the cervix (anteflexion), while the uterus and cervix as a whole lean forward from the upper vagina (anteversion). In about 15% of women the uterus leans backwards towards the sacrum, and is described as retroverted. The cervical os then faces down the long axis of the vagina, rather than at right angles to it. In most instances retroversion is an asymptomatic variant of normality.

It is especially important to distinguish retroversion from anteversion before introducing a sound or similar instrument into the uterine cavity, to avoid perforation of the uterine wall. After the menopause the uterus and cervix gradually become atrophic, and cervical mucus is scanty. The amount of cervix projecting into the vagina also diminishes.

Because the uterus lies immediately behind the bladder, and between the lower parts of the ureters, particular care must be taken not to damage these structures during hysterectomy (Fig. 1.9). The endometrium and uterine cavity

Fundus of anteverted uterus

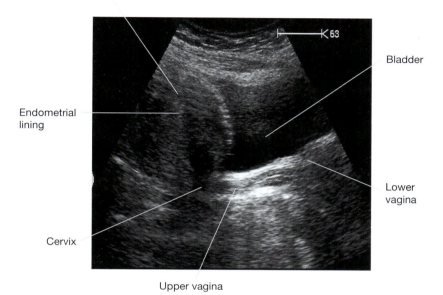

Bladder

Endometrial
lining

Lower
vagina

Cervix

Upper vagina

Fig. 1.9 **Transabdominal scan of the bladder, uterus and vagina.**

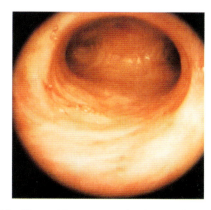

Fig. 1.10 **Normal hysteroscopic view of the endometrial cavity, showing both tubal ostia.**

can be examined by hysteroscopy. The tubal ostia can be seen (Fig. 1.10). Because the anterior and posterior walls are normally in contact, the cavity must be inflated with gas or fluid to obtain an adequate view of the surfaces.

The uterine attachments and supports

Structures attached to the uterus include (Fig. 1.11):

- round ligament
- ovarian ligament
- uterosacral ligament or fold
- cardinal ligament/transverse cervical ligament (of Mackenrodt).

The broad ligament is merely a double fold of peritoneum extending laterally from the uterus towards the pelvic sidewall. The hilum of the ovary arises from its posterior surface. The portion of the fold lateral to the ovary and tube is termed the infundibulopelvic ligament. Between the leaves of this fold, the uterine and ovarian blood vessels form an anastomotic loop. The ovarian ligament forms a ridge on the posterior leaf of the broad ligament, from the cornu of the uterus to the medial pole of the ovary. Developmentally, it is part of the gubernaculum of the ovary, in continuity with the round ligament, which curves round anteriorly from the cornu towards the inguinal canal, through which it passes. The uterosacral ligaments pass upwards and backwards from the posterior aspect of the cervix towards the lateral part of the second piece of the sacrum. In their lower part, they contain plain muscle along with fibrous tissue and autonomic nerve fibres. In their upper part, they dwindle to shallow peritoneal folds. The ligaments divide the pouch of Douglas from the pararectal fossa on each side.

The main ligaments providing support to the internal genital organs are the cardinal ligaments. The traditional name 'transverse cervical ligaments' is a misnomer. The cardinal ligaments are essentially dense condensations of connective tissue around the venous and nerve plexuses and arterial vessels, which extend from the pelvic sidewall towards the genital tract. Medially, they are firmly fused with the fascia surrounding the cervix and upper part of the vagina. They pass upwards and backwards towards the root of the internal iliac vessels. These condensations of fibrous and elastic tissue, together with plain muscle fibres,

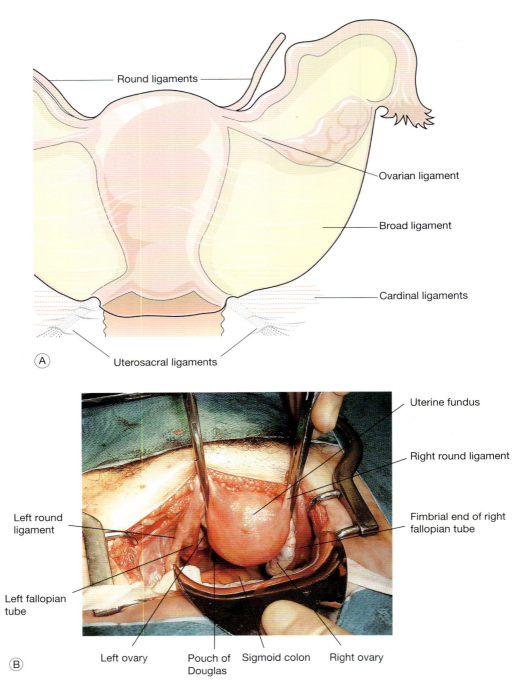

Fig. 1.11 **The uterus and appendages. (A)** Schematic view of the uterine ligaments seen from behind. **(B)** View of the uterus, fallopian tubes and ovaries at abdominal hysterectomy.

are sometimes referred to as the 'parametrium'. They support the upper vagina and cervix, helping to maintain the angle between the axis of the vagina and that of the anteverted uterus. Inferiorly they are continuous with the fascia on the upper surface of the levator muscles.

The pelvic diaphragm

Below the level of the cardinal ligaments, the pelvic organs are supported by a sloping shelf of muscle on each side, formed by the levator ani muscle (Fig. 1.12). The disposition

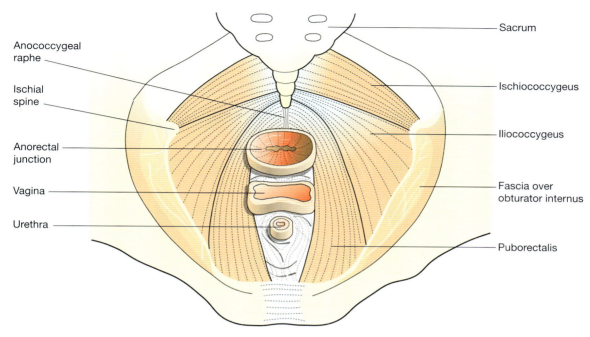

Anococcygeal raphe

Ischial spine

Anorectal junction

Vagina

Urethra

Sacrum

Ischiococcygeus

Iliococcygeus

Fascia over obturator internus

Puborectalis

Fig. 1.12   The urogenital diaphragm from above.

of the muscle bundles is comparable with that of the abdominal musculature. Near to the midline there is a longitudinal muscle bundle, the puborectalis (cf. the rectus abdominis). Laterally, the muscle sheets (iliococcygeus and ischiococcygeus) are oblique/transverse. The most medial fibres of puborectalis are inserted into the upper part of the perineal body. The succeeding fibres turn medially behind the anorectal flexure, and are inserted into the anococcygeal raphe and the tip of the coccyx, along with the fibres of ilio- and ischiococcygeus. Thus all three visceral tubes reach the body surface via a hiatus between the medial margins of puborectalis, and all are supported from behind by the sling action of the muscle when it contracts. Innervation is from the pudendal nerve (S2,3,4). The fascia on the upper surface of the pelvic diaphragm blends with the lower part of the cardinal ligaments. The fascia on the inferior surface of levator ani forms the roof of the ischiorectal fossa.

The main blood supply of the uterus is from the uterine arteries, which are branches of the internal iliac vessels (Fig. 1.13). Each passes medially in the base of the broad ligament above the ureter and ascends along the lateral aspect of the uterus, forming an anastomotic loop in the broad ligament with the ovarian artery (see Fig. 1.4). The uterine veins form a plexus in the parametrium below the uterine arteries, draining into the internal iliac veins. The principal lymph drainage is to iliac and obturator glands on the pelvic sidewall. From the fundus and cornua, lymph drains via the ovarian pathway to aortic nodes, while a few lymphatics in the round ligaments drain into the inguinal nodes (Fig. 1.14). The uterus is supplied by sympathetic and parasympathetic nerves, the exact functional significance of which is uncertain.

Congenital abnormalities of the uterus

Most of the female genital tract develops from the two paramesonephric (Müllerian) ducts, the caudal portions of which approximate in the midline and fuse to form the uterus, cervix and upper part of the vagina. The upper divergent portions of the ducts form the uterine tubes.

Congenital abnormality can result from:

- failure of or incomplete fusion
- failure of canalization
- asymmetrical maldevelopment.

The diagrams in Fig. 3.10 illustrate some of abnormalities that may be encountered. Failures of canalization are likely to present at puberty, as menstrual blood has no way to escape. Incomplete fusion is associated with late miscarriage, pre-term labour and malpresentation. Because of the intimate association during development, congenital abnormality of the female genital tract is commonly associated with abnormality of the urinary tract.

The vulva

The term vulva generally encompasses all the external female genitalia, i.e. the mons pubis, the labia majora and minora, the clitoris, and the structures within the vestibule – the external urinary meatus and the hymen. The mons pubis is a thickened pad of fat, cushioning the pubic bones anteriorly.

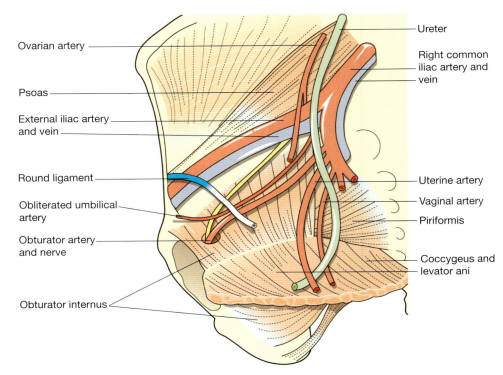

Fig. 1.13 The lateral pelvic sidewall.

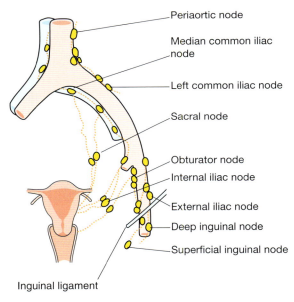

Fig. 1.14 Lymphatic drainage of the uterus. The lymph channels follow the blood supply.

The labia majora contain fatty tissue overlying the vascular bulbs of the vestibule and the bulbospongiosus muscles. The skin of the labia majora bears secondary sexual hair on the lateral surfaces only. There are abundant sebaceous, sweat and apocrine glands. The folds of the labia minora

vary considerably in size, and may be concealed by the labia majora or may project between them. They contain no fat, but are vascular and erectile during sexual arousal; the skin contains many sebaceous glands. Anteriorly, the folds bifurcate before uniting to form a hood above the clitoris and a frenulum along its dorsal surface. Posteriorly, the labia minora are linked by a fine ridge of skin, 'the fourchette'.

The labia minora and the fourchette form the boundaries of the vestibule. Between the fourchette and the posterior part of the hymen there is a crescentic furrow termed the 'navicular fossa'. The urethral meatus lies within the vestibule, close to the anterior margin of the vaginal orifice. There are pairs of small, mucus-secreting paraurethral glands in the lower part of the posterior wall of the urethra. These rudimentary tubules are homologous with the glands in the male prostate. If they become infected and blocked, they may form a paraurethral abscess, cyst or urethral diverticulum. Two mucus-secreting glands, known as Bartholin's glands (or greater vestibular glands), lie posterolateral to the vaginal orifice on each side, embedded in the posterior pole of the vascular vestibular bulb (see Fig. 1.5). Their ducts open near the lateral limits of the navicular fossa. The glands only become palpable, and the duct orifices become visible, if infection is present.

Blood supply

The main sources of the vascularity of the vulva are branches of the internal pudendal arteries. There are also branches from the superficial and deep external pudendal arteries.

Nerve supply

The main sensory supply to the vulva is via the pudendal nerves. Peripheral parts of the vulvar skin are supplied by filaments from the iliohypogastric and ilioinguinal nerves, and from the perineal branches of the posterior cutaneous nerves of the thigh (see Fig. 1.6). The pudendal nerve provides motor fibres to all the muscles of the perineum, including the voluntary urinary and bowel sphincters, as well as the levator ani.

Lymph drainage

The main pathway of drainage is to the superficial inguinal glands, and on through the deep inguinal to the external iliac glands. Some lymphatics from the deeper structures of the vulva pass with vaginal lymphatics to the internal iliac nodes.

The fallopian tubes

The tubes extend on each side from the cornu of the uterus, within the upper border of the broad ligament, for about 10 cm. The tubes and ovaries together are commonly described as the uterine appendages, or adnexa (Fig. 1.15).

The tube can be divided into four parts (Fig. 1.16). The interstitial (intramural) part forms a narrow passage through the thickness of the myometrium. The isthmus, extending out from the cornu for about 3 cm, is also narrow. The ampulla is thin-walled, 'baggy', and tortuous; its lateral portion is free from the broad ligament, and droops down behind it towards the ovary. Near its lateral limit the abdominal ostium is constricted, but opens out again to form the infundibulum. This trumpet-shaped expansion is fringed by a ring of delicate fronds (or fimbriae), one of which is attached to the surface of the ovary.

The walls of the tubes include outer longitudinal and inner circular layers of smooth muscle. The delicate lining (endosalpinx), containing columnar ciliated and secretory cells, has longitudinal folds in the isthmic segment, which change into a highly intricate branching pattern in the ampulla.

Tubal function

At the time of ovulation, the fimbriae clasp the ovary in the area where the stigma (or point of follicular rupture) is forming. Usually, therefore, the ovum is discharged into the infundibulum (funnel) and is carried by tubal peristalsis into the ampulla of the tube, which is where fertilization occurs. Transit of the zygote to the site of implantation in the uterus takes several days.

Sterilization is effected by occluding both tubes, preferably in the narrow isthmic portion, using clips, sutures, rings or diathermy.

Patency of the tubes can be tested by injecting a watery dye (methylthioninium chloride – methylene blue) through the cervix, and observing spill from the abdominal ostia by laparoscopy. The contours of the uterine cavity and tubal lumen may also be demonstrated with radio-opaque fluid during a hysterosalpingogram.

The vagina

The vagina, which links the external and internal parts of the female genital tract, has a dual function: it forms the coital canal, affording access for spermatozoa to reach the cervix, and, with the cervix, it forms the soft-tissue birth canal. It lies in close proximity to the urethra and bladder anteriorly, and to the anal canal and rectum posteriorly. All three canals traverse the pelvic floor, passing between the

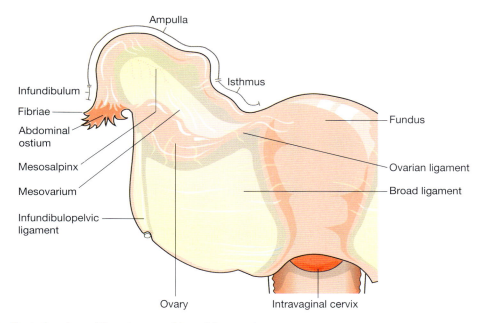

Ampulla
Infundibulum
Fibriae
Abdominal ostium
Mesosalpinx
Mesovarium
Infundibulopelvic ligament
Ovary
Isthmus
Fundus
Ovarian ligament
Broad ligament
Intravaginal cervix

Fig. 1.15 **Posterior view of the uterus and broad ligament.**

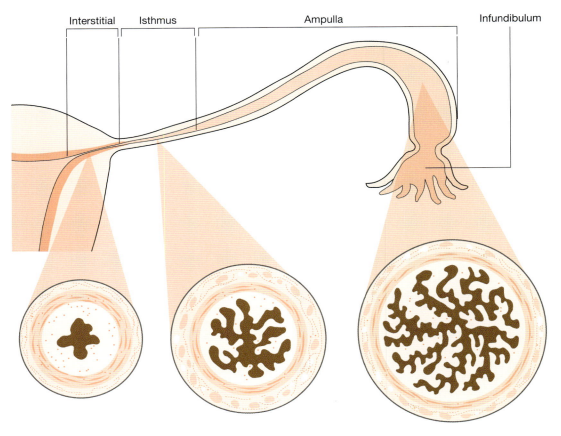

Interstitial Isthmus Ampulla Infundibulum

Fig. 1.16 **The oviduct, showing the structure of the mucosal layer.**

medial (puborectalis) portions of the levator ani muscles. The insertion of these muscle fibres into the anococcygeal raphe creates a sling behind the bowel so that, at the junction of the lower rectum and the anal canal, a sharp angle is created, which is opened when the muscle relaxes. Other muscle fibres are inserted into the perineal body near its apex, creating a similar sling which angulates the axis of the vagina at that level. In turn, the anterior vaginal wall in the area of the bladder neck receives support.

There are differences in the anatomy of the vagina above and below this level. The lower third of the vagina is closely invested by the superficial and deep muscles of the perineum. It:

- incorporates the urethra in its anterior wall
- is separated from the bowel by the perineal body
- has a rich arterial blood supply from branches of the vaginal arteries, and from both external and internal pudendal vessels.

The upper two-thirds of the vagina, above the levator shelf:

- is not invested by muscles, but is wide and capacious
- is in apposition with the bladder base anteriorly, and with the rectum (and, above that, the pouch of Douglas) posteriorly

- is supported laterally and at the vault by the parametrium (cardinal and uterosacral ligaments). During sexual arousal the smooth muscle fibres within the parametrium elevate the vaginal vault and cervix, thereby elongating the vagina and straightening its long axis.

Vaginal structure

The vaginal walls form an elastic fibromuscular tube with a multilayered structure. The lining of stratified squamous epithelium is corrugated into transverse folds (or rugae), which facilitates stretching during childbirth. The epithelium contains no glands, but during the reproductive years the more superficial cells contain abundant glycogen. This polysaccharide is broken down by lactobacilli, which form the normal flora of the vagina, producing lactic acid. This accounts for the low pH in the vaginal lumen (average pH 4.5).

Between the epithelium and the muscle, there is a layer of areolar tissue containing an extensive venous plexus. Vascular engorgement during sexual arousal, analogous to erection in the male, is most marked in the lower part of the vagina, encroaching on the vaginal lumen as the rugae distend. The vasocongestive response also results in increased transudation into the vaginal lumen.

The smooth muscle layers (outer longitudinal, inner circular) are not distinct, and an interlacing pattern is usual. Deep to the muscle, there is another extensive plexus of veins, within the outer vaginal fascia.

The ovary

The ovaries are attached on each side to the posterior surface of the broad ligaments through a narrowed base, termed the 'hilum'. The ovaries are also attached to the cornua of the uterus by the ovarian ligaments. Developmentally, these are the upper portions of the gubernacula ovarii, and they are responsible for drawing the ovaries down into the pelvis from the posterior wall of the abdominal cavity. Typically, each ovary lies in an ovarian fossa, a shallow peritoneal depression lateral to the ureter, near the pelvic sidewall. The position may vary, however, and when the uterus is retroverted, one or both ovaries may lie in the pouch of Douglas.

The ovaries are ovoid in shape, with an irregular surface and a firm, largely solid, stroma, which can be divided indistinctly into an outer cortex and an inner medulla. The surface epithelium of cuboidal coelomic cells forms an incomplete layer, beneath which is a fibrous investment – the 'tunica albuginea'. The germ cells from which the ova are derived are embedded in the substance of the ovaries.

The ovarian blood vessels and nerves enter through the hilum from the broad ligament. The ovarian arteries are direct branches of the aorta. Within the broad ligaments, they form an anastomotic loop with branches of the uterine arteries.

Anatomy of the lower urinary tract

The descending ureters are narrow, thick-walled muscular tubes that cross into the pelvis close to the bifurcation of the common iliac arteries. They lie immediately under the peritoneum of the pelvic sidewall, behind the lateral attachment of the broad ligaments. Curving medially and forwards, they pass through the base of the broad ligaments below the uterine arteries, about 2 cm lateral to the supravaginal part of the cervix, a short distance above the lateral fornices of the vagina.

Approaching the bladder, the ureters pass medially in front of the upper vagina and enter the bladder base obliquely at the upper angles of the trigone.

The wall of the ureter is composed of three elements: an external fibrous sheath, layers of smooth muscle and a lining of transitional epithelium. There may be partial or complete duplication of one or both ureters. An ectopic ureter is one that opens anywhere but the trigone of the bladder, and this may even be into the vagina or the vestibule. Urinary incontinence inevitably results.

The bladder

The urinary reservoir, lined with transitional epithelium, has the shape of a tetrahedron when empty, but the mesh of smooth muscle in the bladder wall can readily distend to contain a volume of half a litre or more. This muscle coat (the detrusor muscle) is thus normally relaxed and capable of considerable stretching without a contractile response. If urinary outflow during micturition is chronically impeded, however, the detrusor muscle becomes irritable and ultimately hypertrophic, producing prominent trabecular bands visible at cystoscopy.

The bladder is covered with peritoneum on its superior surface only. The peritoneum is reflected onto the anterior abdominal wall at a varying level, dependent on the degree of bladder filling. The oblique passage of the terminal part of each ureter through the bladder wall creates a one-way valve, which normally prevents urinary backflow from the bladder. This protects the kidneys from ascending infection. The triangular area within the bladder base defined by the two ureteric orifices and the internal urethral orifice is termed the 'trigone'. Over this area, the epithelium remains smooth, even when the bladder is empty.

The urethra

The female urethra is about 4 cm long. Below the bladder neck it is embedded in the anterior vaginal wall, and the smooth muscle layers of the two structures intermingle. The urethral tissues also reflect the vascularity and turgidity of the vagina itself. Many of the urethral muscle fibres near the bladder neck are longitudinal and continuous with those of the bladder above, forming a funnel that opens out when these fibres contract, flattening the angle between the bladder base and the upper urethra. There are also abundant elastic fibres at this level, whose action helps to restore urethral closure after micturition. Around the lower part of the urethra, there is a fusiform collar of voluntary muscle – 'the external urethral sphincter'. This segment of the urethra passes through the perineal membrane, which keeps it in a stable position. The upper urethra, on the other hand, shares the mobility of the bladder neck. The urethra is lined by transitional epithelium in its upper part, and by squamous epithelium below.

Nerve supply

Apart from the external sphincter, the efferent nerve supply controlling bladder function is from the pelvic parasympathetic system (S2,3,4), which provides the main motor fibres to the detrusor muscle. Afferent fibres conveying the normal sensations of bladder filling also return through the parasympathetic pathway, though some sympathetic sensory fibres convey the feelings of bladder overdistension via the hypogastric plexus. At the level of the second, third and fourth sacral segments of the spinal cord, the sensory and motor parasympathetic nerves form spinal reflex arcs, which are moderated by interaction with higher centres in the brain. Urinary continence depends upon a variety of factors. These include the elastic fibres surrounding the bladder neck, which normally maintain urethral closure; and the tone or reflex contraction of the levator ani muscles, which, through their insertion into the perineal body, elevate the urethrovesical junction, creating an angulation at the junction of the mobile (upper) and fixed (lower) portions of the urethra. The turgidity of spongy tissue underlying the urethral epithelium also assists in occluding the urethra, as does the action of the voluntary sphincter.

Key points

- Without understanding the anatomy of the pelvis, it is impossible to understand the mechanisms of labour.
- The cross-sectional shape of the birth canal is different at different levels. At the pelvic brim it is oval in shape, and the widest part of this oval is in the lateral plane from one side to the other. The outlet is also oval, with the widest part in the anteroposterior plane. The head enters the pelvic brim in the transverse position, as the inlet is widest in this plane, but rotates 90° at the pelvic floor to the anteroposterior plane before delivery. The shoulders also follow the same rotation.

2

History and examination

Introduction

In general, history and examination cannot be divided neatly into different specialties, and questions relating to obstetrics and gynaecology should form part of the assessment of any woman presenting to any specialty. There may be embarrassment and recrimination, for example, when a suspected appendicitis turns out to be a pelvic infection secondary to an unsuspected intrauterine contraceptive device (IUCD). Similarly, not all problems presenting to obstetricians and gynaecologists are obstetrical or gynaecological in nature. It is therefore important to take a full history and perform an appropriate examination in all cases. The key points of gynaecological and obstetrical history and examination are emphasized below.

Gynaecological history

A gynaecological history should follow the usual model for history-taking, with questions about the presenting complaint, its history and associated problems. It should include a past medical history and information about prescription and non-prescription drugs used, and any known allergies. After questions about social circumstances and activities, and family history, the history is completed with a general systemic enquiry. However, during a gynaecological history, there are specific key areas to be expanded upon. These include menstrual, fertility, pelvic pain, urogynaecological and obstetrical histories.

Menstrual history

The pattern of bleeding

The simple phrase 'tell me about your periods' often elicits all the information required. The bleeding pattern of the menstrual cycle is expressed as a fraction, such that a cycle of 4/28 means the woman bleeds for 4 days every 28 days. A cycle of 4–10/21–42 means the woman bleeds for between 4 and 10 days every 21–42 days. Asking the shortest time between the start of successive periods, the longest time between periods, and the average time between periods helps determine the cycle characteristics.

Bleeding too little

Amenorrhoea is the absence of periods. Primary amenorrhoea is when someone has not started menstruating by the age of 16. Secondary amenorrhoea means that periods have been absent for longer than 6 months. Oligomenorrhoea means the periods are infrequent, with a cycle of 42 days or more.

The climacteric is the perimenopausal time when periods become less regular and are accompanied by increasing menopausal symptoms. The menopause is the time after the last ever period, and can only therefore be assessed retrospectively.

Irregular periods, oligomenorrhoea or amenorrhoea, suggest anovulation or irregular ovulation. Specific questions about weight, weight change, acne, greasy skin, hirsutism, flushes or galactorrhoea may help identify the nature of the ovarian dysfunction.

Bleeding too much

It is very difficult to find out how heavy someone's periods are. If menstrual blood loss is accurately measured, an average of 35 mL of blood is lost each month. Heavy menstrual bleeding (previously known as menorrhagia) is defined as loss of more than 80 mL during regular menstruation. Some women will complain of very heavy periods with a normal blood loss, while others will not complain in the presence of heavy menstrual bleeding. Asking how often pads or tampons have to be changed and using pictorial charts can provide more objective information. Whether menstrual loss is excessive, however, is a largely subjective assessment.

Specific symptoms can indicate abnormally heavy menstruation. Although small pieces of tissue are normal, blood clots are not. 'Flooding' is when menstrual blood soaks through all protection. It is both abnormal and distressing. Symptoms of anaemia may also be present. A history of the menstrual cycle since menarche (the first period) can reveal changes in the bleeding pattern. However, an emphasis on the effect on lifestyle and treatments tried previously is particularly important.

Bleeding at the wrong time

It is important to ask specifically about bleeding, brown or bloody discharge between periods (intermenstrual bleeding), or after intercourse (post-coital bleeding). These symptoms can point to abnormalities of the cervix or uterine cavity. Postmenopausal bleeding is defined as bleeding more than 1 year after the last period. Undiagnosed abnormal bleeding requires further investigation. If a woman is postmenopausal, enquiry should be made about past or current use of hormone replacement therapy.

Fertility history

Last menstrual period (LMP)

This question is vital and should be followed with whether that period came at the expected time and was of normal character. As well as alerting to the possibility of pregnancy, the information is important because some investigations need to be performed at specific times of the menstrual cycle.

Contraception

It is useful to establish whether the woman is sexually active, perhaps with something like, 'Are you currently in a physical sexual relationship?' and then, 'Are you using any contraception at present?' A further discussion about fertility issues, unprotected intercourse and risk factors for certain diseases may be appropriate. A contraceptive history should include any problems with chosen contraceptives and why they were stopped. Questions may be followed-up with 'Are you hoping for a pregnancy?' if the situation is not clear.

If there are any infertility issues, their duration and the results of any investigation or treatment may be of relevance.

Cervical smears

Cervical screening programmes vary in different countries but, generally, women between the ages of 20–25 and 60–64 years are invited to participate every 3–5 years. The date of the woman's last smear should be noted, and when it was recommended that she have her next smear. Any previous abnormalities or vaccination should also be noted, and whether she has had any colposcopic investigation or treatment. If she is over 50, it may be relevant to discuss breast screening.

Pelvic pain history

Painful periods

Dysmenorrhoea is a common problem and its effects on lifestyle are important. The cramping pain of primary dysmenorrhoea is at its most intense just before and during the early stages of a period. Young women are particularly affected and the pain has usually been present from the time of the first period. It is not usually associated with structural abnormalities and may improve with age or after a pregnancy. Secondary dysmenorrhoea is when menstruation has not tended to be painful in the past, and is more likely to indicate pelvic pathology. In particular, progressive dysmenorrhoea, where the intensity of the pain increases throughout menstruation, may suggest endometriosis.

Pelvic pain

The relationship of pelvic pain to the menstrual cycle is important. Pain immediately prior to or during periods is more likely to be of gynaecological origin. 'Mittelschmerz' is a cramping pelvic pain that can be midline or unilateral. It occurs 2 weeks before a period and is caused by ovulation. Intermittent discomfort may suggest some scarring or ovarian pathology but it is more commonly non-gynaecological. It is vital to take a urinary and lower gastrointestinal history, as urinary tract infection or irritable bowel syndrome may present with pelvic pain. Any pain is likely to be worse if the person is anxious, stressed or depressed. Chronic pelvic pain is particularly affected by psychosomatic factors, and recognizing this during history-taking is important.

Pain on intercourse

There are two main types of dyspareunia: superficial and deep. They can be differentiated by asking, 'Is it painful just as he begins to enter or when he is deep inside?' Deep dyspareunia is associated with pelvic pathology, such as scarring, adhesions, endometriosis or masses that restrict uterine mobility. Superficial dyspareunia can arise from local abnormalities at the introitus or from inadequate lubrication. It can also be due to a voluntary or involuntary contraction of the muscles of the pelvic floor referred to as 'vaginismus' (see Chapter 19).

Vaginal discharge

Discharge can be normal or be associated with cervical ectopy and, particularly if offensive or irritant, can indicate infection. It can also suggest neoplasia of the cervix or endometrium. Enquire about the duration, amount, colour, smell and relationship to cycle.

Urogynaecological history

Urinary symptoms

A good initial question to ask is, 'Do you ever leak urine when you don't intend to?' If so, find out what provokes it, how it affects her quality of life and how troublesome her symptoms are. Symptoms suggestive of an overactive bladder include – frequency, urgency and nocturia. Incontinence after exercise, coughing, laughing or straining can suggest stress incontinence. It can be difficult to differentiate stress incontinence and urge incontinence, however, as there is often a mixed picture. It is important to ask about fluid intake, and in particular about caffeine and alcohol, which can exacerbate urinary symptoms.

A history of dysuria or haematuria may suggest bladder infection or pathology. 'Strangury' is the constant desire to pass urine and suggests urinary tract inflammation.

Prolapse

Prolapse may be associated with vaginal discomfort, a dragging sensation, the feeling of something 'coming down' and possibly backache. Although the uterus, anterior vaginal wall and posterior vaginal wall can prolapse, it is difficult to separate these by history. Bladder and bowel function should be explored, including a question about the need to digitally manipulate the vagina in order to be able to void.

Gynaecological examination

Signs of gynaecological disease are not limited to the pelvis. A full examination may reveal anaemia, pleural effusions, visual field defects or lymphadenopathy in gynaecological conditions. However, passing a speculum, taking a cervical smear and performing a bimanual pelvic examination are the key skills to acquire. A great deal of sensitivity is required in their use.

Passing a speculum

Preparation

The patient should empty her bladder and remove sanitary protection. The examination room should be quiet and have a private area for the patient to undress. It should contain an examination couch with a modesty sheet and good adjustable lighting. A female chaperone should always be present. The examination requires full explanation and verbal consent.

Stand on the right of the patient with gloves, speculum and lubricating gel immediately to hand. The patient should lie back, bend her knees, put her heels together and let her knees fall apart. The light should be adjusted to give a good view of the vulva and perineum and the modesty sheet should cover the patient's abdomen and thighs.

Inspection

Inspect the hair distribution and vulval skin. Hair extending towards the umbilicus and onto the inner thighs can be associated with disorders of androgen excess, as can clitoromegaly. The vulva can be a site of chronic skin conditions such as eczema and psoriasis, specific conditions such as lichen sclerosis and warts, cysts of the Bartholin's glands, and cancers. Ulceration may imply herpes, syphilis, trauma or malignancy.

Look at the perineum (Fig. 2.1) and gently part the labia to inspect the introitus. Perineal scars are usually secondary to tears or episiotomy during childbirth. A red papule around the urethral opening is usually a prolapsed area of urethral mucosa. A white, plaque-like discharge may suggest thrush, and pale skin with punctate red areas implies atrophic vaginitis. Asking the woman to cough may reveal demonstrable stress incontinence or the bulge of a prolapse.

Speculum examination

Disposable speculums tend to be all one size, but smaller and larger speculums are available if required. Ensure the speculum is warmed, working normally and lubricated with

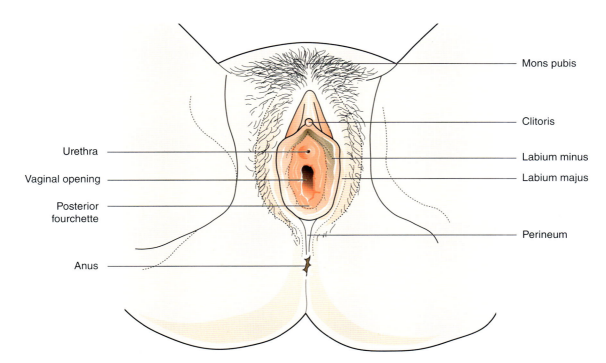

Fig. 2.1 **Inspection of the perineum.**

gel. Hold the speculum so that its blades are oriented in the same direction as the vaginal opening. Part the labia and slowly insert the speculum, rotating it gently until the blades are horizontal (Fig. 2.2).

If the patient is in the lithotomy position at the edge of the couch, the speculum can be turned downwards to avoid pressure on the clitoris. If the patient is lying on the couch itself, it is usually easier to rotate the speculum upwards. It should be inserted fully in a slightly posterior direction, before firmly, but gently, opening to visualize the cervix (Fig. 2.3). The speculum can be closed a little when the cervix pops into view.

If the cervix is not visible, it is often because the speculum has not been inserted far enough before opening. If this is not the case, the cervix is either above or below the blades. As most uteri are anteverted, it is usually below the blades, and the speculum should be angled more posteriorly before reopening. Otherwise, gently insert a finger to determine its position. For removal, the speculum should be opened further and withdrawn beyond the cervix before rotation back again, closure and removal.

Inspect the vagina for atrophic vaginitis and discharge. A creamy or mucousy discharge is normal. A yellow-greenish frothy discharge is seen with *Trichomonas vaginalis* and a grey-green fishy discharge suggests bacterial vaginosis. There may be a purulent cervical discharge with gonorrhoea, and an increased mucousy discharge may occur with chlamydial cervicitis. Swabs, if required, should be taken from the vaginal fornices (high vaginal) or the cervical canal (endocervical).

The cervical os is small and round in the nulliparous and bigger and more slit-like in parous women. Threads from an IUCD may be present. Translucent lumps or cysts around the os are Nabothian follicles, but warts and tumours can sometimes be seen. An ectopy is red, as the epithelium of the cervical canal extends onto the surface of the paler outer cervical epithelium. It varies across the cycle and should be looked on as normal, although it may be associated with contact bleeding or increased discharge.

A bivalve speculum holds open the vaginal walls and obscures any cystocele or rectocele, but a univalve speculum can demonstrate these well. For this, a patient lies in the left-lateral position with her knees drawn up and the lubricated blade of the speculum is used to hold back the anterior vaginal wall. Coughing will show a bulge of the posterior wall if a rectocele is present. When the posterior wall is held back, coughing will demonstrate the bulge of a cystocele and/or uterine descent (Figs 2.5 and 2.6).

Taking a cervical smear

Smears should ideally be performed in the mid- to late follicular phase, not during menstruation and only as part of the screening programme. Confirm the woman's details and ensure you have ascertained all the information required for the request form. Run the speculum under warm water to provide appropriate lubrication and visualize the cervix.

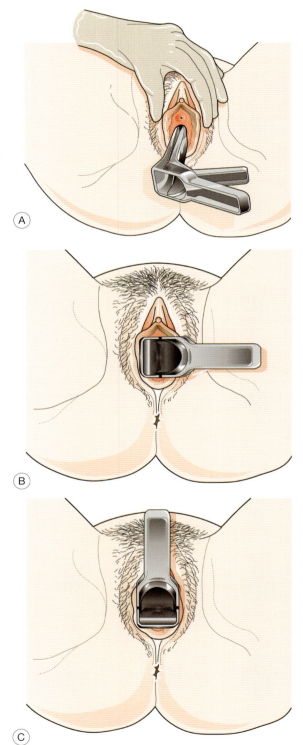

Fig. 2.2 **A–C Insertion of a bivalve (Cusco) speculum.**

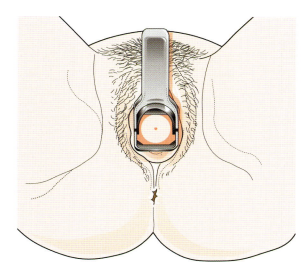

Fig. 2.3 Visualization of the cervix.

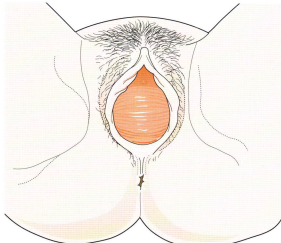

Fig. 2.5 The bulge of a prolapse.

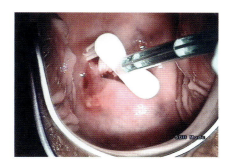

Fig. 2.4 Taking a cervical smear.

The most commonly used technique involves using liquid-based cytology and a broom-type sampling device. Insert the central bristles of the broom-like device into the endocervical canal, deep enough to allow the shorter bristles to fully contact the ectocervix. Push gently and rotate the broom in a clockwise direction five times (Fig. 2.4).

Immediately put the broom into the container of preserving solution and rotate 10 times while pushing against the side of the container. Discard the broom, tighten the lid and label the container with the patient's details. Complete and check the cytology request form, ensuring that all the information required is provided, and marry this, or the computer-generated barcode if the form is completed electronically, to the container for transport to the laboratory. Inform the woman how long the result will take and how it will be delivered.

Pelvic examination

Apply lubricating gel to the gloved fingers of the right hand. Part the labia with the index and middle fingers of the left hand. Gently insert the right index finger into the vagina. If comfortable, insert the middle finger in below the index finger, making room posteriorly to avoid the sensitive urethra.

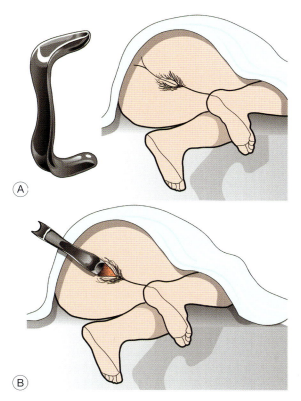

Fig. 2.6 (A,B) Examination with a univalve (Sims) speculum.

The cervix feels like the tip of a nose and protrudes into the top of the vagina (Fig. 2.7).

Feel the cervix and record irregularities or discomfort. 'Cervical excitation' is when touching the cervix causes intense pain and it implies active pelvic inflammation. The dimple of the os can be felt and the firmness of the uterine

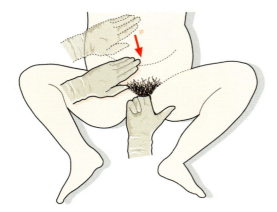

Fig. 2.7   **Digital pelvic examination.**

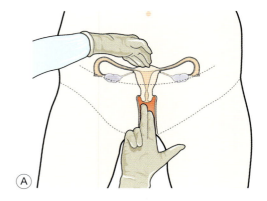

(A)

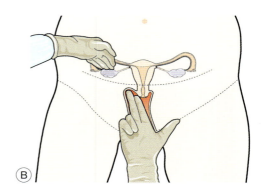

(B)

Fig. 2.9   **(A,B) Examination of the uterus and adnexa.**

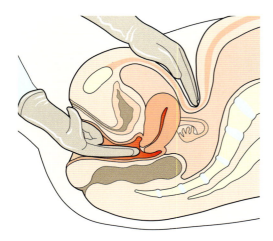

Fig. 2.8   **Bimanual examination.**

body lies above or below the cervix. A vaginal cyst may be an embryological duct remnant, and vaginal nodules may represent endometriosis.

Assess the position of the uterus. It is usually anteverted with the cervix posterior and the uterine body anterior. If the uterus is retroverted, the cervix is anterior and the uterine body lies posteriorly. The fingers should be manipulated behind the cervix to lift the uterus. With the left hand above the umbilicus, feel through the abdomen for the moving uterus (Fig. 2.8). If the uterus cannot be palpated, the hand should be moved gradually down until the uterus is between the fingers (Fig. 2.9A).

Assess the mobility, regularity and size of the uterus. The adhesions of endometriosis, infection, surgery or malignancy fix the uterus and make bimanual examination more uncomfortable. Asymmetry of the uterus may imply fibroids. Uterine size is often related to stage of pregnancy. A normally sized uterus feels like a plum. At 6 weeks, a pregnant uterus feels like a tangerine, at 8 weeks an apple, at 10 weeks an orange and at 12 weeks a grapefruit. At 14 weeks, the uterus can be felt on abdominal palpation alone.

Feel for adnexal masses in the vaginal fornices lateral to the cervix on each side. Push up the tissues in the adnexa and, starting with a left hand above the umbilicus, bring it down to the appropriate iliac fossa, trying to feel a mass bimanually (Fig. 2.9B). In thin women, the ovaries can just be felt, but a definite adnexal mass is abnormal and should be investigated further. As large adnexal masses tend to move to the midline, it can be difficult to differentiate a large ovarian cyst from a large uterus.

Obstetrical history

An obstetrical history follows the usual model for history-taking. However, as with gynaecological histories, there are several unique things to be covered. A history from a pregnant woman starts with calculating the gestation and putting this pregnancy in the context of previous pregnancies. The presenting complaint is next and this encompasses a record of what is happening now, risk factors and symptom progression. It is followed by a complete history of this pregnancy and previous pregnancies. After this, medical, gynaecological, drug, social and family histories are expanded. However, these are often straightforward as pregnant women are usually young and healthy.

Establishment of the estimated day of delivery (EDD)

Term is between 37 and 42 weeks' gestation, but the actual EDD is 40 weeks after day 1 of the LMP. This can cause confusion, as gestation is calculated from the LMP, not conception. When someone is 12 weeks' pregnant, she conceived 10 weeks ago. Phone-based apps or gestational wheel calculators allow the easy calculation of EDD and current gestation from the LMP (Fig. 2.10). In their absence, Naegele's rule can be used. To calculate the EDD, subtract 3 months from the LMP and add 10 days.

These methods assume a regular 4-week cycle. If this is not the case, the EDD may require adjustment. With a regular 5-week cycle, the true EDD will be 1 week later than calculated. An ultrasound scan (USS) is used to confirm the final EDD. However, scans have an associated error that increases with gestation, and in the early second trimester, this is approximately plus or minus 1 week. In general, the EDD from the LMP is used, unless the USS date differs by more than a week.

Obstetrical summary

Parity is a summary of a woman's obstetrical history and two numbers are used to document this. Added together, the numbers give the number of previous pregnancies. Someone who is para 0 + 0 has not been pregnant before. The first number is the total number of live births, plus the number of stillbirths after 24 weeks' gestation. The second number is the number of pregnancies before 24 weeks, in which the baby was not born alive.

A woman who is para 3 + 3 has been pregnant six times. The first '3' might represent a normal term delivery, a live birth at 23 weeks after which the baby died and a stillbirth at 25 weeks' gestation. The other three pregnancies may have been a spontaneous miscarriage at 23 weeks, an early

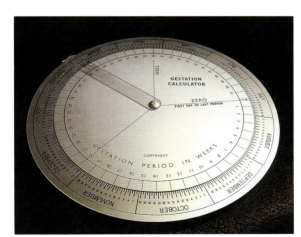

Fig. 2.10 Gestational wheel.

ectopic pregnancy and a first trimester termination. The numbers relate to pregnancies rather than babies, so that the mother of twins would be para 1 + 0. A woman who is primiparous is 'pregnant and para 0'. A parous woman is 'pregnant and para 1' (or more).

What is happening now?

The next stage is the presenting complaint and its history. Assuming there is a specific problem, the history should include when it was first noticed, its progress, management and associated symptoms. It may also be useful to ask about important risk factors, for example a past history of placental abruption, chronic hypertension, smoking or pre-eclampsia.

Remember that there are two patients. The fetus should be assessed by asking about movements, and any recent tests of fetal well-being. Fetal movements are first felt around 20 weeks, a time referred to as the 'quickening' but can be as early as 16 weeks. Concerns about fetal well-being may be established by a reduction in the frequency or change in pattern of fetal movements.

History of this pregnancy

This pregnancy should now be covered in detail. The first thing to ask about is pre-conceptual folic acid, followed by the diagnosis of pregnancy and problems such as bleeding and vomiting or pain in the first trimester. The next thing to ask about is the booking appointment, results of investigations, including dating and anomaly USS, and additional prenatal screening tests. Then cover subsequent antenatal care, including clinics, parentcraft and any day unit assessment. The reason for and outcome of any additional USS should be reported. Any concerns, problems identified or emergency attendance at hospital should be documented, along with plans for the rest of the pregnancy and delivery.

Past obstetric history

Each of the woman's previous pregnancies should be discussed chronologically. Information required includes the date, the gestation and outcome. If the pregnancy ended in the first or second trimester, the diagnosis and management, including any operative procedures, should be recorded. For other pregnancies, information about the method of delivery, the reason for an operative delivery, the sex, weight, health and method of feeding of the baby should be obtained. In particular, any pregnancy and postnatal complication should be highlighted.

Medical history

The medical history should include previous operations, hospitalizations and medical problems. Continuing medical problems are of great importance because they may have an effect on the pregnancy and make complications more likely or complex. In addition, pregnancy may have an effect on medical problems, resulting in their deterioration, improvement or an alteration in management.

Gynaecological history

All or some of the gynaecological topics may be important in the history. Infertility treatment, particularly the use of assisted reproductive technologies, such as egg donation, pre-gestational diagnosis or screening, may suggest the need to modify counselling and tests. The date of the last cervical smear is relevant.

Drug history

It is important to record drugs taken, both over-the-counter and prescribed, and the reasons for their use. The need to continue the drug, or change its dose, as well as any possible teratogenic effects, should be considered.

Family history

In a pregnant woman, it is a family history of fetal abnormalities, genetic conditions or consanguinity that is particularly important. In addition, some obstetrical conditions such as twins, pre-eclampsia, gestational diabetes and obstetric cholestasis may have a familial element.

Social history

It is important to assess the facilities for the forthcoming baby and determine whether further support is required. A woman's occupation and her plans for working during the pregnancy should be noted. It is also important to ask about smoking, drinking and other drugs of misuse.

Systemic enquiry

Often, the systemic enquiry will be covered in the history of the presenting complaint. Remember, however, that many symptoms are more common in pregnancy, including urinary frequency, shortness of breath, tiredness, headache, nausea and breast tenderness.

Low-risk versus high-risk pregnancy

The key to good antenatal care is to recognize which women are more likely to develop problems in pregnancy before they happen. Clearly, all women can develop problems, but women at extremes of age and weight, those with pre-existing medical conditions like diabetes, hypertension and epilepsy, those with significant past or family histories of obstetric problems and those who smoke heavily, misuse drugs or have poor social circumstances are all more likely to develop problems. In these 'high-risk' pregnancies, antenatal care should be tailored to meet the increased needs of the woman and her baby.

Obstetrical examination

In an obstetrical examination, the areas to focus on should be guided by the clinical history. It is only by becoming familiar with examination findings in normal pregnancy that deviations from normal can be fully appreciated. In the hyperdynamic circulation of pregnancy, for example, cardiac murmurs are common. The vast majority of these are flow murmurs, but previously unrecognized pathological murmurs occasionally become apparent. Likewise, in normal pregnancy, skin changes and increasing oedema are common.

A systematic approach is preferable. Starting with the hands and working up to the head and down to the abdomen and legs, will avoid missing important signs. Examination of the skin, sclera, conjunctiva, retina, thyroid, liver and tendon reflexes may reveal important abnormalities that may otherwise be missed. There are three elements of obstetrical examination, however, that are particularly important: blood pressure assessment, abdominal palpation and vaginal examination if indicated.

Blood pressure assessment

The pregnant woman should lie in a semirecumbent position at an approximately 30° angle and time should be taken to ensure that she is relaxed. The room should be quiet, and any tight clothing on her arm removed. The blood pressure should be taken from her right arm, supported at the level of the heart (Fig. 2.11).

An appropriately sized cuff should be used as too small a cuff will overestimate the blood pressure. The best cuffs have an indication of acceptable arm circumference on them. Ideally, the cuff bladder should cover 80% of the arm circumference and the width of the bladder should be 40% of the arm circumference. Problems occur if the bladder length is <67% (this usually means the arm circumference is >34 cm). In such cases, a large or thigh cuff should be used.

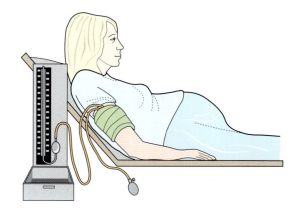

Fig. 2.11   **Blood pressure measurement.**

Abdominal palpation

Ensure the patient has privacy and is comfortable and relaxed. Although pregnant women should avoid lying flat on their back for any period of time, as this can compress major vessels, the woman should be examined in the recumbent position.

Initially, the abdomen is inspected. During inspection, look for the distended abdomen of pregnancy and note asymmetry, fetal movements and tense stretching. The skin may reveal old or fresh striae gravidarum, a midline pigmented linea nigra and any scars from previous surgery. The most common scars to note are the Pfannenstiel scars of previous pelvic surgery, the small subumbilical and suprapubic scars of laparoscopy and the gridiron incision of a previous appendicectomy.

The next stage is palpation. This begins with the symphysis fundal height (SFH) (Fig. 2.12). The uterus is palpated with the palm of the left hand, moving it upwards and pressing with the lateral border. There is a 'give' at the fundus. Hold the end of a tape measure, measuring-side (i.e. centimetre-side) down, at the fundus and mark the tape at the upper border of the pubic symphysis.

At 20 weeks' gestation, the uterus comes up to around the umbilicus and the SFH is ~20 cm. Each week, the uterus grows 1 cm, so that at 28 weeks it is ~28 ± 2 cm and at 32 weeks it is ~32 ± 2 cm. Metric measurement is therefore a reasonable guide to the size for gestation, and is useful in identifying those that are large- or small-for-dates.

The next stage is to feel the uterus using gentle pressure of both hands, noting any irregularities, any tender areas and the two fetal 'poles', head and bottom. The 'lie' of the fetus refers to the axis of the poles in relation to the mother. It is usually longitudinal but can be transverse or oblique. The presentation refers to the part of the baby that is entering the pelvis. Generally, it is the head (cephalic) or the bottom (breech) but it can be the back or limbs (Figs 2.13–2.16). In twins, it should be possible to feel at least three fetal poles.

The 'engagement' of the head refers to how far into the pelvis it has moved (Figs 2.17–2.21). This may be palpated by turning to face the woman's feet and pushing suprapubically, trying to ballot the head between the fingers. The descent can be likened to a setting sun and is recorded as

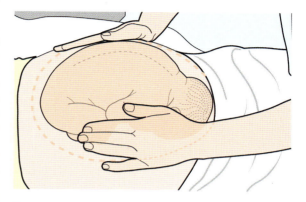

Fig. 2.13 **Palpation of the lie and liquor volume.**

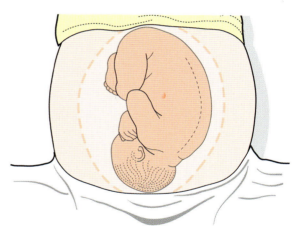

Fig. 2.14 **Longitudinal cephalic.**

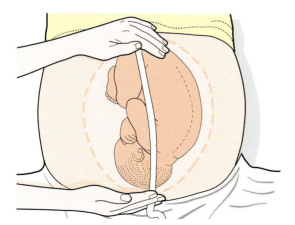

Fig. 2.12 **Measurement of symphysis fundal height.**

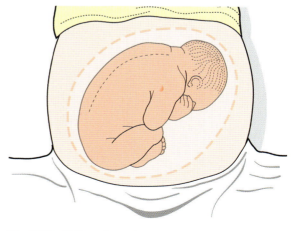

Fig. 2.15 **Oblique breech.**

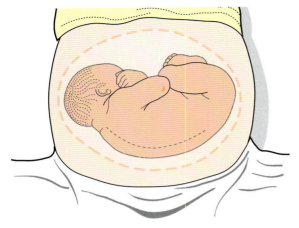

Fig. 2.16 **Transverse (back presenting).**

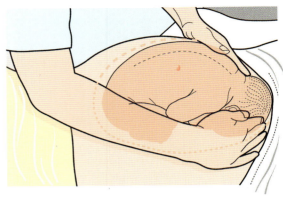

Fig. 2.17 Palpation of the descent of the fetal head.

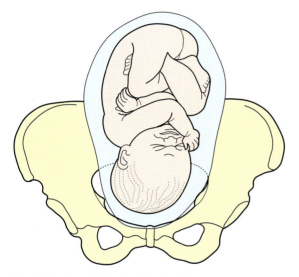

Fig. 2.18 **Head 5/5 palpable (free).**

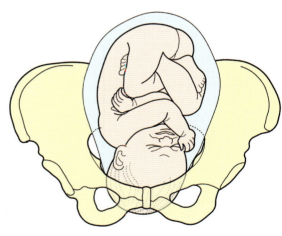

Fig. 2.19 **Head 4/5 palpable.**

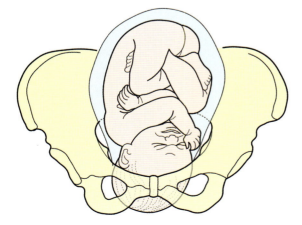

Fig. 2.20 **Head 2/5 palpable (engaged).**

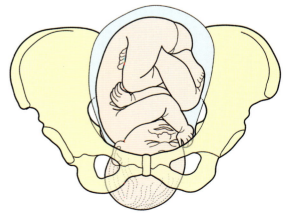

Fig. 2.21 **Head 0/5 palpable (fully engaged).**

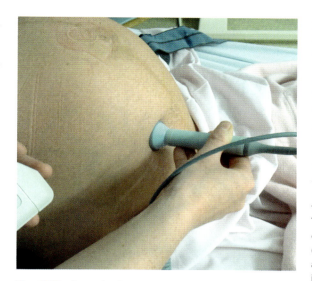

Fig. 2.22 **Auscultation with a Doppler probe.**

'fifths palpable'. It is 'engaged' when the maximum diameter of the fetal head has passed through the pelvic brim. Therefore, at three-fifths (3/5) palpable, it is not engaged but at two-fifths (2/5) palpable it is.

An attempt should be made to get an impression of the liquor volume, particularly if the SFH is abnormal. In oligohydramnios, fetal parts can often be felt easily, while in polyhydramnios the uterus is usually tense and fetal parts are difficult to feel. Also, feel for the back of the fetus. It is firmer than the limbs (the side of most movements) and lies to one side. This helps work out the position of the fetus and where to pick up the fetal heart. To hear the fetal heart, place a USS transducer over the anterior shoulder of the fetus (Fig. 2.22). The rate should be between 100 to 160 bpm and differentiated clearly from the mother's pulse. At the end of the examination, ensure that the woman is comfortable, cover her abdomen and help her to sit up.

Obstetrical vaginal and speculum examination

Speculum and vaginal examination in a pregnant woman should only be performed with a clear clinical indication. Vaginal examination is the cornerstone of intrapartum management. Speculum is used in the diagnosis of antepartum haemorrhage, pre-labour rupture of membranes and to assess pre-labour cervical change.

If the diagnosis of pre-term labour or membrane rupture is suspected from the clinical history, a speculum examination is important for three reasons. The first is to look for evidence of liquor in the vagina. The technique is similar to gynaecological speculum examination, with careful aseptic technique. A pool of fluid, sometimes containing white flecks of vernix, can usually be seen in the posterior vagina or coming from the cervix on coughing. The second is to allow swabs to be taken – either looking for pathogenic bacteria, in particular group B β-haemolytic streptococci, or to test for fetal fibronectin as part of pre-term labour assessment. The third is to allow a visual inspection of the cervix. Digital examination is used to assess the cervical length/effacement (shortening of the cervix), cervical dilatation and descent and position of presenting part. Feel for the cervix and note its position. Is it anterior or posterior and difficult to reach? Note its length. The cervix shortens from 3–4 cm until it is flush with the fetal head and does not protrude into the vagina. This is called effacement. What is its consistency? Is it soft like a cheek or hard like a nose? Feel for the os and how much it is dilated, as determined by how far the fingers can stretch inside it. This may be only 1–2 cm or up to 10 cm at full dilatation. The station of the presenting part is determined relative to the mother's ischial spines. When the biparietal diameter of the fetal head is level with the ischial spines, this is described as station 0. Above this point is -1, -2 etc. and when the head is below the ischial spines it is +1 or +2.

In the early stages of labour and during the induction process, the findings of the cervix can be described using the modified Bishop score (see Table 32.1). As the cervix ripens, it becomes softer, shorter, more anterior and more dilated, and the fetal head descends. As the onset of spontaneous labour approaches, the Bishop score increases.

3

Paediatric gynaecology and disorders of sex development

Normal puberty

Introduction

Puberty should transform a girl into a fertile woman, and its social importance is so great that any deviation from normality may be the cause of considerable embarrassment and anxiety. This chapter describes normal puberty and outlines the management of both precocious and delayed puberty. It will also cover some of the gynaecological conditions which may affect pre- and post-pubertal girls.

Pathophysiology of normal puberty

The onset of pubertal development is heralded by an increase in pulsatile release of gonadotrophin-releasing hormone (GnRH) from the hypothalamus. Following brief activation of the GnRH neurons in the neonatal period, they remain in a dormant state until the onset of puberty. Initially the pulsatile release of GnRH occurs only at night, but as puberty progresses it occurs throughout the day and night. Pulsatile GnRH release causes gonadotropic cells of the anterior pituitary to release luteinizing hormone (LH) and follicle-stimulating hormone (FSH). These gonadotrophins lead to the production of ovarian oestrogen, which initiates the physical changes of puberty.

Pubertal development

The external signs of puberty usually (but not always) occur in a specific order (Fig. 3.1), and are described in five Tanner stages (Figs 3.2 and 3.3). Breast development (thelarche) is usually the first sign of puberty. Pubic and axillary hair (pubarche) normally develops about 6 months later, although one-third of girls' pubic hair may appear before breast development. Breast development occurs as a result of rising oestradiol levels, and pubic and axillary hair by adrenal androgen secretion. Menarche occurs late in puberty, normally corresponding to the end of the growth spurt. Maximal growth velocity usually occurs after the start of breast and pubic and axillary hair development, but in some girls the growth spurt may be the first sign of puberty. The complete process of puberty is usually a slow progression taking a minimum of 18 months.

During puberty the ovaries enlarge and develop multifollicular cysts under the influence of pulsatile gonadotrophin secretion. The uterus also grows steadily through puberty. Due to the relative immaturity of the hypothalamic–pituitary–ovarian axis in the first 2 years following menarche, more than half of menstrual cycles are anovulatory, resulting in irregular cycles. After the first 1–2 years, the capacity for oestrogen-positive feedback on the anterior pituitary develops with the subsequent mid-cycle LH surge and ovulation, resulting in regulation of the menstrual cycle. Anovulatory cycles are often heavy and prolonged, with some girls bleeding for several weeks at a time. This can lead to iron-deficiency anaemia, and in rare cases cardiovascular collapse requiring admission and blood transfusion. Initial anovulatory cycles tend to be pain free, although heavy menstrual loss can result in an element of dysmenorrhoea. When regular ovulatory cycles commence, the periods often become more painful due to the increased levels of circulating prostaglandins.

Age of menarche

Since the late 19th century, there has been a gradual decline in the age of menarche. In the UK, the average age of menarche has fallen from 15 years in 1860 to the current average age of 12.3 years. The onset of puberty will range between individuals, with 95% of girls showing signs of secondary sexual characteristics between the ages of 8.5 and 13 years.

Energy reserves and metabolic conditions play an important role in the timing of pubertal development. Leptin, a hormone released by adipose cells, is known to play a critical role in body weight homeostasis and the metabolic control of puberty. Childhood obesity is consistently associated with an early onset of puberty. Factors which delay the attainment of a critical body weight may delay puberty. These include malnutrition, eating disorders and excessive exercise.

Variations of normal puberty

Premature adrenarche is the secretion of adrenal androgens resulting in the appearance of pubic hair before the age of

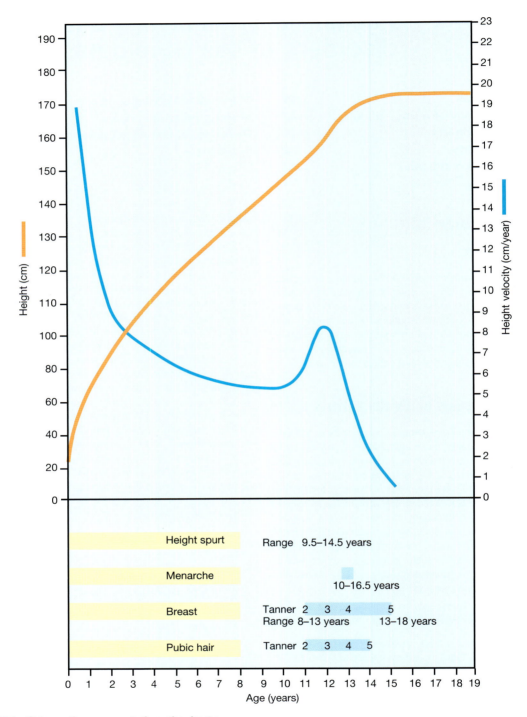

Fig. 3.1 Schematic representation of puberty.

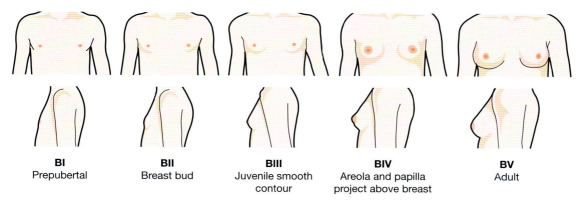

BI	**BII**	**BIII**	**BIV**	**BV**
Prepubertal	Breast bud	Juvenile smooth contour	Areola and papilla project above breast	Adult

Fig. 3.2   **Tanner stages of breast development.**

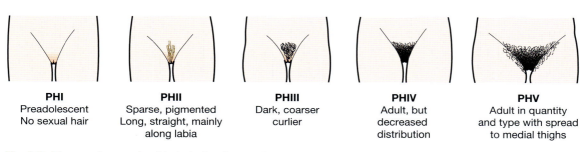

PHI	**PHII**	**PHIII**	**PHIV**	**PHV**
Preadolescent No sexual hair	Sparse, pigmented Long, straight, mainly along labia	Dark, coarser curlier	Adult, but decreased distribution	Adult in quantity and type with spread to medial thighs

Fig. 3.3   **Tanner stages of pubic hair development.**

8 years. Axillary hair, body odour and acne may occur, but other secondary sexual characteristics do not. It can be slowly progressive or stay stable, and puberty usually begins at the normal time. Serum androgen concentrations may be slightly raised or normal. Gonadotrophin levels are prepubertal and bone age is normal.

Premature thelarche is defined as the premature development of breast tissue in the absence of other secondary sexual characteristics before the age of 8 years. The most common age of onset is within the first two years of life but can occur at any age. Progression to precocious puberty can occur in up to a third of girls.

Isolated premature menarche is the occurrence of vaginal bleeding in the absence of other secondary sexual characteristics. It is a diagnosis of exclusion after vaginal and uterine pathology, foreign body and precocious puberty have been ruled out. It can be an isolated event or it can recur. Puberty will be expected to start at the normal time and final adult height will not be affected.

Precocious puberty

The development of secondary sexual characteristics prior to the age of 8 years in girls constitutes precocious puberty and must be investigated. Central (gonadotrophin-dependent) precocious puberty occurs when there is a pituitary or hypothalamic cause, and peripheral (gonadotrophin-independent) precocious puberty occurs when puberty is induced by sex steroids from other courses such as a hormone-secreting tumour. The growth spurt is a striking feature, but frequently it is the occurrence of menstruation which brings the girl to medical attention. In the event of vaginal bleeding, a local cause such as a foreign body or malignancy should always be ruled out. Children with precocious puberty should be under the care of a paediatric endocrinologist.

Causes of precocious puberty

Gonadotrophic-dependent precocious puberty (GDPP)

In 90% of girls with GDPP, no cause is found. In the remaining 10%, causes are intracranial and include encephalitis, meningitis, cranial radiation, hydrocephaly and space-occupying neoplasms, such as optic nerve gliomas. Sexual abuse has been reported as a precipitating cause.

Gonadotrophic-independent precocious puberty (GIPP)

Causes of GIPP include feminizing tumours of the ovary or adrenal, which may give rise to vaginal bleeding without signs of pubertal development. Other causes include hypothyroidism, and the very rare McCune–Albright syndrome, in which cystic cavities develop in the long bones (polyostotic fibrous dysplasia) and café-au-lait skin

Table 3.1	Differential features of delayed puberty			
	Stature	**Gonadotrophins**	**Gonadal steroids**	**Karyotype**
Constitutional delay	Short	Pre-pubertal	Low	Normal
Hypogonadotrophic hypogonadism	Normal	Low	Low	Normal
Primary gonadal failure:				
Turner syndrome and variants	Short	High	Low	XO and variants
Gonadal dysgenesis	Normal	High	Low	XX or XY

pigmentation is evident. Other rare causes include ingestion of exogenous oestrogens.

Investigation and management of precocious puberty

1. Plasma FSH, LH, oestradiol and thyroid function tests
2. X-ray of the hand to determine bone age, which may be advanced
3. Ultrasound scan of the abdomen and pelvis
4. Radiological skeletal survey of the long bones if McCune–Albright syndrome is suspected
5. Cranial computed tomography (CT) or magnetic resonance imaging (MRI) scan.

In the constitutional and cerebral forms, the ovaries may show a multicystic appearance on ultrasound as seen in normal puberty. Ultrasound will also distinguish between a follicular cyst, which will be expected to subside spontaneously, and a predominantly solid oestrogen-secreting granulosa/theca cell tumour of the ovary, which will require surgical removal.

Treatment

With precocious puberty the aims of treatment are to:
1. suppress menstruation and prevent progression of puberty
2. maximize growth potential and
3. achieve psychological well-being.

Not all children need treatment, as symptoms may only be slowly progressive. Treatment prevents progression but does not usually reverse changes that have already happened. If an underlying aetiology is found, this should be treated.

GnRH agonists suppress gonadotrophin secretion. Depot injections are given every 3 months and treatment can be continued for 2–3 years without significant side-effects. Treatment is stopped when an acceptable age for puberty is reached.

Delayed puberty

Delayed puberty in girls is defined as the absence of physical manifestations of puberty by the age of 13 years. Primary amenorrhoea is the absence of menarche and needs to be evaluated in the context of secondary sexual characteristics. The diagnosis may be made by age 15 if a patient has normal secondary sexual characteristics, or if menarche has failed to occur by 2 years post breast budding. In some instances, a girl may enter puberty but the normal progression is not maintained. This is described as 'arrested puberty'.

Causes of delayed puberty

These features of delayed puberty fall into three main categories (Table 3.1).

Constitutional delay

Constitutional delay is the commonest cause of delayed puberty. These girls are normal, but just inherently late at entering puberty. They are usually of short stature, but their height is generally appropriate for their bone age. All stages of development are delayed. They may be considered to be physiologically immature, with a functional deficiency of GnRH for their chronological age, but not for their stage of physiological development. There is frequently a history of delayed menarche in their mothers.

In these patients, bone age shows a better correlation with the onset and progression of puberty than does chronological age. On attaining a bone age of 11–13 years, they can be expected to enter puberty.

Hypogonadotrophic hypogonadism

This is caused by the deficient production, secretion or action of GnRH. It may be associated with:
- conditions affecting body weight, such as chronic systemic disease, malnutrition or anorexia nervosa
- central nervous system tumours – the most common of these rare conditions is craniopharyngioma. Girls may also have associated growth hormone deficiency and, therefore, short stature
- isolated gonadotrophin deficiency. Such patients are generally of appropriate height for chronological age. The association of hypogonadotrophic hypogonadism with anosmia or hyposmia is called Kallmann syndrome, which results from incomplete embryonic migration of GnRH-synthesizing neurons. This occurs in 50% of cases.

Premature ovarian insufficiency (POI)

POI is defined by the loss of ovarian activity before the age of 40. If this happens at a young age, puberty will not occur. There are various different causes of POI, including:

- autoimmune disease (this may also be associated with autoimmune thyroid and adrenal disease)
- chromosomal disorders (Turner syndrome and Fragile X)
- chemotherapy or radiotherapy for a childhood malignancy, as a result of germ cell damage
- metabolic disorders such as galactosaemia
- bilateral oophorectomy.

Other causes

These include hyperprolactinaemia and hypothyroidism. A disorder of sex development may also present with delayed puberty and this is discussed in more detail later.

Investigation of delayed or arrested puberty

The scheme of investigation follows logically from the differential diagnosis discussed previously:

1. plasma FSH, LH, oestradiol, prolactin and thyroid function tests
2. karyotype
3. X-ray for bone age
4. cranial CT or MRI scan.

Management of delayed puberty

Constitutional delay

Often, reassurance and continued observation are sufficient. It is important to reassure the parents as well as the girl herself. Where psychological problems arise as a result of comparison with her peers, induction of puberty may be indicated.

Hypogonadotrophic hypogonadism

In those with low weight, restoration of weight may result in spontaneous onset of puberty. Those with central nervous system tumours require appropriate neurosurgical treatment. Induction of puberty is required, and treatment with hormone replacement is continued until approximately age 50, although 10–20% will have spontaneous return of reproductive function.

Premature ovarian insufficiency

Induction of puberty is required, and hormone replacement is continued until approximately age 50. Pregnancy can be achieved through invitro fertilization (IVF) with ovum donation.

Spontaneous ovulation can occur in this group with a pregnancy risk of approximately 5%.

Induction of puberty

The aim is to ensure normal progress through puberty, and this is achieved by incremental doses of oestrogen, either orally or transdermally. A low dose of oestrogen is commenced and increased gradually over approximately 2 years, in order to maximize breast development. After 2 years of oestrogen therapy, or after the first menstrual bleed, a progestogen is added to avoid unopposed oestrogen stimulation of the endometrium. Commonly, hormone replacement therapy is used, but the combined contraceptive pill is an alternative, preferably on a continuous basis to maximize oestrogen replacement. Bone mineral density should be assessed every 3–5 years, and vitamin D and calcium levels should also be optimized.

Pre-pubertal conditions

Vaginal discharge

Vaginal discharge is the commonest reason for referral to a paediatric gynaecology clinic. The most frequent age of referral is 3–10 years. Non-specific bacterial vulvovaginitis is the most common cause. Vaginal cultures are often non-specific, but organisms commonly found in the rectum or upper respiratory tract are often found, such as group A *Streptococcus* or *Haemophilus influenzae*. Symptoms include discharge, soreness and itching, and these can be chronic and distressing.

Contributory aetiological factors include the hypo-oestrogenic state and neutral pH of the pre-pubertal vagina, the proximity of the vagina and anus, the under-developed flat labia and hygiene. Rarer causes such as a foreign body or tumour must be excluded if symptoms are persistent. Sexual abuse should always be considered but it is not the cause in the majority of cases. Vulval hygiene, with the avoidance of soaps in the genital area and the use of emollients, is the cornerstone of successful management. Threadworms can lead to genital irritation, particularly at night time, so empirical treatment could also be tried.

Vaginal bleeding

Vaginal bleeding in the pre-pubertal girl always needs specialist referral and may require examination under anaesthesia (vaginoscopy and cystoscopy) to rule out local causes such as a foreign body or malignancy. Hormone profile, bone age and pelvic ultrasound should also be performed to look for precocious puberty.

Labial adhesions

Labial adhesions occur due to the hypo-oestrogenic state of the pre-pubertal genitalia. The labia minora fuse together in the midline. There may be a small opening or there may be no visible opening (Fig. 3.4). Typically the labia are apart at birth due to the effect of maternal oestrogens. They then fuse together after a few months. Usually they are asymptomatic, but occasionally urine can get trapped behind them causing post-void dribbling or even urinary tract infections. In most cases, no treatment is required and the parents

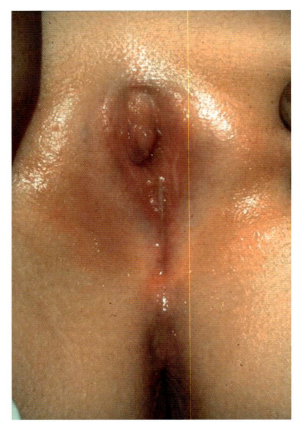

Fig. 3.4   Labial adhesions.

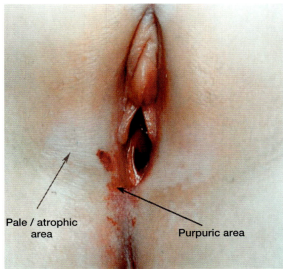

Pale / atrophic area

Purpuric area

Fig. 3.5   Lichen sclerosus.

can be reassured that the adhesions will open up as the girl progresses through puberty. In cases where there are significant urinary symptoms or for maternal reassurance, a low-dose oestrogen ointment can be applied to the adhesions twice daily for 6 weeks. This can cause some breast budding, which will usually disappear after treatment finishes, and the labial adhesions often reoccur. Good hygiene and use of emollients can help to prevent recurrence. In very rare cases, the labia may need to be separated under general anaesthetic.

Lichen sclerosus

Lichen sclerosus is an inflammatory skin condition that occurs in postmenopausal women and pre-pubertal girls. It can affect any part of the body but it most frequently occurs on the genitalia. It can cause itching and discomfort, which can be quite severe. White plaques occur typically in a figure-of-eight pattern around the vulva and anus. There may also be areas of superficial haemorrhage, thickening of the skin and fissures (Fig. 3.5). Diagnosis is usually made by the typical appearance, and biopsies are rarely required. Treatment is with a potent steroid ointment in a reducing regime over a few months. Once it clears up, it may not

recur, or it may flare intermittently, but it will usually (but not always) resolve when the girl goes through puberty. Unlike lichen sclerosus in postmenopausal women, parents can be reassured that it does not increase their risk of malignancy.

Post-pubertal conditions

Adolescent menstrual dysfunction

Menstrual disorders are common in adolescent girls. In up to 25% of girls, it can be quite significant, affecting daily life and resulting in school absence; however, serious pathology is rare. Periods can be irregular, heavy and/or painful, especially in the first few years following menarche. There are many treatment options that are safe to use in adolescents, although the evidence for their use is extrapolated from adult data.

- Tranexamic acid. This is an antifibrinolytic taken during the period, and can reduce blood loss by up to 50%.
- Mefenamic acid. This is a non-steroidal anti-inflammatory that inhibits prostaglandin synthetase. It should be taken regularly, starting the day before menstruation, and can be very effective for dysmenorrhea. It can also reduce blood flow by up to 20%.
- Contraceptive pill. This can be used as first-line management of irregular, heavy and painful periods. It can reduce blood loss by over 40% and reduce menstrual cramping by 50%. The combined contraceptive pill tends to give the best cycle control, but the progestogen only contraceptive pill can also be used, although this can result in irregular bleeding.

The combined pill can be used cyclically, tri-cyclically or on a continuous basis. For girls who are troubled with acne, a more anti-androgenic pill would be appropriate.

■ Oral progestogens. These are commonly used for adolescent menstrual dysfunction. They can be taken continuously to defer or delay menstruation, or cyclically to improve irregular and heavy periods. They should be taken for 21 days, with a 1-week break for menstruation. They have been found to reduce blood loss by over 80%.

■ Levonorgestrel-releasing intrauterine system (Mirena). This is a T-shaped plastic frame that sits in the uterine cavity and releases a small amount of progestogen each day. It can be very useful when first-line treatments have failed or when there are medical contraindications to the use of the contraceptive pill. It can be safely used from menarche onwards and lasts for 5 years. In girls who have never been sexually active, it needs to be inserted and removed under general anaesthetic. It is very effective for both heavy and painful periods. Bleeding can be irregular for the first 3–6 months, but by 12 months 65% will be amenorrhoeic.

Müllerian duct anomalies

Development of the genital tract

The Müllerian ducts begin to develop during the sixth week of embryonic development. The two ducts develop caudally and medially, and then fuse in the midline to create the fallopian tubes, uterus, cervix and upper vagina. The Wolffian ducts regress at around 10 weeks' gestation due to the absence of testosterone. The urogenital sinus forms by week 7. Cells proliferate from the upper portion of the urogenital sinus to form sinovaginal bulbs. These fuse to form the vaginal plate, which extends from the Müllerian ducts to the urogenital sinus. This plate begins to canalize, starting at the hymen, and proceeds upwards to the cervix. This process is complete by 21 weeks' gestation. The Müllerian duct develops in close proximity to the kidneys, and therefore if a Müllerian anomaly is identified, the renal tract should always be assessed.

Imperforate hymen

The hymen is a thin membrane that covers the vaginal opening until late fetal life. It becomes perforate towards term. The incidence of imperforate hymen is approximately 1:1000 live female births. Presentation is usually with increasing cyclical abdominal pain in the absence of menstruation, towards the end of puberty. There may be a palpable abdominal mass, and on gently parting the labia there may be a visible blue bulging membrane (Fig. 3.6). Ultrasound will show a large haematocolpos, where the vagina is filled with blood. Treatment is with incision and

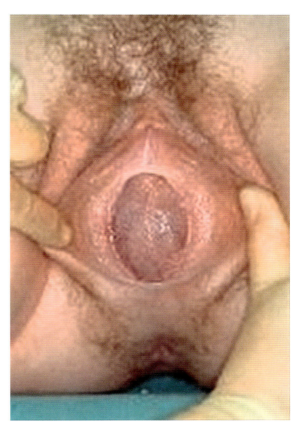

Fig. 3.6 **Imperforate hymen.**

resection of the hymen. If the hymen is not resected, there is a risk of re-obstruction. However, care must be taken not to resect too close to the vaginal mucosa, which may lead to scarring and stenosis at the vaginal introitus.

Transverse vaginal septa

A transverse vaginal septum results from a failure of canalization of the vaginal plate where the urogenital sinus meets the Müllerian duct. They can be perforate and present difficulties with tampons or sex, or they can be imperforate and present with obstructed menstruation. They can vary in their thickness and location within the vagina. On external genital examination, the vaginal opening will look normal. An ultrasound will reveal a haemotocolpos. MRI of the pelvis is essential in order to assess location and thickness of the septum for preoperative planning (Fig. 3.7). Transverse vaginal septa should be referred to a specialist surgeon. Treatment involves surgical resection of the septum with anastomosis of the proximal and distal vaginas. Septa can be resected vaginally, laparoscopically or via an abdomino-perineal approach depending on the classification of the septum. Pregnancy outcomes for low, thin septa are very good. Abdomino-perineal procedures often involve

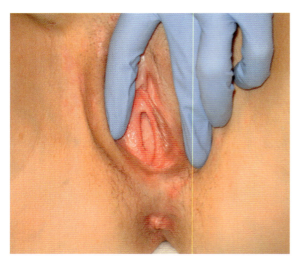

Fig. 3.7 **Haematometrocolpos with a transverse vaginal septum.**

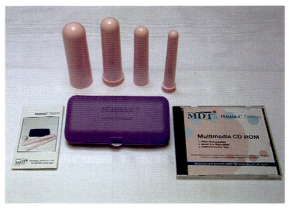

Fig. 3.8 **Dilators can be used to create a vagina, provided the uterus, if present, is non-functioning.**
(Courtesy of Medical Devices Technology International Ltd.)

complex reconstructive surgery, and therefore long-term complications are more common and pregnancy outcomes are poor.

Longitudinal vaginal septa

Longitudinal vaginal septa result from a failure of canalization of the vaginal plate. Septa can be complete, extending from the cervix to the introitus, or they can be partial involving any part of the vagina. They often present with dyspareunia, difficulty with tampons or they may be diagnosed during labour. Over 85% of longitudinal vaginal septa are associated with a uterine anomaly, most commonly a complete septate uterus or uterus didelphys. When there are two separate uteri, one hemivagina can be obstructed, resulting in increasing pain despite normal menstruation. This can be associated with renal anomalies, as in obstructed hemivagina and ipsilateral renal anomaly syndrome. Longitudinal vaginal septa can be resected vaginally.

Mayer-Rokitansky-Küster-Hauser syndrome (MRKH)

This results from interrupted development and failure of fusion of the Müllerian ducts. There is an absent or rudimentary uterus, with vaginal agenesis. It affects 1 in 4500 females. Ovarian function is normal, so it presents with primary amenorrhoea with normal secondary sexual characteristics. Diagnosis is usually made by clinical examination and ultrasound assessment. MRI can be used if there is diagnostic uncertainty. It is possible to create a vagina with regular use of vaginal dilators (Fig. 3.8). This is successful in approximately 85% of cases. If dilation is unsuccessful, vaginas can be created surgically with a traction vaginoplasty or with the use of extravaginal tissues such as bowel. Options for fertility include surrogacy (using

their own eggs through IVF) and adoption. Uterine transplants are being trialed in several countries and although they are still experimental, they are an exciting possibility for the future. Psychological input is essential in the management of girls with MRKH.

Uterine anomalies

Abnormal uterine shapes (Fig. 3.9) are usually asymptomatic but may present with menorrhagia, primary infertility, recurrent pregnancy loss, pre-term labour or abnormal fetal lie. There is no place for surgery with a unicornuate uterus, bicornuate uterus or uterus didelphys. If there is a non-communicating obstructed horn, this will need to be removed laparoscopically. Pregnancy in a rudimentary horn carries a risk of rupture and significant haemorrhage. If a uterine septum is associated with infertility or recurrent pregnancy loss, surgical resection can be considered. Cervical agenesis is a very rare anomaly, which presents with obstructed menstruation. Management is with laparoscopic uterovaginal anastomosis.

Disorders of sex development (DSD)

DSD are a group of conditions where the development of chromosomal, gonadal or anatomical sex is atypical. The incidence of DSD is estimated to be in the region of 1 in 4500 births. Presentation can vary from atypical genitalia at birth, discordance between prenatal karyotype and phenotype at birth, inguinal hernias in childhood, delayed puberty, primary amenorrhoea or virilization in adolescents, or it may be diagnosed following a diagnosis in a sibling. The term DSD was adopted at a consensus conference in 2006; however, it has not been universally accepted by some patients and support groups. Negative aspects of the term DSD include the stigma of having a 'disorder',

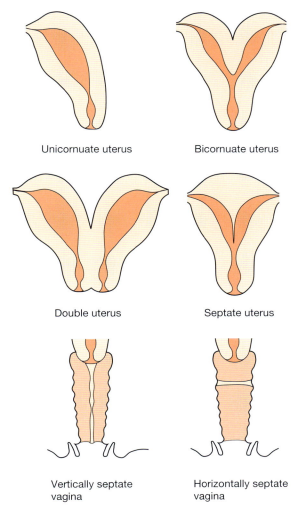

Unicornuate uterus   Bicornuate uterus

Double uterus   Septate uterus

Vertically septate vagina   Horizontally septate vagina

Fig. 3.9   Common genital tract malformations.

and the perception that 'sex' implies sexual behaviour. Some prefer the terms 'intersex' or 'differences/diverse' sex development.

Normal gonadal and genital tract development

The primordial gonads appear during the sixth week of development. Müllerian and Wolffian ducts also begin to develop at this stage. Presence of the *SRY* gene (sex-determiing region of the Y chromosome) in XY embryos stimulates testicular development. Testes produce testosterone, which results in development of the Wolffian structures (the vas deferens, seminal vesicles and epididymis). Peripheral conversion of testosterone to dihydrotestosterone (DHT) requires the enzyme 5-alpha-reductase and causes virilization of the external genitalia. At 12 weeks, the fetus is recognizably male and masculinization of the genitalia is said to be complete by 14 weeks. The penis, similar in size to the clitoris at 14

weeks, enlarges from around 20 weeks until birth. The testes also produce anti-Müllerian hormone (AMH), which causes regression of the Müllerian ducts. Ovarian development was previously considered a 'default' development due to the absence of *SRY*. However, regulatory gene networks are now known to be involved. In the XX gonad, ovarian development is promoted and testicular development inhibited by the expression of specific embryonic genes. The ovarian cortex develops at 12 weeks and by 13.5 weeks primordial follicles are present. The Wolffian structures regress at around 10 weeks, due to the absence of testosterone. As AMH is not produced, the Müllerian ducts develop, and in the absence of testosterone, female external genitalia develop, as previously described.

Turner syndrome

Turner syndrome results from a complete or partial absence of one X chromosome. It is the commonest chromosomal anomaly in females, occurring in 1 out of 2500 female births. Clinical features associated with Turner syndrome include:

- short stature
- POI and infertility
- autoimmune thyroid disease (hypothyroidism)
- diabetes
- inflammatory bowel disease
- sensorineural and conduction deafness
- renal anomalies
- cardiovascular disease, both structural (e.g. aortic root dilatation, bicuspid aortic valve and coarctation) and atherosclerotic
- hypertension
- osteoporosis.

The most common chromosome complement in Turner syndrome is monosomy 45,X or the presence of an abnormal X chromosome such as isochromosome X, a partial deletion or a ring X. Mosaicism is also common and includes 45,X/46,XX and 45,X/46,XY. An accurate karyotype is important as it allows some prediction of clinical severity. Ring karyotype is associated with a more severe phenotype, whereas mosaics generally have a milder phenotype with up to 40% entering spontaneous puberty. If there is a Y chromosome, or fragment of a Y present, then there is a higher incidence of gonadal tumours and the streak gonads should be removed prophylactically. This can be done laparoscopically.

Although the majority of individuals with Turner syndrome are diagnosed during childhood or adolescence, about 10% are not diagnosed until adulthood. The focus of paediatric care is on short stature, whereas adult women are generally more concerned with oestrogen replacement and fertility prospects. Pregnancy is possible, but in general ovum donation and IVF is required. Pre-pregnancy counselling is essential and women should be looked after in a high-risk antenatal clinic. Aortic root dissection can be catastrophic in pregnant women with Turner syndrome.

Women with Turner syndrome should be looked after by clinicians experienced in this condition and regular monitoring for associated problems is essential.

46,XX DSD

Congenital adrenal hyperplasia (CAH)

CAH is the commonest DSD, with an incidence of 1 in 14 000 worldwide. It usually presents with atypical genitalia in the neonate. The name is derived from hyperplasia in the adrenal gland, which arises from the overproduction of steroids (Fig. 3.10). Affected individuals have an enzyme block in the steroidogenic pathway in the adrenal gland, with over 90% being a deficiency in 21-hydroxylase. This enzyme converts progesterone to deoxycorticosterone in the aldosterone biosynthetic pathway, and 17-hydroxyprogesterone (17-OHP) to deoxycortisol in the cortisol biosynthetic pathway. The resultant low levels of cortisol continue to drive the negative feedback loop, leading to increased levels of androgen precursors and, in turn, to elevated testosterone production. 17-OHP levels can be used in the diagnosis and in monitoring control.

Excessive testosterone levels in a female fetus will lead to virilization of the external genitalia. The clitoris is enlarged and the labia are fused and scrotal in appearance. The upper vagina joins the male-type urethra and opens as one common channel onto the perineum. The chromosomes are XX and the ovaries are normal, as are the internal structures, including the fallopian tubes, uterus and upper vagina.

Approximately 75% of children with 21-hydroxylase deficiency CAH will have a 'salt-losing' variety, which affects the ability to produce aldosterone. This represents a life-threatening situation, and those children who are salt-losers often become dangerously unwell within a few days of birth. Affected individuals require lifelong steroid replacement, such as hydrocortisone, along with fludrocortisone for salt-losers. Both under- and over-treatment may result in short stature, and girls may have oligomenorrhoea or amenorrhoea, leading to fertility difficulties.

Traditional management was with feminizing genital surgery during the first year of life to reduce the size of the clitoris and open up the lower vagina. However, childhood clitoral surgery can reduce clitoral sensation and be detrimental to adult sexual function. In addition, vaginal surgery usually needs revising at adolescence. Vaginal surgery is much more successful when performed after puberty when the tissues are oestrogenized. Genital reconstructive surgery in individuals with DSD is highly controversial. Surgical decisions must be made in the context of a multidisciplinary team with involvement of the parents and child (if possible depending on age). Psychological support for the parents and child is imperative.

CAH is an autosomal recessive condition and molecular genetics now allows prenatal diagnosis in families where an affected child has already been born. Prenatal therapy is possible with dexamethasone, as this crosses the placenta and should reduce the drive mediated by low cortisol levels. There are concerns about the effect of antenatal steroid treatment on neurodevelopment of the child, and research into this is ongoing.

46,XY DSD

Complete androgen insensitivity syndrome (CAIS)

CAIS is the most frequently occurring 46,XY DSD, with an incidence of 1 in 40 000 births. CAIS is due to an abnormality of the androgen receptor, which is completely or partially unable to respond to androgen stimulation. In a fetus with CAIS, testes form normally due to the action of the *SRY* gene. These testes secrete AMH, leading to regression of the Müllerian ducts. CAIS women do not therefore have a uterus. Testosterone is also produced; however, due to the inability of the androgen receptor to respond, the

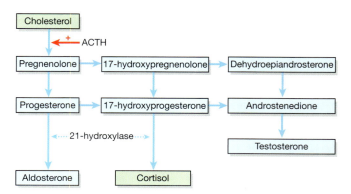

Fig. 3.10 Synthesis of steroid hormones. Deficiency of the enzyme 21-hydroxylase leads to a build-up of precursors, particularly the weak androgens dehydroepiandrosterone and androsterone.

external genitalia do not virilize and instead undergo female development. The result is a female (both physically and psychologically) with no uterus, and testes are found at some point in their line of descent through the abdomen from the pelvis to the inguinal canal. During puberty, breast development will be normal, but the effects of androgens are not seen, and pubic and axillary hair growth is minimal. Around two-thirds of women with CAIS have inherited the androgen receptor gene mutation from their mother (i.e. X-linked inheritance), with the remaining one-third thought to be new mutations.

The commonest presentation is with primary amenorrhoea, although children can also present before puberty with an inguinal hernia found to contain a testis. The diagnosis is made on clinical examination, with typical findings in association with an XY karyotype. However, the genetic mutation responsible can be identified in up to 90% and appropriate referral for genetic testing should be considered. Psychological support is the initial mainstay of treatment, with full disclosure of diagnosis, including karyotype. In the past, the karyotype was often concealed from the patients, leading to secrecy, stigma and isolation. Well-organized patient peer support groups have a valuable role.

Gonadectomy is usually recommended post-puberty due to the small risk of malignancy associated with intra-abdominal testes. After gonadectomy, oestrogen replacement is necessary to maintain bone mineral density and general well-being. The vagina is blind-ending and usually short. Vaginal dilation has good success rates in creating a vagina adequate for intercourse and reconstructive vaginal surgery is rarely required.

Ongoing psychological input from a suitably trained professional who has clinical experience with DSD is a vital part of long-term management.

Partial forms of androgen insensitivity also occur, leading to a spectrum of clinical features. Presentation in this situation is often at birth with atypical genitalia, and careful assessment by a specialist multidisciplinary team is required to determine the most appropriate sex of rearing.

Disorders of testosterone biosynthesis

Rarer DSDs include those resulting from a deficiency in any enzyme required in the biosynthesis or metabolism of testosterone. 5-alpha-reductase converts testosterone to the more active metabolite DHT. Deficiency leads to the development of an undervirilized male (46,XY). The condition is autosomal recessive, and individuals have normal testes. The external genitalia may be ambiguous or phenotypically female. The majority of individuals are reared as female, although subsequent virilization may occur at puberty if the gonads have not been removed. Fertility has been reported in those reared male, but is significantly reduced.

17-beta hydroxysteroid dehydrogenase deficiency occurs when there is an absence or reduction of the enzyme converting androstenedione to testosterone. This condition is autosomal recessive, and results in a 46,XY individual with ambiguous or phenotypically female genitalia. Virilization may occur at puberty.

Ovotesticular DSD

Ovotesticular DSD refers to the presence of both ovarian and testicular tissue in the same individual. The karyotype is 46,XX in over 70% of cases and the gonads may be a separate ovary and/or testes, and/or an ovotestis. The external genital appearance may be ambiguous, with Mül-lerian and Wolffian structures present internally. Asymmetry of gonads and subsequent reproductive tracts and external genitalia may occur. Fertility may be possible depending upon karyotype and phenotype. Ovotesticular DSDs are suspected by excluding other DSDs and are confirmed by histological evidence of both types of gonadal tissue – often a rather major undertaking.

Complete gonadal dysgenesis

This condition is also known as Swyer syndrome. The chromosomes are XY but the gonads are streak and do not function. A total of 10–20% of women with this syndrome have a deletion in the DNA-binding region of the SRY gene. Nevertheless, in approximately 80–90% of cases, the SRY gene is normal and mutations in other testis-determining factors are probably implicated. As the gonads are dysgenetic, no testosterone or AMH is produced and development is phenotypically female. The external genitalia are unambiguously female at birth and the uterus, vagina and fallopian tubes are normal. The condition usually first becomes apparent in adolescence with delayed puberty and amenorrhoea. Women are often taller than may have been expected. A high incidence of gonadoblastoma and germ cell malignancies in the dysgenetic gonad has been reported, and current practice is to proceed to a gonadectomy once the diagnosis is made. Management is otherwise in line with other cases of POI and involves induction of puberty with oestrogen in order to develop secondary sexual characteristics and long-term combined hormone replacement therapy with oestrogen and progesterone. Pregnancy is possible with ovum donation and IVF.

Summary

All individuals with a DSD should be managed by a multi-disciplinary team including an endocrinologist, psychologist, urologist, gynaecologist and geneticist. For children, the surgeon is most commonly a paediatric urologist; at ado-lescence, a gynaecologist may also become involved. Careful clinical assessment is essential and is supported by specialist imaging as well as biochemical and genetic investigation. For newborns with DSD, the decision must be taken as to the most appropriate sex of rearing. Factors taken into consideration will include diagnosis, clinical findings, future fertility potential and the opinions of the family. If the diagnosis is made later in childhood or at adolescence, the sex of rearing is already determined and is not usually reassigned. The diagnosis of CAH in a neonate is a medical emergency due to the risk of a salt-losing crisis. However, the allocation of sex of rearing should not be rushed into and, as noted earlier, birth registration can be deferred until an agreed decision has been made.

Early psychological input provided by a specialist clinical psychologist with experience of supporting people with DSD conditions and their parents is essential. This will enable them to explore their emotions and concerns, manage the period of uncertainty during the diagnostic process, facilitate informed decision making and help with disclosure at an age appropriate level. All adolescents with a newly diagnosed DSD or existing DSD requiring medical or surgical attention should also be routinely offered clinical psychology input.

Controversies

The most controversial aspect of management is the role of feminizing genital surgery in children with atypical genitalia assigned to a female sex of rearing. Parents can be very worried about the immediate appearance and find it difficult to look at the long-term issues. It is important that parents and clinicians are aware of the impact on future sexual function when making a decision about irreversible genital surgery for their child. As previously discussed, surgical decisions must be made in the context of a multidisciplinary team. Psychological support throughout this decision-making process for both the parents and child is imperative.

Key *points*

- Delayed puberty, the absence of physical manifestations of puberty by the age of 13 years, is most commonly a variant of normality referred to as 'constitutional delay'. It may, however, be caused by hypogonadotrophic hypogonadism, Turner syndrome or gonadal dysgenesis. Gonadotrophin levels and a karyotype should be performed.
- Precocious puberty, the appearance of signs of sexual maturation prior to the age of 8 years, may be idiopathic but is also associated with intracranial lesions, feminizing tumours and the very rare McCune–Albright syndrome.
  - Vaginal bleeding in a pre-pubertal girl should always be investigated.
  - Adolescent menstrual dysfunction is common and can be severe enough to affect daily life, but serious pathology is rare.
- If an adolescent girl presents with obstructed menstruation and haematocolpos, and there isn't a blue bulge on examination, it is likely to be a transverse vaginal septum and further imaging with MRI and specialist referral is required.
- If a Müllerian anomaly is found, always assess the renal tract.
- Development of a male requires a Y chromosome, testosterone production and functioning androgen receptors.
- DSD are a group of conditions where the development of chromosomal, gonadal or anatomical sex is atypical.
- Presentation of a DSD can be at birth, or during childhood or adolescence.
- Management of DSD should be undertaken by a multidisciplinary specialist team.

4

The normal menstrual cycle and amenorrhoea

Normal menstrual cycle

Overview of the cycle

The endometrial cycle results from the growth and shedding of the uterine lining – the endometrium. This cycle, the average duration of which is 28 days, is controlled by the hormones from the ovary, and consists of a follicular phase, ovulation and a post-ovulatory (or luteal) phase. During the follicular phase the endometrium thickens (proliferative phase of the endometrium); after ovulation, endometrial growth stops and the endometrial glands become active and full of secretions (the secretory phase of the endometrium).

If the cycle is prolonged, the follicular phase lengthens (longer time to ovulation) but the luteal phase remains constant at 14 days. Fundamental to the normal menstrual cycle are:

- an intact hypothalamo–pituitary–ovarian endocrine axis
- the presence of responsive follicles in the ovaries
- a functional uterus.

Endocrine control of the menstrual cycle

Control of follicular maturation and ovulation is exercised by the hypothalamo–pituitary–ovarian axis (Fig. 4.1). The hypothalamus controls the cycle, but it can itself be influenced by higher centres in the brain, allowing factors such as anxiety or stress to affect the cycle. The hypothalamus acts on the pituitary gland by secreting gonadotrophin-releasing hormone (GnRH), a decapeptide that is secreted in a pulsatile manner approximately every 90 min. GnRH travels through the small blood vessels of the pituitary portal system to the anterior pituitary, where it acts on the pituitary gonadotrophs to stimulate the synthesis and release of follicle-stimulating hormone (FSH) and luteinizing hormone (LH). Although there are two gonadotrophins, there is just a single releasing hormone for both.

FSH is a glycoprotein that stimulates growth of follicles during the 'follicular phase' of the cycle. FSH also stimulates sex hormone secretion, predominantly of oestradiol, by the granulosa cells of the mature ovarian follicle.

LH is also a glycoprotein, and it also stimulates sex hormone production (mainly testosterone, which is subsequently converted by the action of FSH into oestradiol). LH plays an essential role in ovulation. It is the mid-cycle surge of LH that triggers rupture of the mature follicle with release of the oocyte. Post-ovulatory production of progesterone by the corpus luteum is also under the influence of LH.

The cyclical activity within the ovary which constitutes the ovarian cycle is maintained by the feedback mechanisms that operate between the ovary, the hypothalamus and the pituitary. These are described in the next section.

The ovarian cycle

Follicular phase

Days 1–8

At the start of the cycle, levels of FSH and LH rise in response to the fall of oestradiol and progesterone at menstruation. This stimulates development of 10–20 follicles. The follicle that is most sensitive to FSH is the 'dominant' follicle and is the one destined to reach full maturation and ovulation. This dominant follicle appears during the mid-follicular phase, while the remainder undergo atresia. With growth of the dominant follicle, oestradiol levels increase.

Days 9–14

As the follicle increases in size, localized accumulations of fluid appear among the granulosa cells and become confluent, giving rise to a fluid-filled central cavity called the antrum (Fig. 4.2). This transforms the primary follicle into a Graafian follicle, in which the oocyte occupies an eccentric position, surrounded by two to three layers of granulosa cells termed the cumulus oophorus.

Associated with follicular maturation, there is a progressive increase in the production of oestrogen (mainly oestradiol) by the granulosa cells of the developing follicle. As the oestradiol level rises, the release of both gonadotrophins is suppressed (negative feedback), which serves to prevent hyperstimulation of the ovary and the maturation of multiple follicles.

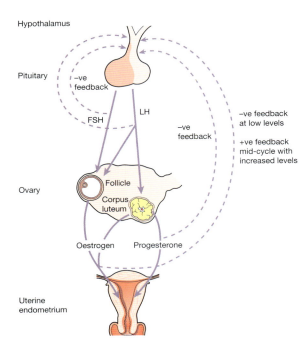

Fig. 4.1   **Hypothalamo–pituitary–ovarian–uterine axis.**

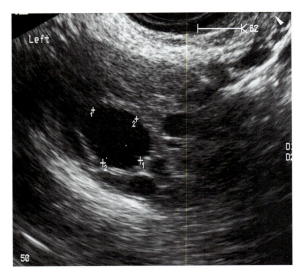

Fig. 4.2   **A dominant follicle on transvaginal ultrasound scan.**

The granulosa cells also produce inhibin. This has been implicated as a factor in the restriction of the number of follicles undergoing maturation.

Ovulation

Day 14

Ovulation is associated with rapid enlargement of the follicle, followed by protrusion from the surface of the ovarian cortex and rupture of the follicle, with extrusion of the oocyte and adherent cumulus oophorus (Fig. 4.3). Some women can identify the time of ovulation because they experience a short-lived pain in one or other iliac fossa. Ultrasound studies have shown that this pain – known as 'mittelschmerz' – actually occurs just before follicular rupture.

The final rise in oestradiol concentration is thought to be responsible for the subsequent mid-cycle surge of LH and, to a lesser extent, of FSH – positive feedback. Immediately before ovulation there is a precipitous fall in oestradiol levels and an increase in progesterone production. Ovulation follows within 18 h of the mid-cycle surge of LH.

Luteal phase

Days 15–28

The remainder of the Graafian follicle, which is retained in the ovary, is penetrated by capillaries and fibroblasts from the theca. The granulosa cells undergo luteinization and these structures collectively form the corpus luteum (Fig. 4.4). This is the major source of the sex steroid hormones oestradiol and progesterone, which are secreted by the ovary in the post-ovulatory phase.

Establishment of the corpus luteum results in a marked increase in progesterone secretion and a second rise in oestradiol levels. Progesterone levels peak 1 week after ovulation (day 21 of the 28-day cycle). Tests of serum progesterone at this time may be used in fertility investigations to confirm the occurrence of ovulation.

During the luteal phase gonadotrophin levels reach a nadir and remain low until the regression of the corpus luteum, which occurs at days 26–28. If conception and implantation occur, the corpus luteum does not regress, because it is maintained by human chorionic gonadotrophin (hCG) secreted by the trophoblast. The detection of the presence of hCG in a sample of urine forms the basis of pregnancy testing. If, however, conception and implantation have not occurred, the corpus luteum regresses, progesterone levels fall and menstruation ensues. The consequent fall in the levels of sex hormones allows the FSH and LH levels to rise and initiate the next cycle.

The uterine cycle

The cyclical production of sex hormones by the ovary induces important changes in the uterus. These involve the endometrium and cervical mucus.

The endometrium

The endometrium is composed of two layers: a superficial layer, which is shed in the course of menstruation, and a basal layer, which does not take part in this process but which regenerates the superficial layer during the subsequent cycle.

The junction between these layers is marked by a change in the character of the arterioles supplying the endometrium.

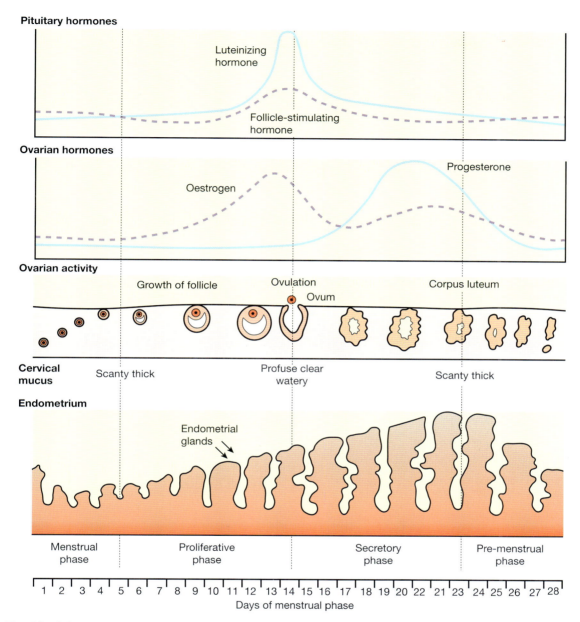

Pituitary hormones

Luteinizing hormone

Follicle-stimulating hormone

Ovarian hormones

Oestrogen

Progesterone

Ovarian activity

Growth of follicle

Ovulation

Ovum

Corpus luteum

Cervical mucus

Scanty thick

Profuse clear watery

Scanty thick

Endometrium

Endometrial glands

Menstrual phase

Proliferative phase

Secretory phase

Pre-menstrual phase

1 2 3 4 5 6 7 8 9 10 11 12 13 14 15 16 17 18 19 20 22 21 23 24 25 26 27 28

Days of menstrual phase

Fig. 4.3 Schematic diagram of ovulation.

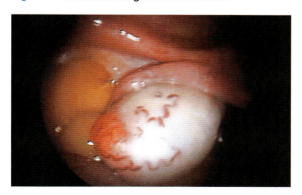

Fig. 4.4 Laparoscopic view of the corpus luteum.

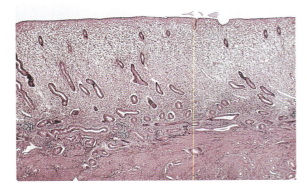

Fig. 4.5 **Proliferative endometrium.**

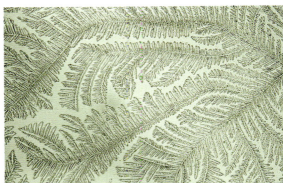

Fig. 4.7 **Cervical mucus – ferning.**

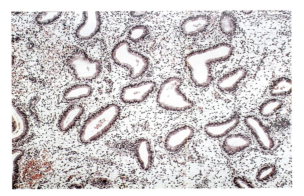

Fig. 4.6 **Secretory endometrium.**

The portion traversing the basal endometrium is straight, but thereafter its course becomes convoluted, giving rise to the spiral section of the arteriole. This anatomical configuration assumes importance in the physiological shedding of the superficial layers of the endometrium.

Proliferative phase

During the follicular phase in the ovary, the endometrium is exposed to oestrogen. After menstruation, the secretion of oestradiol from the ovary brings about repair and regeneration of the endometrium. With ongoing exposure to oestradiol there is ongoing growth and proliferation of glands and blood vessels. At this stage – the 'proliferative' phase – the glands are tubular and arranged in a regular pattern, parallel to each other (Fig. 4.5).

Secretory phase

After ovulation, progesterone production induces secretory changes in the endometrial glands, preparing the endometrium for implantation (Fig. 4.6). This is first evident as the appearance of secretory vacuoles in the glandular epithelium below the nuclei. This swiftly progresses to secretion of material into the lumen of the glands, which become tortuous and their margins appear serrated.

Menstrual phase

Normally, the luteal phase of the ovary lasts for 14 days, at the end of which regression of the corpus luteum is associated with a decline in ovarian oestradiol and progesterone production. This fall is followed by intense spasmodic contraction of the spiral section of the endometrial arterioles, giving rise to ischaemic necrosis, shedding of the superficial layer of the endometrium and bleeding.

The vasospasm appears to be due to local production of prostaglandins. Prostaglandins may also account for the increased uterine contractions at the time of the menstrual flow. The failure of menstrual blood to clot has been ascribed to the presence of local fibrinolytic activity in the endometrial blood vessels, which reaches a peak at the time of menstruation.

Cervical mucus

The glands of the cervix secrete cervical mucus. This changes in quantity and character throughout the cycle in response to sex hormones from the ovary:

- early in the follicular phase the cervical mucus is scant
- later in the follicular phase, the increasing oestradiol levels induce changes in the composition of the mucus (becomes more stretchy). This change is described by the term 'spinnbarkheit'. The water content increases progressively so that just before ovulation occurs the mucus has become watery and is easily penetrated by the spermatozoa. This mid-cycle mucus has a characteristic fern-like pattern when examined microscopically (Fig. 4.7).
- After ovulation, the progesterone secreted by the corpus luteum counteracts the effect of oestradiol and the mucus becomes thick and impermeable. This prevents entry of further spermatozoa. This effect on mucus is one of the ways by which the progestogen-only methods of contraception exert their contraceptive effect.

These changes can be monitored by a woman herself, if she is using the 'rhythm method' of contraception.

Other cyclical changes

Although cyclical changes in ovarian hormones affect the genital tract, these hormones also circulate throughout the body and can affect other organs.

Basal body temperature

A rise in basal body temperature of approximately 0.5°C occurs following ovulation and is sustained until the onset of menstruation. This is due to the thermogenic effect of progesterone acting at the hypothalamic level. Should conception occur, the elevation in basal body temperature is maintained throughout pregnancy. A similar effect can be induced by the administration of progestogens.

Breast changes

The human mammary gland is very sensitive to oestrogen and progesterone. Breast swelling is often the first sign of puberty, in response to the small increase in ovarian oestrogens. Oestradiol and progesterone act synergistically on the breast, and, during the normal cycle, breast swelling occurs in the luteal phase, apparently in response to increasing progesterone levels. The swelling is probably due to vascular changes and is not due to changes in the glandular tissue.

Psychological changes

Some women notice changes in mood during the menstrual cycle, with an increase in emotional lability in the late luteal phase. Such changes may be directly due to falling levels of progesterone, although mood changes are not always closely synchronized with hormonal fluctuations.

Amenorrhoea

Amenorrhoea may be defined as the failure of menstruation to occur at the expected time. It may be considered in two categories:

1. Primary amenorrhoea, when menstruation has never occurred.
2. Secondary amenorrhoea, when established menstruation ceases for 6 months or more.

Primary amenorrhoea

Failure to menstruate by the age of 16 is referred to as 'primary amenorrhoea'. The likely cause of primary amenorrhoea depends on whether secondary sexual characteristics are present or not. If secondary sexual characteristics are absent, then the cause is most likely delayed puberty (see pp. 30–31). If pubertal development is normal, then an anatomical cause should be suspected. The main 'anatomical' causes are:

- congenital absence of the uterus; this is due to a failure of the Müllerian ducts to develop
- imperforate hymen; the menstrual blood is retained within the vagina (a haematocolpos), causing cyclical lower abdominal pain each month at the time of menstruation (cryptomenorrhoea). Inspection of the vulva reveals a distended hymenal membrane through which dark blood may be seen and treatment by incision, usually under anaesthesia, is all that is required (Fig. 4.8).

Failure to menstruate may also be physiological delay; in other words the development is normal but there is an inherent delay in the onset of menstruation. There is often a family history of the same delay in the mother. A progestogen challenge test is useful to identify constitutional menstrual delay. A progestogen (e.g. medroxyprogesterone acetate) is given orally for 5 days, and if the endometrium has been stimulated from endogenous oestradiol then withdrawal of progestogen should lead to a vaginal bleed. If such a bleed occurs, it is reasonable to offer reassurance that spontaneous menstruation is likely to occur. An abdominal ultrasound may be reassuring to confirm that the uterus and ovaries are normal.

Low body weight and excessive exercise are also associated with primary amenorrhoea. The other causes listed in Table 4.1 are rare, although a few are outlined under the 'secondary amenorrhoea', discussion below (see also Chapter 5).

Secondary amenorrhoea

Secondary amenorrhoea means the cessation of established menstruation. It is defined as no menstruation for 6 months in the absence of pregnancy. A full list of causes is given in Table 4.2, but the commonest clinical causes are weight loss, polycystic ovary syndrome (PCOS) and hyperprolactinaemia. The more common conditions are discussed below by system.

Causes

Physiological

The commonest causes of amenorrhoea during the reproductive phase of life are physiological – pregnancy and lactation. Pregnancy should therefore be excluded in all sexually active women presenting with amenorrhoea.

The high postpartum level of prolactin associated with breastfeeding suppresses ovulation and gives rise to lactational amenorrhoea. Amenorrhoea usually persists throughout the time that the infant is fully breastfed, but with the introduction of supplementary feeding and subsequent reduction in the frequency of suckling, prolactin levels fall and ovarian activity is resumed. This hypo-oestrogenic state may lead to atrophic vaginitis, and occasionally to painful intercourse.

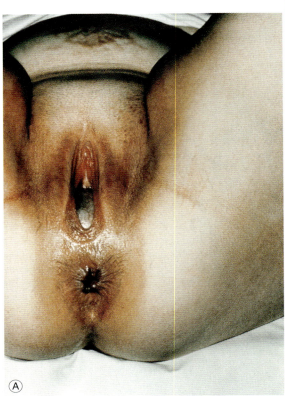
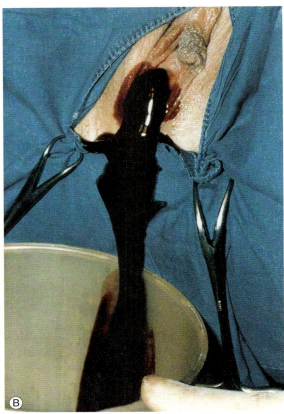

Fig. 4.8   **Imperforate hymen (A) before and (B) after incision.**

Hypothalamic

Hypothalamic amenorrhoea ('hypogonadotrophic hypogonadism') is frequently associated with stress and, in such cases, the condition usually resolves spontaneously. Physical stress in the form of athletic training can also result in suppression of the hypothalamo–pituitary–ovarian axis: there are low levels of pituitary gonadotrophins in association with low levels of prolactin and oestradiol.

The hypothalamus is also sensitive to changes in body weight, and weight loss, even to only 10–15% below the ideal, may be associated with amenorrhoea. Anorexia nervosa should be considered. Restoration of body weight results in the return of ovulatory function, although there may be a significant time interval between the attainment of the ideal body weight and the resumption of ovarian activity. Ovulation induction therapy is not recommended until the restoration of body weight, as pregnancy, if it occurs, carries the risk of growth restriction of the fetus and increased perinatal mortality.

If hypothalamic amenorrhoea is not related to low body weight, treatment will depend on whether or not the woman wants to conceive. If pregnancy is not desired, oestrogen replacement therapy is advisable and is conveniently provided in the form of the oral contraceptive pill. If the woman wishes to become pregnant, ovulation may be induced with pulsatile GnRH therapy or exogenous gonadotrophins.

Pituitary

Prolactin stimulates breast development and subsequent lactation. The secretion of prolactin, a polypeptide hormone produced by the lactotrophs of the anterior pituitary, is inhibited by dopamine from the hypothalamus. High levels of prolactin, which may be either physiological (during lactation) or pathological (see below), in turn suppress ovarian activity by interfering with the secretion of gonadotrophins.

Mildly elevated prolactin levels are common and can be due to stress (e.g. of venepuncture). Sustained higher levels can result in amenorrhoea and galactorrhoea unrelated to pregnancy. Galactorrhoea occurs in <50% of those with hyperprolactinaemia, and <50% of those with galactorrhoea have an elevated prolactin level. The causes of hyperprolactinaemia are given in Box 4.1.

Adenomas occur in the lateral wings of the anterior pituitary and are usually soft and discrete with a pseudocapsule of compressed tissue (Fig. 4.9). If the prolactin level is more than 1000 mU/L, then imaging with computed tomography or (ideally) magnetic resonance imaging (MRI) should be carried out. A microadenoma is <10 mm in diameter and a macroadenoma >10 mm. Visual fields should be checked, as optic chiasma compression may lead to bitemporal hemianopia. One-third of adenomas regress spontaneously and fewer than 5% of microadenomas become macroadenomas. Serum levels correlate well with tumour size, so that if the

Table 4.1	Causes of primary amenorrhoea	
System	**Problem**	**Incidence**
Chromosomal	XO – Turner syndrome	Rare
	46,XY disorders of sex development (DSD)	Rare
	Ovotesticular DSD	Rare
Hypothalamic	Physiological delay	Common
	Weight loss/anorexia/ heavy exercise	Common
	Isolated GnRH deficiency	Rare
	Congenital central nervous system (CNS) defects	Rare
	Intracranial tumours	Rare
Pituitary	Partial/total hypopituitarism	Rare
	Hyperprolactinaemia	Rare
	Pituitary adenoma	Rare
	Empty sella syndrome	Rare
	Trauma/surgery	Rare
Ovarian	True agenesis	Rare
	Premature ovarian failure	Rare
	Radiation/ chemotherapy/ autoimmune	Rare
	Polycystic ovaries	Common
	Virilizing ovarian tumours	Rare
Other endocrine	Primary hypothyroidism	Rare
	Adrenal hyperplasia	Rare
	Adrenal tumour	Rare
Uterine/ vaginal	Imperforate hymen	Not uncommon
	Uterovaginal agenesis	Rare

Table 4.2	Causes of secondary amenorrhoea	
System	**Problem**	**Incidence**
Physiological	Pregnancy	Common
	Lactation	Common
	Menopause	Common
Hypothalamic	Weight loss/anorexia	Common
	Heavy exercise	Common
	Stress	Common
Pituitary	Hyperprolactinaemia	Not uncommon
	Partial/total hypopituitarism	Rare
	Trauma/surgery	Rare
Ovarian	Polycystic ovarian syndrome	Common
	Premature ovarian failure	Uncommon
	Surgery/radiotherapy/ chemotherapy	Uncommon
	Resistant ovary syndrome	Rare
	Virilizing ovarian tumours	Rare
Other endocrine	Primary hypothyroidism	Rare
	Adrenal hyperplasia	Rare
	Adrenal tumour	Rare
Uterine/ vaginal	Surgery – hysterectomy	Common
	Endometrial ablation	Common
	Progestogen intrauterine device	Common
	Asherman syndrome	Rare

Box 4.1

Causes of hyperprolactinaemia

Pituitary adenoma

- microadenomas
- macroadenomas

Secondary to other causes

- primary hypothyroidism
- chronic renal failure
- pituitary stalk compression
- polycystic ovarian syndrome
- drugs (phenothiazines, haloperidol, metoclopramide, cimetidine, methyldopa, antihistamines and morphine)
- idiopathic

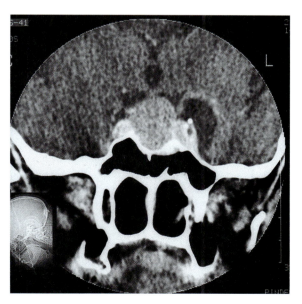

Fig. 4.9 Computed tomography scan of a pituitary macroadenoma.

tumour is relatively large and the prolactin level only modestly elevated, then pituitary stalk compression from a nonsecreting macroadenoma or other tumour (e.g. a craniopharyngioma) is possible. It is possible that apparently idiopathic hyperprolactinaemia may be caused by microadenomas that are too small to be picked up by an MRI scan.

All patients should have pituitary imaging before treatment. This treatment is usually with a dopamine agonist, either bromocriptine or cabergoline, which suppresses the prolactin level and also induces regression of the prolactinoma.

Transnasal transsphenoidal microsurgical excision of an adenoma is only rarely required.

Ovarian

Premature ovarian failure

The menopause (with cessation of ovarian function) normally occurs around the age of 50. The term 'premature ovarian failure' is usually used to describe cessation of ovarian function before the age of 40. As in natural menopause, failure is due to depletion of primordial follicles in the ovaries.

Premature ovarian failure occurs in 1% of women and may be due to surgery, viral infections (e.g. mumps), cytotoxic drugs or radiotherapy. It may also be idiopathic and is occasionally associated with chromosomal abnormality (XO mosaicism or XXX). A low oestradiol level, very high FSH and the absence of any menstrual activity are poor prognostic signs for recovery. Pregnancy by in vitro fertilization with donor oocytes may be possible. There is an association with other autoimmune disorders. Hormone replacement therapy is required to relieve postmenopausal symptoms and minimize the risk of osteoporosis.

Polycystic ovary syndrome

PCOS is associated with menstrual disturbance and is the most common form of anovulatory infertility. It is estimated to affect up to 20% of women in the UK. It is characterized by the presence of at least two out of the following three criteria:

- oligomenorrhoea or amenorrhoea
- ultrasound appearance of large-volume ovaries (>10 cm³) and/or multiple small follicles (12 or more <10 mm) (Fig. 4.10)
- clinical evidence of excess androgens (acne, hirsutism) or biochemical evidence (raised testosterone).

The aetiology of the condition is unknown, but evidence suggests that the principal underlying disorder is one of insulin resistance, with the resultant hyperinsulinaemia stimulating excess ovarian androgen production. Associated with the prevalent insulin resistance, there is a characteristic dyslipidaemia and a predisposition to non-insulin-dependent diabetes and cardiovascular disease in later life. PCOS may therefore be considered to be a systemic metabolic condition rather than one primarily of gynaecological origin (Fig. 4.11).

Treatment depends on whether the presenting problem has been menstrual irregularity, hirsutism or infertility. The combined oral contraceptive pill has been used to regulate the menses. Hirsutism may be treated by cosmetic measures such as waxing or laser treatment. Hirsutism may also be treated with the combined oral contraceptive pill, as it suppresses ovarian androgen production, or with the antiandrogen cyproterone acetate. Women taking an antiandrogen should use effective contraception during, and for at least 3 months after, treatment due to the potential risk of teratogenicity (feminization of a male fetus) with antiandrogen therapy. Clomifene is used to induce ovulation in women with anovulatory infertility (p. 54). If clomifene does not work, ovulation may be induced by

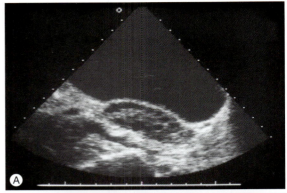

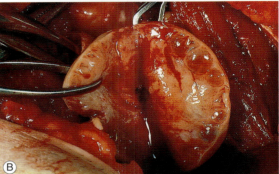

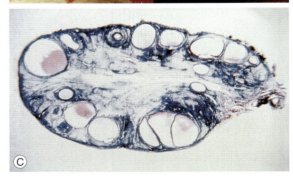

Fig. 4.10 Polycystic ovaries. These are classically bilaterally enlarged with multiple peripherally situated cysts 'like a ring of pearls' in a dense stroma: **(A)** ultrasound scan; **(B)** surgical dissection; **(C)** pathological preparation.

gonadotrophin injections, or by laparoscopic laser or diathermy to the ovary.

The cornerstone to management, however, is weight reduction; this reduces insulin resistance, corrects the hormone imbalance and promotes ovulation. Although initial studies of insulin-sensitizing agents (e.g. metformin) as a therapeutic option in the management of anovulation and other symptoms of PCOS were promising, larger trials have failed to demonstrate benefit.

Individuals may gain benefit from early screening for cardiovascular risk factors, particularly hypertension and glucose intolerance. There is also a longer term increased risk of endometrial hyperplasia and endometrial carcinoma

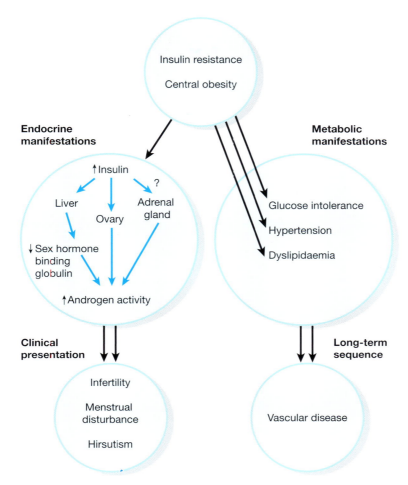

Fig. 4.11 **Pathogenesis of PCOS.** PCOS can be considered to be a disorder primarily of insulin resistance, with the resultant hyperinsulinaemia stimulating excess ovarian androgen production. There may also be dyslipidaemia and a predisposition to later non-insulin-dependent diabetes and cardiovascular disease. ? = uncertain relationship between insulin and the adrenal gland.

as a consequence of the effects of anovulation with unopposed oestrogen stimulation of the endometrium.

Other endocrine causes

These are rare. Women with thyrotoxicosis may have amenorrhoea. Primary hypothyroidism is also associated with amenorrhoea, as thyrotrophin-releasing hormone stimulates prolactin secretion. The most common of the rare adrenal problems is late-onset congenital adrenal hyperplasia. This is usually due to a deficiency of the enzyme 21-hydroxylase, and treatment with a low dose of corticosteroids is usually sufficient to re-establish ovulatory function by suppressing adrenal function. Androgen-secreting adrenal tumours can also occur.

Uterine

Excessive uterine curettage – usually at the time of miscarriage, termination of pregnancy or secondary postpartum

haemorrhage – may remove the basal layer of the endometrium and result in the formation of uterine adhesions (synechiae), a condition known as Asherman syndrome (Fig. 4.12). It may rarely also result from severe postpartum infection. Treatment involves breaking down the adhesions through a hysteroscope with or without inserting an intrauterine contraceptive device to deter reformation.

Summary of clinical management

Initial management:

- exclude pregnancy
- ask about perimenopausal symptoms (e.g. flushings, vaginal dryness)
- take a history, including weight changes, drugs, medical disorders and thyroid symptoms
- carry out an examination, looking particularly at height, weight, visual fields and the presence of hirsutism or

Table 4.3	Further management based on test results	
Ultrasound scan	A scan showing large-volume ovaries (>10 cm^3) and/or multiple small follicles (12 or more <10 mm)	If pregnancy desired, clomifene or gonadotrophins. If pregnancy not desired, consider the combined oral contraceptive pill
Elevated PRL level	If PRL >1000 mU/L on at least two occasions, the diagnosis is hyperprolactinaemia	Arrange MRI or CT of the pituitary. Treat with dopamine agonist
Elevated FSH	If FSH >30 U/L, repeat 6 weeks later. If still elevated and the patient >40 years old, the patient is menopausal. If less than 40, the diagnosis is premature ovarian failure	Consider HRT. Pregnancy with oocyte donation is possible
Abnormal TFTs	If the TFTs are abnormal, treat as appropriate	

CT, Computed tomography; FSH, follicle-stimulating hormone; HRT, hormone replacement therapy; LH, luteinizing hormone; MRI, magnetic resonance imaging; PRL, prolactin; TFTs, thyroid function tests.

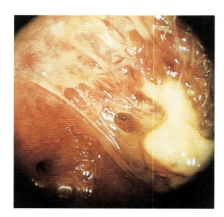

Fig. 4.12 Rarely, adhesions can form within the uterine cavity. If so severe that they obstruct the menstrual flow, the condition is referred to as Asherman syndrome.

virilization; also carry out a pelvic examination, unless this is contraindicated
- check serum for LH, FSH, prolactin, testosterone, thyroxine and thyroid-stimulating hormone (TSH)
- arrange a transvaginal ultrasound scan, looking for polycystic ovaries
- review with the results (Table 4.3).

If the tests listed in Table 4.3 are normal, consider the following causes:
- weight loss
- depression, emotional disturbance or extreme exercise
- Asherman syndrome
- idiopathic amenorrhoea.

In the majority of patients who present with secondary amenorrhoea, investigations will fail to demonstrate any significant endocrine abnormality – idiopathic amenorrhoea. It is probable that there is a disturbance of the normal feedback mechanisms of control. Undue sensitivity of the hypothalamus and pituitary to the negative feedback suppression of endogenous oestrogen may result in impaired gonadotrophin secretion, which is inadequate to stimulate follicular development and results in cycle initiation failure. Those requiring ovulation usually respond well to an anti-oestrogen such as clomifene.

Key *points*

- At the start of the cycle, levels of FSH and LH rise and these stimulate the development of 10–20 follicles. A single dominant follicle matures, secreting oestradiol, and the remainder undergo atresia. As the oestradiol level rises, the release of both gonadotrophins is suppressed (negative feedback), which serves to prevent multiple follicles from maturing and ovulating.
- The very high preovulatory oestradiol level stimulates a positive-feedback mid-cycle surge of LH, which triggers ovulation. The remainder of the ruptured follicle becomes the corpus luteum, and secretes progesterone.
- Progesterone brings about secretory changes in the endometrium that are necessary for successful implantation.
- If conception and implantation occur, the corpus luteum is maintained by hCG secreted by the trophoblast. If, however, conception and implantation have not occurred successfully, the corpus luteum regresses, the levels of sex hormones fall and menstruation ensues.
- The commonest causes of primary amenorrhoea (when menstruation has never occurred) are physiological delay, weight loss, heavy exercise and an imperforate hymen.
- Secondary amenorrhoea is said to have occurred when established menstruation ceases for 6 months or more. Outside pregnancy, lactation and the menopause, the commonest causes are PCOS, stress, weight loss and hyperprolactinaemia.
- PCOS is the commonest cause of anovulatory infertility.

5

Infertility

Introduction

Infertility is a condition that affects approximately one in six couples at some stage in their lives. The cause may be related to a problem with the man, woman or both. In view of the intimate nature of the problem, infertility is often associated with personal distress and embarrassment; effective treatment is available to help an increasing proportion of these couples.

Definitions

Infertility is defined by the World Health Organization (WHO) as the inability of the couple to achieve a clinical pregnancy within 12 months of beginning regular unprotected sexual intercourse. A couple can have primary infertility – no previous pregnancies within the relationship – or secondary infertility, where the couple has had at least one pregnancy.

Infertility is rarely absolute, and most couples have a degree of subfertility. Around 84% of the normal fertile population will conceive within 1 year, and 92% by the end of 2 years. However, the older the couple are when they start trying to conceive, the lower the chance of success, particularly if the couple wish to have more than one child. Cumulative pregnancy rates and live birth rates are the terms used to express the chance of conception within a given time interval. Fig. 5.1 illustrates the relationship between female age at which couples start building a family and their chance of realizing a family with one child, with and without use of in vitro fertilization (IVF) (similar figures can be generated for family sizes of two and three children).

Fecundability is the percentage of women exposed to the risk of a pregnancy for one menstrual cycle, who will subsequently produce a live-born infant (normal range 15–28%). Fecundability usually diminishes slightly with each passing month of not conceiving.

Age and fertility

Normal fertility declines as the woman's age increases. A woman is born with a finite number of oocytes; around 1 million. This falls to approximately 250 000 at puberty, and by the time the menopause is reached, the number of oocytes has fallen to below 1000. During her reproductive life, a woman will release only 500 mature oocytes – a form of pre-conceptual natural selection – while the remaining oocytes undergo atresia or apoptosis. The rate of oocyte loss is a dynamic process, with the rate of follicular recruitment increasing from birth to age 14 years and then progressively decreasing until the menopause. At the menopause, which occurs at an average age of 51 years, there are no functioning oocytes.

The decline in fertility is directly related to the declining oocyte population and the eggs' inherent quality. There is a small fall in monthly fecundity rates from the age of 31 years, a more pronounced decrease from the age of 36 years, and a very steep decline from the age of 40 years. In assisted conception procedures, this decline is also observed with a gradual decline in success rates from age 34 years. In addition, in both natural and assisted conception pregnancies, there is a substantial increase in rates of miscarriage with advancing maternal age. Although older men are less fertile, the effect of age on men's fertility is less pronounced than for women.

Causes of infertility

The causes of infertility can be categorized in a simple manner, but in reality more than one problem can often be identified in a couple. Causes include: ovulation disorders (25%); male factor (25%); unexplained (25%) and tubal factors (15%). Remaining causes include endometriosis-related infertility.

Diagnosis

The diagnosis of infertility is a process of exclusion, identifying couples where the cause is clear, those in whom there is a possible cause and those in whom the cause is unexplained. The aim of investigation should be to reach a diagnosis as soon as possible, using only tests that are of proven value.

Table 5.1	Examination of a woman
Examination	**Reason**
Height and weight to calculate BMI	High or low BMI associated with lower fertility
Body hair distribution	Hyperandrogenism
Galactorrhoea	Hyperprolactinaemia
Uterine structural abnormalities (most usefully determined by transvaginal ultrasound)	May be associated with infertility
Immobile and/or tender uterus	Endometriosis or pelvic inflammatory disease, associated with tubal damage

Table 5.2	Examination of a man
Examination	**Reason**
Scrotum	Varicocele
Size (volume) of the testes	Small testes associated with oligospermia
Position of the testes	Undescended testes
Prostate	Chronic infection

Box 5.1

Initial investigations

Female:

- early follicular phase luteinizing hormone (LH), follicle-stimulating hormone (FSH), oestradiol, anti-Müllerian hormone (AMH)
- rubella (offer vaccination if not immune)
- luteal phase serum progesterone (to assess ovulation)
- test of tubal patency (laparoscopic hydrotubation, hysterosalpingo-contrast sonography [HyCoSy] or hysterosalpingography [HSG])

Male:

- semen analysis × 1

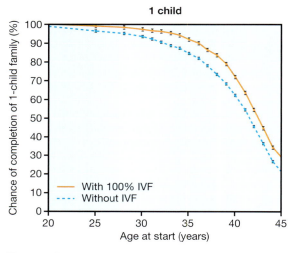

1 child

Fig. 5.1 Relationship between the female age at which couples start building a family and the chance of realizing a family with one child, with and without use of IVF (with permission from J. Dik F. Habbema et al.; Realizing a desired family size: when should couples start?; Human Reproduction, Vol. 30, No. 9, pp. 2215–2221, 2015).

History and examination

Factors that provide clues to the aetiology are outlined in Tables 5.1 and 5.2. Other important factors to be noted are the woman's age and the duration of infertility – generally, the older the woman is and the longer the period of infertility, the poorer the prognosis. The order in which the investigations are performed varies, depending on whether the couple has primary or secondary infertility, with an earlier assessment of tubal patency in the latter. Early assessment is also indicated if a specific abnormality is suspected from the history, and for an older patient.

Examination of the woman

Height and weight should be recorded and used to calculate the body mass index (BMI). The normal range is between 19 and 25. A change of weight of >10% in the preceding year may cause a disturbance of the menstrual pattern and anovulation. A BMI at either extreme is detrimental to fertility (see later).

Increased body hair is associated with hyperandrogenism, most commonly due to polycystic ovary syndrome (PCOS). Breast examination may demonstrate galactorrhoea, which is associated with hyperprolactinaemia. Pelvic examination is important, to look for signs of structural abnormalities, infection and pathological processes, such as endometriosis or pelvic inflammatory disease.

Examination of the man

Examination of the man is not essential in the absence of any relevant history. If, however, the semen analysis is abnormal, examination of the genitalia may be helpful, looking specifically at size (volume); consistency and position of the testes; the outline of the epididymis (for the presence of the vas deferens); and finally, the scrotum, for evidence of swellings.

Investigations and their interpretation

The investigations should be arranged in a logical manner with reference to the history, along with appropriate general health screening (Box 5.1). Additional tests may be necessary, depending on the clinical circumstances (Box 5.2).

Additional investigations to be performed selectively

Female:

- pelvic ultrasound scan for ovarian morphology and uterine abnormalities
- laparoscopy for diagnosis of endometriosis, may be combined with tubal patency test
- hysteroscopy for intrauterine anomalies
- prolactin and thyroid function tests
- testosterone, androstenedione, 17-hydroxyprogesterone and sex hormone-binding globulin (SHBG, in order to calculate the Free Androgen Index, when raised is an indicator of hyperandrogenism)

Male:

- sperm function tests (see text), if initial test is consistently abnormal
- mixed agglutination reaction test or immunobead test for antisperm antibodies
- FSH, LH, testosterone if low sperm count (oligospermia) (raised FSH if testicular failure, low if central nervous system cause)
- transrectal ultrasound for suspected abnormalities of the seminal vesicles and prostate

Male factors

Classification

Male factor infertility can be a problem of sperm production, sperm function or sperm delivery. Sperm production may be completely absent (azoospermia) in, for example, testicular failure. More commonly there is a reduced count of sperm of normal appearance (oligospermia). Additionally, a high proportion of the sperm may be poorly motile, lacking the normal forward progressive movement (asthenospermia) or may appear morphologically defective (teratospermia) with abnormalities of the head, midpiece or tail.

Normal sperm function – the ability of the sperm to reach, bind and fertilize the oocyte – is more difficult to demonstrate. At present, there are no reliable methods of measuring sperm function, other than monitoring the proportion of sperm moving and assessing the speed of their progress. Antisperm antibodies can affect sperm motility.

Problems with sperm delivery may be caused by absence or blockage of the vas deferens or epididymis. It may also be related to impotence, premature ejaculation or a physical inability to have normal sexual intercourse.

Semen analysis

This provides information about spermatogenesis and an aspect of sperm delivery, but gives little information about sperm function. The WHO has produced a normal range of values for semen, based upon semen analyses performed upon samples obtained from men with a time to pregnancy interval of up to 12 months (Table 5.3). The values, however, are empirical and do not reflect a cut-off point below which pregnancy will not occur. Rather, there is an increase in probability of conception with increasing numbers of sperm

Table 5.3 WHO criteria for semen analysis (2010)

Parameter	Lower limit of reference range
Volume	1.5 mL
Concentration	15×10^6/mL
Total motility	40%
Progressive motility	32%
Normal forms	4%
Vitality	58%

Reproduced with permission from WHO (with permission from WHO laboratory manual for examination and processing of human semen; 5th ed., 2010 © WHO)

and motility up to 40 million/mL and 40%, respectively, with a relative plateau thereafter.

An individual man's sperm count varies considerably, and in the presence of one abnormal result, a second count should be arranged. As spermatogenesis takes approximately 3 months to complete, the samples ought to be produced at least 3 months apart. Samples should be produced by masturbation or after intercourse into a non-lubricated condom after a period of abstinence of between 3 and 5 days. The sample should be analysed in an accredited laboratory and according to WHO guidelines.

Tests of sperm function

Sperm function tests are no longer used in routine clinical practice, with more emphasis now placed on the identification of the number of abnormal/normal sperm as part of the routine analysis. Some sperm function tests, such as the ability of sperm to swim through culture medium, are employed in specialized reproductive medicine units, where more complicated treatment may be contemplated.

The post-coital test involves asking the couple to have sexual intercourse timed to the woman's mid-cycle. Then, 6–12 h later, a sample of endocervical mucus is taken, looking for the presence or absence of sperm. Some studies have shown a positive correlation between the finding of motile sperm in the mucus and the chance of subsequent pregnancy. The use of this test, however, is controversial, as other studies have shown that the finding of a positive or negative result does not alter the chance or timing of a pregnancy. As a result, most centres have abandoned this procedure.

Antibodies can develop against sperm in response to injury or infection of the testis and epididymis. Men who have had a vasectomy and attempted reversal are the commonest group in whom antisperm antibodies are identified. The antibodies can be serum (IgG) or bound (IgA), and attach principally to the tail, midpiece or head of the sperm. Tests used to detect antisperm antibodies include the mixed agglutination reaction test and the immunobead test. Levels between 17% and 49% are likely to be associated with a fall in fertility, and levels greater than 50% significantly affect fertility.

Female factors

Ovulation

Ovulation is an 'all or nothing' phenomenon, with usually one oocyte released per ovulatory cycle.

Causes of anovulation

Ovarian failure is found in about 50% of women with primary amenorrhoea, and 15% of those presenting with secondary amenorrhoea. Most women with primary amenorrhoea will have an established diagnosis before presenting to an infertility clinic. The cause may be genetic, e.g. Turner syndrome (45,XO), or autoimmune. In those presenting with secondary amenorrhoea and ovarian failure, there may be an obvious cause, such as previous ovarian surgery, abdominal radiotherapy or chemotherapy. There will also be a proportion of women in whom no reason can be identified – idiopathic premature menopause.

Weight-related anovulation Weight plays an important part in the control of ovulation. A minimum degree of body fat (considered to be around 22% of body weight) is needed to maintain ovulatory cycles. Substantial weight loss leads to the disappearance of the normal 24-h secretory pattern of gonadotrophin-releasing hormone (GnRH), which reverts to the nocturnal pattern seen in pubescent girls. As a result, the ovaries develop a multifollicular appearance on ultrasound. Prolonged exercise can, by increasing the muscle bulk and decreasing the body fat, have the same effect, and it is not uncommon for women athletes or ballerinas to be amenorrhoeic. Excessive weight can also have an adverse effect on ovulation. This probably results from excess oestrone, generated in the adipose tissue by conversion from androgens, interfering with the normal feedback mechanism to the pituitary gland.

Excess weight has a profound effect on female fertility, with a significant reduction in the chance of a successful pregnancy: it reduces the chance of conception, increases the risk of miscarriage, as well as substantially increasing the risk of obstetric complications during the pregnancy and at delivery. The distribution of the fat is important, with central (visceral) fat having a bigger impact than peripheral fat distribution. The waist–hip ratio, which more reliably picks up visceral fat distribution, seems a more reliable guide to the impact of fat on fertility than the BMI.

Polycystic ovary syndrome Of the women presenting with anovulatory infertility, 50% will have PCOS (see Chapter 4).

Luteinized unruptured follicle syndrome In certain patients, the oocyte may be retained following the luteinizing hormone (LH) surge, the so-called 'luteinized unruptured follicle syndrome'. Repeated pelvic ultrasound scans fail to show the expected collapse of the follicle at ovulation, and the follicle persists into the luteal phase. As no longitudinal studies have shown this to be a persistent finding in the same woman, there is uncertainty regarding its relevance to fertility.

Hyperprolactinaemia Hyperprolactinaemia is diagnosed in 10–15% of cases of secondary amenorrhoea. About one-third of these women will have galactorrhoea, and occasionally, there may be some evidence of visual impairment (bitemporal hemianopia) due to pressure on the optic chiasma from a pituitary adenoma.

Tests of ovulation

Only a pregnancy categorically confirms ovulation. However, there are a number of investigations that imply that ovulation has taken place:

- history – over 90% of women with regular menstrual cycles will ovulate spontaneously
- urinary LH kit – this picks up the mid-cycle surge of LH that starts the cascade reaction leading to ovulation
- mid-luteal phase progesterone – this is the most commonly used test of ovulation. A luteal phase progesterone value of >28 nmol/L is found in conception cycles and, as a result, this value is generally regarded as evidence of satisfactory ovulation. However, it is important to time the blood sample carefully – between 7 and 10 days before the next menstrual period. This can only be determined with some knowledge of the length of the patient's normal menstrual cycle; the information is inevitably retrospective.

Other tests

Less commonly employed tests include serial ultrasound scans to monitor the growth and subsequent disappearance of a Graafian follicle. A luteal phase endometrial biopsy looking for appropriately timed secretory changes is no longer considered of value. Basal body temperature was previously considered to be of value as there is a rise of 0.5°C if ovulation has occurred (due to the thermogenic effect of a rise in serum progesterone), but, in practice, this is now rarely used.

Testing ovarian reserve

Ovarian reserve is defined as the number of viable oocytes in the ovary. This is particularly important in women contemplating more complex fertility treatment, and may provide a guide to their response to treatment. Determining the level of follicle-stimulating hormone (FSH) at the beginning of the menstrual cycle is a commonly employed test. A raised FSH taken between days 2 and 5 of the menstrual cycle indicates impaired ovarian reserve, and a likely poor response to ovarian stimulation. Other methods that appear to be more reliable include:

- measuring the antral follicle count by ultrasound – the number of small developing follicles seen in the ovary
- measuring the ovarian volume – this is an indication of ovarian activity, as ovaries decrease in size with advancing age and the decline in oocyte numbers
- measuring the concentration of anti-Müllerian hormone (AMH). AMH is produced in small developing follicles and, unlike FSH, can be usefully measured throughout the menstrual cycle.

Although tests of ovarian reserve may be important in identifying women who may not respond well to fertility treatment or will have a shorter reproductive lifespan, they have limited value in predicting overall natural fertility if the woman has a regular menstrual cycle and is ovulating.

Further investigations

Pelvic ultrasound is useful in defining ovarian morphology, and is more reliable than pelvic examination in identifying potentially relevant pelvic pathology such as fibroids, ovarian cysts and endometrial polyps.

Chlamydia serology has been used as a screening test for tubal pathology. Those with a positive antibody titre are more likely to have tubal pathology because of the association between chlamydial infection and salpingitis.

Serum testosterone measurement is indicated if there is evidence of hirsutism to exclude more sinister disorders, such as androgen-secreting tumours of the ovary or adrenal gland. In women with elevated testosterone, measurement of 17-hydroxyprogesterone is relevant in order to exclude late-onset congenital adrenal hyperplasia. Thyroid function tests are commonly performed, as approximately 7% of women in this age group will have a thyroid disorder, which may have an impact on a pregnancy if not appropriately treated.

A progestogen challenge test may be useful in women with a history of amenorrhoea and normal levels of FSH and prolactin. It is used to determine whether the woman is clinically oestrogenized. This acts as a guide to what would be the most appropriate medication to use to induce ovulation. If the bleeding is normal following 5 days of an oral progestogen, the patient is well oestrogenized, whereas if it is absent or scanty, the woman is relatively poorly oestrogenized. The presence of a withdrawal bleed also demonstrates the presence of endometrium and the patency of the genital tract. The ability to visualize and measure the endometrial thickness by transvaginal scanning can also inform the progesterone challenge test, as a thick and therefore adequately oestrogenized endometrium can be seen on scan.

Tubal patency

Classification

The fallopian tube can be blocked distally – at the fimbrial end – or, less commonly, at the proximal end – the cornu. In addition, the tubo–ovarian relationship may be disrupted by peritubal adhesions. Fimbrial disease has varying degrees of severity:

- agglutination of the fimbria to produce a narrowed opening – known as a phimosis
- complete agglutination to form a hydrosalpinx (fluid-filled tube).

In addition, tubal damage can also involve the endosalpinx, with intraluminal adhesions and flattening of the mucosal folds. Microsurgery to relieve tubal blockage, therefore, may not restore tubal function.

The important features for fertility prognosis appear to be:

- degree of dilatation of the fallopian tube
- extent of the fibrosis of the wall of the tube
- damage to the endosalpinx
- if one or both tubes are affected.

Tests of tubal patency

In the absence of a positive history suggestive of pelvic pathology, a negative physical examination and a negative *Chlamydia* antibody titre, the least invasive method for assessing tubal patency should be employed.

Hysterosalpingography (HSG) HSG is widely employed in the assessment of tubal patency. It involves inserting a cannula into the cervix and passing radio-opaque fluid into the uterine cavity and fallopian tubes, demonstrating their outline (Fig. 5.2). The test is performed under X-ray screening on an outpatient basis. If the HSG is normal, this finding can be relied upon in 97% of cases. However, if the

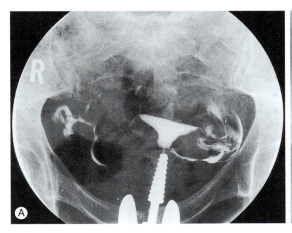 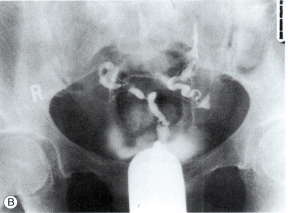

Fig. 5.2 **HSG of (A) normal uterus and (B) abnormal uterus.** In **(B)** the radio-opaque dye does not flow through the fallopian tubes, thus indicating blockage.

HSG is abnormal, the diagnosis can only be relied upon in 34% of cases (false positive rate 66%), and a laparoscopy is required to confirm the nature of the abnormality.

Hysterosalpingo-contrast sonography (HyCoSy) This technique involves a pelvic ultrasound scan at which galactose-containing ultrasound contrast medium is inserted into the uterine cavity, outlining any abnormalities such as submucosal fibroids and endometrial polyps, before passing down the fallopian tubes to confirm tubal patency. The technique offers a similar level of diagnostic accuracy to HSG.

Diagnostic laparoscopy with dye hydrotubation Diagnostic laparoscopy ('lap and dye') remains the 'gold standard' investigation. It provides a direct view of the pelvic organs, and also offers the possibility to treat minor pathology discovered during the investigation. Methylthioninium chloride (methylene blue) dye is inserted through a cannula in the cervix to demonstrate tubal patency. Hysteroscopy is often carried out at the same time in order to examine the uterine cavity. The diagnostic laparoscopy requires admission to hospital, usually as a day case, and a general anaesthetic. As such, it is the most invasive and expensive investigation of tubal patency, so most specialists undertake a HyCoSy or HSG as the first-line assessment.

Selective salpingography If HSG or laparoscopy detects a proximal blockage, further investigation may be considered. The blockage could simply be due to spasm of the muscle of the uterine cornua or to genuine pathology. A fine guidewire is inserted into the internal tubal ostium under direct fluoroscopic control or by direct vision using a hysteroscope. This may dislodge a small plug of amorphous debris, restoring patency. This technique appears to increase the likelihood of pregnancy in women with proximal tubal damage.

Salpingoscopy More detailed investigation of the interior of the fallopian tube is possible but is only really necessary if the question of pursuing tubal surgery is raised. A fine telescope, called a salpingoscope, can be passed down an operating laparoscope and inserted into the ampullary portion of the fallopian tube. Approximately 50% of patients with macroscopically damaged fallopian tubes will have fine intratubal adhesions. If present, these adhesions adversely affect the outcome of subsequent tubal surgery.

Falloposcopy Advances in fiberoptics have allowed the development of a very fine instrument, a falloposcope, with a diameter of <1 mm, which can be inserted into the fallopian tube via the uterine cavity. Falloposcopy appears to be effective in detecting tubal pathology and can be performed on an outpatient basis. The equipment is fragile and expensive, however, and its use is limited to a small number of centres, mainly as a research tool.

It is important to note that all of these techniques are useful in demonstrating patency, but none is capable of directly assessing tubal function.

Treatment

Approximately one-fifth of couples with infertility conceive spontaneously during investigation or while awaiting treatment. However, the probability of this is related to the age of the woman, how long the couple has been trying to conceive for, whether they have been pregnant before, tubal patency and sperm motility. Consequently, these factors must be taken into account when considering conservative treatment, with early referral to assisted conception services generally appropriate for most couples after the initial investigations have been completed. The couple should be counselled about general health matters such as smoking, alcohol intake and diet. It is appropriate to recommend folic acid to the woman as routine prevention of neural tube defects. Where the diagnosis is established, specific treatments can be employed.

Anovulation

There are various ways of inducing ovulation, depending on the underlying cause. Successful ovulation induction should be continued for long enough to give the optimum chance for conception – generally 12 months.

Hyperprolactinaemia is treated with a dopamine agonist, either bromocriptine or cabergoline.

Excess or decreased body weight should be managed by dietary adjustments. Although ovulation can generally be induced by exogenous gonadotrophins, this should be avoided, particularly if the woman is underweight or obese, as there is an increased risk of pregnancy complications. Women with moderate obesity often show resistance to treatment with clomiphene citrate and gonadotrophins, requiring much higher doses to induce ovulation.

Anovulation in oestrogenized patients

Most of these women have PCOS (85% of patients presenting with oligomenorrhoea and 25% of those with amenorrhoea). First-line treatment in this condition is oral anti-oestrogen therapy, usually with clomiphene citrate or letrozole.

Clomiphene citrate's mode of action is to increase the plasma FSH concentration, mainly by competitively blocking the negative feedback effects of endogenous oestradiol on the hypothalamus (FSH is the principal hormone responsible for follicular recruitment and development). Letrozole suppresses oestrogen-negative feedback centrally and does not have the anti-oestrogenic effects on the endometrium that are observed with clomiphene.

Initially, a dose of 50 mg daily of clomiphene citrate for 5 days is given at the beginning of a cycle (days 2–6 inclusive). If there is no response (judged by luteal phase progesterone estimations), the dose is increased to a usual maximum of 100 mg daily for 5 days. Rarely, in obese patients, the dose may be increased to 150 mg daily for 5 days. Clomiphene may induce multiple follicles, and consequently there is a 10% chance of a multiple pregnancy. The alternative approach of 5 mg daily of letrozole for 5 days from day 2 of the cycle is a more successful treatment, but letrozole is not licensed for ovulation induction.

Ovulation can be achieved successfully in approximately 80% of cycles, with cumulative pregnancy rates of up to 30% after 6 months' treatment.

Side-effects while using clomiphene citrate include:

- vasomotor symptoms (hot flushes) (11%)
- pelvic discomfort (7%)
- nausea (2%)
- breast discomfort (2%).

These are seldom severe, and simple explanation and reassurance are usually all that is required. More significant problems include visual disturbances (1.5%) and cholestatic jaundice (rare). In both these situations, the drug should be discontinued and not used again. Some women do not respond to oral ovulation–induction agents such as clomiphene or letrozole; these patients will require treatment with exogenous gonadotrophins.

Exogenous gonadotrophins are derived from two sources: extracted from postmenopausal women's urine or, more recently, created *in vitro* by genetically engineered mammalian cells. Although the original urinary-derived gonadotrophins contained an equal mixture of FSH and LH, refinement of the extraction techniques has resulted in highly purified FSH compounds (>99% of protein content is FSH). The recombinant genetically engineered FSH preparations attain similar levels of purity.

All these medications require administration by subcutaneous injection. Around 4% of women undergoing gonadotrophin treatment will develop ovarian hyperstimulation syndrome (OHSS) and this will be severe in 0.5%. The incidence of multiple pregnancy with gonadotrophin treatment is around 20%, although with careful monitoring and 'step up' of the dose, this can be reduced to <5%. The aim is to achieve development of a single follicle using a low-dose regimen, starting at one ampoule daily for 10 days, and then increasing the dose, if necessary, by small increments until satisfactory follicular growth occurs. Response is monitored by ovarian ultrasound, sometimes combined with serum oestradiol measurement.

When the follicle reaches maturity, ovulation is induced by administering human chorionic gonadotrophin (hCG), which replaces the physiological LH surge. Gonadotrophin therapy is highly successful in restoring normal fertility to women with hypothalamic amenorrhoea (see later), or PCOS. For women with unexplained infertility, clomiphene and exogenous gonadotrophins have not been shown to improve the chance of conception and referral for IVF is appropriate.

If standard ovulation–induction treatment fails in patients with PCOS, laparoscopic ovarian diathermy can be offered. The ovarian capsule is pierced four times for 5 seconds with a needle point diathermy. Encouraging results have been reported, with spontaneous ovulation returning in up to 71% of cycles without the risk of hyperstimulation or multiple pregnancy. In women where spontaneous ovulation does not occur, most become more responsive to clomiphene or gonadotrophin therapy. Unfortunately, the effect is time limited, with chronic anovulation returning in 50% of women within 2 years. There is also the risk of iatrogenic adhesion formation and reduction in the ovarian reserve, leading to premature menopause if diathermy is used excessively.

Metformin, an oral antidiabetic drug, is of value in helping to induce ovulation in obese women with PCOS; metformin may be used either alone or in combination with clomiphene, but the overall effect is inferior to letrozole.

Anovulation in oestrogen-deficient women

Women who have a low FSH, normal prolactin, and either a low serum oestradiol or a negative progestogen withdrawal test (hypogonadotrophic hypogonadism), require exogenous gonadotrophins in order to ovulate (see previously).

Tubal disease

There are two treatment options in the presence of tubal disease, namely surgery and IVF.

Tubal surgery

Surgery used to be the principal treatment for occlusive tubal disease but, as the results of IVF have improved, tubal surgery is performed less frequently.

Selection of women

Women considered for tubal surgery need to be carefully selected, taking into consideration:

- the woman's age
- the site and extent of the tubal damage
- other factors that might influence fertility.

As with other treatments, age has an important effect on the outcome and IVF may be a better option for women in their late 30s or their 40s. Distal tubal occlusion carries a poorer prognosis than proximal disease and surgery should be reserved only for cases in which damage is relatively minor. In women with minor damage, the live birth rate after surgery is around 40% over a period of 18 months. Women with a moderate-to-severe distal abnormality, and those with damage at more than one site on the same tube, have a poor prognosis and IVF is more appropriate. With limited proximal damage, pregnancy rates of nearly 50% can be achieved after tubal surgery.

Techniques

Conventionally, tubal surgery has been performed by laparotomy, through a low transverse incision, with microsurgical techniques used to restore tubal patency. However, tubal surgery is now largely performed laparoscopically. Even completely occluded tubes have been opened successfully laparoscopically, using either a CO_2 laser or electrodiathermy. In skilled hands, the results compare very favourably with conventional tubal surgery using an operating microscope.

More recently, selective salpingography (passing a fine catheter through the uterus and along the fallopian tube under X-ray screening) has been used successfully to treat some women with proximal obstruction caused by a plug of amorphous debris.

Risks of tubal surgery

Women who have undergone tubal surgery have a 10-fold increased risk of having an ectopic pregnancy and should be advised to undergo an ultrasound scan at around 6 weeks' gestation to confirm the site of a subsequent pregnancy.

Endometriosis

Endometriosis is discussed in Chapter 8. There is no evidence that treating minimal peritoneal endometriosis with drugs improves natural fertility. Indeed, medical treatment of endometriosis often involves creating anovulation for up to 6 months and this effectively delays the couple trying for a pregnancy. However, there is some evidence to suggest that surgery to ablate the endometriotic lesions and to divide adhesions that may have formed from endometriosis increases the chance of natural conception. Similarly, prior to IVF, treatment of endometriosis with GnRH analogues for 3 months may significantly improve the likelihood of pregnancy.

If the endometriosis involves the ovary or the fallopian tube, surgical treatment appears to be beneficial by correcting the anatomical defect. The results of surgery, even where the endometriosis is quite severe, appear to be quite encouraging. However, if pregnancy does not occur within 6 months, IVF should be considered.

Male factor problems

Azoospermia and a raised serum FSH

Azoospermia and a raised serum FSH signify spermatogenic failure (non-obstructive azoospermia). This can be confirmed by testicular biopsy. Occasionally, islands of spermatogenesis can be identified and sperm can be extracted from a testicular biopsy and used for intracytoplasmic sperm injection (ICSI) as part of IVF treatment (see later). If no sperm is identified at surgical sperm retrieval, the only remaining option is the use of donor sperm.

Donor insemination (DI)

Men who donate sperm do so for altruistic reasons and, within the UK, sperm donors are no longer anonymous. All potential donors are screened for a family history of medical and genetic conditions, and for infection, particularly human immunodeficiency virus, and hepatitis B and C. For the latter reason, semen is frozen in straws and quarantined for a minimum of 6 months. The donor is screened again for infection at the end of this period, and only if this second screen is negative is the sperm used for treatment.

Semen is inserted into the woman's uterus at the time of ovulation (see later). Ovulation is usually predicted by serial pelvic ultrasound scans or by the detection of the LH surge using a urinary assay. The chance of conception in the first cycle of treatment is 18.8%, falling rapidly to around 6% per cycle for the next 12 months.

Azoospermia and a normal FSH

Azoospermia in the presence of a normal FSH signifies a block of the vas deferens or epididymis. The most common group of men in this category are those who have had a vasectomy. Using microsurgical techniques, the vas can be re-anastomosed (vasovasostomy) or attached to the epididymis (vasoepididymostomy), depending on the site of the obstruction. Although good anatomical results can be achieved, pregnancy rates are often disappointing, partly because the build-up of pressure distal to the obstruction may have damaged the delicate epididymis, and partly because antisperm antibodies may have formed. The time from the original vasectomy to the reversal procedure provides a useful guide to prognosis. With good surgical technique, pregnancy rates are approximately 60%, but fall to 30% if the interval from vasectomy to re-anastomotic surgery is >10 years.

Men in whom spermatogenesis is normal but surgery is not possible may be suitable for epididymal sperm aspiration in combination with IVF and ICSI. The sperm can be obtained under local anaesthesia by placing a needle percutaneously into the epididymis, or using more conventional microsurgical techniques under a general anaesthetic. As the sperm sample is usually of poor quality, direct ICSI into the oocytes is necessary (see later).

A significant proportion of men who have congenital absence of the vas have been found to carry a variant of cystic fibrosis. They have compound heterogenicity, where each chromosome 7 carries a different mutation at the site of the transmembrane conductance regulator gene, which is responsible for cystic fibrosis. These couples therefore need careful screening for the common cystic fibrosis mutations. If his partner is found to be a carrier of one of the mutations there is a one in four chance of their child being affected with cystic fibrosis.

Hypogonadotrophic hypogonadism

Hypogonadotrophic hypogonadism is rare but can be treated successfully with exogenous gonadotrophins (FSH and hCG) or by using a GnRH infusion pump.

Idiopathic oligospermia

This is the most common diagnosis in male factor infertility. A wide range of oral treatments have been employed to improve fertility but there is no firm evidence that the use of any oral medication can improve conception rates. Multivitamins have been associated with an improvement in sperm parameters and are recommended for all men whose partners are trying to conceive. The mainstay of treatment is ICSI using sperm prepared in culture medium.

Varicocele

There is ultrasound evidence of a varicocele in 15% of the general male population. Surgery to correct the defect is not justified in the absence of symptoms and in the presence of a normal semen analysis. Even in the presence of oligospermia, there is no evidence that the sperm count (or the conception rate) can be improved with surgery, and therefore surgery is no longer recommended in otherwise asymptomatic men.

Unexplained infertility

If no cause can be found, then the main treatment would be to proceed to IVF, although conservative management is always an option.

Assisted conception

'Assisted conception' techniques are those in which gametes, either sperm or eggs, are manipulated to improve the chance of conception (Table 5.4).

Intrauterine insemination (IUI)

IUI was historically used to treat couples with unexplained infertility, a 'mild' male factor infertility and mild endometriosis, but is now mainly restricted to those with coital difficulties and couples requiring donor sperm (DI). Sperm is prepared in a culture medium, separating the seminal fluid, poorly motile sperm and other cellular debris in the ejaculate, and producing a clean sample of highly motile sperm. This is then placed directly into the uterine cavity via a fine plastic catheter. IUI is used alone, with the insemination timed to natural ovulation, or in conjunction with controlled ovarian stimulation. The latter involves ovulation–induction agents, such as clomiphene or gonadotrophins, which are used to recruit up to two mature follicles. When the follicles reach an appropriate size, around 17 mm, ovulation is induced with hCG, and the prepared sperm is inserted into the uterine cavity.

In the UK, in 2014, 4675 cycles of DI were performed. Overall, the live birth rates following unstimulated DI are around 11.2% per cycle, increasing to 14.6% for stimulated DI. One complication of controlled ovarian stimulation is the high rate of multiple pregnancy, which in some older studies has been as high as 29%. For this reason, careful dosing, monitoring and a willingness to cancel the cycle due to an excessive response of the ovaries to ovulation induction are required.

In vitro fertilization

The term 'in vitro fertilization' refers to the mixing of sperm and egg outside the body.

Indications

IVF was originally developed for women with tubal disease. However, the indications for IVF have expanded considerably and now include:

- male factor infertility
- severe endometriosis
- failed ovulation induction
- unexplained infertility
- preimplantation diagnosis for genetic disease
- surrogacy
- egg donation.

Technique

Hormonal regimen

The aim of the treatment is to recruit, or rescue, a cohort of antral stage follicles, and support their growth through to maturity (superovulation). This is achieved by the administration of exogenous FSH, given by intramuscular or subcutaneous injection. In addition, most modern protocols use some form of pituitary suppression, either a GnRH agonist or an antagonist, principally to block an inappropriate LH surge. As the release of LH is blocked, hCG, which has a similar action, is used as a substitute, given approximately 36 h before oocyte recovery.

Oocyte collection

During superovulation treatment, each ovary enlarges to the size of a tennis ball and they generally lie within 1 cm of the posterior vaginal fornix (Fig. 5.3). This allows the oocytes to be collected using a needle passed through the vaginal vault, guided by a vaginal ultrasound probe, whilst the woman is sedated. The oocytes, with their cumulus cell mass, are identified easily (Fig. 5.4) and after removal are placed in an incubator.

Table 5.4	Assisted conception techniques		
Name	**Technique**	**Advantages**	**Disadvantages**
Superovulation with IUI	Mild ovarian stimulation. Prepared sperm injected through the cervix	For women who are not ovulating. Chance of success 10% per cycle	Risk of multiple pregnancy
IVF	Ovaries are superovulated, eggs retrieved and mixed with sperm before intrauterine transfer	Effective for a number of indications, including 'unexplained' infertility	Risks of superovulation (OHSS) and multiple pregnancy. Small increase in incidence of congenital anomalies amongst offspring. Expensive
ICSI	Stimulation and oocyte retrieval as for IVF, but sperm injected directly into the oocyte	Can be used to treat the majority of male factor infertility	Risks of superovulation (OHSS) and multiple pregnancy. Increased incidence of imprinting disorders in offspring. Expensive

Fertilization and incubation

On the morning of oocyte retrieval, the man collects a sperm sample by masturbation. After preparation in culture medium, the sperm are added to the test tubes containing the oocytes. The tubes are inspected 16 h later for the characteristic signs of fertilization, the presence of a male and female pronucleus (see Fig. 5.5). The pronucleate embryos are returned to the incubator for a further 24 or 48 h, with surplus embryos being frozen at this stage.

Embryo transfer

Embryos can be transferred to the uterus at 48 or 72 h after the oocyte collection, at the 4- or 8-cell stage, respectively (Fig. 5.6), or on day 5 at the blastocyst stage. Transferring at the blastocyst stage appears to provide the best chance of pregnancy. Although a maximum of two embryos is transferred to the uterus in women under 40, there is a move in the UK to select out those women most at risk of a twin pregnancy, and electively transfer a single embryo (eSET). An eSET policy is widely used in Europe and is associated with a significant reduction in the incidence of multiple pregnancies. In contrast, women over the age of 40, who are more likely to have aneuploid embryos, can have up to three embryos transferred, although this has not been associated with a higher live birth rate than when just two embryos are transferred.

Luteal support

As the pituitary gland has been desensitized (and so will not be producing LH), the luteal phase has to be supported with progesterone suppositories for 14 days, until the result of the pregnancy test is known.

Results

In the UK, in 2011, 48 147 women had a total of 61 726 cycles of IVF or ICSI, with an overall live birth rate of 24.5% per cycle started.

Interpreting success rates

There is considerable variation in success rates from clinic to clinic, depending on the clinic's experience and the mixture of couples treated. In the UK, the Human Fertilisation and Embryology Authority (HFEA, see later), have produced a patient guide providing information on outcomes in each clinic licensed for IVF. The most significant factor in determining an individual couple's chance of success is the woman's age, with a dramatic fall in pregnancy rates as age advances (Box 5.3). Success rates gradually decline from 34 years old, so that by the age of 45 the chance of pregnancy with a woman's own oocytes is approximately 1%.

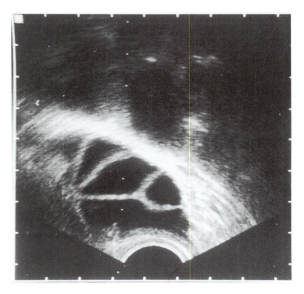

Fig. 5.3 Vaginal ultrasound illustrating superovulated ovary at egg collection.

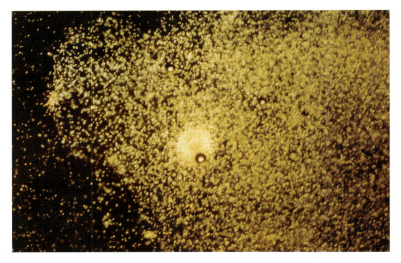

Fig. 5.4 Oocyte–cumulus cell complex identified at egg collection.

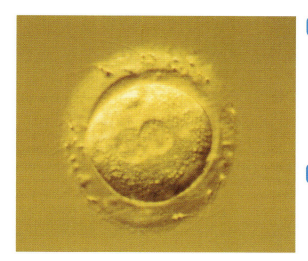

Fig. 5.5 **Fertilized egg showing male and female pronucleus.**

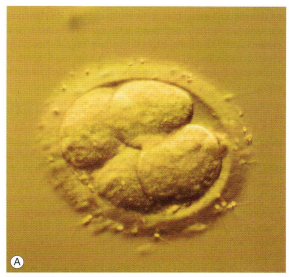

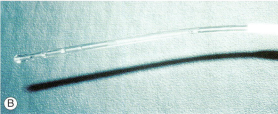

Fig. 5.6 **Embryo transfer. (A)** A 4-cell embryo ready for transfer into the uterus. **(B)** Loaded embryo transfer catheter.

The live birth rates quoted represent the chance of success in a single cycle. The first cycle of treatment gives the couple the highest chance of success, but the pregnancy rate in subsequent cycles s not dissimilar. The cumulative pregnancy rate in women under the age of 40 is 68.4% after six attempts.

Box 5.3

Main factors negatively affecting IVF success

The main factors are:

- increasing age of the woman
- increasing duration of infertility
- number of previous unsuccessful treatments
- absence of previous pregnancies
- low ovarian reserve
- hydrosalpinges (ideally are surgically treated prior to IVF)

Box 5.4

Indications for ICSI

- Requirement for sperm aspiration:
  - congenital absence of the vas deferens
  - obstructive azoospermia: post-infection or iatrogenic
- semen analysis below reference ranges for any parameter
- Repeated failed fertilization with standard IVF.

Embryo freezing

Approximately 25% of couples have 'spare' embryos left over after the initial treatment. These can be frozen in liquid nitrogen and replaced during a subsequent natural or artificial cycle, to give a further chance of a pregnancy. With careful selection of embryos for freezing, the live birth rate following frozen embryo transfer can be equivalent to those of 'fresh' transfer.

Gamete intrafallopian tube transfer (GIFT)

This also involves the use of superovulation using the same protocols as described for IVF, followed by oocyte collection by vaginal ultrasound-guided needle aspiration. Thereafter, the two techniques differ. With GIFT, the 'best' three oocytes are selected and a laparoscopy is performed. The fallopian tube is cannulated and the selected oocytes, along with approximately 100 000 sperm, are returned to the tube. Fertilization then occurs in the fallopian tube. However, due to the poor success rates of this strategy compared with IVF, very few centres now offer this technique.

Intracytoplasmic sperm injection

This technique has revolutionized the treatment of male factor infertility. The indications for ICSI are outlined in Box 5.4. If there are no sperm in the ejaculate and none in the epididymis, sperm can still be retrieved from testicular biopsies in approximately half of the men.

Technique

Oocytes are collected in the standard IVF fashion and then prepared for ICSI by removing their surrounding cumulus cells. A smooth-ended glass pipette is used to hold the oocyte still, while a sharp ultrafine pipette pierces the egg and deposits one sperm along with a tiny amount of culture medium. Prior to injection the selected sperm needs to be immobilized to avoid damaging the delicate structure of the oocyte. The subsequent embryo is transferred to the uterus or frozen, as per IVF.

Results

The pregnancy outcomes following ICSI are comparable to that of conventional IVF (live birth rate of 26.5% per cycle). An increased risk of genetic and developmental defects in post-ICSI pregnancies has been reported. Furthermore, a proportion of male factor infertility has a genetic basis, and by performing ICSI the genetic abnormality may be passed on to the next generation (whereas otherwise it would not). The significance of these findings is limited, with the majority of ICSI offspring being completely normal.

Egg donation

Women with primary ovarian failure will require treatment involving oocyte donation (Box 5.5). This treatment is also increasingly being used for 'older' women. Another indication for egg donation (or for DI where the disorder is in the male partner) is genetic disease. Egg donation is more complicated than sperm donation, as the donors have to undergo IVF treatment to the stage of oocyte collection. Some centres offer an 'egg-sharing' programme, whereby an infertile couple who cannot afford treatment agrees to go through an IVF cycle but donate half the harvested eggs to a recipient who funds both couples' treatment. This concept clearly raises ethical and moral concerns, although early research suggests that both parties benefit.

Results

This is a successful treatment, with pregnancy rates generally higher than conventional IVF, and maintained even in women over the age of 40. This is largely due to the young age of the egg donors (on average 25 years old) and illustrates the fact that the quality of the oocyte is the most significant factor in the age-related decline of fertility.

Host surrogacy

Some women have functional ovaries but no uterus, due to either a congenital abnormality or previous hysterectomy. Such a woman could undergo IVF treatment, with the embryos then being transferred to another woman (a 'host surrogate') whose uterus has been suitably prepared by hormone treatment. The 'host' will carry the pregnancy and then return the baby to the commissioning couple after delivery. According to English law, the 'mother' is the woman who delivers the child, therefore the commissioning couple is required to adopt the child or have a parental order, even though it may be genetically theirs.

Preimplantation genetic diagnosis (PGD)

Couples who have a history of repeated pregnancy failure due to genetic disease or who have had a child with a specific genetic abnormality may benefit from PGD. The couples undergo a conventional IVF treatment cycle, generally using ICSI as the means of fertilization. The embryos are left until day 5, by which stage they have divided to the blastocyst stage. Generally, 5 trophectoderm cells out of the approximately 250-cell blastocyst are removed and analysed for specific chromosomal abnormalities using next-generation sequencing. Unaffected embryos are replaced by embryo transfer in the usual manner. This allows the couple to start a pregnancy knowing that the child is unaffected by the specific genetic condition generating the concern.

Results

The overall chance of success is slightly lower than for conventional IVF, but greater than 25% per treatment cycle.

Side-effects of assisted conception

Globally, approximately 25% of all IVF pregnancies are twin pregnancies and there remain some triplet pregnancies as a consequence of IVF. The introduction of elective eSET is aimed at reducing the multiple pregnancy rate to less than 10%, but in 2013 it was 15.3%.

OHSS is a condition where the ovaries over-respond to the gonadotrophin injections:

- more than 30 follicles may start to mature, resulting in ovarian enlargement and abdominal discomfort
- very high concentrations of oestradiol and progesterone make the woman feel nauseated
- if the condition is severe, protein-rich ascites can accumulate, and more rarely, pleural effusion may result
- the sudden shift in fluid can result in hypovolaemia, with resulting renal and thrombotic problems; untreated, the condition can be fatal.

The incidence of severe OHSS is low (<1%) and it only occurs if the hCG injection is given during superovulation. Women with polycystic ovaries are the most vulnerable and they have a risk of around 5%. Once a diagnosis is made, treatment is supportive with fluid replacement, generally with protein-rich fluids rather than simple crystalloid solutions. Serum electrolytes are monitored because hyperkalaemia and/or hyponatraemia can develop. Thromboprophylaxis is required because of the risk of venous thromboembolism.

Box 5.5

Indications for egg donation
- Premature ovarian failure
- Gonadal dysgenesis
- Iatrogenic – surgery, radiation and chemotherapy
- Carriers of genetic disease
- Failed IVF – poor response, inaccessible ovaries, repeated failure to fertilize (with woman's own eggs)

Hyperstimulation usually occurs in women who conceive and can last throughout the early first trimester. If the woman does not conceive, the condition is self-limiting and resolves spontaneously.

Fetal abnormality

Approximately 3% of all infants are diagnosed with a congenital anomaly. IVF is associated with a 30–40% increased risk of major congenital anomalies compared with natural conceptions. Notably, this risk is not attributable to the increased risk of congenital anomalies associated with multiple birth, since the excess risk remains among singletons. It appears that the increased risk is partly attributable to the underlying infertility or its determinants, since couples who take longer than 12 months to conceive also exhibit an increased risk of anomalies (hazard ratio: 1.20). The principal anomalies which occur in IVF pregnancies include a range of gastrointestinal, cardiovascular and musculoskeletal defects, and specifically septal heart defects, cleft lip, oesophageal atresia and anorectal atresia. While the relative risk of congenital anomalies amongst IVF pregnancies is increased, the absolute risk remains low.

The UK Human Fertilisation and Embryology Act

This Act, passed by the UK Parliament in 1990, brought about the formation of a regulatory body, known as the HFEA. Further powers were given in the revision of the Act in 2008. The HFEA regulates research on human embryos, the storage of gametes and embryos, and the use in infertility treatment of donated gametes and of embryos produced outside the body. The HFEA came into operation in August 1991, with the principal aim of ensuring that human embryos and gametes are used responsibly and that infertile couples are not exploited. Assisted conception treatment can only be legally performed in a centre licensed by the HFEA. This license is renewed on an annual basis.

All women and men who donate gametes (either sperm or eggs) or receive assisted conception treatment have to be registered with the HFEA. The outcome of treatment is also recorded. The HFEA also requires all couples considering assisted conception to be offered counselling by a trained counsellor. Paramount in the HFEA's philosophy is the welfare of the potential child.

Key points

- Infertility is defined as the inability to conceive after 12 months of regular unprotected coitus. It affects approximately one in six couples.
- The commonest causes of infertility are ovulatory problems, semen abnormalities and blockage of fallopian tubes, but for many it is unexplained. Other causes include coital difficulties and endometriosis.
- Investigation involves semen analysis, tests of ovulation and tests for tubal patency.
- Treatment of anovulation may include anti-oestrogens (particularly clomiphene or letrozole) or exogenous gonadotrophins.
- ICSI combined with IVF offers a treatment option to couples with male factor infertility.

6

Early pregnancy care

Miscarriage

Miscarriage is common, occurring in as many as 20% of all pregnancies. It is very upsetting for the parents, and considerable sensitivity is required. Clinical management should ideally take place in an early pregnancy unit and be founded on two important principles:

1. Until the diagnosis of a non-continuing pregnancy is confirmed, a wait and see approach should be adopted, remembering that dates may be incorrect.
2. There should be a low threshold of suspicion for ectopic pregnancy. The absence of an ectopic pregnancy on ultrasound scanning does not mean that there is not an ectopic pregnancy.

Definition

In the UK, miscarriage is defined as the loss of a pregnancy at <24 weeks gestation, where there are no signs of life. If there are signs of life with subsequent death at any gestation, the baby must be registered as a live birth and neonatal death. From ≥24 weeks, a baby born with no signs of life is registered as a stillbirth.

A threatened miscarriage is where bleeding occurs but the pregnancy may continue, whereas in an inevitable miscarriage, the pregnancy will not continue. The cervix may be dilated.

The diagnosis should be confirmed by ultrasound scan unless the patient is clinically in shock, requiring immediate surgery.

Miscarriage can be further divided into the following categories:

- *incomplete*: passage of some, but not all of the pregnancy tissue
- *complete*: all pregnancy tissue has been expelled from the uterus
- *delayed/missed (silent)*: where the pregnancy is not continuing, but there are no symptoms of miscarriage; 'anembryonic pregnancy' is a type of 'missed' miscarriage, in which embryonic development fails at a very early stage in the pregnancy
- *septic*: a complication of incomplete miscarriage or therapeutic (sometimes illegal) abortion in which intrauterine infection occurs
- *recurrent*: three or more consecutive miscarriages.

Incidence

As noted earlier, the incidence of miscarriage is about 20%, and is highest in early pregnancy, falling to <1% after the end of the first trimester. Evidence from studies of human chorionic gonadotrophin (hCG) assays performed in very early pregnancy and from assisted conception units suggest that rates of very early miscarriage may be as high as 50–60%.

The incidence of miscarriage increases with maternal age, rising by a factor of 10 after the age of 40 years compared with before 35 years. Once the fetal heart is seen on an ultrasound scan, the chance of a successful outcome is high (<5% risk of miscarriage).

Aetiology

There are a number of conditions recognized as causing sporadic and/or recurrent miscarriage.

Fetal chromosomal abnormalities

About half of all clinically recognized first-trimester losses are chromosomally abnormal, with 50% of these being autosomal trisomy, 20% 45XO monosomy, 20% polyploidy and 10% other abnormalities. In second-trimester miscarriage, the incidence of chromosomal abnormality is lower, at about 20% overall.

Immunological causes

Autoimmune disease

Approximately 15% of women who are investigated for recurrent miscarriage are found to be positive for antiphospholipid antibodies (lupus anticoagulants, anticardiolipin antibodies or both). Untreated, they have a subsequent rate of fetal loss approaching 70–80%. Effective treatment can be provided with low-dose aspirin (although some would recommend avoiding this in the first trimester of pregnancy) and low-molecular-weight heparin. These antibodies are also associated with arterial and venous thrombosis, fetal growth restriction, pre-eclampsia and thrombocytopenia, and this should be borne in mind for later pregnancy management. Lupus anticoagulant is not synonymous with systemic lupus erythematosus (SLE), as it is present in only 5–15% of patients with SLE and the majority of women who are LA or ACA positive do not have SLE.

Alloimmune disease

It is possible that recurrent miscarriage is caused by some immunological problem at the interface between trophoblastic cells and maternal cells, although the exact nature of this proposed problem has not been clearly elucidated. There has been interest in endometrial natural killer cells, which were originally thought to be the cause of miscarriage, but a more recent hypothesis suggests that they might have a role in rejecting abnormal embryos and allowing normal ones to thrive. There is a suggestion that steroids may be of benefit in treating this condition, although further research is required.

Endocrine factors

Women with polycystic ovary syndrome have an increased incidence of both sporadic and recurrent miscarriage. Although this has been attributed to high circulating levels of luteinizing hormone in the follicular phase of the cycle, there is no evidence of any effective therapy.

Inadequate luteal function has been reported in association with recurrent miscarriage in 20–60% of cases, but a recent study has shown no convincing evidence to support the use of artificial progestogens.

In women with diabetes mellitus who have poor control around the time of conception, the incidence of miscarriage is around 45%. Women whose control is good are no more likely to have a miscarriage than those who do not have diabetes.

There is no clear association between thyroid dysfunction and miscarriage unless it is poorly controlled, although the role of thyroperoxidase antibodies is currently being explored.

Uterine anomalies

It is possible that structural uterine anomalies such as bicornuate or septate uteri cause miscarriage, but this causation is not proven with certainty. Uterine fibroids may also interfere with early pregnancy growth, but the extent to which they cause miscarriage is difficult to determine because of other associated factors, such as age, hormonal dysfunction and subfertility.

Infections

Any serious maternal infection causing high fever at any time in pregnancy may adversely affect the fetus and lead to pregnancy loss. There are also a number of specific infectious agents, such as Zika virus, rubella virus and cytomegalovirus, which can cross the placenta and may lead to miscarriage, as well as to later fetal abnormality and neonatal illness. Malaria, trypanosomiasis, mycoplasma pneumonia, listeriosis and syphilis have also all been implicated in early pregnancy loss. These are unlikely to cause recurrent loss.

Environmental pollutants

Cigarette smoking (both active and passive) and high alcohol consumption are associated with slightly higher rates of sporadic and recurrent miscarriage.

Unexplained

At least 50% of miscarriages, either sporadic or recurrent, have no identifiable cause.

Clinical presentation and management

Presentation

There is usually a history of bleeding per vaginam (PV) and lower abdominal pain. The passage of tissue is sometimes reported (Fig. 6.1). The bleeding can vary from being life-threateningly severe, requiring urgent

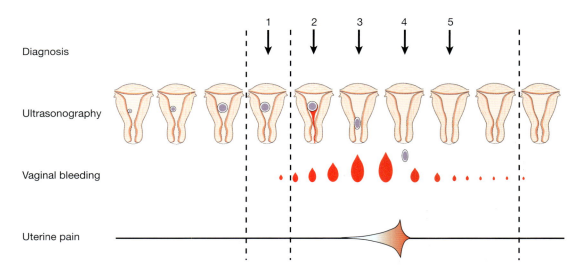

Fig. 6.1 Clinical and ultrasound features of a miscarriage. 1. Ultrasound may show fetal heart activity, or the pregnancy may appear non-viable. 2. Vaginal bleeding and pain begin. 3. The cervical os is open – an inevitable miscarriage. 4. The gestational sac is extruded. 5. Pain and bleeding usually settle rapidly.

and aggressive resuscitation, to the lightest brown spotting.

In a missed or delayed miscarriage, there may be no symptoms at all. It is seldom possible to make a reliable diagnosis based on clinical examination alone, and management is largely based on ultrasound scan findings (Table 6.1). Transvaginal scans (TVS) provide superior images compared with abdominal scans.

Viable intrauterine pregnancy

If a fetal heart is seen following a threatened miscarriage, the prognosis is good, and the parents can be offered reasonable reassurance (Fig. 6.2). If there are recurrent bleeds, however, the pregnancy may be considered as high risk.

Empty gestational sac

If TVS shows an empty gestational sac with an average diameter >25 mm, the pregnancy is very likely to be non-continuing (Fig. 6.3). A second opinion should be sought to confirm. If the sac is <25 mm, the UK National Institute for Health and Care Excellence (NICE) guidelines advise repeating a scan in 1 week to confirm the diagnosis. Although this waiting time creates anxiety, it is essential to confirm if the pregnancy is not continuing.

A true gestational sac should be differentiated from a 'pseudosac', which may be found in an ectopic pregnancy (Fig. 6.4). A pseudosac is caused by fluid secreted in response to the hCG produced by the ectopic pregnancy, and it lacks the 'double decidual ring' outline seen with a true sac (see Figs 6.3 and 6.5).

Table 6.1	The first 9 weeks		
Days	Weeks	Clinical features	Scan features
0	0	Menses	
7	1		
14	2	Conception	
21	3		
28	4	Pregnancy test positive (menses due)	Empty uterus
	5		Gestational sac (hCG >2000 IU/L)
	6	Nausea	Yolk sac
		Breast tenderness	Fetal heartbeat on transvaginal scan
			Fetal pole 4 mm
	7		Fetal pole 10 mm
	8		Fetal heartbeat on transabdominal scan
			Fetal pole 14 mm
	9		Fetal pole 22 mm

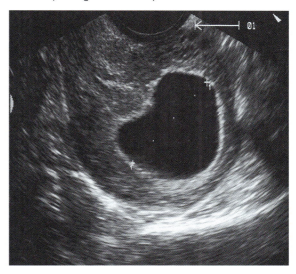

Fig. 6.3 An empty gestational sac at 8 weeks' gestation. This pregnancy was an anembryonic, sometimes referred to as a 'silent' miscarriage.

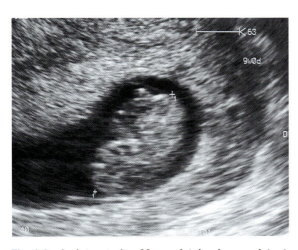

Fig. 6.2 An intrauterine 22-mm fetal pole, consistent with 9 weeks' gestation. Fetal heart activity was seen.

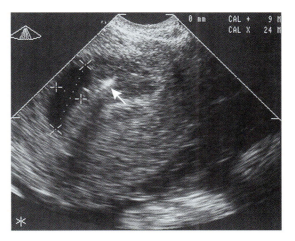

Fig. 6.4 A pseudosac and intrauterine contraceptive device (arrow) in the presence of an ectopic pregnancy.

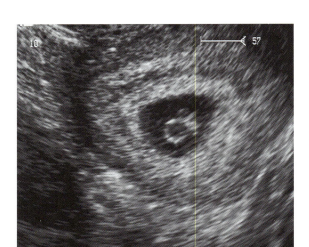

Fig. 6.5 Intrauterine gestational scan containing a 6-mm fetal pole with a yolk sac. No fetal heart activity was detected by transvaginal scan. Note the double decidual ring consistent with intrauterine pregnancy.

Fetal pole with no fetal heartbeat

A fetal heartbeat is usually seen on a TVS if the fetal pole is more than 2–3 mm, but should always be seen by the time the pole is 7 mm (Fig. 6.5) (a length of 15 mm is appropriate for a transabdominal scan). Re-scanning should be arranged in the next 7–10 days before confirming a non-continuing pregnancy, or a second opinion sought if confirming that day.

Empty uterus

There has been a complete miscarriage, the pregnancy is very early or there is an ectopic pregnancy. An ectopic pregnancy must be excluded before diagnosing a complete miscarriage. An intrauterine sac will usually be seen on TVS if the hCG is >1000 IU, and its absence raises the possibility of an ectopic pregnancy. Serum levels of hCG should rise by more than 63% in 48 h if the pregnancy is continuing and intrauterine; a smaller rise suggests an ectopic pregnancy (see Fig. 6.7). If the level doubles and the woman remains well, the ultrasound scan should be repeated in 1 week to ensure that the pregnancy is intrauterine and ongoing. If the level rises but does not double, is static or is only slightly reduced, an ectopic pregnancy should be considered. Management of ectopic pregnancy and pregnancy of unknown location (PUL) is discussed later.

Gestational trophoblastic disease

See Chapter 15.

Management of early pregnancy loss

This should ideally take place in an early pregnancy unit run by dedicated caring staff. Once a diagnosis has been established and explained to the woman, providing there is no ongoing heavy vaginal bleeding, the options of expectant, medical or surgical management under general or local anaesthetic with manual vacuum aspiration can be discussed. Surgical management of miscarriage (SMM) and medical management of miscarriage with or without the antiprogestogen drug mifepristone (depending upon gestation) and a synthetic prostaglandin (misoprostol) are technically analogous to the methods employed in the therapeutic termination of pregnancy (Chapter 20). Many units offer outpatient medical management of early miscarriages. Misoprostol may be administered, after which the woman is allowed to return home and asked to perform a pregnancy test in 3 weeks. If this remains positive, she should be reviewed to exclude an ectopic pregnancy, molar pregnancy or retained pregnancy tissue. Expectant management should be considered as an option, but the woman needs to be warned that the onset, duration and magnitude of vaginal bleeding and pain are unpredictable. The benefits and risks of all options should be discussed prior to consent being obtained. In patients who opt for expectant management, a pregnancy test should be performed after 3 weeks.

Recurrence risk

About 1% of couples will experience three or more consecutive losses. Only a very few women have a specific recurring cause. Where no specific abnormalities are found, counselling and reassurance of women with recurrent miscarriage are the mainstays of successful management: 60–75% of women who have suffered three consecutive miscarriages and who have no apparent underlying cause will have a successful pregnancy at their next attempt. Research into therapies is ongoing, and the use of unproven treatments should be resisted.

Mid-trimester loss

Following mid-trimester loss, the possibility of cervical weakness should be considered. The diagnosis is supported by a history of relatively painless cervical dilation, and there may be a history of cervical surgery. There is no single diagnostic test for cervical weakness, which makes reliable diagnosis impossible. Inserting a cervical suture (cervical cerclage) may be of benefit, but infection can develop after insertion (Fig. 6.6). Transabdominal cerclage is used when a vaginal approach is not technically possible due to the short length of the cervix or when a vaginally placed suture has failed.

Rhesus isoimmunization

Confusion remains about the need for anti-D immunoglobulin administration in the first trimester of pregnancy. Current NICE guidelines recommend that all non-sensitized rhesus-negative women should be offered anti-D immunoglobulin

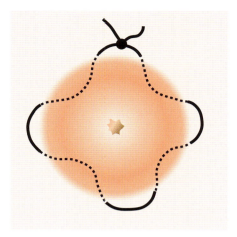

Fig. 6.6 **A cervical suture.**

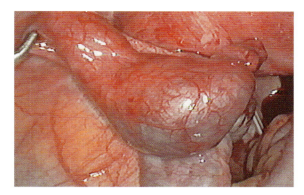

Fig. 6.7 **An ectopic pregnancy in the ampulla of the fallopian tube.**

where SMM or ectopic pregnancy is undertaken, or when a miscarriage is confirmed with a fetal pole at ≥12 weeks. Anti-D immunoglobulin should also be offered to rhesus-negative women with a threatened miscarriage at ≥12 weeks.

After a miscarriage

Miscarriage is a bereavement; the emotional trauma experienced will vary from one couple to the next, but the negative impact of a miscarriage should not be underestimated. Information about support groups, such as 'the Miscarriage Association' and 'the Ectcpic Pregnancy Trust', should be given to all women at the time of pregnancy loss.

Sepsis

Fortunately, this is rare. It is most frequently encountered after termination of pregnancy in countries where abortion is illegal, but sometimes occurs after a spontaneous miscarriage, especially in the presence of retained pregnancy tissue. There is usually pyrexia, tachycardia, malaise, abdominal pain, marked tenderness and a purulent vaginal loss. Endotoxic shock may develop, which has a significant rate of maternal mortality. The responsible organisms include Gram-negative bacteria, streptococci (haemolytic and anaerobic) and other anaerobes (e.g. *Bacteroides*). Sepsis should be treated in a timely manner, by administering appropriate antibiotics and ensuring that the uterus is empty of any retained pregnancy tissue.

Ectopic pregnancy

Although non-intrauterine pregnancies can be ovarian, cervical, Caesarean scar or intra-abdominal, the majority are tubal (Fig. 6.7). The incidence of ectopic pregnancy is 11 per 1000, and ectopic pregnancy remains one of the major causes of maternal mortality.

The history and examination should include the date of the last menstrual period, the date of positive pregnancy test and symptoms suggesting pelvic infections. Symptoms of PV bleeding, abdominal pain, shoulder tip pain and bowel upset are important. Pelvic examination should be gentle to avoid tubal rupture. If the pregnancy test is positive and the woman is not in shock, an ultrasound scan (ideally transvaginal) will be helpful in distinguishing between ectopic pregnancy, miscarriage and a continuing intrauterine pregnancy. A pseudosac can be confused with an intrauterine gestation sac in 20% of ectopic pregnancies. A serum beta hCG level that does not increase by over 63% in 48 h increases the likelihood of ectopic pregnancy.

Management depends on the overall clinical picture, the scan result and the serum level of hCG. Tubal pregnancy can be managed by laparoscopy, laparotomy, medical management or expectant management in selected cases. Management must be tailored to the clinical condition and future fertility preferences of the woman (Fig. 6.8).

- If the woman is in shock on admission and a pregnancy test is positive, urgent surgery should be undertaken. Resuscitation (and sometimes blood transfusion) will be required.
- In a haemodynamically stable woman, a laparoscopic approach is preferable to an open approach. In the presence of a healthy contralateral tube, there is no clear evidence that salpingotomy should be preferred to salpingectomy. Postoperative tracking of serum hCG is necessary following salpingotomy to identify the small number of cases complicated by persistent trophoblast.
- Surgery should be considered for women who have an adnexal mass >35 mm, an ectopic pregnancy with a positive fetal heartbeat, significant free fluid in the Pouch of Douglas, serum hCG >5000 IU/L (depending upon local guidelines) or symptoms consistent with pain or bleeding from an ectopic pregnancy.
- In a well woman with a positive pregnancy test and an empty uterus on TVS, a serum hCG level assay is performed and repeated after 48 h. If

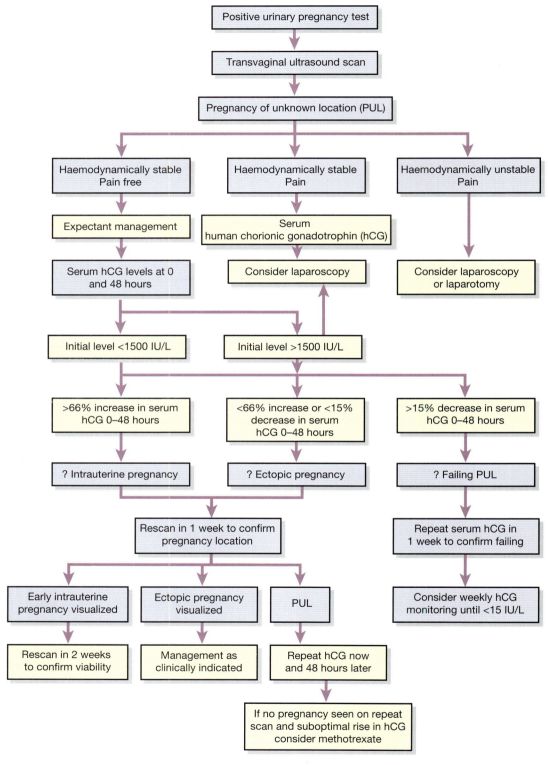

Fig. 6.8 **Algorithm for managing suspected ectopic pregnancy.** hCG, human Chorionic Gonadotrophin; PUL, Pregnancy of Unknown Location.

an ectopic pregnancy is likely and the woman remains asymptomatic, medical management with methotrexate ($50\,mg/m^2$) may be considered. If medical therapy is offered, women should be given verbal and written information about the possible need for further treatment, the need to avoid pregnancy for 3 months after the last dose of methotrexate and adverse effects following treatment. Women should be able to return easily for assessment during follow-up.

■ Expectant management is an option for clinically stable asymptomatic women with an ultrasound diagnosis of ectopic pregnancy and a serum hCG level of less than 1500 IU/L.

On occasion, a PUL is diagnosed where there is no evidence of an ectopic or intrauterine pregnancy, but the hCG level remains elevated. As mentioned previously, a PUL may be managed expectantly, medically or surgically, depending upon symptoms and level of hCG.

Intervention is required in 20–30% of cases of PUL. If women are managed expectantly, serial serum hCG measurements should be performed until hCG levels are <15 IU/L. In addition, women selected for expectant management of PUL should be given clear information about the importance of compliance with follow-up, and should be within easy access of the unit treating them.

Rarely, a heterotopic pregnancy is diagnosed. This is a combination of an ectopic pregnancy and an intrauterine pregnancy. It is more common after in vitro fertilization, but can occur spontaneously.

Anti-D immunoglobulin should be offered to non-sensitized women who are undergoing surgery for an ectopic pregnancy.

Key *points*

- Miscarriage is the loss of a pregnancy before 24 weeks' gestation.
- Management is centred on accurate diagnosis, counselling and minimizing complications.
- Care must be taken to avoid uterine evacuation if there is any possibility of a continuing pregnancy. A wait and see approach must be adopted until the diagnosis is certain.
- There should be a low threshold of suspicion for ectopic pregnancy.
- Ideally, care should be undertaken in an early pregnancy unit with TVS capability.
- An empty uterus and a positive pregnancy test suggest an ectopic pregnancy, until proven otherwise.

7 Heavy menstrual bleeding, dysmenorrhoea and pre-menstrual syndrome

Heavy menstrual bleeding

Heavy menstrual bleeding (HMB) is defined, for clinical purposes, as bleeding that has an adverse impact on the quality of life of a woman; it may occur alone or with other symptoms. Menstrual blood loss can be measured, but this is usually only performed for research purposes. HMB was often called 'menorrhagia' in the past, but this term is better avoided, as it means different things to different people (e.g. the definition in the USA is different from that in the UK). HMB is the commonest cause of iron-deficiency anaemia in women in well-resourced countries.

Menstrual problems are becoming more prevalent, as women experience more periods in their lifetime now than their predecessors did 100 years ago (approximately 400 vs 40 periods). This is because women have fewer children and breastfeed less (leading to lactational amenorrhoea). Only 50% of women who complain of excessive heavy bleeding, however, actually suffer from blood loss that falls outside the normal range for women not complaining of any menstrual abnormality (>80 mL/month).

The medical and surgical treatment of HMB represent an appreciable burden to health service resources. HMB is a common indication for hysterectomy, although the number of these procedures performed has fallen in the last two decades with the introduction of effective alternative treatments. Although a commonly performed operation, hysterectomy is a major surgical procedure, and its use needs to be balanced against the potential associated mortality and morbidity. Satisfaction rates with hysterectomy are, however, very high.

Causes of HMB

The causes are summarized in Table 7.1.

Uterine pathology

HMB is associated with both benign pathology (e.g. uterine fibroids, endometrial polyps, adenomyosis, pelvic infection) and, extremely rarely, malignant pathology (e.g. endometrial cancer). Over half of women with an excessively heavy blood loss of >200 mL/period will have fibroids. With the advent of high-quality ultrasound that is readily available in outpatient clinics, pathology is identified in a greater proportion of women.

Endometrial polyps are common benign localized overgrowths of the endometrium. They consist of a fibrous tissue core covered by columnar epithelium, and it is believed that they arise as a result of disordered cycles of endometrial apoptosis and regrowth. Although it is uncertain that they cause HMB, it is likely that intrauterine endometrial polyps do increase the likelihood of irregular bleeding (Fig. 7.1). It is unlikely, however, that small endocervical polyps detected at the time of a routine cervical smear have the same effect. Malignant transformation of such polyps is very rare.

Uterine fibroids (leiomyomas) are benign tumours of the myometrium that are present in approximately 20% of women of reproductive age. They are well-circumscribed whorls of smooth muscle cells and collagen, and may be single or multiple (Fig. 7.2). Size varies from microscopic growths to tumours that weigh as much as 40 kg, and they are more common in women of Afro-Caribbean origin. Submucous fibroids project into the uterine cavity, intramural fibroids are contained within the wall of the uterus, and subserosal fibroids project from the surface of the uterus; cervical fibroids arise from the cervix.

Many are asymptomatic, but when symptoms do occur, they are often related to the site and/or size of the fibroid. Presenting symptoms include menstrual dysfunction, infertility, miscarriage, dyspareunia and pelvic discomfort. The mechanism by which fibroids adversely affect reproduction is unclear, but may be related in part to distortion of the uterine cavity, affecting implantation. Fibroids that do not distort the cavity are unlikely to have an adverse impact. Fibroids may also present because of pressure effects on surrounding organs, such as increased frequency of micturition as a result of pressure on the bladder, or even hydronephrosis due to ureteric compression. Growth of fibroids is mediated by sex steroids, and they therefore grow during pregnancy and shrink after the menopause. Occasionally, necrosis of the fibroid ('red degeneration') leads to acute abdominal pain during pregnancy. The incidence of malignant change (leiomyosarcoma) in fibroids is considered to be extremely low (0.1%).

HMB in the absence of pathology

This was known in the past as 'dysfunctional uterine bleeding', but again, this term should be avoided. HMB in the absence of recognizable pelvic pathology or systemic disease is a diagnosis of exclusion, and is probably the commonest

Table 7.1	The main causes of HMB
1. Uterine pathology, e.g. fibroids	Common
2. No apparent cause	Very common
3. Medical disorders, including clotting defects	Very rare

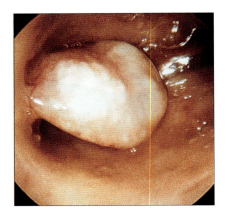

Fig. 7.1 Hysteroscopic view of intrauterine polyp.
(Courtesy of Karl Storz Endoscopy (UK) Ltd.)

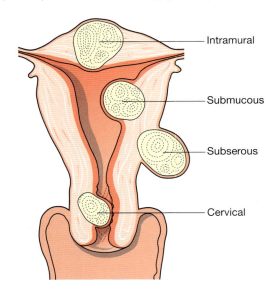

Intramural

Submucous

Subserous

Cervical

Fig. 7.2 Sites of fibroids throughout the uterus.

'diagnosis' reached after investigating women with HMB. Some HMB with no pathology may be 'anovulatory' or 'ovulatory', although this is not an important distinction clinically, as treatment is the same in both cases. The underlying cause is likely to reside at the level of the endometrium, although the precise nature of the vascular and endocrine abnormality remains elusive.

Medical disorders and clotting defects

Very rarely, HMB is associated with medical problems such as thyroid disease (both hypo- and hyperthyroidism), hepatic disease and renal disease (although the majority of women with end-stage renal failure are amenorrhoeic). Other symptoms of the underlying medical disorder are likely to be present.

Certain coagulation abnormalities (e.g. von Willebrand disease) and platelet defects (e.g. thrombocytopenia) are associated with an increased incidence of HMB.

Assessment of HMB

History

The number of sanitary towels used, duration of bleeding and passage of clots seem to have little correlation with the actual volume of blood lost. However, complaints of 'flooding' (leakage of heavy blood loss onto clothing) and having to use 'double sanitary protection' (pad and tampon) to prevent leakage of blood onto clothes are indicative of HMB, and are likely to have a negative impact upon the woman's quality of life. It is important, therefore, to ask about the degree of inconvenience experienced, such as time lost from work, or becoming housebound during menses owing to fear of social embarrassment from an episode of flooding in public.

A history of irregular bleeding, dyspareunia, pelvic pain or intermenstrual or post-coital bleeding may raise the suspicion of underlying pathology, and often requires additional investigation. These can be termed 'red flag' symptoms.

The woman should also be questioned about symptoms suggestive of anaemia, such as fatigue and light-headedness. A history suggestive of systemic disease such as a thyroid disorder or a clotting abnormality would signal that further investigation for such causes is required. The woman should also be questioned about risk factors for endometrial cancer, such as unopposed oestrogen use, tamoxifen use, polycystic ovary syndrome or family history of endometrial or colon cancer. It is also important to establish if she has a history of thromboembolism, as many medical treatments for HMB are hormonal, and thus their use may be relatively or absolutely contraindicated.

Examination

The woman should be examined for signs of anaemia. Abdominal, bimanual and speculum examinations should be considered; however if the history suggests HMB without structural or histological abnormality, pharmaceutical treatment can be started without carrying out a physical examination or other investigations at initial consultation in primary care. An enlarged, 'bulky' uterus suggests uterine fibroids, and tenderness suggests endometriosis, pelvic inflammatory disease or adenomyosis.

Investigations

Laboratory tests

A full blood count should be carried out in all women to diagnose/exclude anaemia. Thyroid function tests and coagulation tests should be performed only if there are features in the history. No other endocrine tests are routinely indicated.

Ultrasound

Ultrasound is the first-line diagnostic tool for identifying structural abnormalities, and a pelvic ultrasound scan should be performed if either history or examination suggests structural uterine pathology. Imaging should also be undertaken in women in whom pharmaceutical treatment has failed, or if it is not possible to assess the uterus clinically because of obesity. The site and size of abnormalities such as fibroids can be determined, together with assessment of the ovaries (Fig. 7.3).

Endometrial assessment

This should be performed in all women aged >45 years, as well as in younger women with persistent HMB in spite of medical treatment, red flag symptoms such as irregular bleeding or risk factors for endometrial cancer. This can take the form of an endometrial biopsy or a hysteroscopy, both of which can be carried out either as an outpatient or inpatient procedure (Fig. 7.4) and p. 125.

Cervical cytology

This should be performed if it is due, or if the cervix looks suspicious.

Treatment of causes of HMB

Focal uterine pathology

Benign intrauterine polyps will usually be removed by polypectomy using hysteroscopic techniques. If malignant pathology is detected, then this should be treated as appropriate.

Fibroids may be treated medically or surgically.

Medical

Pharmaceutical treatment should be considered where fibroids measure less than 3 cm and cause no distortion of the uterine cavity. If contraceptive and/or hormonal treatments are acceptable, the following treatments can be offered:

- levonorgestrel-releasing intrauterine system (LNG-IUS)
- tranexamic acid, non-steroidal anti-inflammatory drugs (NSAIDs) or combined oral contraceptive (COC)
- norethisterone (15 mg) daily from days 5 to 26 of the menstrual cycle, or;
- injected long-acting progestogens.

Unfortunately, the symptoms caused by fibroids respond poorly to medical treatments used where there is no pathology; therefore, in women with fibroids measuring 3 cm or more, or with fibroids causing distortion of the uterine cavity, ulipristal acetate should be offered. The drug is started when menstruation has occurred, and should be taken as one 5-mg tablet daily for a treatment course of up to 3 months, up to a maximum of four intermittent courses.

Ulipristal acetate is a progesterone receptor modulator, a class of drugs that represents an exciting development in the treatment of fibroid-related HMB and possibly also of HMB in the absence of pathology. Treatment with this class of drugs leads to a rapid decrease in bleeding in 80%

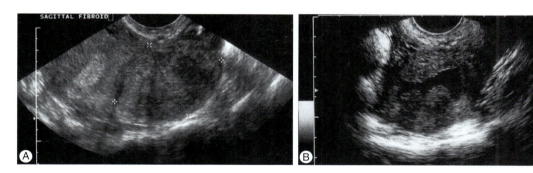

Fig. 7.3 **Uterine fibroids. (A)** A large intramural fibroid. **(B)** Two submucous fibroids projecting into the cavity of the uterus, which contains a small amount of fluid (saline infusion ultrasound scan).

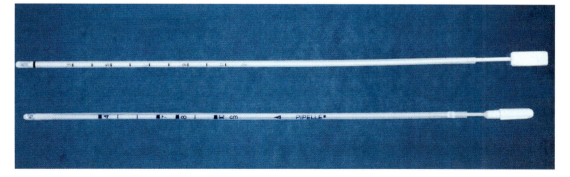

Fig. 7.4 **Two varieties of endometrial samplers.**

of women, without leading to hypo-oestrogenism or inhibiting ovarian cyclicity. They are very well tolerated. The duration of their use is currently restricted, as they cause unique changes in the endometrium that are difficult to interpret. However, further clinical trials are ongoing.

Since growth of fibroids is hormone dependent, gonadotrophin-releasing hormone (GnRH) analogues (which result in hypo-oestrogenism) may be used to shrink fibroids. GnRH analogues are derivatives of natural GnRH, with modifications that confer greater potency and longer activity. Depot injection of GnRH analogues, however, leads to pituitary downregulation with hypo-oestrogenism. Fibroids shrink by approximately 50% over 3 months of treatment, but regrowth occurs upon cessation of treatment. During treatment, hypo-oestrogenism can result in symptoms such as hot flushes, and may also cause bone loss. In view of concerns about osteoporosis, GnRH analogues are limited to short-term use (<6 months). 'Add-back' hormone replacement therapy (HRT) is required to minimize the risk of osteoporosis and other side-effects.

Surgical

Hysteroscopic resection of small submucous fibroids is often possible, and can lead to improved fertility and relief of menstrual problems. Endometrial ablation in the presence of small fibroids is possible (see later).

Myomectomy involves incision of the fibroid pseudocapsule, enucleation of the bulk of the tumour and closure of the resulting defect. The operation is usually performed as an open abdominal procedure, although laparoscopic techniques are sometimes employed. Myomectomy is associated with a similar degree of morbidity to hysterectomy. There is a risk of haemorrhage (due to the vascularity of fibroids), and a small possibility that an emergency hysterectomy may need to be performed during surgery to arrest uncontrollable bleeding. Furthermore, there is a risk of adhesion formation, which could compromise fertility (as a result of tubal obstruction), and the possibility that residual seedling fibroids may grow, leading to the recurrence of fibroids. GnRH analogues are often used preoperatively to shrink fibroids, with associated decreased intraoperative blood loss. Pregnancies after myomectomy are frequently delivered by planned caesarean section because of concerns regarding uterine rupture during labour.

Uterine artery embolization (UAE), which is performed by interventional radiologists, is an effective and safe technique. It involves interruption of the blood supply to the fibroid by blocking the uterine arteries with coils or foam delivered through a catheter placed in the femoral artery. The healthy myometrium revascularizes immediately, owing to the development of collateral circulation from vaginal and ovarian vessels. Fibroids, however, do not appear to revascularize, and shrink by about 50%, a reduction which appears to be sustained. Pain following occlusion of the vessels is often severe, and usually requires opiate analgesia. Potential complications include infection, fibroid expulsion and adverse effects due to exposure of the ovaries to ionizing radiation. The incidence of these is low, and immediate morbidity is less than that following hysterectomy, although pain and fever from post-embolization syndrome is not uncommon, and deaths (though rare) have occurred.

UAE, myomectomy or hysterectomy should be considered in cases of HMB where large fibroids (greater than 3 cm in diameter) are present and bleeding is having a severe impact on a woman's quality of life. Women should be informed that UAE or myomectomy may potentially allow them to retain their fertility, but studies are underway to improve our understanding of this. There is evidence that a successful pregnancy is possible following UAE, and even after failed myomectomy, although rates of miscarriage may be higher and rates of caesarean section and postpartum haemorrhage may be higher. There are also reports of transient or permanent ovarian failure after UAE in up to 5% of cases. This occurs most often in women over the age of 45, but there have been case reports of ovarian dysfunction in younger women.

If childbearing is complete and the woman is experiencing severe symptoms as a result of her fibroids, then hysterectomy may be considered (see later).

HMB with no pathology

In the majority of cases of HMB, no specific cause is found. Sometimes a woman is seeking reassurance that there is no pathology, and does not necessarily wish treatment. Most women, however, request treatment. The following treatments may be considered.

Medical treatment

Intrauterine progestogens. The LNG-IUS delivers progestogen directly to the uterus (Fig. 7.5), and is a first-line treatment for HMB that is particularly suitable for women requiring contraception as it is a highly effective reversible method of contraception and can stay in place for up to 5 years. After 12 months, menstrual blood loss is reduced by around 95%, and many women are amenorrhoeic. The

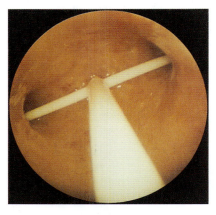

Fig. 7.5 **An intrauterine progestogen-releasing system in the uterus.** (Courtesy of Karl Storz Endoscopy (UK) Ltd.)

main problems with the LNG-IUS are the high incidence of irregular bleeding, particularly within the first 3–6 months after insertion, and an expulsion rate of 5%.

Prostaglandin synthesis inhibitors. NSAIDs taken during menstruation reduce menstrual blood loss by around 25% by reducing endometrial prostaglandin concentrations. The NSAID most commonly used for treatment of HMB is mefenamic acid, although other NSAIDs have similar efficacies. Side-effects include gastrointestinal complaints, dizziness and headache. These drugs are also of benefit for treating dysmenorrhoea.

Antifibrinolytics. Antifibrinolytics, such as tranexamic acid, work by inhibiting plasminogen activator, thereby reducing the fibrinolytic activity in the endometrium. This increases clot formation in the spiral arterioles and reduces menstrual blood loss. Taking tranexamic acid during menstruation reduces blood loss by around 50%. Gastrointestinal side-effects, nausea and tinnitus can occur. The drug should not be taken by women who are predisposed to thromboembolism.

NSAIDs and antifibrinolytics are the best options for women wishing to conceive, as they are only taken during menstruation and do not suppress ovulation.

Combined oral contraceptive pill. This reduces blood loss by approximately 50%. Its mechanism for doing so is thought to be due to suppressive effects on the endometrium. There is no age restriction on the use of the COC in women at low risk of cardiovascular complications (see p. 132).

Systemic progestogens. Oral progestogens are widely prescribed for HMB, but well-designed trials of this therapy do not demonstrate a meaningful reduction in menstrual blood loss. Taken in a cyclical fashion, however, oral progestogens are often useful in regulating otherwise irregular cycles. If the depot injectable progestogen (medroxyprogesterone acetate) is administered for long enough, amenorrhoea frequently results. During the initial months of use, however, bleeding can be unpredictable and heavy. Side-effects of progestogens include nausea, bloating, headache, breast tenderness, weight gain and acne.

GnRH analogues. Amenorrhoea occurs as a result of pituitary downregulation, which leads to inhibition of ovarian activity. However, women may experience problems associated with the resultant hypo-oestrogenism – particularly hot flushes and vaginal dryness. GnRH analogues are usually reserved for short-term use only (up to 6 months), and add-back HRT is usually prescribed to relieve symptoms of hypo-oestrogenism.

Danazol. This is a synthetic androgen with anti-oestrogenic and anti-progestogenic activity that reduces menstrual blood loss but is no longer recommended because of its poor side-effect profile, which includes irreversible virilization.

Surgical treatment

Endometrial ablation. Using a number of different techniques, it is possible to destroy most or all of the endometrium, thereby lessening or stopping menstrual blood loss altogether. Because the endometrium regenerates from the basal layer, it is essential to ablate to the endomyometrial border. Endometrial ablation offers a safer method of symptom control, much shorter hospital stay and shorter recovery period than hysterectomy. Early techniques involved a hysteroscopic procedure under general anaesthesia, during which the endometrium was treated under direct visualization by laser, diathermy or by resection. Newer, nonhysteroscopic procedures included ablation with a heated balloon and bipolar radiofrequency impedance-controlled endometrial ablation (e.g. NovaSure), and other approaches are being developed all the time (Fig. 7.6). These newer procedures carry fewer risks than the hysteroscopic resections, and some can be performed under local anaesthesia.

The success rates of the different ablative techniques are broadly similar. All are associated with a 70–80% overall satisfaction rate, and an amenorrhoea rate of 20% for balloon treatment and around 50% for impedance-controlled ablation. Complications are rare, but include uterine perforation, hyponatraemia and infection. Pregnancy is contraindicated after an ablation procedure, and women are urged to use a reliable, if not permanent, form of contraception.

Hysterectomy. This is the only treatment that guarantees amenorrhoea, and as a consequence, it is associated with a high level of satisfaction. Hysterectomy is performed via the abdominal or vaginal route, the latter with or without laparoscopic assistance (laparoscopically assisted vaginal hysterectomy, or LAVH). Abdominal hysterectomy involves a laparotomy incision, which is usually transverse; a vaginal hysterectomy involves an incision through the vaginal wall. The choice between the two procedures depends on the size of the uterus, the degree of uterine descent, whether the ovaries will be removed (which is difficult by the vaginal route) and the skills and preferences of the surgeon (Table 7.2). In current practice, hysterectomy is increasingly carried out entirely laparoscopically (either by LAVH or by total laparoscopic hysterectomy). The decision to proceed with laparoscopic hysterectomy will depend on the experience of the surgeon, the presence of other gynaecological conditions or disease, the size of the uterus, the presence and size of fibroids and the history of previous abdominal surgery (including caesarean section).

Complications of hysterectomy include haemorrhage, bowel trauma, damage to the urinary tract, infection, postoperative thromboembolism and risk of vaginal prolapse in later years. Complications are more common in those with uterine fibroids. Women undergoing a vaginal procedure recover more quickly from the operation than do those undergoing an abdominal hysterectomy, but the incidence of major complications, although low, is slightly higher with the vaginal route.

For women with no pathology who are undergoing an abdominal hysterectomy and who have a history of normal cervical cytology, there is the choice of having a 'subtotal' hysterectomy. This involves removing the body of the uterus but leaving the cervix behind. The advantages of a subtotal hysterectomy compared with a 'total' hysterectomy are that the operation is quicker and entails less risk of damage to structures surrounding the cervix (bowel and urinary tract) (Fig. 7.7). It has also been reported (though not proven) that

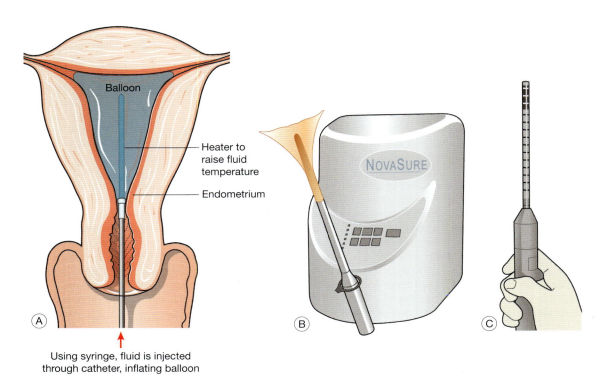

Balloon

Heater to
raise fluid
temperature

Endometrium

(A)

(B)

(C)

Using syringe, fluid is injected
through catheter, inflating balloon

Fig. 7.6   Conservative surgical treatments for menorrhagia. (A) A thermal balloon; **(B)** impedance-controlled
ablation; **(C)** microwave endometrial ablation.

Table 7.2	Pros and cons of different hysterectomy methods	
	Pros	**Cons**
Total abdominal hysterectomy (TAH)	Cervix is removed, therefore no further need for smears and no further risk of cervical malignancy (thus particularly suitable for those with a history of abnormal cytology) Good access to ovaries	Increased surgical morbidity
Subtotal abdominal hysterectomy	Fewer complications than TAH (↓bleeding, ↓infection, ↓bladder injury, ↓ureteric damage) Good access to ovaries	Risk of cervical cancer remains as before
Vaginal hysterectomy	May be lower incidence of bladder and bowel injury in straightforward cases (compared with abdominal hysterectomy) No painful abdominal wound	Limited ovarian access Contraindicated with: • large uterus • restricted uterine mobility • limited vaginal space • adnexal pathology • cervix flush with vagina

these advantages include less postoperative disruption to bowel, bladder and sexual functioning. If the cervix is left intact, the surgeon must be careful to remove any residual endometrium in the cervical canal at the time of surgery, to minimize the small risk that menses would continue from the endometrium in the cervical canal. The disadvantages of a subtotal hysterectomy are that the woman must continue the cervical cytology screening programme. The risk of cervical cancer arising in the stump of the cervix is extremely small (<0.1%), provided that cervical cytology was normal prior to the operation.

Whether the ovaries are removed at the time of abdominal hysterectomy depends on several factors, including the woman's preferences, her age, her family history of breast or ovarian carcinoma and her attitude towards HRT. Removal of healthy ovaries at the time of hysterectomy should not routinely be undertaken, and in women under age 45 considering hysterectomy for HMB with other symptoms that may be related to ovarian dysfunction (e.g. pre-menstrual syndrome [PMS]), a trial of pharmaceutical suppression for at least 3 months should be used as a guide to the need for oophorectomy. If removal is being considered, the impact

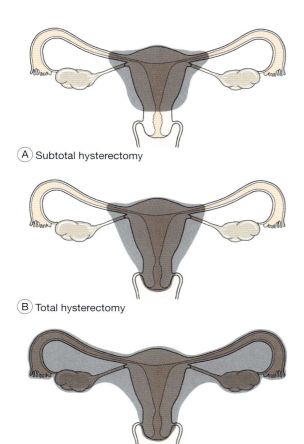

(A) Subtotal hysterectomy

(B) Total hysterectomy

(C) Total hysterectomy with bilateral salpingo-oophorectomy

Fig. 7.7 **Types of abdominal hysterectomy. (A)** Subtotal abdominal hysterectomy; **(B)** total abdominal hysterectomy; **(C)** total abdominal hysterectomy with bilateral salpingo-oophorectomy.

of this procedure on the woman's wellbeing and need for HRT should be discussed preoperatively. Women with a significant family history of breast or ovarian cancer should be referred for genetic counselling prior to a decision about oophorectomy. There is no doubt that removal of ovaries at the time of hysterectomy will reduce the risk of later development of ovarian cancer (lifetime risk 1 in 52 in the UK), but recent data suggest that women aged 35 to 45 years who have a hysterectomy with ovarian conservation are at lower risk of all-cause mortality and have lower death rates from ischaemic heart disease and cancer compared with women whose ovaries are removed at the time of hysterectomy. It has therefore been suggested that removal of this biologically active organ may have harmful effects in the long term. Women should, however, also be informed about the risk of possible loss of ovarian function even if ovaries are retained during hysterectomy. It may therefore be appropriate to discuss 'routine' oophorectomy in women over 45 and ovarian conservation in women under 45.

The decision must remain, however, a very individualized consideration.

Medical disorders and clotting defects

Referral should be made to the appropriate physician/haematologist to institute further investigation and treatment of the underlying condition.

Dysmenorrhoea

Excessive menstrual pain (dysmenorrhoea) is a significant clinical problem. It characteristically involves cramping lower abdominal pain that may radiate to the lower back and legs and may be associated with gastrointestinal symptoms or malaise. It has been estimated that dysmenorrhoea affects 30–50% of menstruating women. It is also one of the most frequent causes of absenteeism from school and days taken off work. As with HMB, dysmenorrhoea may be idiopathic (primary dysmenorrhoea) or due to pelvic pathology (secondary dysmenorrhoea).

Primary dysmenorrhoea

This generally begins with the onset of ovulatory cycles, typically within the first 2 years of the menarche. Pain is usually most severe on the day of or the day prior to the start of menstruation. There is good evidence that prostaglandins are involved in the aetiology, as higher concentrations of PGE_2 and $PGF_{2\alpha}$ are found in the menstrual fluid of women who suffer from dysmenorrhoea than those who do not. $PGF_{2\alpha}$ increases the contractility of the myometrium and can lead to the dysmenorrhoea.

Management of primary dysmenorrhoea

Pelvic examination may not be helpful in primary dysmenorrhoea, and is not appropriate when dealing with an adolescent. A transabdominal ultrasound scan will reveal normal pelvic organs and provide considerable reassurance to a young woman and her family. Discussion and reassurance are an essential part of the management. If dysmenorrhoea is unresponsive to standard medical therapy (see later), then consideration should be given to the possibility of underlying pathology, and appropriate investigation instituted.

Treatment of primary dysmenorrhoea

Prostaglandin synthesis inhibitors. NSAIDs reduce the uterine production of $PGF_{2\alpha}$, and thus dysmenorrhoea. Most NSAIDs have been shown to be effective treatments, but mefenamic acid and ibuprofen are preferred in view of their favourable efficacy and safety profiles.

COC. Suppression of ovulation with the combined contraceptive pill is highly effective in reducing the severity of dysmenorrhoea.

Depot progestogens. The injectable progestogen-only contraceptive suppresses ovulation, and thus may be a useful treatment in alleviating dysmenorrhoea.

Levonorgestrel-releasing intrauterine system (LNG-IUS). In addition to reducing menstrual blood loss, the LNG-IUS is effective at reducing dysmenorrhoea. However, insertion of the device may be difficult in women who have never been pregnant.

Secondary dysmenorrhoea

This is, by definition, associated with pelvic pathology. Its onset usually occurs many years after the menarche. Common associated pathologies are endometriosis, adeno-myosis, pelvic infection and fibroids. It may also be associated with the presence of an intrauterine contraceptive device. In contrast, however, the LNG-IUS is associated with reduced dysmenorrhoea.

Management of secondary dysmenorrhoea

Women who have no complaints other than dysmenorrhoea and who have no abnormalities upon abdominal, pelvic or speculum examination may be safely treated without further investigation. Swabs from the genital tract, however, are helpful in excluding active pelvic infection, particularly *Chlamydia trachomatis*.

If pelvic masses such as fibroids are suspected, a pelvic ultrasound may be helpful. A laparoscopy is indicated if endometriosis or pelvic inflammatory disease is suspected, or in those women for whom standard medical therapy has been ineffective. Treatment is dependent on the underlying pathology (see Chapter 8 for the management of endometriosis).

Pre-menstrual syndrome

PMS can usefully be defined as 'a condition manifesting with physical, behavioural and psychological symptoms in the absence of organic or psychiatric disease, which regularly occurs during the luteal phase of each ovarian cycle and which disappears or significantly regresses by the end of menstruation'. PMS is considered severe if it impairs work, relationships or usual activities. Some observers note that as many as 40% of women suffer mild symptoms, and of these, 5–8% have symptoms severe enough to disrupt their lives, principally in the 2 weeks leading up to the start of menstruation.

Over 150 symptoms have been attributed to PMS, but particularly:

- mood changes/irritability
- abdominal bloating
- breast tenderness (cyclical mastalgia)
- headaches.

Aetiology

The exact aetiology of PMS remains unknown, although ovulatory cycles are generally considered to be a necessary prerequisite. There are suggestions that it is the changing patterns of hormone levels, rather than the absolute levels, that are important. Coupled with this, some women may be sensitive to progesterone and/or progestogens. A second theory involves the neurotransmitters serotonin and gamma-aminobutyric acid (GABA). The levels of both have been associated with the occurrence of PMS symptoms. GABA levels are altered in women with PMS symptoms, whilst selective serotonin reuptake inhibitors (SSRIs) improve PMS symptoms.

Clinical presentation

As there are no specific biochemical tests for PMS, the diagnosis is dependent on a prospective charting of symptoms over a minimum of two cycles to confirm that there is a true exacerbation in the luteal phase when compared with the follicular phase of the cycle (Fig. 7.8). A simple calendar record of the presence or absence of a woman's principal symptoms and days of menstruation is appropriate. There are numerous specific criteria, although many of them are research tools that are not necessarily always applied strictly to clinical practice. An example of one of these tools is shown in Box 7.1. A symptom diary should be completed prior to commencing treatment, especially if this involves medication.

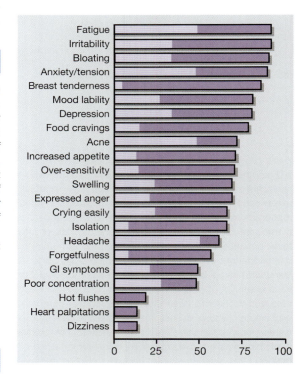

Fig. 7.8 Reported incidence (cycles, %) of individual symptoms in the follicular phase of the cycle (open bars) and the luteal phase of the cycle (filled bars) in 170 women. GI, Gastrointestinal.

Box 7.1

Example of a set of diagnostic criteria for PMS

1. The presence, by self-report, of at least one of the following somatic and affective symptoms during the 5 days before menses in each of the three previous cycles

Affective symptoms:	Somatic symptoms:
Depression	Breast tenderness
Angry outbursts	Bloating
Irritability	Headache
Anxiety	Swelling
Confusion	
Social withdrawal	

2. Relief of the above symptoms within 4 days of the onset of the menses, without recurrence until day 12 of the cycle
3. Presence of the symptoms in the absence of any pharmacological therapy, hormone ingestion or drug or alcohol misuse
4. Reproducible occurrence of symptoms during two cycles of prospective recording
5. Identifiable dysfunction in social or economic performance by one of the following criteria:
   - discord in relationship confirmed by partner
   - difficulties in parenting
   - poor work or school performance
   - increased social isolation
   - legal difficulties
   - suicidal ideation
   - medical attention sought for somatic symptoms

From Mortola et al. 1990, Obstet Gynecol 76:302.

Differential diagnosis

Symptoms that can be worse in the follicular phase are not attributable to PMS. Other conditions such as endometriosis, migraine headaches, depression and anxiety disorders are exacerbated premenstrually, but again should not be confused with the more specific diagnosis of PMS. Peri-menopausal mood changes are usually non-cyclical, and in these circumstances, a serum follicle-stimulating hormone (FSH) measurement should be considered. A normal FSH level does not exclude the menopause, but the investigation may be of particular value in women who have had a hysterectomy with ovarian conservation (since there is no menstruation) or in those who are using a progestogenic method of contraception. The breast pain associated with PMS is usually cyclical, bilateral and poorly localized, and commonly involves 'lumpiness'. By contrast, noncyclical breast pain is precisely localized and rarely bilateral.

In those with abdominal bloating, it is important to consider intra-abdominal pathology such as ovarian cysts, ascites or irritable bowel syndrome. The abdominal bloating associated with PMS is rapidly relieved by the onset of menstruation, perhaps owing to the relaxing effect of pro-gesterone on smooth muscle or to the comparative stasis of the gut in response to morphine-like endorphins. Hypothyroidism and anaemia should be considered in those complaining predominantly of fatigue. The characteristics of endogenous depression are different to those of the mood

Box 7.2

Possible treatments for PMS

Probably effective
- SSRIs
- psychological approaches, including cognitive behavioural therapy
- suppression of ovulation
- oophorectomy

May be effective
- diet
- exercise
- vitamin B_6
- complementary therapy
- evening primrose oil

Probably not effective
- progesterone

changes and irritability commonly observed in PMS, but, as both conditions are relatively common, it is not unusual to encounter both in the same woman.

Management

Women with mild PMS do not usually need medical treatment, and may be helped by reassurance and information. General health measures should be encouraged in all women, such as improved diet with a low glycaemic index, increased exercise, self-relaxation, and reducing smoking and drinking. Some women find self-help groups supportive, while others choose yoga or hypnosis.

Symptomatic treatment

A number of symptomatic treatments are in use, although the evidence supporting their effectiveness is limited. Women with pre-menstrual bloating can be treated in the same way as those with irritable bowel syndrome, and those with oedema may respond to a diuretic such as spironolactone. Breast tenderness can also be treated with diuretics, evening primrose oil or low-dose danazol. Women should be counselled regarding the potential irreversible virilizing effects of low-dose danazol. Effective contraception must also be used at the same time. Mood changes are considered in more detail later.

Treatment aimed at the hypothesized underlying cause

A wide variety of medical treatments for PMS have been considered, many of which are still in current use. Close scrutiny, however, reveals that only a limited number of these are of proven value, and the treatment modalities are classified accordingly in Box 7.2. The 'probably effective' group consists of treatments demonstrated to be effective by good-sized trials, usually randomized placebo-controlled trials. The use of a placebo arm is particularly important in PMS research, as most placebo treatments demonstrate symptom improvements of around 30%. Treatments classified as 'probably not effective' have also been examined in well-conducted studies, and no significant benefit has been demonstrated over placebo. The 'may be effective' group includes therapies for which studies have been inconclusive, often because of small patient numbers. These three groups will be considered in more detail below.

Probably not effective

Progesterone or progestogens

The rationale for the use of progesterone or progestogens in the management of PMS is based on the unsubstantiated premise that the condition is due to a progesterone deficiency. Although initial data suggest that women with PMS have serum concentrations of progesterone metabolites (pregnenolone and allopregnanolone), there is no consistent evidence that these women have low concentrations of progesterone. In addition, systematic reviews of randomized trials do not suggest any useful clinical benefit of treatment with these hormones. However, intramuscular or subcutaneous depot administration of medroxyprogesterone may be helpful, due to its anovulatory effect.

May be effective

Diet

Diet should be altered so that more of the meals consumed have a low glycemic index. It is suggested that an increased carbohydrate intake increases serotonergic activity, which in turn improves symptoms.

Exercise

Aerobic activity leads to increased endorphin levels, which is known to improve mood, and several studies suggest that this may be of some benefit in the treatment of PMS.

Complementary therapy

Studies have explored the use of homeopathy, relaxation, massage, reflexology, chiropractic therapy and biofeedback. While there were some positive findings, there is no compelling evidence to support the regular use of any of these therapies. Despite the lack of an evidence base, these complementary therapies should be discussed as possible treatment options, as part of an integrated holistic treatment plan.

Food supplements

Similar to complementary therapies, there are mixed results in randomized, placebo-controlled trials.

Vitamin B$_6$ (pyridoxine)

Pyridoxine is involved in the metabolism of dopamine and serotonin, low levels of which lead to high levels of prolactin and aldosterone, possibly explaining the fluid retention experienced by women with PMS. It may also account for some of the psychological symptoms attributable to alterations in neurotransmitter levels.

Vitamin B$_6$ can be taken on a continuous basis or during the second half of the menstrual cycle. Owing to safety concerns (i.e. the peripheral neuropathy that may result from taking high doses), a maximum dose of 10 mg/day is recommended.

Evening primrose oil

This contains essential fatty acids, including gamolenic acid. Trials demonstrate some clinical improvement, principally in the relief of mastalgia. Other supplements with mixed reviews include *agnus castus* Vitex, *Ginkgo biloba* and magnesium.

Probably effective

Psychological approach

Techniques aimed at reducing stress may be beneficial. Cognitive behavioural therapy (CBT), which encourages relaxation, and the use of 'coping skills' can be helpful and should be considered as a first-line option for women with severe symptoms.

Selective serotonin reuptake inhibitors

PMS often presents with symptoms similar to those of anxiety and depression, and this association has resulted in treatment with a variety of antidepressants. Reduced platelet uptake of serotonin and reduced levels of serotonin in the blood of women with PMS during the luteal phase suggest that there is a role for SSRIs in PMS treatment. Meta-analysis shows that SSRIs are effective, with around 60% of women with severe PMS reporting a reduction in physical and behavioural symptoms compared with around 30% of controls. This effectiveness is often apparent after only one or two cycles. Side-effects include insomnia, gastrointestinal disturbances, fatigue and loss of libido, but may be acceptable at the recommended low dose. Intermittent use in the luteal phase is as effective as continuous daily dosing, and may help to limit side-effects. A gradual rather than abrupt withdrawal is appropriate if the SSRI has been taken on a continuous basis, in order to avoid symptoms of withdrawal. SSRIs can be offered as a first-line treatment option, but should be stopped before and during a pregnancy, as there is a possible association with congenital malformations.

Ovarian suppression

Because the majority of PMS symptoms can be attributed to cyclical ovarian hormone production, the suppression of ovulation is a logical treatment option. The effectiveness of second-generation combined hormonal contraceptives (CHCs) for the treatment of PMS is uncertain; some research suggests an improvement in symptoms, whereas other research suggests symptom exacerbation. There is now evidence to support the use of CHCs containing drospirenone. This can be attributed to its antimineralocorticoid and anti-androgenic properties. Recent results suggest that more benefit is obtained from continuous rather than cyclical administration. Depot medroxyprogesterone, a long-acting injectable progestogen, may also be helpful.

The synthetic androgen danazol suppresses ovulation, and a relatively low dose of 200 mg twice daily is effective in improving the symptoms of mastalgia. Use of danazol is limited by its potential for irreversible virilization, and effective contraception should be used to avoid virilization of a female fetus.

Transdermal oestrogen (100–200 µg/day), by way of patches designed for HRT, is associated with an improvement in PMS symptoms. If the woman has not had a hysterectomy, a progestogen is required to avoid endometrial stimulation, hyperplasia and possible malignant transformation. The lowest dose of progestogen needed for endometrial protection is recommended; micronized progesterone taken orally or vaginally for 10–12 days during each cycle should be considered first-line treatment. The LNG-IUS is also particularly suitable, since the serum level of progestogen is very low, thus minimizing the risk of progestogenic side-effects (which may mimic/exacerbate PMS), and it also provides contraceptive cover. Any unscheduled bleeding in women taking high-dose transdermal oestrogen should prompt early investigation.

GnRH analogues are a highly effective way of suppressing ovarian function, and are therefore an effective treatment for severe PMS. As oestrogen is suppressed to postmenopausal levels, the PMS symptoms may be replaced by menopausal ones, including hot flushes and increased risk of osteoporosis. These can be minimized with the use of add-back HRT, either tibolone or a continuous combined preparation. A therapeutic trial of GnRH analogues with add-back HRT is often beneficial in clarifying the diagnosis if the symptom diary is not conclusive. It also helps to establish that the woman can tolerate an HRT preparation, should oophorectomy become appropriate. Use of GnRH analogues for more than 6 months must include add-back HRT and regular measurement of bone density, for example annual dual-energy X-ray absorptiometry scanning. Although generally accepted as a treatment option, GnRH analogues are not specifically licensed for use in women with PMS.

Bilateral oophorectomy

This is an effective treatment for PMS. It is, however, a surgical procedure, and therefore not without significant short-term surgical risks. The procedure can usually be undertaken laparoscopically. There are also longer-term risks of premature menopause if HRT is not taken postoperatively. This surgical option is therefore only suitable for those very likely to benefit from it, as suggested by a definite response to a GnRH analogue, and only in those who have completed their family. It is reasonable not to opt for this procedure if the natural menopause is likely to be occurring in the near future.

Individual management strategy

Given the large number of treatments advocated, it can be difficult to determine which is the best approach for a specific patient. As PMS is usually a chronic condition, it is important to consider the side-effect profile of treatments that may be used over many years. Once the diagnosis is established by prospective symptom diary-keeping, it seems sensible to try those treatments with fewest significant side-effects, which should initially include diet modification, regular aerobic exercise and techniques aimed at stress reduction. A significant proportion of women will benefit from trying these three together, and drug therapy can then be considered for those who do not improve sufficiently.

Appropriate first-line therapy includes CBT, low-dose SSRI or a drospirenone-containing CHC. The next stage is high-dose SSRI, oestrogen patches or ovarian suppression with a GnRH analogue. Successful symptom improvement, however, can pose a dilemma, as continuous treatment may not be appropriate. Long-term suppression with medroxyprogesterone acetate administered every 3 months intramuscularly or subcutaneously should be considered as an alternative. Bilateral oophorectomy should be reserved for the severest cases, with a preoperative trial of GnRH analogue essential beforehand.

Key *points*

- HMB can be classified as being related to structural uterine pathology (e.g. fibroids) or not. Very rarely, HMB may be secondary to some specific medical disorders, including clotting defects.
- Medical treatment includes prostaglandin synthesis inhibitors, antifibrinolytics, the COC pill, systemic progestogens, intrauterine progestogens, GnRH analogues and danazol. With the exception of GnRH analogues, these treatments are less successful in the presence of fibroids. Endometrial ablation and hysterectomy are the two surgical options.
- Dysmenorrhoea may be idiopathic (primary dysmenorrhoea) or due to pelvic pathology (secondary dysmenorrhoea). Treatment is with prostaglandin synthesis inhibitors, the combined contraceptive pill or depot injection of intrauterine progestogens.
- PMS can be defined as a regular pattern of symptoms occurring before menstruation, with a lessening of symptoms soon after the start of bleeding.
- The aetiology of the condition is poorly understood, and diagnosis is dependent on prospectively charting the symptoms to confirm that there is a true cyclical variation.
- Only a limited number of treatments are more effective than placebo; these are listed in Box 7.2. Initial treatment should include dietary advice, regular aerobic exercise and techniques aimed at stress reduction. An SSRI is the most appropriate first-line drug; if unsuccessful, it may be appropriate to institute a trial of ovarian suppression. Long-term suppression with medroxyprogesterone acetate or surgical oophorectomy may be considered.

8

Pelvic pain and endometriosis

Pelvic pain

Physiological pelvic pain with menstruation or childbirth is almost universal, but many women present with pelvic pain for other reasons. Pelvic pain can be acute (commonly associated with a miscarriage, an ectopic pregnancy or appendicitis), or it can be chronic, lasting for many months or years.

With acute pain, there is usually a well-defined pathological cause that either resolves spontaneously or can be effectively treated. It is important to recognize that chronic pelvic pain (CPP) is a symptom, not a diagnosis. CPP presents in primary care as frequently as does migraine or lower back pain. Aiming for accurate diagnosis and effective management from the first presentation may help to improve the woman's quality of life, and may avoid a seemingly endless succession of referrals, investigations and operations.

Pelvic pain is considered under the two headings of 'acute' and 'chronic', and there is often significant overlap. Although there are many gynaecological causes of pelvic pain, the non-gynaecological causes are also important; therefore, a multidisciplinary approach, particularly for women with CPP, is required.

Pain is a subjective phenomenon. Many of the factors affecting pain are centrally mediated, so pelvic pain is often made worse by psychological, psychiatric or social distress. The organs within the peritoneal cavity (the viscera) are sensitive to inflammation, chemicals and stretching or distortion caused by specific stimuli (for example, adhesions or gaseous distension). The sensitivity of different organs to varying stimuli is an important factor influencing pelvic pain. For example, the cervix and uterus are relatively insensitive, whereas the fallopian tubes are exquisitely sensitive. Crushing of the bowel is associated with minimal discomfort, whereas stretching and distension cause severe pain. Unlike painful cutaneous stimuli, it is often very difficult to localize visceral pain.

History

The history is arguably the most important factor in determining how quickly the diagnosis is reached and appropriate treatment is instigated. Particular attention should be given to the time of onset of the pain; the characteristics, radiation, severity of the pain; exacerbating and relieving factors; cyclicity; and analgesic requirements. Associated symptoms of gastrointestinal, urological or musculoskeletal origin should be sought. It is also important to take a detailed menstrual history; in particular, the frequency and character of vaginal bleeding, any intermenstrual bleeding or vaginal discharge and their relationship to the pain. A sexual history may be of help, particularly superficial or deep dyspareunia, contraception and sexually transmitted infections (STIs). There may be a family history of gynaecological disorders (for example, endometriosis). A cervical cytology history should be recorded.

With chronic pain, there is often value in taking a detailed family and social history, including marital or relationship problems, pressure at work, financial worries and problems in childhood or adolescence, such as sexual abuse. Listening is centrally important to the history-taking, and may in itself be therapeutic for some women. It is useful to ask some open-ended questions such as: 'What do you think the cause of your pain might be?' and 'How is the pain affecting your life?' to give the woman an opportunity to tell you about aspects of the problem that might not be apparent from a more systematic history.

If the history suggests there is a non-gynaecological component to the pain, referral to the relevant healthcare professional, such as a gastroenterologist, urologist, genitourinary medicine physician, physiotherapist, psychologist or psychosexual counsellor, should be considered.

Examination

The examination is most usefully undertaken when there is time to explore the woman's fears and anxieties. The examiner should be prepared for new information to be revealed at this point. Observation of the woman's general demeanor is important when assessing the severity of pain. Eye-witness accounts from other health professionals and friends or family may also be helpful. The temperature, pulse and blood pressure should be recorded.

Abdominal examination should include inspection for distension or masses, palpation for tenderness, rebound, guarding and abdominal auscultation if gastrointestinal obstruction or ileus is suspected. Permission should be sought to perform a vaginal and rectal examination. Inspection of the vulva and vagina at speculum examination may reveal abnormal discharge (suggestive of infection) or bleeding. A bimanual examination may reveal uterine or adnexal enlargement suggestive of a pelvic mass, fibroids or an ovarian cyst. Cervical excitation (pain associated with digital displacement of the cervix) is associated with ectopic pregnancy and pelvic infection. Tenderness or pain elicited by bimanual palpation of the pelvic organs themselves is suggestive of an ongoing inflammatory process, which may be infective (e.g. *Chlamydia*) or non-infective (e.g. endometriosis). A fixed immobile uterus suggests multiple adhesions from whatever cause, and nodularity within the uterosacral ligaments (sometimes palpable only by combined rectovaginal examination) can be a feature of endometriosis.

Acute pelvic pain

There are many causes of acute pelvic pain, but the most important gynaecological conditions are ectopic pregnancy, miscarriage, pelvic inflammatory disease and torsion or rupture of ovarian cysts (Box 8.1). If the urine pregnancy test (UPT) is negative, a high vaginal swab, endocervical swab and full blood count should be performed for evidence of infection. All sexually active women below the age of 25 years who are being examined should be offered opportunistic screening for *Chlamydia*. An ultrasound scan is helpful in identifying ovarian cysts, but non-gynaecological causes of pain should not be forgotten.

While waiting for the results of the investigations, it is important to continue monitoring the patient's vital signs and to provide analgesia. If the diagnosis is unclear and the pain is not resolving, a diagnostic laparoscopy may be warranted.

The management of miscarriage, pelvic inflammatory disease and ovarian cysts is discussed in the appropriate chapters. Pain experienced mid-cycle with ovulation, the so-called 'mittelschmerz', is an innocent cause of pain. This pain is usually sudden in onset, can be quite severe and, if persistent in each cycle, will respond to ovulation suppression with the combined oral contraceptive.

Box 8.1

Causes of acute pelvic pain
- *Gynaecological*: ectopic pregnancy, miscarriage, acute pelvic infection, ovarian cysts
- *Gastrointestinal*: appendicitis, constipation, diverticular disease, IBS
- *Urinary tract*: urinary tract infection, calculi
- *Other causes*: musculoskeletal

Chronic pelvic pain (CPP)

Healthcare costs associated with CPP are very considerable, and do not take into consideration the disability and suffering of the woman and loss of earnings to both the individual and employer. CPP can lead to loss of employment, family and marital discord, divorce, medical misadventures and litigation. Among high-quality studies, the rate of dysmenorrhoea was 16.8–81%, that of dyspareunia was 8–21.8% and that of non-cyclical pain was 2.1–24% worldwide.

The definitions of CPP are numerous, but one suitable definition is 'intermittent or constant pain in the lower abdomen or pelvis of at least 6 months' duration, not occurring exclusively with menstruation or intercourse and not associated with pregnancy'. A comparison between acute pelvic pain and CPP is shown in Table 8.1.

The management of CPP is particularly challenging, as there are many possible causes and contributory factors (Box 8.2). Association with dysmenorrhoea, dyspareunia, irregular menstruation, abnormal vaginal discharge, cyclical pain and infertility may all be helpful in suggesting an underlying gynaecological problem. Altered bowel habits, excess flatulence or flatus, constipation or diarrhoea, on the other hand, point to a gastrointestinal problem, particularly irritable bowel syndrome (IBS). However, these bowel symptoms can also be associated with the presence of

Table 8.1	Comparison of acute and CPP
Acute	**Chronic**
Well-defined onset	Ill-defined onset
Short duration	Unpredictable duration
Rest often helpful	Rest usually not helpful
Variable intensity	Persistent
Anxiety common	Depression common
Disease symptom	May not be possible to identify an underlying disease process

---

Box 8.2

Differential diagnoses for women with CPP
- *Gynaecological*: endometriosis, adhesions (chronic pelvic infection), adenomyosis, leiomyoma, pelvic congestion syndrome, ovarian cysts
- *Gastrointestinal*: adhesions, appendicitis, constipation, diverticular disease, IBS
- *Urinary tract*: urinary tract infection, calculus, interstitial cystitis
- *Skeletal*: degenerative joint disease, scoliosis, spondylolisthesis, osteitis pubis
- *Myofascial*: fascitis, nerve entrapment syndrome, hernia
- *Psychological*: somatization, psychosexual dysfunction, depression
- *Neuropathic*: pudendal nerve entrapment, spinal cord neuropathies

gynaecological pathology such as endometriosis. Psychiatric, urological and musculoskeletal causes of chronic pain are further possibilities. Physical and sexual abuse can also predispose women to CPP.

Known gynaecological causes of CPP include endometriosis, adhesions and pelvic varices. Adhesions can cause pain if there is associated organ distension or stretching or increased vascularity. Dense vascular adhesions on division have been shown to relieve pain. Symptoms suggestive of IBS or interstitial cystitis are often present in women with CPP. These conditions may be the primary cause of or a component of CPP.

Up to 40% of women with CPP, however, do not have an identifiable cause, despite extensive investigation. It is therefore important to plan which investigations are necessary. In gynaecology, such investigation often involves a diagnostic laparoscopy. Further management then depends on whether a pathological cause has been identified or not; this is considered below. Again, there is some overlap between the two groups (Fig. 8.1).

Pelvic infection

Chronic pelvic infection is associated with a high incidence of tubal damage, and consequently an increased incidence of ectopic pregnancy, infertility or CPP. It may occur due to relapse of infection after inadequate treatment, reinfection from an untreated partner, post-infection tubal damage or further acquisition of STIs. The severity of the problem is related to the number of episodes of pelvic inflammatory disease and the extent of pelvic adhesions.

Endometriosis

See in the section of Endometriosis.

Ovarian cysts

The majority of ovarian cysts are benign, particularly those presenting with acute pain. Pain may occur because of cyst torsion, cyst rupture or bleeding into a cyst. Management depends on the presenting clinical situation, but suspected torsion necessitates surgical intervention.

Other causes

If investigations are negative and there remains significant diagnostic doubt about gynaecological origin of pain, it may be worth considering a 3-month trial of ovarian suppression with a gonadotrophin-releasing hormone analogue (GnRHa). In around three quarters of women who experience a dramatic reduction of symptoms following suppression and recurrence after treatment stops, a hysterectomy may lead to long-term improvement. Many, however, may not wish to have or may not be suitable for such radical surgery, and others will experience no improvement despite the hysterectomy.

No identifiable pathological cause for the pain

Treating a woman with CPP without a specific diagnosis is particularly difficult because of the problems involved in choosing an appropriate therapeutic intervention. In these cases, CPP syndrome is considered a disease entity in its own right, and strategies are required to relieve the physical, psychological and social distress that it causes.

Management options include psychosocial therapy, analgesia management (including use of anticonvulsants like gabapentin), hormonal treatments, antidepressants (like amitriptyline), complementary therapies, surgery (including surgical excision of nerves, or uterine nerve ablation) and, rarely, pelvic clearance. Communication with the woman should include sharing of information and an honest and realistic discussion of the treatment options.

Encouragement to lead as normal a life as possible whilst investigation and treatment are instigated is acknowledged to be very important. This includes encouraging return to work, exercise, maintaining a healthy diet, avoiding the inappropriate use of analgesia and looking for alternatives to analgesia where possible. Complementary therapies such as reflexology, homeopathy and acupuncture may be helpful.

The risks of medical misadventure associated with CPP can be minimized by adopting a sympathetic and caring multidisciplinary approach, or by referral to healthcare professionals with special interest and expertise in managing this condition. A multidisciplinary team approach should ideally include expertise in pain management, gastroenterology, gynaecology, neurology, psychiatry and psychology. Specific psychological approaches to the management of CPP, with input from psychologists and liaison psychiatrists, may be helpful to many women. These approaches include behavioural therapy, cognitive behavioural therapy, group therapy and pharmacological therapy. Pharmacological therapy (e.g. antidepressants and anxiolytics) may be particularly valuable for those individuals with depression as a secondary consequence of CPP.

Endometriosis

Gynaecological causes of CPP include endometriosis and adenomyosis.

Endometriosis is the presence of endometrial-like tissue outside the uterus, which induces a chronic inflammatory reaction. This tissue usually lies within the peritoneal cavity, predominantly in the pelvis and commonly on the uterosacral ligaments behind the uterus (Fig. 8.2). Rarely, it can also be found in distant sites such as the umbilicus, abdominal scars, perineal scars and even the pleural cavity and nasal mucosa. Like the true endometrium, it responds to cyclical hormonal changes and bleeds at menstruation. Such bleeding may cause symptoms.

Adenomyosis occurs when there is endometrial tissue within the myometrium of the uterus. The uterus is enlarged

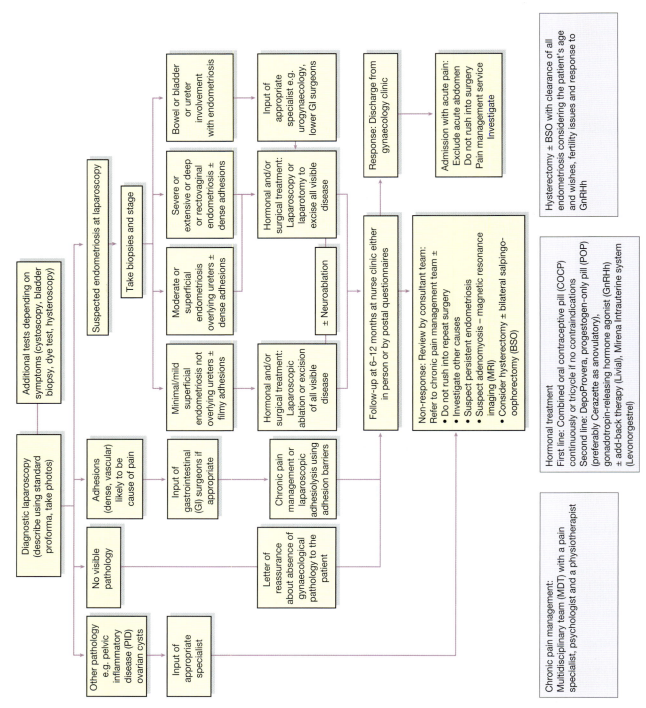

Fig. 8.1   An example of a management pathway for patients with CPP following laparoscopy.

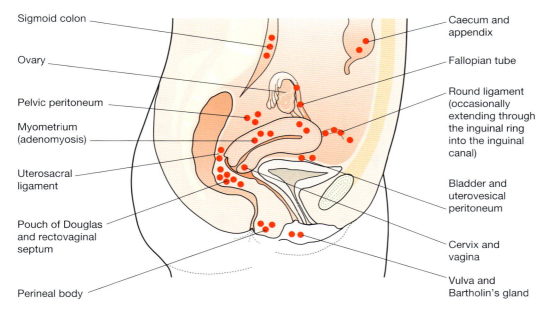

Sigmoid colon

Ovary

Pelvic peritoneum

Myometrium
(adenomyosis)

Uterosacral
ligament

Pouch of Douglas
and rectovaginal
septum

Perineal body

Caecum and
appendix

Fallopian tube

Round ligament
(occasionally
extending through
the inguinal ring
into the inguinal
canal)

Bladder and
uterovesical
peritoneum

Cervix and
vagina

Vulva and
Bartholin's gland

Fig. 8.2 **Common sites for endometriotic deposits in the pelvis.**

and feels 'boggy'. There is painful and heavy menstruation. Previously, adenomyosis was difficult to diagnose clinically, and was diagnosed only with histological examination of the uterus after hysterectomy. With advances in imaging technology, adenomyosis can be identified on ultrasound scan or by magnetic resonance imaging (MRI) of the pelvis. It is commonly considered to be a separate entity from endometriosis, occurring in a different population and having a different aetiology.

Incidence

The reported incidence of endometriosis varies widely; for example, among asymptomatic fertile women undergoing laparoscopic sterilization procedures, the incidence of endometriosis ranges from 4–43%. Endometriosis is more commonly identified in infertile women. Most cases of endometriosis are diagnosed in women aged 25–35 years, although the symptoms of endometriosis can present as early as the onset of puberty. As it is oestrogen-dependent, it is rarely diagnosed postmenopausally, but recurrence has been associated with the use of hormone replacement therapy.

Aetiology

The precise aetiology of endometriosis remains unclear, with no single explanation reliably explaining all its features. Sampson's 'implantation' theory postulates that endometrial fragments flow in a retrograde manner along the fallopian tube during menstruation, 'seeding' themselves on the pelvic peritoneum. In support of this theory is the fact that it is

sometimes possible to see blood flowing from the fimbrial end of the fallopian tube if a laparoscopy is carried out during menstruation – it is believed that retrograde menstruation occurs in 90% of menstruating women. Seeding onto scars (such as after caesarean section or on perineal scars after delivery) has been observed. In some animal models, endometrial tissue has been surgically implanted directly onto the peritoneum to mimic endometriosis. In other animal studies that involved the surgical creation of retrograde menstruation, endometriosis developed in 50% of cases.

This theory, however, cannot be the only mechanism of endometriosis formation, as endometriosis has been reported in women with congenitally obstructed fallopian tubes. Meyer's 'coelomic metaplasia' theory proposes that cells of the original coelomic membrane transform to endometrial cells by metaplasia, possibly as a result of hormonal stimulation or inflammatory irritation. This could explain the presence of endometriosis in nearly all the distant sites, although it is also possible that spread from the uterus to these distant sites occurs by venous or lymphatic microembolism.

In some instances, the presence of endometriosis may be explained by neoplasia. This is particularly true in the ovary, where a solitary ovarian endometrioma is sometimes included in the classification of ovarian neoplasia as the benign counterpart of endometrioid carcinoma.

The question remains why endometriosis becomes established in some, but not all, women, and it is possible that there is some genetic or immunological predisposition that accounts for such wide variation. Endometriosis is significantly more common in first-degree relatives of women with the disease, and twin studies also support a genetic basis.

Box 8.3

The common presenting symptoms of endometriosis
- Severe dysmenorrhoea
- Chronic pelvic pain
- Deep dyspareunia
- Pain during ovulation
- Cyclical or perimenstrual symptoms (e.g. bladder or bowel), with or without abnormal bleeding or pain
- Chronic fatigue
- Pain on defecation (dyschezia)
- Infertility (especially with dysmenorrhoea)

Clinical presentation

In most instances, clinical presentation occurs because of pelvic disease. Endometriosis is the commonest cause of secondary dysmenorrhoea. There is usually continuous non-spasmodic pain that is worse immediately before and throughout menstruation, and colicky dysmenorrhoea may also occur in association with heavy menstrual loss and the passage of clots. In addition, there may be dyspareunia, which may relate to endometriotic deposits in the pouch of Douglas or to ovarian endometriomas. Typically, this pain settles when the period ends, but some women also describe continuous lower abdominal pain that is not specifically related to their cycle or to sexual activity. The common presenting symptoms of endometriosis are outlined in Box 8.3.

One of the puzzles regarding endometriosis is the lack of correlation between the severity of these symptoms and the extent of the disease. Extensive deposits leading to the obliteration of the pouch of Douglas and involving the ovaries, fallopian tubes and other pelvic organs may be completely asymptomatic; conversely, women with peritoneal lesions only a few millimetres across may be debilitated by pain.

Menstrual disturbances may be associated with endometriosis, and in particular with adenomyosis. Where there is also significant ovarian involvement, the menstrual cycle may become erratic. Rarely, post-coital bleeding is experienced in the presence of endometriosis involving the ectocervix, or where deposits in the pouch of Douglas penetrate into the posterior fornix.

Endometriosis at distant sites is rare, but may generate local symptoms, such as cyclical epistaxes with nasal deposits, pneumothoraces with pleural deposits ('catamenial pneumothorax') or headaches and/or seizures due to endometriosis in the brain. Monthly rectal bleeding may occur if the bowel mucosa is affected, or haematuria with bladder involvement.

Examination

The clinical diagnosis of endometriosis is aided by the following findings:

Table 8.2	Possible mechanisms by which endometriosis may reduce fertility	
System	**Mechanism**
Coital function	Dyspareunia, leading to reduced frequency of coitus
Sperm function	Inactivation of spermatozoa by antibodies
	Phagocytosis of spermatozoa by macrophages
Tubal function	Fimbrial damage
	Reduced tubal motility with prostaglandins
Ovarian function	Anovulation
	LUF syndrome
	Luteolysis caused by prostaglandin $F_{2\alpha}$
	Altered release of gonadotrophins

1. blue nodules seen in the posterior vaginal fornix upon speculum examination
2. a fixed (immobile) retroverted uterus
3. thickened pelvic ligaments, particularly the uterosacral ligaments, which may be nodular
4. tenderness in the lateral and posterior fornices with applied pressure on the uterosacral ligaments
5. ovarian enlargement if there is an endometrioma.

Nodules are most reliably detected when clinical examination is performed during menstruation. Attempts to move the uterus may also provoke pain. This pain often resembles the presenting symptom, particularly when this was dyspareunia.

With the exception of visualizing endometriotic nodules, none of these features is diagnostic of endometriosis; and conversely, their absence does not exclude the disease. There are many other causes of pelvic pain, such as IBS and recurrent urinary tract infection, which can confuse the differential diagnosis. In particular, chronic conditions such as pelvic inflammatory disease and adhesions mimic many features of endometriosis. Laparoscopy is therefore usually necessary to make the diagnosis.

Endometriosis and infertility

Endometriosis is commonly diagnosed in women who are undergoing laparoscopic investigations for infertility but who do not have specific symptoms. Although endometriosis and infertility are associated more frequently than can be explained by chance, the exact mechanism of their inter-relationship is uncertain (Table 8.2).

Severe disease can cause infertility by forming periovarian and peritubular adhesions and by affecting ovarian tissue (due to the formation of ovarian cysts called endometrioma/chocolate cysts); however, the association between mild endometriosis and infertility is less clear. Theoretically, high prostaglandin production from endometriotic tissue could impede tubal motility, or the spermatozoa may be affected by adverse immunological factors.

Another possibility is that infertility caused by some unrelated factor may predispose women to endometriosis simply because, in the absence of pregnancy and lactational amenorrhoea, the affected woman will have more periods. Other theories suggest that both endometriosis and infertility are manifestations of a third, unidentified problem. An association with luteinized unruptured follicle (LUF) syndrome, in which follicular development proceeds along apparently normal lines but oocyte release does not occur, provides another explanation. As endometriosis is more common in women with this condition, it has been proposed that failure to release follicular fluid mid-cycle may result in an environment that promotes the establishment of endometriosis.

Investigation

Transvaginal ultrasound can detect gross endometriosis involving the ovaries (endometriomas/chocolate cysts) and occasionally the rectum, and MRI can delineate the extent of active endometriotic lesions greater than 1 cm in diameter in deep tissues, e.g. the rectovaginal septum. Laparoscopy remains the traditional standard diagnostic method (Fig. 8.3). Active endometriotic lesions are classically described as red, puckered and inflamed, or as 'burnt match heads' (cigarette burns). Inactive lesions look like scars. The endometriotic lesions can be superficial, or deep and infiltrating. The degree to which laparoscopic visualization alone may be adequate, however, has been questioned (see Box 8.4), and it has been proposed that clinicians should confirm a positive laparoscopy by histology of biopsies.

Little is known about the rate of progression of low-grade endometriosis, but a proportion of untreated patients may deteriorate over as little as 6 months. The prompt return of symptoms after treatment, seen in many patients, may represent re-extension of uneradicated residual disease.

It is impossible to guarantee a cure after treatment. Routine repeat laparoscopy after completion of treatment, therefore, has limited prognostic value, and is probably best reserved for those patients with recurrent symptoms.

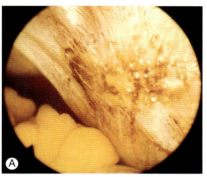

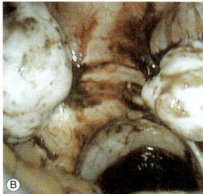

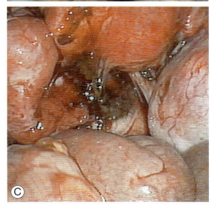

Fig. 8.3 Peritoneal appearances of endometriosis.
Laparoscopic views show: **(A)** clear blisters ('sago' granules), 'blood blisters', yellow-brown patches, 'powder burns', atypical vascularity and telangiectasia; **(B)** bilateral endometriomas; **(C)** severe endometriosis with adhesions. (Parts **(B)** and **(C)** courtesy of Karl Storz Endoscopy (UK) Ltd.)

Box 8.4

Laparoscopic and histological appearance of endometriotic lesions

- Haemosiderin deposits covered with peritoneum resemble the classical appearance of endometriosis, but may arise from local haemorrhage of any origin. Most often, the typical chocolate cysts that are seen in the ovary are endometriomas; however, sometimes the histological examination shows that these have arisen from haemorrhage into a follicular or corpus luteum cyst.
- A wide range of subtle peritoneal changes, such as clear 'sago' blisters, glandular papillae, white opacified patches, red flame-like lesions and circular peritoneal defects may prove on biopsy to be a result of endometriosis.
- Even more perplexing is the finding that normal peritoneum, when biopsied and studied with scanning electron microscopy, may contain endometrial-type cells. These may be more common in patients with proven disease elsewhere, but can also be found in apparently normal women.
- As many as 52% of patients with pelvic pain but no visible endometrial deposits in the peritoneum have been found on histological examination to harbour lesions deep in the uterosacral ligaments.

While the tumour marker of serum cancer antigen 125 (CA 125) may be elevated in endometriosis, measuring serum CA125 levels has no value as a diagnostic tool.

Management

Medical treatment with non-steroidal anti-inflammatory drugs and/or simple analgesics is widely employed, and many women will be taking these prior to diagnosis. Medical treatment with ovulation suppression is most useful for symptomatic relief, but is of no value for the treatment of endometriosis in patients wishing to conceive. Treatment duration is usually limited to between 3 and 6 months. Surgical treatment may be conservative, with laser or diathermy ablation/excision of lesions, or radical, involving hysterectomy and oophorectomy.

Medical treatment

Medical treatment is founded upon the observation that endometriosis improves during both pregnancy and the menopause; so creating a 'pseudo-pregnancy' with progestogens or combined oral contraceptives and a 'pseudo-menopause' with GnRHa analogues is appropriate and frequently effective. Ovulation suppression limits the likelihood of conception, but nonetheless, it is still advisable for women to use barrier methods of contraception (unless using the combined oral contraceptive as their treatment method). To avoid inadvertent administration during pregnancy, all therapies should be initiated within the first 3 days of the start of a menstrual period.

For symptomatic endometriosis, continuous progestogen therapy (e.g. medroxyprogesterone acetate 10 mg twice daily for 90 days or a progesterone-only contraceptive pill) is most cost-effective, has fewer side-effects and is more suitable for long-term use compared with more expensive alternatives. Progestogens act directly on the endometrial target tissue by binding to progestogen receptors. This produces decidualization of the endometrial tissue, subsequent thinning of the endometrium and no menses. The combined oral contraceptive pill is also an appropriate alternative; it is usually taken continuously or in a tricycle regimen in order to reduce the frequency of menstrual cycles. The usual risk factors for the suitability of using the combined pill should be evaluated, but if its use is appropriate and symptoms are alleviated, it can be continued for several years or even longer. The levonorgestrel-releasing intrauterine system (Mirena) is an effective option used to reduce endometriosis-associated pain. It is also useful in preventing the recurrence of endometriosis after surgical treatments.

Second-line drugs are the GnRHa analogues (which can be administered by nasal spray, implants or injection) or the orally administered androgen danazol. GnRHa analogues bind to GnRHa receptors in the pituitary gland. They initially stimulate gonadotrophin release, but the pituitary gland becomes rapidly desensitized to GnRHa stimulation, thereby suppressing gonadotrophin release and, in turn, ovarian steroid secretion. The profound hypo-oestrogenic state that is thus produced not only affects endometrial tissue, but also causes side-effects mimicking the menopause. Therapy is limited to 4–6 months, and it is routine to prescribe 'add-back' hormone replacement therapy (e.g. Tibolone) to alleviate the predictable menopausal side-effects and negative effects on bone density. The use of add-back therapy does not reduce the effect of treatment on pain relief. Danazol combines androgenic activity with anti-oestrogenic and anti-progestogenic activity. It has a relatively high incidence of androgenic and perimenopausal side-effects, and is therefore rarely used in current practice.

Medical treatment can also be used as a diagnostic tool. If amenorrhoea and symptom relief are achieved, then it is extremely likely that the symptoms were due to endometriosis. If symptoms persist, a review of the diagnosis is necessary, and other causes of pelvic pain must be considered.

Surgical treatment

When continued fertility is required, conservative surgery is appropriate. This is usually carried out laparoscopically, and includes diathermy destruction, laser vaporization, helium beam coagulation or excision of endometriosis deposits. It may bring about symptom relief, and has a role in subfertile women. Recurrence risks following conservative surgery are as high as 30%. Cystectomy, rather than drainage and coagulation, should be performed for an ovarian endometrioma >3 cm in diameter.

Hysterectomy with bilateral oophorectomy for women who have completed their childbearing can be curative. Hormone replacement will be needed; although this may activate residual disease, this possibility can be minimized by using a combined preparation rather than an oestrogen-only form.

The surgical management of deep infiltrating endometriosis is complex, and should be undertaken in an expert centre with the appropriate multidisciplinary expertise.

Fertility treatment

There is no evidence that medical treatment of endometriosis is of any value in the management of subfertility. Surgical ablation or excision of minimal and mild endometriosis does improve fertility, but whether surgery has a role in moderate and severe endometriosis is less clear. Surgical treatment of large ovarian endometriotic cysts probably enhances spontaneous pregnancy rates, and will improve transvaginal access if in-vitro fertilization (IVF) is considered. In cases of moderate and severe endometriosis, assisted reproduction techniques should be considered as an alternative to surgery or following unsuccessful surgery.

Complications, prognosis and long-term sequelae

Depending upon the severity of the disease, adhesions and fibrosis may distort the bowel, bladder, ureters and other neighbouring viscera, leading to chronic problems with these systems. The physical and psychological morbidity from long-term pain can be considerable.

Key points

- Acute pelvic pain and CPP have numerous, occasionally overlapping, causes (Boxes 8.1 and 8.2).
- Many women present because they want to seek medical opinion. Often, they already have a theory or a concern about the origin of the pain. These ideas should preferably be discussed in the initial consultation.
- The multifactorial nature of CPP should be discussed and explored from the start. The aim should be to develop a partnership between clinician and patient to plan a management programme.
- In the past, diagnostic laparoscopy has been regarded as the 'gold standard' in the diagnosis of CPP. It may be better seen as a second line of investigation if other therapeutic interventions fail. Transvaginal scanning and MRI are useful tests for diagnosing adenomyosis.
- Women with cyclical pain should be offered a therapeutic trial using the combined oral contraceptive pill, progesterone-only pill or a GnRHa analogue for a period of 3–6 months before having a diagnostic laparoscopy.
- Women with symptoms suggestive of IBS should be offered a trial of antispasmodics and should try amending their diet to control symptoms.
- Women should be offered appropriate analgesia to control their pain, even if no other therapeutic manoeuvres are yet to be initiated. If pain is not adequately controlled, consideration should be given to referral to a pain management team or a specialist pelvic pain clinic.
- While the commonest causes of CPP are endometriosis and chronic pelvic infection, over one-third of women with CPP will have no identifiable pathology. It is important to avoid unnecessary investigations by accepting the 'CPP syndrome' as a disease entity in its own right.
- Endometriosis is caused by the presence of endometrium-like tissue outside the uterine cavity. Endometrium-like tissue growing within the uterine wall is referred to as adenomyosis, and may be a different pathological entity.
- Endometriosis may be caused by the seeding of endometrial cells when menstrual blood flows in a retrograde direction along the fallopian tubes. Other possible aetiological mechanisms are coelomic metaplasia and venous or lymphatic spread.
- Clinical endometriosis is a common gynaecological problem, and the incidence is higher among women with subfertility. Symptoms include secondary dysmenorrhoea, dyspareunia, lower abdominal pain and heavy menstrual bleeding. There may be ovarian enlargement, thickening of uterosacral ligaments, fixed retroversion of the uterus and tenderness on pelvic examination.
- Definitive diagnosis of endometriosis required laparoscopy.
- Medical management of clinical endometriosis is achieved by the administration of progestogens, the combined oral contraceptive pill or GnRHa analogues, or the use of the Mirena intrauterine system. Surgical management may involve laparoscopic ablation or excision of deposits, ovarian cystectomy or hysterectomy with bilateral oophorectomy.

9

The menopause and hormone replacement therapy

Introduction

Human female fertility terminates relatively abruptly in middle-age. The reasons for this are unclear as, in evolutionary terms, those genes that 'favour' giving birth to as many offspring as possible would be expected to proliferate. In other words, the genes of mothers who continued giving birth to children for as many years as they could, would be expected to be successful. Human children, however, remain dependent on their mothers for many years after birth, and if mothers continued to reproduce until the end of their lives they would be less able to support the later children to independent maturity. The incidence of congenital abnormality also increases with maternal age. This would be a waste of personal resources without genetic benefit, and would also limit the support such a mother could offer to her grandchildren, in whom she has a quarter-part genetic investment.

The flaw in this otherwise reasonable teleological argument, however, is that previously the vast majority of women died long before reaching the current average age of menopause, thus diluting the role of longevity in the evolutionary process. The true reasons behind this process of ovarian failure, the menopause, are therefore not yet fully elucidated.

Menopause literally means 'last menstrual period' and the definition is 12 months of absent menses in a woman with a uterus who is not pregnant or taking hormones that might induce amenorrhoea. The years leading up to the menopause are known as the perimenopause and are associated with fluctuating levels of oestrogen that result from declining ovarian function, which lead to changes in a number of systems and may give rise to significant symptoms. Although physiological, the menopause has important adverse long-term effects on health (Table 9.1), which can, in part, be offset by the use of hormone replacement therapy (HRT). The pros and cons of this treatment will be discussed in more detail and need to be carefully considered on an individual basis before treatment is started.

Physiology

The perimenopause (or climacteric) may begin months or years (average 4 years) before the last menstrual period, and symptoms may continue for years afterwards. The median age at menopause in the UK is 50.8 years and it occurs when the supply of oocytes becomes exhausted. A newborn girl has over half a million oocytes in her ovaries; one-third of these disappear before puberty and most of the remainder is lost during reproductive life. In each menstrual cycle some 20 or 30 primordial follicles begin to develop and most become atretic. As only about 400 cycles occur during an average woman's lifetime, most oocytes are lost spontaneously through ageing, rather than through ovulation.

In premenopausal women oestradiol is produced by the granulosa cells of the developing follicle, but as the menopause approaches this production becomes very variable. The proportion of anovulatory menstrual cycles increases and progesterone production declines. Pituitary production of follicle-stimulating hormone (FSH) and luteinizing hormone (LH) rises because of diminishing negative feedback from oestrogen and other ovarian hormones such as inhibin, but other pituitary hormones are not affected. Serum levels of FSH over 30 IU/L, when associated with irregular or absent periods, can be used clinically to clarify the diagnosis of the menopause (see later), although levels begin to rise significantly around the age of 38 in normally cycling women. Anti-Müllerian hormone is a better marker of follicular reserve than FSH and is used particularly to assess the response to ovarian stimulation during assisted conception.

Circulating androstenedione, mainly of adrenal origin, is converted by fat cells into oestrone, a less potent form of oestrogen than oestradiol. After the menopause, this is the predominant circulating oestrogen, rather than ovarian oestrogens.

Signs and symptoms (Table 9.1)

Vaginal bleeding

Irregular periods before the menopause are usually the result of anovulatory menstrual cycles, and if irregular bleeding persists, endometrial assessment may be required to exclude the possibility of endometrial carcinoma. The menopause itself can be recognized only in retrospect after 1 year of amenorrhoea (see earlier). Further vaginal bleeding after this timeframe is 'postmenopausal' and investigations may be required. Approximately 10% of those with postmenopausal bleeding have a gynaecological malignancy.

Table 9.1	The consequences of oestrogen deficiency	
Short Term Problems	Vasomotor Symptoms	Hot Flushes
	(80% of women in Western countries	Night sweats
		Headaches
		Palpitations
		Insomnia
	Psychological	Irritability
		Poor concentration
		Poor short-term memory
		Depression/ Low Mood
		Lethargy
		Decreased self confidence
	Sexual Problems	Decreased libido
		Dyspareunia
	Musculoskeletal	Joint aches
Intermediate Term	Urogenital	Atrophic Vaginitis
		Vaginal dryness
		Urethral symptoms
		Urge incontinence/ frequency
Long term problems	Circulation	Cardiovascular disease
		Cerebrovascular disease
	Skeletal	Osteoporosis
		Hip Facture
		Vertebral Fracture

Hot flushes

A 'hot flush' is an uncomfortable subjective feeling of warmth in the upper part of the body, usually lasting around 3 min. Approximately 50–85% of menopausal women experience such vasomotor symptoms, although only 10–20% seek medical advice. Flushes are sometimes accompanied by nausea, palpitations and sweating and may be particularly troublesome at night leading to severe insomnia. They are thought to be of hypothalamic origin and may in some way be related to LH release. It is thought that a fall in oestrogen levels affects central neurotransmitters such as alpha-adrenergic or serotonergic systems, which in turn affect central thermoregulatory centres and LH-releasing neurons.

About 20% of women begin experiencing flushes while still menstruating regularly. Flushes usually improve as the body adjusts to the new low oestrogen concentrations, but in approximately 25% of women, they continue for more than 5 years and can be extremely distressing, impairing quality of life. Exogenous oestrogen administration, in the form of HRT, is effective in relieving these symptoms in about 90% of cases.

Genitourinary atrophy

The genital system, urethra and bladder trigone are oestrogen dependent and undergo gradual atrophy after the menopause. Thinning of the vaginal skin may cause dyspareunia and bleeding, and loss of vaginal glycogen causes a rise in pH, which can predispose to local infection. Urgency of micturition may result from atrophic change in the trigone. Unlike flushes, these atrophic symptoms may appear years after the menopause and do not improve spontaneously, although they respond well to a short course of local or systemic oestrogen.

Other symptoms

Some studies have suggested that many symptoms, including irritability and lethargy, can be improved by hormone therapy more effectively than by placebo. However, many investigators feel that although low mood may be associated with menopause and can be relieved by HRT, the same may not be true for clinical depression, which is not usually caused directly by oestrogen withdrawal. The response to oestrogen in this situation is therefore uncertain and may depend on the presence of other symptoms such as vasomotor symptoms or insomnia.

Long-term effects

The menopause alters a woman's susceptibility to breast cancer, cardiovascular disease (CVD) and osteoporosis.

Breast cancer

Although the risk of breast cancer increases with increasing age, the rate of increase slows after the menopause. The risk of breast cancer is decreased if the menopause is premature and increased if it occurs late, such that a woman who has had a menopause in her late 50s has double the risk of breast cancer when compared with a woman who has had a menopause in her early 40s.

Cardiovascular disease

A premenopausal woman's risk of developing coronary artery disease is less than one-fifth of that of a man of the same age, a sex difference that disappears with increasing age. The incidence of CVD rises exponentially in both sexes, but the risk factors for CVD differ between the sexes, as does the impact of preventative measures. Epidemiological studies and the known physiological effects of oestrogen support a protective effect against vascular disease, although the difference in risk factors referred to previously may also be contributory.

Studies looking at the effect of postmenopausal oestrogen therapy on CVD suggest that unopposed oestrogen treatment

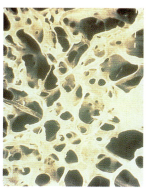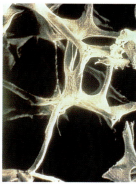

Fig. 9.1 **Normal (left) and osteoporotic (right) bone.** (Reproduced with permission from Dempster D et al. American Journal of Bone and Mineral Research 1: 15–21.)

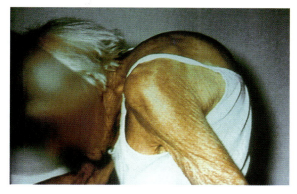

Fig. 9.2 **Severe osteoporosis of the spine.** (Reproduced with permission from slide set, A woman's guide to osteoporosis, produced by Wyeth Laboratories.)

may reduce the risk of ischaemic heart disease. However, more recent studies looking at the incidence of subsequent myocardial infarction have found no protective effect overall. Starting combined HRT at the time of the natural menopause (i.e. around 50 years) does not seem to be associated with an increased incidence of cardiovascular events and may even be associated with a decrease. However, the impact in women over 60–65 years of age at initiation of HRT is less clear.

Osteoporosis

Bone resorption by osteoclasts is accelerated by the menopause (Fig. 9.1). Oestrogen receptors have been demonstrated on bone cells, and oestrogens have been shown to stimulate osteoblasts directly. Calcitonin and prostaglandins may also be involved as intermediate factors in the link between oestrogen and bone metabolism.

In the first 4 years after the menopause there is an annual loss of 1–3% of bone mass, falling to 0.6% per year thereafter. This leads to an increased rate of fractures, particularly of the distal radius, the vertebral body and the upper femur, and one or more of these fractures will affect 40% of women over 65 years. Wedge compression fractures of the spine leading to the so-called 'dowager's hump' affect 25% of white women over 60 years of age (Fig. 9.2), and fractures of the hip have occurred in 20% of women by the age of 90 years. Women who are underweight have a higher risk of osteoporosis, which may in part be caused by reduced peripheral conversion of androgens to oestrogen. Women of Afro-Caribbean origin have a smaller risk of osteoporosis than white or Asian women, as they have a greater initial bone mass.

Osteoporosis has important consequences for women and for health services. In the UK, over 35 000 postmenopausal women suffer femoral fractures every year and 17% of them die in hospital. HRT has a very significant benefit in reducing the incidence of osteoporosis and osteoporotic fractures.

Administration of oestrogen decreases fracture risk; however, it is not recommended as a first-line treatment, as the long-term risks (particularly stroke) are considered to outweigh the benefits.

Diagnosis

The menopause may be confused with pre-menstrual syndrome, depression, thyroid dysfunction, pregnancy and, rarely, phaeochromocytoma or carcinoid syndrome. Vasomotor symptoms may be caused by calcium antagonists and by antidepressive therapy, especially tricyclics.

The diagnosis of post-menopause is clinical and can only be made in retrospect after 12 months of amenorrhoea (possibly 6 in women under 40 years of age). If there is clinical confusion, such as in a younger woman, the serum FSH level should be measured, which should be >30 IU/L postmenopausally. In younger women (<40 years) two FSH levels should be measured 6 weeks apart, as levels of FSH often fluctuate considerably during the perimenopause. Therefore perimenopausally, the level may be in the premenopausal range, and it should be noted that FSH levels peak physiologically in mid-cycle, making it worth re-checking apparently high levels a second time. If there is diagnostic doubt about whether a woman is perimenopausal, especially over 45 years of age, a therapeutic trial of HRT may be considered. Absence of a satisfactory response suggests that symptoms are unrelated to low levels of oestrogen.

Hormonal therapy

Oestrogen supplementation is the basis of replacement therapy. Although progestogens may have a small role in relieving vasomotor symptoms, they are added to oestrogen to protect the endometrium and reduce the hyperplasia that would otherwise result. The oestrogens may be systemically administered as daily oral tablets, twice-weekly or weekly transdermal patches, or subcutaneous implants administered every 6–8 months. Daily nasal sprays, skin creams and 3-monthly vaginal rings are available in some countries.

Whatever the route of administration, women who have not undergone hysterectomy should be placed on a regimen which includes a progestogen, to minimize the risk of endometrial cancer associated with unopposed oestrogen therapy, as mentioned earlier. This advice also applies to women who have undergone endometrial resection. Women who have had a hysterectomy do not require a progestogen.

Oral preparations

The oral route may have a more beneficial effect than parenteral therapy on lipid profiles, leading to higher high density lipoprotein (HDL), which is non-atherogenic, and lower Low density lipoprotein (LDL) levels that is atherogenic, but it is potentially more thrombotic. Tablets may be given as an oestrogen-only preparation for those who have had a hysterectomy, or as a combined oestrogen–progestogen preparation for those who have not. The combined form may be administered cyclically or continuously.

Cyclical preparations, which usually lead to monthly withdrawal bleeds, are used perimenopausally, and the continuous combined preparations, the so-called 'no-period' HRT, are an option from more than 2 years after the last menstrual period. This continuous combined therapy is more convenient for the 80+% who do not suffer unscheduled bleeding, but erratic bleeding beyond the first 6 months of treatment warrants further investigation.

Alternatives to these oestrogen–progesterone preparations are tibolone and raloxifene. Tibolone is a synthetic steroid with weak oestrogenic, progestogenic and androgenic effects, which may be started 2 years after periods have ceased in a similar way to the continuous combined preparations. Raloxifene, a synthetic selective oestrogen receptor modulator (SERM), has oestrogenic effects on bone and lipid metabolism, but has a minimal effect on uterine and breast tissue. It is therefore ineffective for controlling perimenopausal symptoms, but it has a useful role in protecting against osteoporosis and it does not cause vaginal bleeding.

New preparations are under development, and recently a combination of oestrogens and the SERM bazedoxifene in combination has reached the market.

Transcutaneous administration

Transdermal patches are available as an unopposed oestrogen form, or as cyclical or continuous oestrogen–progestogen combinations. Skin reactions, ranging from hyperaemia to blisters, affect a small percentage of users.

The clinical advantage of transcutaneous administration is that it does not increase the risk of thrombosis since it minimizes the effect on hepatic production of coagulation factors. It may also avoid gastrointestinal side-effects and changes in lipoprotein levels. Patches are usually applied to the buttock, and each patch lasts for between 3 and 7 days, depending on the formulation. This method appears to be as effective as oral preparations in treating symptomatic women and for the prevention of osteoporosis.

Percutaneous oestrogen gels are also available. A measured dose is rubbed into the skin and avoids the prolonged skin contact of patches. The same contraindications apply as for other unopposed oestrogens.

Subcutaneous implants

Oestradiol may be implanted in subcutaneous fat, usually in the lower abdomen, at intervals of no less than 5 or 6 months. The oestradiol level does not always fall away to baseline before symptoms recur and there is a risk of tachyphylaxis (persistent symptoms despite ever-increasing oestradiol levels) unless strict dose control is observed. Providing that pre-implant oestradiol levels are monitored, the risk of tachyphylaxis is minimized. Testosterone implants can be used where there is low libido.

Vaginal preparations

These include oestradiol tablets, low-dose oestradiol-releasing silastic ring pessaries, and oestriol vaginal pessaries and vaginal cream. Low-dose preparations are all useful in the treatment of atrophic vaginitis since the systemic absorption is very small after the first few weeks of administration.

Risks and side-effects of hormone treatment

General

Nausea and breast tenderness occur in about 5–10% of patients. Uterine bleeding is common, particularly with low-dose regimens, and in general, the lowest dose that controls symptoms should be used. Irregular bleeding should be investigated as appropriate. There is a slight risk of cholelithiasis with oral preparations. Diabetes control is improved and the incidence is lower in those taking HRT.

Endometrial carcinoma

Unopposed therapy (i.e. oestrogen only) increases the incidence of endometrial cancer four-fold, and it should therefore be used only for those who have had a hysterectomy. The incidence is reduced to a relative risk of <1.0 with opposed therapy (i.e. with the addition of progesterone for at least 10 days per cycle). The levonorgestrel-releasing intrauterine system (Mirena) protects the endometrium effectively when used in conjunction with oestrogen-only HRT in postmenopausal women.

Breast cancer

A link between sex hormone treatment and breast cancer is biologically plausible because of the connection between late menopause and breast cancer, as noted earlier. There is a small increase in likelihood of being diagnosed with breast cancer with combined HRT after 5 years of use, although oestrogen alone in hysterectomized women does not have this adverse effect. It would thus seem likely that it is the progestogen that causes the increase in the incidence of breast cancer. There is no increased risk in those who stopped taking HRT more than 5 years previously. It may be that breast cancer diagnosed while on HRT is more curable.

Other cancers

The evidence of any adverse effect on other cancers, such as ovarian, is equivocal and any effect is likely to be very small. The incidence of colon cancer is decreased in those taking HRT.

Venous thromboembolic disease

There is an increased risk of venous thromboembolic disease in the first year of oral HRT treatment, with a relative risk of approximately 4.0 in the first 6 months and 3.0 in the second 6 months (baseline risk 1.3/1000 per year). This increased risk is largely confined to the first year of use. There is apparently no increased risk in those taking transdermal HRT. Routine pre-treatment screening for thrombophilia is not recommended, but it should be carried out in those with a personal or family history of venous thromboembolic disease. It is not known whether transcutaneous administration of oestrogen is associated with an increased risk of secondary venous thromboembolism (VTE) and it should therefore be avoided in those who have had a prior thrombotic episode.

Stroke

There is a significant increase in the likelihood of stroke in all age groups with oral HRT, although the impact is small in younger menopausal women, as the baseline risk of stroke is so low.

Contraindications to hormone treatment

Pregnancy, venous thromboembolic disease and a history of recurrent venous thromboembolism are recognized contraindications to HRT, as are liver disease and undiagnosed vaginal bleeding. Treated hypertension and other cardiovascular risk factors are not contraindications if effectively managed.

Use of oestrogen-containing HRT is widely considered to be contraindicated following breast carcinoma (including

intraductal carcinoma) and following advanced endometrial carcinoma. There are also theoretical reasons why it should be avoided in those who have had ovarian cancer.

Duration of hormone replacement therapy

When oestrogens are given for vasomotor symptoms, they are generally continued for 2 or 3 years and then stopped. Whether to continue therapy beyond this time depends on whether symptoms recur and on a weighing up of the risks of osteoporosis against the potential side-effects, including breast cancer, for that particular individual.

Non-hormonal treatment

Drugs

Vasomotor symptoms may be reduced by clonidine, which acts directly on the hypothalamus, but in practice it is of limited value as it is no more effective than placebo in randomized controlled trials. The selective serotonin reuptake inhibitors have also been shown to be effective. Palpitations and tachycardia may be improved by beta-blockers. Sedatives, hypnotics and antidepressants may be helpful in the treatment of non-vasomotor symptoms.

Herbal preparations are taken by many women, but conclusive evidence of their benefit is lacking.

The first-line treatment for osteoporosis in women over 60 is currently a bisphosphonate, and oestrogen is used only for those where this is inappropriate. In younger women, prevention and treatment are not recommended unless there is a history of fracture. In elderly women, supplementation with calcium, calcitonin and vitamin D reduces the risk of hip fractures. Moderate exercise may slow the rate of bone loss, though compliance with exercise programmes is often poor.

Psychological support

Since menopausal symptoms often resolve with time, some women with menopausal symptoms need only reassurance. Others may have particular stresses at this time of life, such as children leaving home, which may accentuate their perimenopausal symptoms and can severely compromise quality of life. The marked placebo benefits in various studies show the importance of psychological support and a sympathetic ear.

Key points

- The average age of women experiencing spontaneous menopause in the western world is 51 years.
- Menopause is defined as 1 year of amenorrhoea in the presence of a uterus and in the absence of another cause such as low body mass or excess exercise.
- The menopause is caused by ovarian failure as the supply of oocytes is depleted. FSH rises as oestrogen production falls, and an FSH of >30 IU/L is suggestive of postmenopausal status.
- Cessation of periods is often preceded by irregular bleeding. A vaginal bleed more than a year after menopause usually warrants investigation.
- Vasomotor symptoms, such as hot flushes, affect around two-thirds of women and may continue for more than 5 years after the menopause. They can severely affect quality of life and should not be dismissed. Other symptoms include genitourinary atrophy and, possibly, some psychological symptoms.
- Long-term health risks of the post-menopause include CVD and osteoporosis. Fractures of the radius, vertebral body or femoral neck affect 40% of women over the age of 65 years.
- HRT is offered to treat menopausal symptoms and to reduce long-term hypo-oestrogenic side-effects. If the woman still has a uterus, opposed HRT (oestrogen and progesterone) is necessary to avoid the risk of endometrial carcinoma. Oral, transcutaneous and vaginal preparations are available, in addition to subcutaneous implants.
- Side-effects of HRT include an increased incidence of breast carcinoma with combined HRT and venous thromboembolic disease with oral preparations.

10

Pelvic organ prolapse

Introduction

Pelvic organ prolapse (POP) is described as the descent of one or more of the pelvic organs into the vagina. It can affect any of the compartments of the vagina: anterior (bladder), posterior (bowel) or apical (uterus/cervix or vault if patient has already had a hysterectomy). Although prolapse in a single compartment can happen, typically more than one compartment will be involved (e.g. bladder and uterine prolapse coexisting).

These organs are supported in the pelvis by the muscles, ligaments and fascia of the pelvic floor. If the pelvic floor is damaged or weakened, for example as a result of childbirth, the organs descend down into the vagina, causing prolapse. A third of women who have had children will develop a symptomatic prolapse; the lifetime risk of requiring surgery for prolapse is around 11% for women. Stress urinary incontinence (SUI) has the same aetiology and can coexist with prolapse in any compartment.

Aetiology

POP is caused by injury to the pelvic floor. The injury can be to the muscles (levator ani) or the fascial supports, including many important ligaments (e.g. the uterosacral and cardinal ligaments). The most likely time to injure the pelvic floor is during childbirth; however, chronic constipation and other factors, which lead to an increase in intra-abdominal pressure, can contribute.

Childbirth

Childbirth results in trauma to the pelvic floor and loss of support to the female pelvic organs. Direct trauma, such as avulsion of the levator ani or ligaments, can happen at the time of vaginal delivery, especially with forceps deliveries. Pelvic nerve damage also plays a part. The pudendal nerve is crushed against the bony pelvis during labour and the longer the woman is in labour, the worse the damage is likely to be. Forceps deliveries also increase the risk of levator ani damage. A prolonged labour, in particular a prolonged second stage with a large baby and subsequent instrumental delivery consequently increase the risk of prolapse even further.

Menopause

The menopausal state, characterized by oestrogen deficiency and loss of connective tissue strength, has been implicated as a contributing factor in the development of prolapse. However, prolapse can also occur in young women before the menopause, so simply being menopausal is not always implicated.

Congenital

Congenital weaknesses, or neurological deficiency of the tissues, account for prolapse in a very small proportion of women as can connective tissue disorders (e.g. Ehlers-Danlos syndrome). Very rarely, children may be born with congenital cloacal abnormalities, which result in abnormal genitalia.

Gynaecological surgery

Although surgery is often used to treat prolapse, it can be responsible for some types of prolapse. A colposuspension, an operation done for SUI (see Chapter 11), alters the anatomy of the vagina. The bladder neck is lifted up behind the symphysis pubis to support the bladder, but this results in gravitational effects on the posterior vaginal wall that can then lead to posterior wall prolapse in up to 25% of women who undergo this operation. Vaginal vault prolapse is a recognized sequelae of hysterectomy.

Genetic

Genetic factors have been implicated in the development of prolapse. It is uncommon, for example, in the African population, possibly related in some way to the different collagen content of tissues.

Types of prolapse

The main types of prolapse, and the main symptoms, are summarized in Table 10.1.

It is important to remember that a single prolapse is very rare, with most patients having *multicompartment* prolapse, i.e. more than one of these listed below.

Table 10.1	Types of POP	
Compartment	**Prolapse**	**Symptoms[a]**
Anterior	Urethrocele Cystocele	SUI Poor bladder emptying, residual urine, frequency and urinary infection
Apical	Uterine (procidentia) Vault (enterocele)	Bleeding and/or discharge from ulceration in association with procidentia Backache
Posterior	Enterocele Rectocele	Pressure, backache Difficulty in bowel emptying

[a]In addition to the general symptoms of discomfort, dragging, the feeling of a 'lump' and, rarely, coital problems.

Urethrocele

The term 'urethrocele' is occasionally used to describe descent of the part of the anterior vaginal wall over which the urethra sits. This is approximately the lower 3–4 cm of the anterior wall. Descent here leads to urethral hypermobility, which can disrupt the urethral continence mechanism, predisposing to SUI. This is not treated by prolapse surgery but by SUI surgery (see Chapter 11).

Cystocele

The bladder rests on the anterior vaginal wall and its supporting mechanisms. A cystocele occurs when there is descent in the anterior compartment and the bladder prolapses into the vagina (Fig. 10.1).

Uterine prolapse

The cervix, with the uterus on top, normally sits in the upper third of the vagina. When apical supports are lost it descends and is called a uterine prolapse (Fig. 10.2).

Rectocele

Weakening of the tissue that lies between the vagina and rectum (rectovaginal fascia) allows the rectum to protrude into the lower posterior vaginal wall, causing a rectocele (Fig. 10.3). Laxity of the perineum may also be present, which gives a gaping appearance to the fourchette (the posterior margin of the introitus).

Enterocele

An enterocele occurs in the upper vagina (Fig. 10.4). Weakness in the support mechanism here leads to descent of the vagina and a peritoneal sac, potentially containing small bowel or omentum. Enteroceles are apical prolapses, i.e.

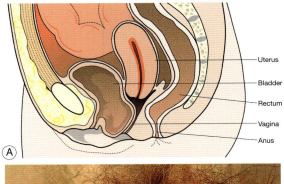

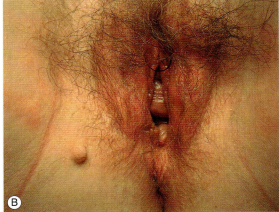

Fig. 10.1 **(A,B) Cystocele.**

the top of the vagina. Therefore they are commonly found with uterine prolapses, or if the patient has had a hysterectomy, the top of the vagina descends with an enterocele in it. This is called a vault prolapse.

Prolapse staging

Many different classification systems have been described to attempt to stage (size) POP, and these are shown in Fig. 10.5. The universally recommended tool is the pelvic organ prolapse quantification system (POP-Q). This system describes location in addition to the size of prolapse. The simplified staging system shown in Table 10.2 is the one commonly used in clinical practice. Procidentia is a term used when the cervix, uterus and vaginal wall have completely prolapsed through the introitus, i.e. stage 4 prolapse.

Symptoms

Prolapse is often asymptomatic and it may only be detected when women attend for a cervical smear test. The only real symptom of POP is that of feeling a lump or swelling coming from the vagina. Patients will describe it in different ways. The commonest description used by patients is of 'something coming down', and this is usually accompanied by discomfort

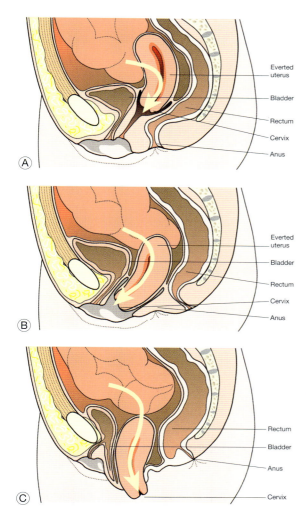

Fig. 10.2 **Uterine prolapse. (A)** Stage I; **(B)** stage II and **(C)** stage III.

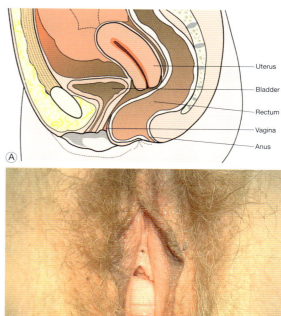

Fig. 10.3 **(A,B) Rectocele.**

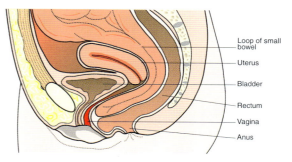

Fig. 10.4 **Enterocele.**

and a dragging sensation. Some will describe a lump that they can see or feel, others will describe a swelling that either 'hangs out', 'pops in/out' or they need to push in themselves. The feeling of things coming down will sometimes cause a sensation of pulling.

Patients sometimes describe backache, which improves when lying down, although this can often be for other reasons, e.g. arthritis and not the prolapse. If the POP is protruding outside the vagina it may rub on the woman's clothes and this may lead to ulceration of the cervix and thickening of the vaginal mucosa, which can bleed and be sore. Prolapse itself however *does not* cause pain. Women who are in a lot of pain may have a prolapse, but it is not the cause of their pain.

Coital difficulties are an uncommon presenting symptom, but a common one to find. Although sex is usually possible with a POP, women are worried they should not have sex because of concern that they may make things worse or because they often feel embarrassed by their perceived appearance of their vagina.

Although a very large POP that protrudes outside the vagina can lead to urethral kinking, which may lead to voiding difficulties or problems emptying their bowels, it is very rare for this to occur. However, functional bladder and bowel symptoms (i.e. urinary or faecal incontinence, constipation, difficulty passing urine or urine infections) will coexist in most patients with POP. This is not because they are necessarily caused by the POP, but because they have the same aetiology. Taking a history must include asking for these symptoms so that these problems can be addressed, but managing the prolapse alone will not improve these symptoms in most patients.

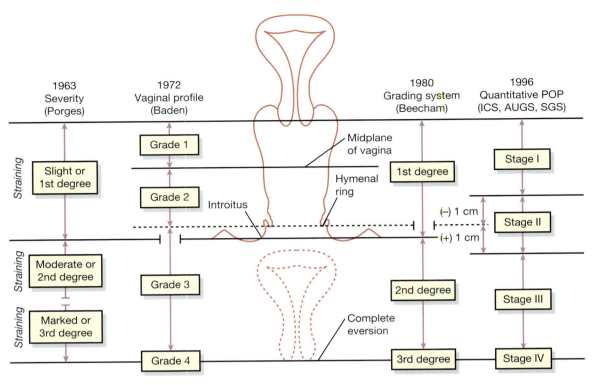

Fig. 10.5 Classification systems that have been used to stage (size) POP.

Table 10.2	The simplified staging system commonly used to stage POP
Pelvic organ prolapse quantification system (POP-Q)	
Stage 0	No prolapse demonstrated
Stage I	The most distal portion of the prolapse is more than 1 cm above the level of the hymen
Stage II	The most distal portion of the prolapse is 1 cm or less proximal or distal to the plane of the hymen
Stage III	The most distal portion of the prolapse is more than 1 cm below the plane of the hymen but protrudes no further than 2 cm less than the total vaginal length in cm
Stage IV	Essentially complete eversion of the total length of the lower genital tract is demonstrated

Signs

Examination for prolapse forms part of the general gynaecological examination. Abdominal examination, although historically done to detect a pelvic mass that may be pushing the pelvic organs downwards, is in fact more likely to detect a palpable bladder, which if found after voiding is a sign of urinary retention.

Pelvic examination is then performed, initially with the patient supine. The woman is asked to abduct her legs. On inspection of the vulva one may note atrophic changes (scanty hair, thinning of the labia). Vaginal atrophy may be seen, suggesting the need for oestrogen treatment. Urinary leakage should be looked for on coughing, and an assessment of the perineum is made. By gently parting the labia majora with the thumb and index finger of the left hand, prolapse may be seen appearing at the introitus. The woman should be asked to strain or cough to push down any prolapse, making it easier to identify. A bimanual examination may then be performed, and may give a useful indication of uterine size and possibly descent.

Examination in the left lateral position can also be helpful (see Fig. 2.6). This allows a systematic examination of the entire vagina, exerting gentle traction with the speculum on the posterior vaginal wall. Sponge forceps are occasionally used during this examination to reduce a large prolapse or to enable the examiner to distinguish the anatomy. The speculum can then be slowly withdrawn along the posterior wall of the vagina and the full extent of any rectocele will come into view. If a prolapse is not apparent with the woman lying down, it may sometimes be necessary to examine her in the standing position.

Management

As with many conditions, POP can be managed surgically or non-surgically. Non-surgical management is termed 'conservative management' and in the case of POP should be tried before resorting to surgery.

Conservative management

No treatment

If a POP is not causing symptoms and the woman is unaware of it, then she does not require any treatment. Simply because a doctor notices a prolapse within the vagina does not mean that it requires management.

Many women are aware of the presence of a POP; however, it may not be troubling them or interfering with their quality of life or daily activities. It is perfectly reasonable to reassure these women that they do not have serious pathology and that no further management is required.

Lifestyle advice

Patients should be advised about weight reduction and smoking cessation. Fluid and dietary advice will also be helpful for concomitant bladder and bowel symptoms.

Pelvic floor exercises

Supervised pelvic floor muscle exercises by trained physiotherapists have been proven to improve symptoms in stage I–II prolapse, reducing the need for surgery. The key word here is *supervised*. Simply giving the patient a leaflet about pelvic floor exercises and telling her to go and do them, although unlikely to do any harm, is also unlikely to produce any benefit. Sending an enthusiastic patient to an enthusiastic physiotherapist, however, can produce cure/improvement rates of 60–70%.

Pelvic floor physiotherapy is of less proven benefit in women with stage III–IV POP, but it still has a role in the treatment of associated urinary and bowel symptoms.

Vaginal pessaries

These are devices specifically made for women to wear in their vagina. Pessaries do not cure prolapse but provide support while the women is wearing it, thereby relieving POP symptoms. They are commonly used. Pessaries come in various shapes and sizes and some are shown in Fig. 10.6.

The mostly commonly used pessary is called a 'Ring' pessary. It is an inert plastic ring, which is placed in the vagina so that one edge of the ring is behind the symphysis pubis and the other is in the posterior fornix (Figs 10.7 and 10.8). The ring stretches the vault of the vagina and thus supports the uterus. Traditionally once a pessary is fitted, arrangements are usually made to change it every 4–6 months by a healthcare professional. At this examination, the vagina is inspected thoroughly for atrophic changes and ulceration due to pressure necrosis. The pessary is either washed and reused, or replaced depending on the type. Many of the newer pessaries are amenable to self-management and the patients remove it themselves, choosing when to wear it. Sexual activity is therefore possible with pessary use and

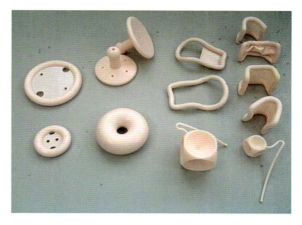

Fig. 10.6 A selection of the commonly used vaginal pessaries.

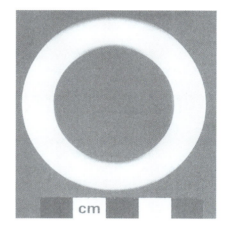

Fig. 10.7 Ring pessary (50 mm diameter).

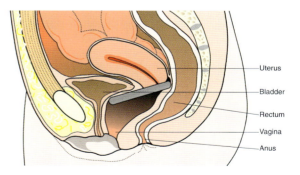

Fig. 10.8 Ring pessary in situ. Note that the anterior vaginal wall is elevated to reduce the cystocele and the uterine prolapse has been corrected.

sexually active women should not be excluded from this treatment option.

Complications from pessaries may include urinary symptoms (frequency, infection), vaginal discharge, bleeding, or, very rarely, fistula formation (if the pessary is neglected).

Vaginal oestrogen therapy

If atrophy of the lower genital tract is noted, with or without association with POP, topical oestrogen therapy (commonly administered topically as a cream) may help. Systemic absorption of oestrogen is negligible and is safe to use in most women. It improves vaginal tissue thickness, quality and sensitivity, and may therefore improve many symptoms the patient may be experiencing that are not necessarily caused by the POP. It can also help decrease the incidence of vaginal pessary complications in postmenopausal women.

In some women it may also be sensible to use preoperatively to help improve vaginal skin.

Surgical management

The choice of surgical procedure will depend on the patient's age, type and stage of prolapse, if they are sexually active, any comorbidities including raised body mass index (BMI), and ultimately the patient's wishes.

Complications can occur with all types of surgery, not just prolapse surgery. These include infection, bleeding and organ injury, which could be life threatening. Chronic pain can also occur with all surgery, including prolapse surgery. Prolapse surgery can result in vaginal scarring and narrowing, making having sex difficult and sometimes impossible.

Recurrence of prolapse after surgical correction is common, with up to 30% of women having vaginal prolapse repairs requiring a second operation within 5 years. Careful counselling of patients must therefore not only be about what operation to have but also about complications and risk of recurrence, and thus the importance of trying conservative treatments first.

Operations can be performed via the vaginal route, abdominally or laparoscopically.

The following procedures can be considered, either in isolation or performed in combination. It may also be appropriate in some patients to combine them with surgery for SUI (see Chapter 11).

Anterior repair (colporrhaphy)

This is a vaginal operation performed to treat a cystocele. The principle of an anterior repair is to make a midline incision through the vaginal skin and to reflect the underlying bladder off the vaginal mucosa. Once this is achieved, supporting sutures are placed into the fascia in order to elevate the bladder.

The remaining redundant vaginal skin that has been 'ballooning' down is excised, and the vaginal skin is then sutured closed.

Posterior repair (colporrhaphy)

This is a vaginal operation performed to treat rectoceles. The principles of a posterior repair are similar to those of an anterior repair. An incision is made in the posterior vaginal wall and the rectum is separated from the vagina (Fig. 10.9). Supporting sutures are placed in the disrupted rectovaginal fascia to reduce the prolapse. The lax vaginal skin is then excised and the incision closed. This operation can be combined with a repair of the perineal body to support the perineum (perineoplasty). Again, particular care must be taken not to narrow the vagina and cause dyspareunia.

Vaginal hysterectomy

Vaginal hysterectomy is performed for uterine prolapse. The aim is not simply to remove the uterus, i.e. the prolapsing organ, as all that will simply happen is that the vaginal vault will descend instead. Once the uterus is removed the supporting uterosacral ligaments are shortened and reattached to the vaginal vault to support the upper vagina.

Manchester repair

Manchester repair (also called 'Fothergill repair') has a role in treating a woman with cystocele and a uterine prolapse,

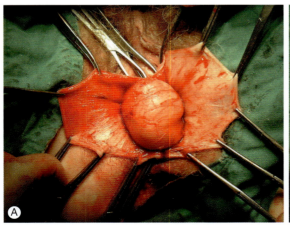 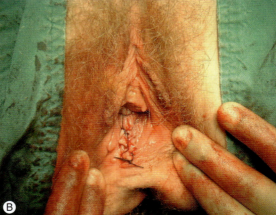

Fig. 10.9 **Posterior colporrhaphy. (A)** The posterior wall is opened in the midline to expose the rectum. **(B)** The posterior wall is closed after reducing the prolapse.

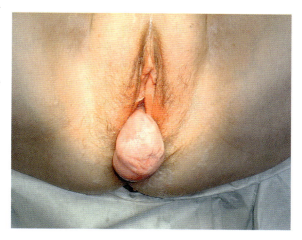

Fig. 10.10 **Vault prolapse.**

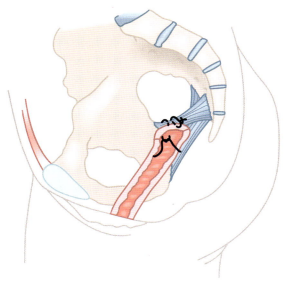

Fig. 10.11 **Sacrospinous ligament fixation (for post-hysterectomy vault prolapse).**

but is not commonly performed. A vaginal approach is used. The skin around the cervix is incised. The uterosacral and transverse cervical (cardinal) ligaments are divided and shortened, the cervix is amputated, and the shortened ligaments are approximated anterior to the cervical stump. The anterior repair is performed and completed as before.

Sacrospinous ligament fixation

This is a vaginal operation performed for apical prolapse, typically post-hysterectomy vault prolapse (Fig. 10.10), but it can also be performed for a uterine prolapse.

The procedure requires the surgeon to suture the top of the vaginal vault, or uterus (hysteropexy), to the sacrospinous ligament, a ligament that runs from the base of the sacrum to the ischial spine in the lower back/buttocks (Fig. 10.11).

Vaginal implant repairs

Colporrhaphy procedures can be supported with the use of an implant. These were thought to add to the strength of the repair and potentially decrease recurrence. Implants can be biological (e.g. porcine dermis) or synthetic (e.g. polypropylene mesh similar to those used in abdominal hernia repairs), absorbable or non-absorbable. Implants and synthetic meshes in particular have been associated with an increased risk of complications (e.g. vaginal exposure and organ perforation), however, without much proven benefit. They are therefore currently not routinely used for primary prolapse surgery.

Sacrocolpopexy (sacrohysteropexy)

This operation for prolapse is done abdominally, either open via an incision or laparoscopically. It is performed for apical or multicompartment prolapse involving the vaginal apex (vault or uterus), and has a higher success rate with lower recurrence rates than vaginal apical procedures.

Sacrocolpopexy involves suturing the vaginal vault to the body of the sacrum indirectly by using a polypropylene mesh interposed between the two structures. If the uterus is still in place, a hysterectomy may be required first to be able to attach the mesh to the anterior vagina. In women wishing to conserve their uterus (e.g. patient preference, family not complete) the mesh can be wrapped around the cervix instead. This is called a sacrohysteropexy.

Key *points*

- POP is the descent of the pelvic organs (urethra, bladder, uterus and bowel) into the vagina.
- The biggest risk factor is childbirth. Obesity, the menopause, gynaecological surgery or age. Conditions increasing intra-abdominal pressure also contribute.
- Prolapse can be the following: anterior compartment (urethrocele or cystocele – urethra or bladder prolapse, respectively); apical (uterus or vaginal vault post-hysterectomy); or a posterior (rectocele and enterocele – prolapse of the rectum or small bowel, respectively). Prolapse is rarely found in isolation and most women have a combination of the above.
- Women with prolapse tend to present with a 'something coming down' discomfort, but may also have urinary or bowel symptoms.
- Asymptomatic prolapse does not need to be treated.
- Treatment should first be conservative (i.e. pessaries, pelvic floor exercises) before resorting to surgical repair.
- Surgical options can be either vaginal or abdominal and may often need to be combined.

11

Female urinary incontinence

Introduction

Urinary incontinence (UI) is defined as any involuntary loss of urine which is a social or hygienic problem.

UI is common – it is reported by 46% of women attending UK primary care clinics but is often underdiagnosed and undertreated. UI increases with age, with the incidence of an overactive bladder (OAB) as high as 50% or more in institutionalized elderly females. UI is a major quality of life (QOL) issue because it causes significant distress and can have negative physical and psychological impacts.

Types of urinary incontinence

The commonest types of UI in women are:

- stress urinary incontinence (SUI)
- overactive bladder (OAB)
- mixed incontinence (SUI and OAB)
- retention with overflow
- fistula.

SUI is the commonest cause of UI, accounting for 40% of cases. It is defined as involuntary loss of urine on effort or physical exertion, including sporting activities, or on sneezing or coughing, in the absence of any detrusor contraction. 'Activity-related incontinence' might be the preferred term in some languages to avoid confusion with psychological stress.

An **OAB** accounts for about 30% of cases of female UI. Women complain of a sudden, compelling desire to pass urine which is difficult to defer (urgency). This is usually associated with daytime urinary frequency (more than previously deemed normal for the woman) and, as the problem tends to be both day and night, women can have nocturia (interruption of sleep one or more times because of need to micturate), and, in severe cases, enuresis (bed wetting). Urge urinary incontinence (UUI) is a severe form of OAB.

In **mixed urinary incontinence (MUI)** women complain of incontinence associated with both urgency and physical exertion. This accounts for around 30% of cases.

Retention with overflow is common in elderly female patients with an underactive bladder or in those with a

neurological problem. The bladder continues to fill until it simply spills over, resulting in leakage.

A **fistula** is an abnormal communication between two epithelial surfaces and, in the UK, usually results as a complication of surgery. In under-resourced countries, obstructed labour is a common cause. Any communication between the lower urinary tract (ureter, bladder or urethra) and the genital tract (uterus and vagina) will result in continuous dribbling UI. Fistulae account for only 1 in 1000 cases of incontinence in women in the UK.

The mechanism of continence

Normally, continence is maintained at the level of the bladder neck.

1. **Proximal urethral sphincter mechanism** is present in the region of the bladder neck and the proximal urethra is a water-tight seal, which maintains the pressure in the urethra greater than the pressure in the bladder. The anatomical basis of that seal is considered to be a series of arteriovenous anastomoses within the wall of the proximal urethra. They allow some degree of turgor pressure to be exerted circumferentially around the urethra, which results in the formation of a hermetic seal by keeping the urethra occluded. The effect of any pressure exerted around the periphery of a hollow tube is to occlude that tube. If the pressure is exerted in numerous places around the circumference of the tube, then the tube will simply close.
2. **Distal urethral sphincter mechanism** – the pressure in the proximal urethra exceeds that in the bladder; the greatest pressure difference exists at the mid-urethra. This is made of striated muscle within the wall of urethra and is innervated by nerve roots S2–4 via the pudendal nerve.
3. **Supporting tissues around urethra** include the pubourethral ligaments, derived from the fascia of the pelvic floor, and, to a lesser degree, the pelvic floor musculature, namely the levator ani muscle. They maintain the proximal urethra in an intra-abdominal position and any rise in intra-abdominal pressure is

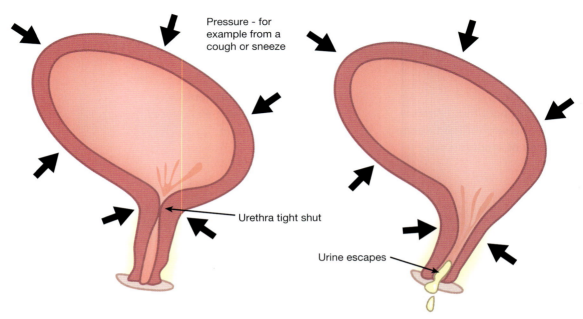

Pressure - for example from a cough or sneeze

Urethra tight shut

Urine escapes

1) Normal
The bladder neck is well supported and the muscle sphincter squeezed tight shut. A rise in abdominal pressure acts evenly on squeezing the bladder and sealing the urethra – no leakage of urine

2) Stress incontinence
The bladder neck has fallen and the muscle sphincter is strained. So a rise in abdominal pressure acts more by squeezing the bladder than sealing the urethra – urine escapes

Fig. 11.1 Aetiology of stress urinary incontinence.

transmitted equally to the bladder and the proximal urethra; the pressure difference will not change and continence will therefore be maintained. Weakness or damage to the supporting tissues can make the urethra hypermobile and any rise in intra-abdominal pressure makes it move outside the abdomen, leading to unequal distribution of pressure, which may predispose to SUI (Fig. 11.1).

There is also the concept of bladder stability. The bladder muscle, the detrusor, should relax during bladder filling and contract during micturition. This involves a complex interaction between the structural/anatomic parts of the urinary tract and between nervous control systems. Patients with OAB have involuntary bladder (detrusor) contraction. If the contraction is modest, then the woman will appreciate the contraction as urinary urgency, but if the contraction is strong enough to elevate the pressure in the bladder above that in the urethra, then there will be associated UUI.

Aetiology of incontinence

Stress urinary incontinence

SUI clearly requires some degree of weakness of one or both of the proximal and distal urethral sphincter mechanisms and/or supporting tissues around the urethra. While no single

aetiological factor exists in all women with SUI, there are a series of predisposing factors that often explain the condition. These include:

■ pregnancy and vaginal delivery
■ prolapse
■ menopause
■ collagen disorder
■ obesity.

Pregnancy

Vaginal delivery may cause direct damage of the pelvic floor or denervation of the pudendal nerve (pudendal neuropathy), thus predisposing to SUI. Pregnancy itself can cause some irreversible pelvic floor damage.

The first vaginal delivery causes maximum damage to the pelvic floor and all subsequent vaginal births can worsen the damage. Elective caesarean section therefore may have some protective role in preventing the occurrence of SUI. Some women develop SUI during pregnancy owing to raised intra-abdominal pressure related to uterine contents together with the smooth muscle–relaxant effect of progesterone.

Prolapse

Prolapse and SUI coexist in over 50% of cases. While these conditions are often concurrent, one may be mild or asymptomatic. The relationship relates to pelvic floor dysfunction, which is the main aetiology of both conditions.

Menopause

Many women date the onset of their symptoms from the menopause. There is evidence that lack of oestrogen weakens the urethral sphincter complex and reduces maximal urethral closure pressure (intrinsic sphincter deficiency), leading to SUI. The effect of this pressure reduction is that a smaller rise in intra-abdominal pressure will result in SUI.

Collagen disorder

Collagen is a major component of the pubourethral ligaments. There are several different types of collagen within the body and there is evidence that there are different types of collagen in varying proportions in the pubourethral ligaments of women who become incontinent compared with the pubourethral ligaments of those who do not.

Overactive bladder

In most women, the aetiology of an OAB is unknown (idiopathic). Neurological conditions, typically multiple sclerosis, stroke or spinal cord injury, are known to be a cause of overactivity. There is also a link between psychological upset and OAB, with such patients having a higher incidence of anxiety and neuroses.

Voiding difficulty

Voiding difficulties in women are mainly due to an underactive detrusor (hypotonia in 90% of cases) and less commonly (10%) due to anatomical obstruction (due to previous surgery or increased urethral sphincter activity). The aetiology of the detrusor hypotonia is either due to ageing, with the natural reduction in muscle fibres and muscle strength, or pregnancy and childbirth, due to nerve damage (pudendal neuropathy). There is some evidence that young women who put off voiding during their adult life ('infrequent voiders') are more prone to this problem. Women with neurological disease can have voiding difficulty due to either detrusor hypotonia or obstruction; in the latter case secondary to inappropriate contraction of the urethral sphincter or incoordination (dyssynergia) between bladder and urethral sphincter complex.

Clinical presentation

This will depend on the underlying cause for UI. Patients can complain of symptoms related to OAB, for example frequency, urgency, nocturia with or without associated UUI and enuresis, or UI associated with exertion or constant leakage. It is important to enquire about voiding symptoms, for example, hesitancy, straining to void, poor or intermittent urinary stream and post-micturition symptoms, such as

Table 11.1	Effect of urinary incontinence upon QOL
Emotions	Feelings of stigma and humiliation. Social and recreational withdrawal. Fear and anxiety related to being incontinent in public
Relationships	Reduced intimacy, affection and physical proximity. Marriage breakdown and subsequent divorce
Employment	Absence from work. Loss of concentration. Interruption of work for toilet breaks
Sleep	Nocturia is common and quality and amount of sleep is affected. Tiredness the next day. Risk of falls especially in the elderly
Exercise and sport	A barrier to exercise
Travel and holidays	Reluctance to visit new places. Need to pack protective materials

sensation of incomplete emptying and post-micturition dribbling. Accompanying 'red flag' symptoms, such as haematuria, persistent bladder or urethral pain, or recurrent urinary tract infection (UTI), warrant urological assessment of lower and upper urinary tracts.

Nearly half of women with SUI have coexisting pelvic organ prolapse, and therefore an enquiry about symptoms and impact on QOL is essential. Bowel dysfunction can be associated with UI and must be explored. A full medical history and drug history will allow assessment of whether these problems are contributory to the patient's incontinence.

UI is a major QOL issue and can prevent a woman from socializing and cause limiting or restricting of physical activity (Table 11.1). In severe cases, it can have a significant psychological impact leading to depression, loss of self-esteem and anxiety, resulting in a detrimental effect on personality. It can also have a significant negative impact upon a woman's sex life, and incontinence during intercourse can lead to avoidance of sexual activity and intimacy. Nocturia can affect concentration and working. Nocturia in the elderly also carries the risk of falls, with fractured neck of femur a common outcome. It should be noted that in the elderly, UI is the second most common reason for a patient being unable to return to independent living. It is therefore essential to assess to what degree the woman's symptoms are impacting on her lifestyle.

Diagnostic evaluation

Clinical examination

All women should undergo an abdominal and pelvic examination. Abdominal examination may reveal a palpable bladder suggesting urinary retention, and, infrequently, an otherwise unsuspected pelvic mass. Pelvic examination may reveal

Table 11.2	Bladder diary (frequency-volume chart)										
Patient A			**Patient B**			**Patient C**			**Patient D**		
Time	V. (mL)	I.	Time	V. (mL)	I.	Time	V. (mL)	I.	Time	V. (mL)	I.
0800	500		0800	400	x	0800	450		0800	150	
1200	300		1000	200		1000	400		1000	150	
1600	200		1030	50	xx	1300	350		1200	150	
		x	1100	50		1430	400		1400	150	
1900	350		1400	250		1600	500		1600	150	
2300	200		1700	250		1900	350		1800	150	
			1900	75		2100	400		2000	150	
0400	250		1930	50	x	2300	400		2200	150	
			2230	300					0000	150	
			0300	100					0200	150	
			0400	50					0400	150	

pelvic organ prolapse or vaginal atrophy. Useful observations during your assessment include:

SUI (clinical stress leakage): observation of involuntary leakage from the urethra synchronous with effort or physical exertion, or on sneezing or coughing.

Extra-urethral incontinence: observation of urine leakage through channels other than the urethral meatus – for example, fistula or ectopic ureter.

Focused neurological examination, if appropriate. This may include assessment of cognitive function, ambulation and mobility, hand function and lumbar and sacral spinal segment function.

- **Per rectal examination:** if symptoms of anal incontinence are present, the anal sphincter tone should be determined by digital examination.

Investigations

Urinalysis

Every woman presenting with lower urinary tract symptoms should have a urinalysis performed. The presence of leucocytes and nitrites suggests a UTI and this may be causing or worsening the patient's symptoms. If the patient is symptomatic of UTI, treatment with a broad-spectrum antibiotic is started and a mid-stream specimen of urine sent. Recurrent UTI and presence of haematuria should prompt cystoscopy, and ultrasound of the upper renal tracts. The presence of glycosuria may suggest diabetes, which can predispose to recurrent UTIs and urinary frequency.

Frequency-volume chart (bladder diary)

Bladder diaries should be used in the initial assessment. Patients should be encouraged to complete a minimum of 3 days of the diary, covering variations in their usual activities, such as both working and leisure days. The patient should record the amount, type and timing of fluid intake along with the timing and amount of voiding and episodes of UI. It is a simple, non-invasive tool to assess urinary frequency, urgency, diurnal and nocturnal cycles, functional bladder capacity and total urine output. Fluid intake and pad changes can give an indication of the severity of wetness. This may also be used for monitoring the effects of treatment and act as feedback. Table 11.2 shows an example from four patients.

- Patient A has normal frequency but is incontinent when not needing the toilet. This is likely to represent SUI.
- Patient B has a normal bladder capacity (400 mL) but is emptying her bladder with as little as 50 mL in it, and this is typical of an OAB. In addition, she is wet when going to the toilet; further evidence of OAB.
- Patient C is over-drinking and this is giving her urinary frequency and high urinary output.
- Patient D has a small capacity bladder – probably inflammatory in nature.

Cystoscopy

This is not required for initial investigation of UI. Cystoscopy is indicated if women have haematuria or recurrent UTIs.

Ultrasound measurement of post-void residual

This is a simple non-invasive test and should be performed if incomplete emptying, voiding dysfunction or recurrent UTI are suspected, to check for post-void residual volume.

Pelvic ultrasound (to assess the pelvic organs) has a limited role in evaluation of women with UI other than if pelvic masses are suspected.

Quality-of-life questionnaires

There are several disease-specific validated QOL questionnaires for subjective assessment of lower urinary tract symptoms in women, including sexual dysfunction. This should be a part of the assessment of every woman both before and after treatment, along with an impression of what she expects from treatment; shared goals will improve patient satisfaction.

Box 11.1

Indications for urodynamic studies
1. Symptoms of OAB leading to a clinical suspicion of detrusor overactivity
2. Symptoms suggestive of voiding dysfunction
3. Anterior compartment prolapse
4. Previous surgery for stress incontinence

Table 11.3	Difference in patients' symptoms with OAB, SUI and MUI		
Symptoms	**OAB**	**SUI**	**MUI**
Urgency (strong, sudden desire to void)	Yes	No	Yes
Frequency with urgency (>8 times/24 h)	Yes	No	Yes
Leaking during physical activity, e.g. coughing, sneezing, lifting, etc.	No	Yes	Yes
Amount of urinary leakage with each episode of incontinence	Large (if present)	Small	Variable
Ability to reach the toilet in time following urge to void	Often no	Yes	Variable
Waking to pass urine at night	Usually	Seldom	Maybe

Urodynamic studies

These tests are a dynamic assessment of the lower urinary tract and offer objective information about bladder and urethral function. They are, however, invasive, expensive and time-consuming, and some women find them embarrassing. Furthermore, they are not foolproof in providing a diagnosis. The indications for urodynamic studies are listed in Box 11.1.

Treatment

Initial assessment is aimed at ruling out 'red flags' that warrant referral and further investigations and trying to categorise predominant symptoms – for example, SUI predominant (Table 11.3). If a patient is thought to have MUI, treatment should be directed towards the predominant symptom.

Treatment depends on the type of incontinence and should start with conservative treatment, and this usually includes two distinct approaches: lifestyle interventions and bladder retraining by a continence advisor or clinical nurse specialist.

Lifestyle interventions

The patient needs to be educated about what she can do to improve things herself without any potential side-effects (Box 11.2).

Box 11.2

Lifestyle interventions
■ Normalize fluid intake (1.5 L per day). Many women drink too much, worsening frequency and incontinence, though many people with OAB over-restrict the amount of fluid they drink, increasing the risk of bladder irritation
■ Cut down alcohol and restrict caffeine. These drinks should constitute no more than a third of the total daily fluid intake
■ Lose weight if body mass index (BMI) >30
■ Stop smoking
■ Avoid carbonated drinks
■ Treat chronic constipation and chronic cough

Bladder retraining

This involves analysis and alteration of the patient's behaviour and her environment to alter her maladaptive voiding pattern, and should be offered for a minimum of 6 weeks. The objective is to re-establish cortical control over voiding. The woman's bladder diary is reviewed and based on this, the time interval between voids is increased to achieve a normal micturition pattern. To aid bladder retraining, various techniques are used, such as distraction techniques, doing something that requires concentration or pelvic floor squeezes.

Physiotherapy

A trial of supervised pelvic floor muscle training by a physiotherapist for at least 3 months is the first-line treatment for women with SUI and MUI. Treatment involves muscle training using pelvic floor exercises (Kegel exercises), which are repetitive voluntary contractions and relaxations of the pelvic floor muscles. The aim is to increase the strength of the voluntary pelvic floor muscle contraction and teach voluntary contraction of the muscles before increases in abdominal pressure (counter brace).

Biofeedback can be used as an adjunct to physiotherapy. It allows the patient to recognize the strength of an appropriate pelvic floor muscle contraction by verbal feedback during digital palpation, or electromyogenic feedback using vaginal electrodes.

Cones can be inserted vaginally for short periods to produce contractions to retain them. Patients exercise daily with increasing weights, retaining the cone for 10–20 min each time. There is no evidence that biofeedback or the use of vaginal cones is better than supervised pelvic floor exercises. However, in women who cannot actively contract their pelvic floor muscles it may aid motivation and adherence to treatment.

Drug therapy

Overactive bladder

There are several pharmacological treatments for UI, but anticholinergic medication remains the mainstay of medical treatment for the OAB. There are several preparations available with comparable effectiveness but they vary in their dosage, frequency side-effects, tolerability and cost. Some of the available anticholinergics are as follows:

- fesoterodine (Toviaz)
- solifenacin (Vesicare)
- oxybutynin (Lyrinel XL, Ditropan, Kentera)
- darifenacin (Emselex)
- tolterodine (Detrusitol and Detrusitol XL)
- trospium (Regurin XL)
- propiverine (Detrunorm XL).

They are effective in about 50% of women who will have up to 50% improvement. The main side-effects include dry mouth, dizziness, nausea and constipation, and may result in the woman discontinuing treatment. If treatment is not effective or well tolerated, then either the dose can be changed, an alternative anticholinergic drug can be offered or the drug can be administered transdermally.

Mirabegron is a beta-3 adrenoreceptor agonist that works by relaxing the bladder and helping the bladder to fill and store more urine. It is currently indicated in women in whom anticholinergics are contraindicated, ineffective or have unacceptable side-effects.

Stress urinary incontinence

Medical therapy for SUI comprises vaginal topical oestrogen and Duloxetine.

Vaginal oestrogens should be prescribed to all women with UI who are postmenopausal and have signs of vaginal atrophy, even if they are taking a systemic hormone replacement therapy.

Duloxetine is a combined serotonin and noradrenaline reuptake inhibitor licensed for use in moderate to severe SUI. Blockade of serotonin and noradrenaline reuptake in the spinal cord stimulates pudendal motor neurons, increasing stimulation of urethral striated muscles in the sphincter and enhancing contraction. Duloxetine improves SUI by increasing urethral closure pressure and electrical activity of the sphincter. Adverse effects are related to increases in noradrenaline and serotonin, and include gastrointestinal disturbances, dry mouth, headache and, rarely, suicidal ideology.

Surgery

Surgical treatment of SUI and OAB are entirely different, with the former condition usually responding to minimally invasive procedures. OAB, however, requires major surgery with significant risk of complications, and here, surgery is very much a last resort.

Surgery for SUI

There are various surgical procedures for SUI. The National Institute for Health and Clinical Excellence (NICE) currently recommends offering one of the following procedures:

1. MUS – mid-urethral sling (tension-free transvaginal tape)

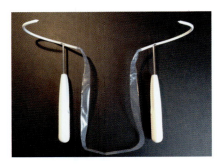

Fig. 11.2   Polypropylene mesh (tape).

2. Colposuspension
3. Autologous fascial sling
4. Bladder neck injections.

MUS is minimal access surgery that involves the passage of a small strip of tape (Fig. 11.2) through either the retropubic or obturator space, with entry or exit points at the lower abdomen or groin. The tape can be of different types depending on entry and exit wounds.

1. Retropubic tape (TVT)
2. Trans-obturator tape (TVT-O / TOT)
3. Mini sling

The tape is artificial non-absorbable synthetic material made of polypropylene and is microporous. The tape is left under the mid-urethra (between the urethra and vagina) without tension, being held by its serrated polypropylene edges into one or other part of the patient's connective tissue. Although the tape is effective from day 1, it takes several weeks before the tape is invaded by fibroblasts and then connective tissue is laid down in and around the tape, making it permanently fixed into the tissues. This forms a hammock which then prevents urethral hypermobility with increase in abdominal pressure, thus preventing leakage. For this reason, it is essential that the patient avoids any straining, heavy lifting or any other causes of increased intra-abdominal pressure for up to 10–12 weeks.

Retropubic tape (tension-free vaginal tape [TVT] – top bottom, bottom top)   This was the first tape to be developed and used clinically. It was introduced to UK practice in 1998. The tape is inserted vaginally, bypasses the bladder neck and bladder in the retropubic space and exits suprapubically (Fig. 11.3).

Trans-obturator tape (TVTO inside out or TOT outside in)   This procedure was first described in 2002. Here, after the same insertion point in the vagina, the tape is passed through the obturator membrane on either side and out towards the adipose tissue of the thigh (Fig. 11.4). TOT has the advantage over TVT of less risk of damage to the internal organs and voiding dysfunction but has significantly higher incidence of thigh pain (see Table 11.4).

Single incision tapes – 'mini tapes'   The first 'mini tape' was introduced with the proposed benefit of less likelihood of damage to vessels, nerves and pelvic organs, as passage through tissues was less.

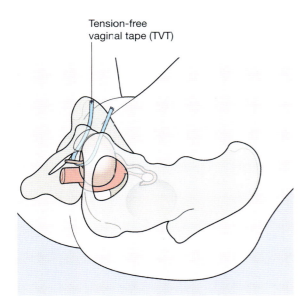

Tension-free
vaginal tape (TVT)

Fig. 11.3 **Tension-free vaginal tape.**

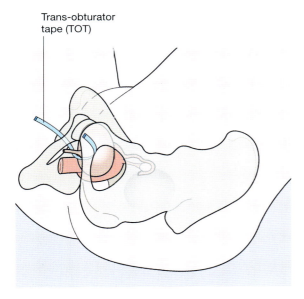

Trans-obturator
tape (TOT)

Fig. 11.4 **Trans-obturator tape.**

The tape is inserted through a similar vaginal incision but then anchored into the patient's tissues without exiting through the skin, hence the name 'single incision slings/tapes.'.

Overall success rates with tape procedures for SUI is 85–90%. Tapes are widely studied and are relatively safe procedures. Complications are infrequent and different for different types of tape (Table 11.4).

Women experiencing complications have raised concerns about the safety of tape devices. The current recommendation is to offer women all the options and appropriate treatment (tape and non-tape), as well as appropriate information

Table 11.4	Complications with MUS
Failure to cure SUI	10–15% (short term)
De novo OAB	5–15%
Voiding difficulty	5–10% short term (higher with TVTs)
	1–2% long term
Urinary infection	5%
Vaginal tape exposure	2–3%
Thigh pain	5–10% (higher with TOTs)
Operative blood loss	Higher with retropubic tapes
Bladder injury	5–8% (more with retropubic tapes)
Urethral trauma	1%

(patient information leaflets) to make informed choices. When surgery that involves the use of a tape is contemplated, the retropubic approach is recommended.

Open (Burch) colposuspension This is an abdominal operation (open or laparoscopic) where the bladder neck and base are elevated by suturing the upper lateral vaginal walls to the iliopectineal ligaments (Cooper's ligament).

The success is similar to MUS (85–90%) but it has higher complication rates, mainly short-term morbidity with a longer hospital stay and longer recovery, higher voiding difficulties (10–15%), detrusor overactivity and genitourinary prolapse (posterior vaginal wall prolapse). This procedure was commonly performed for SUI before MUS were introduced. However, with the recent controversies regarding the use of mesh for surgery for SUI, more women are now opting to have this procedure.

Biological sling surgery Sling procedures can be performed using either autologous or allograft material. When using autologous material (autologous fascial sling), a strip of rectus fascia is harvested from the abdominal wall or fascia lata from thigh, and is placed in a sling under the bladder neck, causing urethral closure when the sling is stretched.

Bladder neck injections The procedure involves injecting bulking agents composed of synthetic materials, bovine collagen, or autologous substances to augment the urethral wall at the level of proximal urethra to achieve better coaptation of urethral mucosa to increase urethral resistance to urinary flow (Fig. 11.5). This is a minimally invasive procedure and can be performed under local anaesthesia as a day case procedure. These are less effective than the other definitive procedures (66% success) and give temporary improvement in the symptoms, and hence injections need to be repeated after a few months. They are a good treatment choice for young women who have not completed their family, women not keen for definitive surgery or older women with several comorbidities who might not be fit for anaesthetic.

Surgery for an overactive bladder

If medical treatment fails, then the patient can be offered either intravesical Botox (botulinum toxin type A) or sacral nerve root stimulation. These are specialized procedures

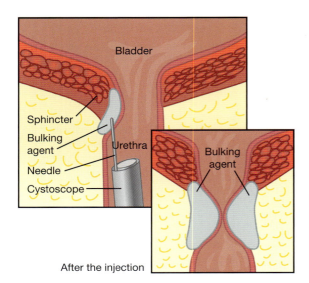

Bladder

Sphincter

Bulking agent

Needle

Cystoscope

Urethra

Bulking agent

After the injection

Fig. 11.5 Bladder neck injection.

and are performed by the urologist or a specialist urogy-naecologist. Rarely patients with OAB with small-capacity neurogenic bladder may require extensive surgery like urinary diversion, detrusor myomectomy or augmentation cystoplasty.

Treatment of voiding disorders

The treatment of voiding difficulty irrespective of underlying cause is clean intermittent self-catheterization (CISC) or an indwelling catheter (urethral or suprapubic) in women who are unable to perform CISC.

Treatment of genitourinary fistulae

If a period of indwelling catheterization fails to close the fistula, surgical correction will be required.

Key points

- Female UI is a common problem and is a major QOL issue.
- History taking and examination is the key step in patients' management as this helps to clinically diagnose the type of UI, which will help to direct initial treatment.
- Lifestyle advice is an essential starting point in the management of incontinence.
- The patient's expectation from treatment should be explored to increase patient satisfaction.

12

Ovarian neoplasms

Introduction

A neoplasm (tumour) is an abnormal mass of tissue that can be either benign or malignant (cancer). Ovarian neoplasms are classified into a wide range of benign and malignant groups, as well as an intermediate group termed borderline. Structurally they are found to be cystic (fluid filled), solid or mixed in appearance.

Ovarian cancer is the second most common of the gynaecological malignancies in most affluent countries (endometrial cancer being more common). In the UK, there are around 7000 newly diagnosed cases each year and approximately 4300 women annually die of the disease. The overall 5-year survival is around 40%.

Ovarian cancer occurs predominantly in the fifth, sixth and seventh decades of life, with the peak age being around 75 years. There are many histological types and subtypes of ovarian cancer, but epithelial ovarian cancer represents 90%.

Natural history

Unlike, for example, cervical cancer, there is no clearly defined precancerous ovarian lesion. Benign, borderline and invasive tumours are recognized, but these are distinct pathological entities and there is little evidence of progression from one to the other (Fig. 12.1). Indeed, there is even controversy about whether malignant epithelial tumours, which are the most common, arise from the ovary and then metastasize or arise as multicentric disease de novo. The multicentric theory is supported by the fact that ovarian-like tumours can arise in the peritoneum of women who have previously had both ovaries removed. Cancer in this case is called primary peritoneal cancer.

Aetiology

It is entirely possible that the different types of ovarian neoplasm have differing aetiologies, particularly as germ cell tumours, which account for 25% of ovarian neoplasms, occur in much younger women than do the epithelial tumours.

Reproductive history

Reproductive history is an important determinant of epithelial ovarian cancer risk. Nulliparous women have a higher risk than parous women and the risk is inversely correlated with parity (Fig. 12.2). Additionally, breast feeding reduces this risk. It is thought that the number of ovulation events in a woman's reproductive life is the main risk factor.

Exogenous oestrogens

Oral contraceptives

Overwhelming evidence now exists that women who have used the combined oral contraceptive pill at some stage in the past have a reduced risk of developing ovarian cancer. The longer the use, the lower the risk. This is again thought to be through the reduction in the number of ovulation events.

Hormone replacement therapy (HRT)

In postmenopausal women, the effect of oestrogen replacement therapy has been investigated because of a reported increased risk in women who received diethylstilboestrol (a non-steroidal oestrogen) early in life. The balance of evidence, however, suggests that HRT has no significant effect on ovarian cancer risk.

Repeated (incessant) ovulation

It has been suggested that the more often a woman ovulates, the greater the risk of ovarian carcinoma. The apparently protective effects of both pregnancy and the combined oral contraceptive pill further support this theory. The mechanism is uncertain, but it may be that repeated monthly repair of the ovarian epithelium after ovulation predisposes to malignant change. Despite this plausible theory, however, it is likely that ovarian carcinogenesis is multifactorial.

Genetic factors

It is now accepted that a genetic predisposition exists in at least a proportion of ovarian cancer cases. Although overall

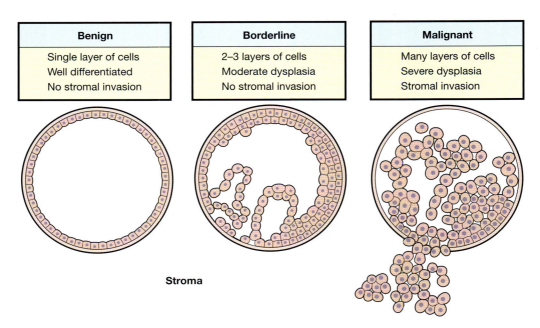

Benign	Borderline	Malignant
Single layer of cells	2–3 layers of cells	Many layers of cells
Well differentiated	Moderate dysplasia	Severe dysplasia
No stromal invasion	No stromal invasion	Stromal invasion

Stroma

Fig. 12.1 **Morphology and behaviour of surface epithelium–derived neoplasms.**

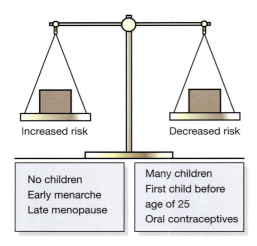

Increased risk   Decreased risk

No children	Many children
Early menarche	First child before age of 25
Late menopause	Oral contraceptives

Fig. 12.2 **Risk factors in ovarian cancer.**

there is a slightly increased risk of ovarian cancer in those with a family history, the risk is small for most categories, except for those of early onset and those with more than one affected first-degree relative. If one affected primary relative has ovarian cancer and the cancer was diagnosed when she was <50 years old, a woman's risk of developing ovarian cancer is around 5%. If there are two primary relatives under the age of 50 years with the disease, the risk is approximately 25%.

Only 5–10% of cases of ovarian carcinoma, however, have a direct genetic association. Of particular significance in this small group are the breast–ovarian cancer tumour suppressor genes *BRCA1* and *BRCA2*, as these are associated with a 10–50% lifetime risk of developing ovarian carcinoma. Mismatch repair genes associated with cancer of the colorectum, endometrium, stomach, urinary tract and small bowel are also responsible for a small proportion of this hereditary group. Women with such a history may warrant regular screening, and it is reasonable to consider bilateral oophorectomy after completion of their family. Such an operation will substantially reduce the risk but will not prevent primary peritoneal carcinoma.

Other factors

There has been controversy about the possible role of talcum powder in the aetiology of ovarian cancer. Insufficient evidence in the form of case–control studies exists to completely dismiss reported associations. Similar problems beset the assessment of smoking, diet and alcohol consumption. Endometriosis is thought to increase the risk.

Pathology

Neoplasms can arise from any of the elements that comprise a mature ovary, including its surface serosal or mesothelial elements (Fig. 12.3). A number of simpler themes can be drawn from a wide diversity of tumour types, namely: epithelial tumours, which are by far the most common (70% of primary ovarian tumours [benign and cancerous]); sex cord/stromal tumours; germ cell tumours; and secondary metastatic tumours (Table 12.1). Most of the epithelial tumour types can be further broadly classified as benign, borderline or malignant.

Table 12.1	Pathology of ovarian tumours		
Type	**Subtype**		
Epithelial	Serous	Common	Benign and malignant
	Mucinous	Common	Benign and malignant; associated with pseudomyxoma peritonei
	Endometrioid	Uncommon	Usually malignant
	Clear cell	Uncommon	Usually malignant
	Urothelial-like (Brenner)	Uncommon	Rarely malignant
	Borderline	Common	Separate clinical entity; do not invade
Sex cord/stromal	Granulosa cell	Rare	Low grade; often secrete sex hormones
	Thecoma/fibroma	Uncommon	Rarely malignant; may secrete sex hormones; Meigs syndrome
	Sertoli/Leydig	Rare	May secrete sex hormones
Germ cell tumours	No differentiation	Rare	Dysgerminoma; may secrete hCG
	Extra-embryonic differentiation	Rare	Yolk sac tumours (endodermal sinus tumours), malignant ovarian choriocarcinoma
	Embryonic differentiation (teratoma)	Common	Mature teratomas (benign) may contain epithelium, hair, teeth and greasy white sebum; immature (malignant) are rare
Metastases		Common	Especially endometrial, gastrointestinal tract and breast

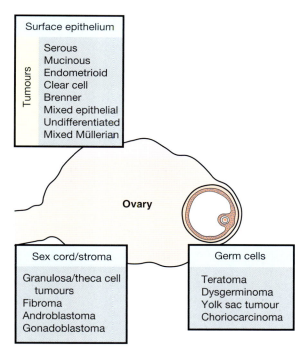

Surface epithelium

Tumours

Serous
Mucinous
Endometrioid
Clear cell
Brenner
Mixed epithelial
Undifferentiated
Mixed Müllerian

Ovary

Sex cord/stroma

Granulosa/theca cell tumours
Fibroma
Androblastoma
Gonadoblastoma

Germ cells

Teratoma
Dysgerminoma
Yolk sac tumour
Choriocarcinoma

Fig. 12.3 **Ovarian neoplasms arise from three basic tissue components.**

Borderline tumours

The term 'borderline' is reserved for tumours that display some of the characteristics of malignant tumours but show no evidence of stromal invasion. Women with borderline ovarian tumours have a much better prognosis than those with frankly malignant tumours. Nevertheless, long-term survival is by no means as high as might be expected and late recurrence up to 20 years after removal of the primary tumour can occur. Despite lacking the features of invasion, these tumours may present at an advanced stage, raising the possibility of multicentric origin. The treatment of these is predominantly surgical as they tend to be resistant to chemotherapy.

Epithelial tumours

These arise from the surface epithelium of the ovary.

Serous tumours

Serous tumours are the most common ovarian neoplasm, accounting for almost 50% of ovarian cancers. They also account for 20% of all benign ovarian tumours, and these cases occur primarily in women of reproductive age. Serous cystadenomas (benign) are usually unilocular cysts filled with straw-coloured (serous) fluid and are of variable size (Fig. 12.4). They are bilateral in 20% of cases. Serous cystadenocarcinomas involve both ovaries in over 50% of cases and may have both cystic and solid components. Psammoma bodies, concentrically laminated calcified concretions, are a frequent histological finding.

Mucinous tumours

These comprise 20% of all ovarian tumours and less than 10% are malignant. Benign tumours are usually unilateral and only 20% of malignant tumours are bilateral. Mucinous tumours are usually multiloculated and contain mucinous fluid of variable viscosity. They are generally the largest of the common epithelial tumours. Uncommonly, concomitant pseudomyxoma peritonei may be present. This is

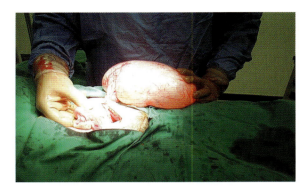

Fig. 12.4 **A unilateral benign cystadenoma.**

characterized by a characteristic gelatinous tumour within the peritoneal cavity. It is unclear to what extent pseudo-myxoma peritonei truly arises from the ovary rather than from a primary mucinous tumour of the appendix.

Endometrioid tumours

Endometrioid tumours are usually malignant and closely mimic endometrial cancer in histological appearance. In around 30% of cases there is a coexistent second primary in the endometrium.

Clear cell tumours

These are virtually all malignant and may be a variant of endometrioid tumours. They are the most frequent epithelial tumour found in association with ovarian endometriosis. It must be emphasized, however, that ovarian cancer developing from endometriosis is uncommon.

Urothelial-like tumours

Urothelial-like or Brenner tumours are uncommon, usually unilateral and rarely malignant. They in part comprise epithelium of urothelial type but their main component is ovarian stroma. A rare aggressive variant is the urothelial or transitional cell carcinoma.

Sex cord/stromal tumours

This is a group of rare neoplasms that comprise <5% of all ovarian tumours.

Granulosa cell tumours

These are functional, low-grade cancers and account for around 5% of ovarian malignancies. Three-quarters secrete sex hormones, most commonly oestrogen, which in turn may lead to precocious pseudopuberty, irregular menstrual bleeding or postmenopausal bleeding, depending on the age of presentation. They tend to recur late but can be monitored with serum oestradiol measurements. Characteristically they contain cells with 'coffee bean' nuclei and 'gland-like' spaces called Call–Exner bodies, which are pathognomonic.

Thecoma/fibroma

These tumours are usually unilateral and rarely malignant. They contain cells ranging from theca cells to fibroblastic-type cells. Tumours containing the former are oestrogenic, although they are less common than granulosa cell tumours. Rarely, ovarian fibromas may present with non-malignant ascites and pleural effusion, which resolve after removal of the tumour (Meigs syndrome).

Sertoli/leydig cell tumours

These are among the rarest ovarian tumours, accounting for <1% of such. They occur in young women, the mean age being in the mid-20s. They are almost invariably unilateral and are commonly androgenic, though many are nonfunctional and only a few are oestrogenic. They contain either Sertoli cells or Leydig cells, and in the case of the latter, may be accompanied by stroma-derived fibroblasts.

Germ cell tumours

This heterogeneous group of tumours affects mainly children and young women, and comprises 20–25% of all ovarian tumours. Only around 4% are malignant. However, they represent the majority of ovarian tumours in children, where around one-third are malignant.

Teratoma

Teratomas are colloquially known as ovarian dermoid cysts, and these are almost always benign and are very common. They characteristically contain elements from all three embryonic germ cell layers and are thought to occur via parthenogenesis, a form of reproduction in which the ovum develops without fertilization. Mature teratomas may contain epithelium, hair, teeth and greasy white sebum, and constitute 20% of all ovarian neoplasms. They are commonest in women in their 20s but account for 50% of ovarian neoplasms in females under 20 years. Malignant change, usually squamous cell, is rare (<1%) and usually occurs in postmenopausal women.

Immature teratomas are rare, characteristically occurring in children under 15 years of age. Specialized tissue derivatives from a single germ layer are found in 3% of teratomas, notably among those with predominantly thyroid tissue (struma ovarii) and carcinoid tumours.

Dysgerminoma

Dysgerminoma is the most common malignant germ cell tumour, comprising at least 50% of this group. Nevertheless, it is relatively uncommon and represents only 3% of all ovarian cancers. Some 75% occur in females aged 10–30 years, the median being 22 years, and it is the most frequently encountered ovarian malignancy in pregnancy. It is also the malignancy most likely to be associated with gonadoblastoma in gonadal dysgenesis. At least 10% are bilateral and there may be a raised serum human chorionic gonadotrophin (hCG) level.

Endodermal sinus or yolk sac tumour

This is the second most common malignant germ cell tumour of the ovary but comprises only 1% of all ovarian cancers. It rarely affects women over 40, the median age being 19 years. Presentation is commonly with a sudden onset of pelvic symptoms and a pelvic mass. Elevated serum levels of alpha-fetoprotein are found with normal hCG levels. Coexistent teratomas are found in 20% of patients.

Choriocarcinoma

These secrete hCG and may present with precocious pseudopuberty. They have a poor prognosis and do not respond well to chemotherapy (unlike uterine trophoblastic disease).

Metastatic tumours

Secondary tumours in the ovaries are surprisingly common. Cervical cancer only rarely metastasizes to the ovaries, but spread from endometrial cancer is far more frequent. Breast cancer may also metastasize to the ovaries, and patients presenting with single or bilateral ovarian masses should be examined carefully to exclude a breast lesion.

Cancers of the gastrointestinal tract also metastasize to the ovary, and in the case of gastric cancer give rise to the so-called Krukenberg tumour. This contains mucin-producing 'signet ring' adenocarcinoma cells. Such tumours may elicit a stromal response in the ovary, which may cause hormone production; as a result, virilization may be a presenting complaint. In such cases, confusion with sex cord/stromal tumours is possible, although these, unlike Krukenberg tumours, are usually unilateral.

Spread

Ovarian cancer spreads trans-coelomically, whereby a tumour is 'seeded' within the peritoneal cavity onto the surfaces of the intraperitoneal structures and organs. Those who die usually do so from intestinal obstruction and cachexia as a consequence of widespread intraperitoneal disease. Malignant pleural effusions are seen, and para-aortic lymph node metastases are found in up to 18% of cases where the disease appears otherwise to be confined to the ovary.

Presentation

As a rule, ovarian cancer tends to present at a late stage. Occasionally, ovarian cancers are diagnosed incidentally during pelvic or abdominal palpation for another reason. This mode of presentation, however, is the exception rather than the rule. In general the symptoms are diverse and non-specific. As a result, patients often do not recognize the sinister nature of their symptoms, and the disease

Table 12.2	Symptoms in ovarian cancer
Symptom	**% of patients**
Pain (late symptom)	50–60
Abdominal swelling (persistent bloating)	50–65
Anorexia	20
Nausea and vomiting	20
Weight loss	15
Abnormal vaginal bleeding	15
Frequency	10
Malaise	5
Change in bowel habit	5
Virilization	Rare
Precocious puberty	Rare

Table 12.3	Signs of ovarian cancer
Sign	**% of patients**
Pelvic mass	70–80
Abdominal mass	60–70
Ascites	30–40
Pleural effusion	10–15
Hepatomegaly	<5
Cervical lymphadenopathy	<5

progresses insidiously until they develop gastrointestinal complications or bowel obstruction secondary to widespread intraperitoneal malignancy. This is the reason for a new guideline from the National Institute for Health and Care Excellence (NICE) emphasizing the importance of investigating persistent non-specific symptoms.

The varied nature of these symptoms results in many cases being referred to inappropriate specialties for investigation. The most frequent complaint is abdominal distension due either to ascites or masses (Table 12.2). The most common clinical signs are an abdominal or pelvic mass and ascites (Table 12.3).

Investigation and staging

Adopting a low index of suspicion, investigation is often with ultrasound and tumour markers. The risk of malignancy index (RMI) aids in the differentiation of benign from malignant lesions (RMI = ultrasound score × menopausal score × CA125). If the index of suspicion is high, then computed tomography (CT) or magnetic resonance imaging can be used in addition to the tumour markers to examine the pelvis, and to look for peritoneal spread, ascites, liver metastases and ureteric obstruction. An X-ray or CT scan of the chest is important to look for pleural effusions or macroscopic chest disease. An open mind needs to be kept, as a proportion of these patients will have cancers other than ovary, such as bowel, pancreatic, etc. Until a

Table 12.4 Staging of ovarian cancer

Stage	Definition	5-year survival
I$_A$	One ovary	
I$_B$	Both ovaries	60–70%, but can be 95% for I$_A$
I$_C$	I$_A$ or I$_B$ with ruptured capsule, tumour on the surface of the capsule, positive peritoneal washings or malignant ascites	
II$_A$	Extension to uterus and tubes	
II$_B$	Extension to other pelvic tissues, e.g. pelvic nodes, pouch of Douglas	50%
II$_C$	II$_A$ or II$_B$ with ruptured capsule, positive peritoneal washings or malignant ascites	
III$_A$	Pelvic tumour with microscopic peritoneal spread	
III$_B$	Pelvic tumour with peritoneal spread <2 cm	20%
III$_C$	Abdominal implants >2 cm ± positive retroperitoneal or inguinal nodes (Fig. 12.5)	
IV	Liver parenchymal disease. Distant metastases. If pleural effusion, must have malignant cells	6%

Additional sources
www.cancerresearchuk.org

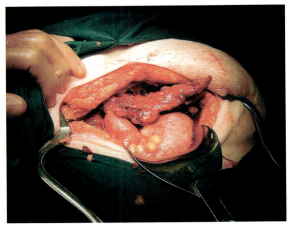

Fig. 12.5 **The omentum in this stage III$_C$ cystadenocarcinoma is almost completely replaced with tumour.** Optimal debulking was not achieved.

mass has been assessed histopathologically, it is never possible to be certain of its exact nature. Across the UK any suspected ovarian cancer should be referred to a specialist gynaecological-oncology team, who will assess the potential diagnosis and decide upon appropriate management through a multidisciplinary meeting. This team comprises gynaecological surgeons, oncology physicians, radiologists and pathologists, among other specialists such as nurse specialists. It is through this process that the management of all gynaecological cancers will be determined.

Ovarian cancer is staged surgically according to the International Federation of Gynecology and Obstetrics system (Table 12.4).

Tumour markers

Around 80% of epithelial ovarian cancers are associated with elevated levels of a tumour marker (blood test) called CA125. This marker is of value in the assessment of patients presenting with pelvic masses, as well as in sequentially monitoring the response to treatment and to help identify presymptomatic relapse during follow-up. However, CA125 may also be elevated in the serum of women with benign conditions, such as endometriosis, or where peritoneal irritation has taken place. It can also be elevated in cardiac failure (particularly right-sided), hepatic failure and some systemic inflammatory conditions. A positive result, therefore,

while suggestive of ovarian cancer, is not diagnostic. Conversely, a negative result for tumour markers does not exclude a diagnosis of ovarian cancer, as 50% of stage 1 (confined to the ovary) ovarian cancers will have a normal CA125.

About 65% of ovarian germ cell tumours produce elevated serum levels of hCG, alpha-fetoprotein or both. These markers can again, if elevated, be very useful in monitoring response to therapy and in detecting tumour recurrence after completion of therapy.

Treatment

Benign tumours

Benign tumours require either excision or possibly drainage under laparoscopic control. There may be difficulties in deciding whether a cyst is benign or malignant. In general, ovarian cysts in young women tend to be benign and the risk of malignancy increases with age. A cyst is often assumed at surgery to be benign if it is unilateral and unilocular with smooth external and internal surfaces, and no solid elements (Fig. 12.4). Although not conforming to this rule, teratomas are benign and the diagnosis is usually obvious when they are opened after removal.

Epithelial cancers

Most patients with epithelial ovarian cancer present late and the overall survival is poor (Fig. 12.5). Because of this and because of new developments, particularly with chemotherapeutic agents, the modern approach to treatment is to consider ovarian cancer as a chronic disease. This means that the tumour is primarily treated with the aim of achieving remission but accepting that the tumour will probably become active again in the future. When this occurs, further treatment to achieve control will be given. In this way, while most patients will not be cured in the conventional sense, many patients will have a prolonged period of good-quality life.

Treatment is usually a combination of surgery and chemotherapy. Traditionally, this has been in the form of aggressive surgery attempting to remove all areas of the tumour and including removal of both ovaries, the uterus and omentum. Complete removal of the tumour is often unrealistic, however, and the concept of surgical debulking has arisen. This is where the tumour deposits are removed as far as possible, aiming to reduce the size of deposits to below 1 or 2 cm in dimension. Chemotherapy will almost certainly be used as well. In this setting, it is called 'adjuvant chemotherapy'. There are many active chemotherapeutic agents that can be used in ovarian cancer. In the first-line setting, the current standard is platinum based. This is usually carboplatin, which will usually be combined with a taxane. This chemotherapy is given over six cycles and usually in the outpatient setting.

Recently, in many cancer centres, a different approach has been adopted for the most advanced cases of ovarian cancer. These patients are frequently unfit and, with the advent of CT imaging, it is easier to identify patients in whom surgery will achieve little. In these cases, after histological confirmation with image-guided needle biopsy, chemotherapy is used first of all rather than surgery. Surgery will usually be considered midway through the chemotherapy treatment. The effect of this is a more rapid control of the cancer and a reduction in the surgical-related morbidity. This approach of neoadjuvant chemotherapy followed by surgery has been evaluated by randomized trial and reduces postoperative morbidity and mortality without compromising overall cancer survival.

Most patients with advanced ovarian cancer will relapse at some point after primary treatment. In this situation, further chemotherapy will usually be considered. The specific type of chemotherapy will depend upon the chemotherapy that has been used in the past, as well as the interval since chemotherapy was last used. In the case of the first relapse, if the interval since treatment is significant, then a further challenge with carboplatin will frequently be tried. Other drugs include the taxanes, topotecan and Caelyx, and, more recently, Avastin. Ideally, patients should be considered for entry into clinical trials, as the evidence suggests that patients who are entered into trials tend to have better outcomes. Many patients will have several lines of chemotherapy over a number of years before eventually dying of their disease. As most patients will eventually die of their disease progression, it is important to consider formal palliative care when appropriate.

In young women who wish fertility to be preserved and in whom the disease appears confined to one ovary, it is reasonable to consider conservative surgery. The other ovary and omentum, a common site for metastases, should be

biopsied and a thorough inspection made of all peritoneal surfaces.

Non-epithelial tumours

These tumours frequently occur in young women where preservation of fertility is an important consideration. It is also clear that many of these tumours, especially those of germ cell origin, are exquisitely sensitive to chemotherapy, and radical surgery is therefore inappropriate. Extremely good survival can be achieved with limited surgery and subsequent combination chemotherapy.

Survival

It is difficult to accurately estimate survival and the rate depends upon methodology and definitions. Overall 5-year survival (all stages) is in the order of 40% (Table 12.4). Although the overall prognosis from ovarian cancer is poor, the 5-year survival has improved markedly over the past three decades. A better prognosis can be expected for women with malignant germ cell tumours, where the reported 5-year survival from most studies is in excess of 75%.

The only real prospect for improving survival in epithelial cancers is either detection at an early stage or development of better chemotherapy. Screening is still the subject of research, with trials involving the combination of tumour markers (such as CA125) and ultrasound. At present, it seems unlikely that screening and early detection of low-risk groups is going to be a useful proposition.

Key points

- Ovarian cancer is the second commonest gynaecological cancer. There are around 7000 newly diagnosed cases each year in the UK. The 5-year survival is about 40%.
- Unlike cervical cancer, there is no recognized premalignant stage and most new cases present with advanced disease (stage III or IV).
- Genetic factors have been identified (e.g. the *BRCA1* and *BRCA2* tumour suppressor genes), which identify a small proportion of women at risk. Other risk factors include low parity. Use of the oral contraceptive pill protects against ovarian cancer.
- Presentation is usually with vague abdominal symptoms, pelvic mass and malaise. Treatment is primarily surgical, although advances have been seen recently in chemotherapy, particularly with platinum-based drugs, taxanes and Avastin. Patients with advanced disease at presentation will often have histological confirmation followed by chemotherapy and then surgery.
- Research strategies are directed towards earlier diagnosis and improved chemotherapies. Currently available tests do not fulfil the criteria for a screening programme aimed at low-risk women.

13

Uterine neoplasia

Introduction

The uterus consists of both the cervix and the body (or 'corpus' of the uterus). For many reasons, including their causative factors and their treatment, tumours arising from the corpus and the cervix are usually regarded as originating from two separate organs. This chapter will consider cancers arising from the uterine body; cancers arising from the cervix are discussed in Chapter 14.

The majority of malignancies arising from the uterine body arise from the endometrium. The endometrium consists of both glandular and supporting (or 'stromal') elements, and it is possible for either to undergo malignant change. The majority of uterine malignancies are adenocarcinomas arising from the endometrial glands (Figs 13.1 and 13.2A). Sarcomas of the muscle of the uterus, the myometrium or the stromal tissues of the endometrium are much rarer (Fig. 13.2B).

Incidence

In the UK, the incidence of endometrial cancer has been increasing and it is now the fourth most common cancer in women after breast, bowel and lung cancers. There are around 9000 cases diagnosed in the UK annually.

Approximately 90% of cases will be diagnosed after the menopause whereas only around 1% of endometrial carcinomas will develop in women under the age of 40. There is evidence that the incidence is rising in developed countries.

Aetiology

The majority of endometrial cancers are associated with conditions in which there are prolonged high levels of oestrogen production, and it is therefore postulated that oestrogen has a role in the development of the disease (Box 13.1).

High levels of oestrogen may be physiological, as with obesity (due to the aromatization in body fat of peripheral androgens to oestrogens), or with conditions such as polycystic ovarian syndrome (due to long-term anovulation) and late menopause. It is thought that a third of cases are related to obesity. Being obese increases one's risk several-fold. The relationship between diabetes/hypertension and endometrial cancer is possibly a result of the increased incidence of obesity in these groups of women, although the role of insulin has been questioned. Nonphysiological causes of increased oestrogen include unopposed (without progesterone to protect the endometrium) oestrogen hormone replacement therapy (HRT), which increases the risk four-fold. This risk is reduced to a relative risk of <1.0 with opposed HRT (i.e. with the addition of progestogen for at least 10 days per cycle). Tamoxifen, a drug with oestrogenic characteristics that is commonly used in the treatment of breast cancer, also increases the risk. Oestrogen-secreting tumours, which are rare, also increase the risk of endometrial carcinoma.

Endometrial cancer is also seen less frequently in women who have used the combined oral contraceptive pill, probably because it administers progestogens throughout the cycle. Women who smoke, and are therefore likely to reach an earlier menopause, also have a lower than expected incidence of the disease.

The more common and oestrogen-dependent type of endometrial cancer is sometimes called type I disease and is seen in women around the time of the menopause or soon after. It is generally diagnosed at an earlier stage and as a result has a better prognosis. There may be premalignant change (see Endometrial hyperplasia, later) and the tumour cells of type I disease usually have oestrogen and progesterone receptors. This form of the cancer has characteristic growth factor alterations that distinguish it from normal endometrium.

Type II endometrial cancer is probably not related to oestrogen production. It is seen in older women, progresses more rapidly and is not associated with a hyperplastic or in situ phase. The chances of surviving 5 years with this type of cancer are considerably lower than for the type I form, even with early-stage disease.

Clinical features and diagnosis

Abnormal uterine bleeding is the cardinal symptom of endometrial carcinoma. The bleeding is most commonly

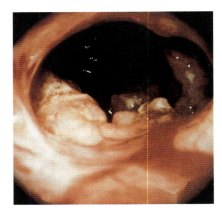

Fig. 13.1 **A hysteroscopic view of an endometrial carcinoma arising from the posterior uterine wall.** (Courtesy of Karl Storz Endoscopy (UK) Ltd.)

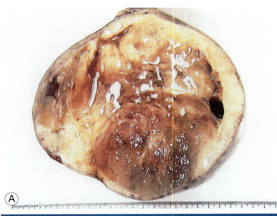

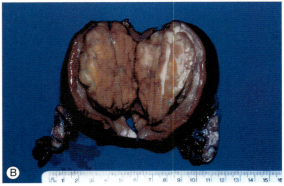

Fig. 13.2 **Macroscopic picture of (A) endometrial carcinoma and (B) endometrial sarcoma.** (Courtesy of Dr N Wilkinson, Department of Pathology, Leeds.)

postmenopausal, and women with this symptom should be regarded as having malignancy until proven otherwise. Around 5% of women with postmenopausal bleeding will have a primary or secondary malignancy, most commonly endometrial cancer (80%), cervical cancer or (rarely) an

---

Box 13.1

Risk factors for endometrial carcinoma

Increase risk

- Obesity, especially upper body obesity
- Nulliparity
- Late menopause
- Unopposed oestrogen therapy, including tamoxifen
- Oestrogen-secreting tumours (granulosa/theca cell ovarian tumours)
- Carbohydrate intolerance
- Polycystic ovary syndrome
- Personal history of breast or colon cancer
- Family history of breast, colon or endometrial cancer

Decrease risk

- The combined oral contraceptive pill
- Progestogens

---

ovarian tumour. As the condition can occur in premenopausal women, any irregular uterine bleeding in those over 40 years of age should also be investigated, especially if the patient is obese or has other risk factors

A less common mode of presentation in the postmenopausal group is that of vaginal discharge – either blood stained, watery or purulent. Pain is rarely associated with early disease and usually indicates metastatic spread. Endometrial carcinoma can also present with abnormal cells on a smear consistent with endometrial origin.

Mode of spread is principally direct and will usually involve the myometrium to a greater or lesser degree. The cervix, fallopian tubes, as well as the local supporting tissues (parametrium) can also become involved with more locally advanced cases. Lymphatic and haematogenous spread may also occur.

There are four main methods of investigation, listed as follows. The method chosen depends on the patient's risk factors and the local facilities. In current practice, most patients will be investigated through dedicated clinics with pre-defined investigative protocols. In many cases, these clinics will be 'one stop', where all investigations are performed in one sitting.

Ultrasound

Transvaginal scanning, often a first-line investigation, can be used to measure the endometrial thickness and character in postmenopausal women (Fig. 13.3). If the thickness is less than 4 mm and the endometrium smooth and regular, endometrial cancer is very unlikely.

Endometrial biopsy

An outpatient biopsy can be obtained using one of a number of samplers, for example the Pipelle (Fig. 13.4). The Pipelle is a thin (3 mm diameter) plastic tube with a plunger that is withdrawn to suck a sample of tissue into the tube for subsequent histological analysis. The Pipelle is passed through the cervix to obtain a sample of endometrium.

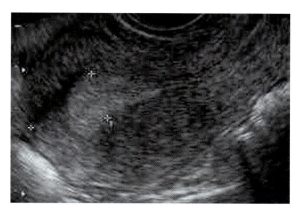

Fig. 13.3   Transvaginal ultrasound image demonstrating thickened endometrium. (Courtesy of Dr C Hardwick, Glasgow.)

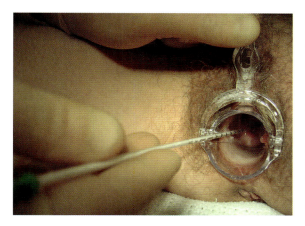

Fig. 13.4   Pipelle endometrial biopsy.

Dilatation and curettage

This procedure is usually carried out under general anaesthesia and is combined with hysteroscopy. The cervix is dilated sufficiently to allow the introduction of a sharp curette, an instrument that scrapes off the endometrium for histological analysis. This used to be standard of care but is now being superseded by less invasive methods. It is rarely used alone now, being combined with hysteroscopy in cases where additional investigations are required.

Hysteroscopy

The inside of the uterine cavity can be visualized directly using a hysteroscope (fine telescope), which can be introduced with or without anaesthesia depending on the instrument and the local facilities (Fig. 13.1). Biopsy or curettage (see previously) can also be performed at the same time. Hysteroscopy with biopsy is considered to be the 'gold standard' investigation.

Pathology

Endometrial pathology can be divided into hyperplasia, carcinoma or sarcoma.

Endometrial hyperplasia

Prolonged endometrial hyperplasia is a potential risk factor that is thought to result from persistent and prolonged oestrogenic stimulation of the endometrium. Hyperplasia is characterized by an increased number of endometrial cells due to proliferation and this results in a thicker endometrium. The nomenclature of this condition is confusing and the terms 'simple hyperplasia', 'glandular hyperplasia', 'cystic glandular hyperplasia' and 'endometrial hyperplasia' are synonymous. There have been many revisions, but since 2014 the World Health Organization has suggested simplifying to a binary classification on the basis of the presence or absence of cellular atypia: viz. hyperplasia without atypia and hyperplasia with atypia. The atypia may be severe enough to create difficulty in distinguishing the hyperplastic state from a well-differentiated carcinoma.

To diagnose hyperplasia histologically, there should be an increase in the gland-to-stromal ratio. The glands may vary in size and shape or they may branch abnormally. Cytological atypia includes a loss of polarity of cells within the glands, an increase in the nuclear–cytoplasmic ratio and nuclear irregularity with hyperchromatic changes, chromatin clumping and prominent nucleoli. This atypia is the only feature distinguishing benign endometrial lesions from those with invasive potential.

Atypical hyperplasia with cytological atypia coexists with endometrial carcinoma in 5–30% of cases, and many will progress to carcinoma. This progression depends on the severity of atypia and it is thought that about 10–20% will develop carcinoma within 10 years.

Hyperplasia is usually discovered by endometrial biopsy as part of the investigation of abnormal uterine bleeding. 'Simple' hyperplasia without atypia often occurs in anovulatory teenagers and in the perimenopausal years. It is common to treat hyperplasia with progestogens in young women. The Mirena intrauterine device, which delivers progesterone to the endometrium, is often used to manage abnormal uterine bleeding in premenopausal women and is likely to have a protective effect in those with endometrial hyperplasia. Hysterectomy is the usual recommendation in those with atypical hyperplasia.

Endometrial carcinoma

Endometrial adenocarcinoma can have a variety of histological appearances depending upon whether it is purely glandular or has areas of squamous differentiation (which may appear malignant or benign), or whether it demonstrates a papillary or clear cell pattern. The latter two forms are associated with a poorer prognosis.

Endometrial sarcoma

Endometrial sarcoma is very rare. It tends to be a locally aggressive tumour that metastasizes early and is generally characterized by a poor prognosis.

Prognostic factors

Endometrial cancer is falsely regarded as a less aggressive tumour than other gynaecological malignancies, but this is simply because it more commonly presents at an earlier stage (Table 13.1). Stage-for-stage, endometrial cancer has a prognosis similar to that of cancer of the cervix. There are many factors that affect the prognosis, the most obvious being the stage of disease. This is an indication of how far the cancer has spread, as well as how aggressive the tumour is. The histological type of endometrial cancer is also important. Papillary serous cancer, which is more common in older women, spreads in a manner similar to cancer of the ovary and is associated with a significantly poorer prognosis. Other factors that affect the prognosis are outlined in Box 13.2.

Table 13.1	FIGO staging of endometrial carcinoma
Carcinoma of the endometrium FIGO 2009 scheme	
IA	Tumour confined to the uterus, no or $<\frac{1}{2}$ myometrial invasion
IB	Tumour confined to the uterus, $>\frac{1}{2}$ myometrial invasion
II	Cervical stromal invasion, but not beyond uterus
IIIA	Tumour invades serosa or adnexa
IIIB	Vaginal and/or parametrial involvement
IIIC1	Pelvic node involvement
IIIC2	Para-aortic involvement
IVA	Tumour invasion bladder and/or bowel mucosa
IVB	Distant metastases including abdominal metastases and/or inguinal lymph nodes

Uterine sarcomas were staged previously as endometrial cancers, which did not reflect clinical behaviour. Therefore, a new corpus sarcoma staging system was developed based on the criteria used in other soft tissue sarcomas.

Box 13.2

Prognostic factors in endometrial cancer
- Histological type
- Histological differentiation
- Stage of disease
- Myometrial invasion
- Peritoneal cytology
- Lymph node metastasis
- Adnexal metastasis

Treatment

Endometrial carcinoma is staged using the International Federation of Gynecology and Obstetrics (FIGO) scheme (Table 13.1). This is a surgico–pathological system based on histology results from the excised uterus, tubes, ovaries and lymph nodes. Before operating, most patients will be investigated with cross-sectional imaging, usually in the form of a magnetic resonance imaging (MRI) scan. This is to determine the degree of involvement of the local tissues as well as to allow an assessment of the lymph nodes. Sometimes computed tomography scanning is used, but MRI gives a better indication of local infiltration (Fig. 13.5).

The mainstay of treatment is surgical, in the form of hysterectomy and bilateral salpingo-oophorectomy. This procedure is often performed laparoscopically, which reduces length of stay and improves recovery time. Usually peritoneal cytology is sent, although this is not currently part of the FIGO staging. There is debate as to whether the pelvic lymph nodes should be removed, sampled or left alone. The balance is the trade-off between potential complications and the additional information (positive or negative) that each option brings. Having certainty of a negative lymph node status can reduce or limit the extent of adjuvant radiotherapy. If, during the preoperative investigations or at the time of laparotomy, the disease is discovered to have

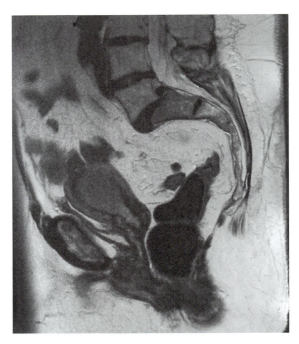

Fig. 13.5   A sagittal image through the uterus, showing the endometrial cavity distended by tumour. The tumour extends into the endocervical canal and is invasive posteriorly at the fundus. (Courtesy of Dr S Swift, Department of Radiology, St James's Hospital, Leeds.)

spread beyond the uterus, treatment should be individualized and is often focused upon gaining control of the local tumour. Treatment of disease in the fallopian tubes or ovaries is with surgery, followed with adjuvant treatment. More widespread tumour, however, should be managed depending on the degree and location of spread and the condition of the patient.

The treatment of those with endometrial cancer after surgery is related to the stage of the disease (Table 13.1). Radiotherapy may be used as an adjuvant (postoperative) treatment if the tumour invades the myometrium deeply, as there is a statistically higher risk of extrauterine disease. Local radiotherapy to the vault of the vagina (brachytherapy) may prevent recurrence developing in this area. Radiotherapy to the whole pelvis (external beam radiotherapy) will also prevent local disease recurring in this area but, surprisingly, does not improve overall survival. An argument for performing formal lymphadenectomy is that if the nodes are free of tumour, then radiotherapy can be avoided in cases that might otherwise have been irradiated.

Radiotherapy may be used for treatment of local disease if the patient is medically unfit for major surgery. However, this is becoming less common as most patients' comorbidity can be optimized for surgery. For more advanced lesions whole-pelvic radiotherapy may be used.

If disease is widespread, chemotherapy may be considered. The drugs most helpful in this situation are cisplatinum and doxorubicin. Once again, their influence on survival is controversial, as response rates to measurable disease are only in the order of 20%.

In a patient who is unfit or unable to undergo surgery, high-dose progestogens can be used to slow the progression of the disease, as these tumours are often hormone sensitive. Use of progestogens, however, is becoming less common.

Recurrence

In most patients treated for endometrial cancer, the cancer will not recur and the prognosis will be good. Most relapses occur early (i.e. within 2 years of primary treatment) and recurrence is commonest in the vault of the vagina and, less commonly, in the lymph node chains, lungs, bone and liver. It should be remembered that 80% of those with distant recurrent disease will die within 2 years and care should be taken to maximize the quality-of-life over this time, rather than subject the patient to treatments with high morbidity and a slim chance of success.

Those with a recurrence, especially an isolated vault recurrence, who have not received radiotherapy should be considered for this treatment. For the remainder, the choice is between hormonal therapy and chemotherapy. The main

hormonal option is high-dose progestogens, which may give a response (slowing the disease) in around 30% of patients. This aims to slow the progression of the disease. Chemotherapy can produce tumour shrinkage in some cases but toxicity is considerable, not least because these patients are often frail and have severe coexistent medical disorders.

Summary

Endometrial cancer is often considered to be easily treatable and usually is, but, stage for stage, its survival approximates that of other gynaecological cancers. It is fortunate that most women present with postmenopausal bleeding in the early stages of the disease.

To ensure the best possible outcome, women who present with bleeding 6 months or more after their last menstrual period should be referred urgently for a gynaecological opinion. From there, referral to a cancer centre specializing in the treatment of gynaecological cancer is likely to be beneficial.

Key *points*

- Endometrial cancer is the most common gynaecological cancer in the UK, and is generally a postmenopausal disease.
- The aetiology is not fully known, but exposure to unopposed oestrogens is known to increase the risk of developing the disease.
- Endometrial cancer classically presents with postmenopausal bleeding or irregular premenopausal bleeding. Less commonly, the presentation can be with vaginal discharge.
- Diagnosis is made by biopsy of the endometrium. The cavity can be directly visualized with a hysteroscope, and the tissue sampled by curettage or using an outpatient sampling device. Postmenopausally, endometrial carcinoma is very unlikely if the transvaginal endometrial thickness is <4 mm.
- Treatment is generally surgical (hysterectomy and removal of the ovaries), and in some cases, lymphadenectomy may be advisable. In advanced or recurrent disease, radiotherapy is the treatment of choice.

Additional electronic sources

www.cancerresearchuk.org/.

www.rcog.org.uk/globalassets/documents/guidelines/ green-top-guidelines/gtg_67_endometrial_ hyperplasia.pdf.

Cervical neoplasia

Introduction

Cervical cancer is the most common cancer among women in many developing countries, and worldwide there are over 450 000 cases each year. The overall lifetime risk is about 5% in parts of Africa, India and Latin America compared with 1% in Europe and North America. About 3100 cases of cervical cancer are presently diagnosed each year in the UK, and 1300 of these women will die from the disease. In the UK, cervical cancer is relatively uncommon, representing around 2% of female cancers. It is, however, the most common cancer in young females.

Fortunately, cervical cancer has a premalignant phase and many of the criteria for a suitable screening programme are fulfilled. The aim of this screening is to detect premalignant cervical disease by means of a 'smear test' and to treat the premalignant disease before invasion occurs. Both the incidence and mortality have fallen considerably since the introduction of this screening programme. In many affluent countries, the introduction of the human papillomavirus (HPV) vaccine aims to reduce this further still.

Cervical intraepithelial and cervical cancer screening

Transformation zone

Cervical intraepithelial neoplasia (CIN) develops in the 'transformation zone' of the cervix. Understanding the transformation zone is the key to understanding cervical cancer screening. The endocervix is lined by columnar epithelium and the ectocervix by squamous epithelium. Under the influence of oestrogen, part of the endocervix everts, thereby exposing the columnar epithelium to the chemical environment of the upper vagina (Fig. 14.1). The change in pH, along with other factors, causes the delicate columnar epithelium cells to transform into squamous epithelium through the process of metaplasia. The transformation zone is this area of the cervical epithelium that has undergone the change and is consequently more unstable. CIN can develop in this transformation zone and it is this area that is sampled cytologically.

Cells shed from the surface may be sampled by a variety of devices, so that cells from both the endocervix and ectocervix can then be examined microscopically for cytological abnormalities termed dyskaryosis. Cellular abnormalities are classified into different degrees of 'dyskaryosis'; mild (low grade), moderate and severe (both high grade). Although dyskaryosis is a cytological diagnosis (Fig. 14.2), the degree of dyskaryosis correlates, to some extent, with the degree of CIN, which is a histological diagnosis (Figs 14.3 and 14.4). The difference being that cytology looks at individual cells, whereas histology examines the cells as a tissue and therefore has architecture. As well as examining the desquamated cervical cells, cervical smear reports may also identify infection such as candidal, trichomonal or wart virus infection. Rarely, they may identify cells from other parts of the genital tract, such as malignant endometrial or ovarian cells.

The precise rates of progression and spontaneous resolution of the disease are unknown. Roughly one-third of lesions will progress to the next stage (CIN I–II, CIN II–III, etc.), a third will remain unchanged and a third will regress. The duration of progression to invasive carcinoma is variable, but the average is perhaps around 10 years.

Screening recommendations

In the UK, there is an organized systematic population-based computerized screening programme, with national recommendations to screen from the ages of 25–65 years.

Colposcopy

Significant dyskaryosis on a cervical smear is an indication for further assessment with colposcopy. This is a procedure by which the cervix is examined in more detail using a type of binocular microscope referred to as a 'colposcope' (Fig. 14.5). Although moderate and severe dyskaryosis are absolute indications for colposcopy, controversy exists as to whether it is required for mild dyskaryosis. Currently the National Health Services (NHS) screening programme tests for high-risk HPV type when a low-grade dyskaryotic smear is identified. If high-risk HPV is identified the patient will be referred to colposcopy, whereas if it is negative the risks are very low, and the patient remains on routine screening. The indications for colposcopy are listed in Box 14.1.

The patient is placed in the lithotomy position and a bivalve speculum is then inserted to allow visualization of

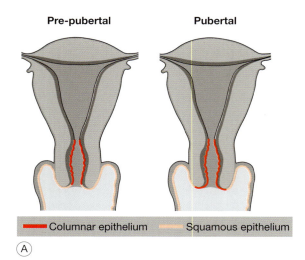

Pre-pubertal **Pubertal**

Columnar epithelium   Squamous epithelium

(A)

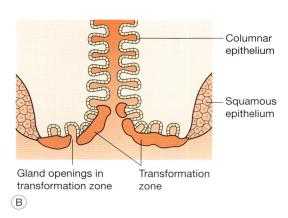

Columnar epithelium

Squamous epithelium

Gland openings in transformation zone   Transformation zone

(B)

Fig. 14.1 **The transformation zone. (A)** The cervix everts at puberty, exposing the columnar epithelium of the endocervical canal. **(B)** This epithelium, referred to as the transformation zone, gradually undergoes metaplasia to squamous epithelium.

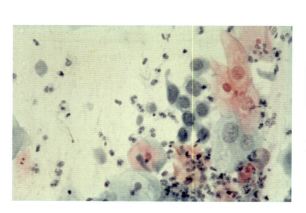

Fig. 14.2 **Slide prepared from a cervical smear.** There is moderate dysplasia with hyperchromasia, irregular nuclei and multinucleation. This slide also shows *Trichomonas vaginalis*, leucocytosis and a spermatozoon.

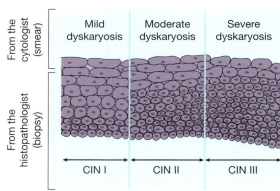

From the cytologist (smear)

| Mild dyskaryosis | Moderate dyskaryosis | Severe dyskaryosis |

From the histopathologist (biopsy)

CIN I   CIN II   CIN III

Fig. 14.3 **The CIN grading system.**

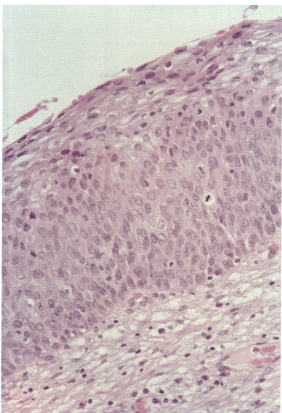

Fig. 14.4 **CIN II in a biopsy specimen.** There are abnormal cells arising from the basal layer, but not extending to the full thickness of the epithelium.

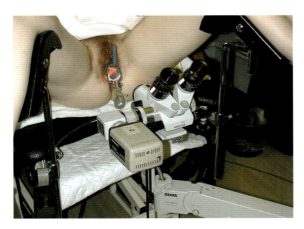

Fig. 14.5 Colposcopy, using a high-powered microscope, allows detailed examination of the cervix.

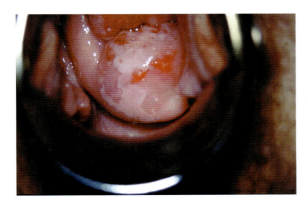

Fig. 14.6 Acetic acid coagulates protein, and the abnormal cells, which have more protein, appear 'aceto-white'.

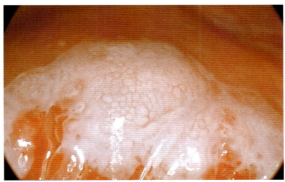

Fig. 14.7 Patches of aceto-white may be separated by areas of blood vessels, creating a mosaic pattern.

Box 14.1

The indications for colposcopy

Abnormal cervical cytology

Smear result	Action
High-grade (severe) dyskaryosis	Colposcopy
High-grade (moderate) dyskaryosis	Colposcopy
Low-grade dyskaryosis (or borderline) with high-risk HPV type positive	Colposcopy
Low-grade dyskaryosis (or borderline) and high-risk HPV negative	Return to screening
Glandular dyskaryosis	Colposcopy

the cervix. It is important to identify the squamocolumnar junction. Abnormal epithelium, such as CIN, contains an increased amount of protein and lower levels of glycogen than normal epithelium. If acetic acid is applied to the cervix, the protein coagulates and the abnormal cells appear white: 'aceto-white' (Fig. 14.6). There may also be a 'mosaic' pattern with patches of aceto-white separated by areas of red vessels (Fig. 14.7). Some of the vascular patterns may appear

'punctated' if the vessels are viewed end-on. The inter-vessel distance increases with more severe lesions, and bizarre branching with coarse punctation and atypical vessels suggests invasive disease. Lugol's iodine (Schiller's iodine) stains glycogen mahogany brown, and the abnormal cells, which have less glycogen and therefore take up less iodine, can also be viewed in this way.

Treatment of cervical intraepithelial neoplasia

High-grade CIN (CIN II and III) requires treatment. With CIN I there is more controversy and generally a period of cytological surveillance will be employed, as many of these lesions will spontaneously resolve. If high-grade CIN is suspected colposcopically, the options are to treat immediately (termed 'see-and-treat') using an excisional method (e.g. large loop excision of the transformation zone, LLETZ) or to biopsy to confirm high-grade CIN and treat thereafter. This depends on the certainty of the colposcopic findings and the likelihood that the patient will attend for the follow-up.

The cervix is infiltrated directly with local anaesthetic, and a loop diathermy excision is performed (Fig. 14.8). The alternative of ablating the area has the disadvantage that the histological assessment is less complete (see Table 14.1). As smoking is an aetiological factor, its cessation should be discussed with the patient.

Follow-up

This is defined by the national screening guidelines. Any woman who has had CIN, whether treated or not, continues to be at risk of developing cervical cancer due to either incomplete treatment of her CIN or the development of new disease. Follow-up is therefore important to consider and this is usually carried out cytologically by repeating smears. Colposcopy can also be used. National protocols vary but, in England, a smear with HPV testing ('test of cure') is performed in primary care at 6 months. If this is negative with no evidence of high-risk HPV type then the patient is returned to routine screening. If not, the patient returns to colposcopy for assessment.

Success of the UK cervical screening programme

The aim of screening is to identify women at high risk of cervical cancer to enable intervention at a time that allows treatment to substantially reduce this risk. The NHS screening programme in England is thought to save 4500 lives per year. Although successful, it will not be able to prevent all cervical cancers. It is estimated that for the UK cervical screening programme, for women aged between 25 and 49 years, 3-yearly screening prevents 84 cervical cancers out of every 100 that would develop without screening.

Cervical cancer

Aetiological factors

Cervical cancer arises from areas of CIN, as noted earlier. At least 30% of patients with CIN III, if left untreated, will

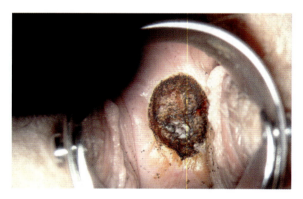

Fig. 14.8   An area of CIN II has been excised using a loop (Table 14.1). The cauterized area heals spontaneously.

probably go on to develop invasive disease over a period of 5–20 years.

Sexual behaviour

Cervical cancer is usually a disease of sexually active women and has been linked mainly to HPV. Women with cervical cancer are likely to have had more sexual partners and to have started intercourse earlier, and are less likely to have used barrier methods of contraception, compared with other women. The sexual behaviour of their partners is also important. The disease is more frequent in parous women.

Human papillomavirus

A strong association has been observed between HPV serotypes 16 and 18 (and others), pre-invasive disease and invasive cervical cancer. It is believed that certain serotypes of HPV are important cofactors in the development of cervical cancer and may act by producing proteins (E6/7) that affect the action of the p53 gene product. The p53 gene is important in repairing DNA, and, if damaged, may predispose to malignant change. HPV is present in around one-third of all women in their 20s in the UK. This is the basis for both HPV triage in the screening programme as well as for HPV vaccination.

The combined oral contraceptive pill

Studies have shown that prolonged use of the oral contraceptive pill increases the risk of cervical cancer up to four-fold, but only in women who carry HPV. It can be argued that this effect is attributable to differences in sexual behaviour, rather than to the pill itself.

Smoking

Women who smoke are also at increased risk of developing cervical cancer. This may be due to alterations in immune function in the cervical epithelium or chemical carcinogenesis.

Table 14.1	Treatment modalities for CIN		
Method	**Summary of method**	**Pros**	**Cons**
Loop excision of the transitional zone	Wire loop with high-frequency current	Easy outpatient procedure. Tissue is available for pathology	Small association with cervical incompetence and stenosis
Laser vaporization	Destruction with CO_2 laser	Easy outpatient procedure. Known depth of tissue destruction	No tissue available for pathology
'Cold' coagulation	Heating to approx. 120°C	Easy outpatient procedure	No tissue available for pathology. Depth of tissue destruction not known
Cone biopsy	Surgical excision, often under anaesthesia	Large specimen obtained. Tissue is available for pathology	Often needs general anaesthesia. Associated with cervical incompetence and stenosis

Future prevention

As certain subtypes of HPV are now known to be the main aetiological factors associated with the development of cervical cancer, there has been significant effort to develop a vaccine for these virus subtypes and it is likely that there will be new products in the near future. Two separate vaccines have been developed with the aim of protecting an individual from the common oncogenic HPV subtypes. Cervarix and Gardasil have now passed through clinical trials and are available in many countries. More recently, Gardasil-9 has been developed, which aims to prevent cervical, vulval, vaginal and anal cancer, as well as genital warts caused by HPV 6 and 11. It is thought that for these vaccines to be most effective, girls should be inoculated before they have become sexually active. Routine inoculation of girls at the age of 12–13 has commenced in the UK with Gardasil (HPV 6, 11, 16 and 18). The intended benefit is to reduce the incidence of cervical carcinoma by 70%. Additionally, this will reduce the incidence of vulval and anal cancers as well as warts. As not every cervical cancer will be prevented, however, it is important that cervical screening continues.

Presentation

Patients with cervical cancer may present with post-coital bleeding, intermenstrual bleeding, menorrhagia or an offensive vaginal discharge. It should be noted that in younger women these symptoms are common and are more likely to be related to physiological ectropion, menstrual irregularity, breakthrough bleeding and chlamydia infection. In early cases there may be no symptoms, and the diagnosis is made only as an incidental finding after abnormal cervical cytology is discovered. Other symptoms such as backache, referred leg pain, leg oedema, haematuria or alteration in bowel habit are usually associated with advanced-stage disease, when the cancer has begun to infiltrate adjacent anatomical structures. General malaise, weight loss and anaemia are also late features.

Three categories of clinical appearance are described.
1. The most common is an exophytic lesion (Fig. 14.9). It usually arises on the ectocervix, often producing a large friable polypoid mass which bleeds easily. It can also arise from within the endocervical canal so that the canal becomes distended and 'barrel shaped'.
2. An infiltrating tumour shows little ulceration or exophytic growth but tends to produce a hard, indurated cervix.
3. An ulcerative tumour erodes a portion of the cervix and vaginal vault, producing a crater with local infection and seropurulent discharge.

Pathology

The majority of cervical cancers are squamous, and may be of keratinizing (the commonest), large cell, non-keratinizing

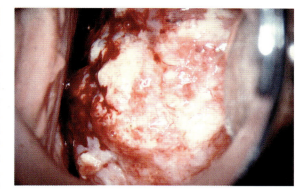

Fig. 14.9 **This squamous cell carcinoma was stage II$_A$.**

and small cell subtypes. Around 10–25% are adenocarcinomas. There may also be coexistent squamous metaplasia or neoplasia (adenosquamous carcinoma).

Spread

Cervical cancer spreads by direct extension into adjacent structures and via the draining lymphatics. Blood-borne metastases are rare. Direct invasion beyond the cervix is usually into the parametrium, upper vagina and pelvic sidewall, and this tumour may lead to ureteric obstruction. There may also be invasion of the bladder and rectum.

There is no predictable pattern of lymphatic spread, with paracervical, parametrial and both internal and external iliac nodes potentially involved. There may also be a spread to the common iliac, para-aortic and left supraclavicular area.

The risk of lymph node metastases correlates with both stage and tumour volume. Around 5–10% of patients with apparent stage I disease have pelvic node involvement. The incidence of para-aortic node involvement is less, at around 5% of patients with stage I disease and 25% with stage III disease.

Staging, investigation and prognostic factors

By definition cervical cancer is staged (International Federation of Gynecology and Obstetrics [FIGO]) by clinical examination (Table 14.2), which is often carried out under anaesthetic, and the diagnosis confirmed histologically by biopsy. The examination should include a rectovaginal examination to assess parametrial involvement. The stage is 'not altered' by subsequent radiological (e.g. magnetic resonance imaging [MRI] or computed tomography [CT]) or surgico–pathological findings (although in early disease, the histological dimensions of the tumour are important). Although this may seem inconsistent, it is to maintain consistency with other parts of the world where the disease is more common but where 'high tech' imaging is not always available. However, in clinical practice staging is based upon

Stage	Invasion	Prognosis 5-year survival	Treatment
I$_{A1}$	Depth of invasion ≤3 mm and width ≤7 mm (includes early stromal invasion of up to 1 mm)	98–99%	Local excision; if margins of a LLETZ/cone clear (i.e. no residual tumour or CIN) then conization is adequate, with no need for pelvic lymphadenectomy
I$_{A2}$	Depth of invasion 3.1–5 mm and width ≤7 mm	95%	Simple hysterectomy and pelvic lymphadenectomy. If fertility sparing required, large cone and lymphadenectomy
I$_{B1}$	Tumour confined to cervix and diameter <4 cm	90–95%	Radical hysterectomy (and lymphadenectomy)
I$_{B2}$	Tumour confined to cervix and diameter >4 cm	80%	Chemo–radiotherapy
II$_A$	Upper two-thirds of vagina	70–90%	Chemotherapy & radiotherapy
II$_B$	Upper two-thirds of vagina plus parametrial disease	60–70%	Chemo–radiotherapy
III$_A$	Lower-third of vagina	30–50%	Chemotherapy & radiotherapy
III$_B$	Pelvic sidewall and/or hydronephrosis		Chemo–radiotherapy
IV$_A$	Bladder, rectum	20%	Chemo–radiotherapy
IV$_B$	Beyond pelvis		

Table 14.2 FIGO staging of cervical cancer

the best assessment of the disease. The use of MRI and CT scanning has replaced the use of cystoscopy and intravenous urography. Positron emission tomography/CT is now being more widely used to assess the extent of lymph node involvement and this allows more individualized radiotherapy. If nodes are radiologically suspicious, for example, it is likely to be more appropriate to avoid surgery and treat with chemotherapy and radiotherapy.

Although in developed countries a greater proportion of cases present with stage I disease, in worldwide terms, the majority (>75%) of women with cervical cancer present with advanced stage (stage III/IV) disease. The prognosis for patients with early-stage disease is relatively good (Table 14.2), but the prognosis for patients with advanced-stage disease is poor.

Management

Stage I$_{A1}$–I$_{A2}$

Stage I$_{A1}$ can be cured by simple excision. If preservation of fertility is required, a cone biopsy with close cytological follow-up may be adequate treatment; where preservation of fertility is not important, simple hysterectomy can be preferable. With stage I$_{A2}$ there is around 5% chance of nodal involvement. In these patients, local excision, as above, would be combined with formal pelvic lymphadenectomy. If these nodes are positive, adjuvant radiotherapy would be required too.

Stage I$_B$–II$_A$

The choice between radical hysterectomy and radical radiotherapy is determined by the size and distribution of the cancer as well as the clinical condition of the patient.

There is no difference in survival between the two methods but there are significant differences in morbidity.

Radical hysterectomy and pelvic lymphadenectomy involve total hysterectomy, excision of the parametria, upper vagina and paracolpos, as well as dissection and removal of the pelvic lymph nodes. The key surgical principle is to obtain a satisfactory surgical margin and to be able to histologically assess the draining lymphatics. Oophorectomy may be performed if appropriate, but the ovaries are rarely the site of metastatic spread and usually can be safely conserved. The operative mortality is <1%, although potential morbidity includes infection, thromboembolic disease, haemorrhage and ureteric fistulae. There are also medium-term problems with reduced bladder sensation and voiding difficulties, together with long-term problems of high residual urinary volumes, recurrent urinary infections, stress incontinence and lymphocyst formation.

Radical radiotherapy usually consists of external beam therapy (teletherapy) to the pelvis and local vaginal therapy (brachytherapy). There is good evidence that combining this with cisplatin chemotherapy increases the survival rate and combined chemo–radiotherapy has become the standard of care. Teletherapy is delivered in fractions over a number of weeks to treat the pelvic lymphatics, whereas with brachytherapy a vaginal delivery system is inserted and left in situ for 12–18 h to irradiate central disease. In the UK, brachytherapy is now in the form of high-dose radiotherapy, which results in much shorter treatment times. The radiation dose that can be given is limited by the size of the lesion and the proximity of the bladder and bowel, both of which are particularly susceptible to radiation damage. Radiation side-effects are described as early and late. Initially there is often radiation cystitis and diarrhoea from proctitis. Late effects include fibrosis causing vaginal stenosis and sexual dysfunction, amongst others. As this morbidity often gets worse with time, surgery is considered to be more suitable for those patients who are younger. In those found to have positive pelvic nodes postoperatively, it is usual to offer adjuvant chemotherapy and radiotherapy (chemo–radiotherapy).

Patients with stage I_{B1} will be offered either surgery or chemo–radiotherapy. In most modern cancer centres, patients will be extensively imaged. If there is a suggestion of extension outwith the cervix, then chemo–radiotherapy would be advised rather than surgery. There are two reasons for this: first, the morbidity associated with radical surgery plus chemo–radiotherapy is significantly greater than with the latter alone and second, if the cervix has been removed, it is not possible to give the high doses, via brachytherapy, that are required to achieve local control.

Similarly, for patients with stage I_{B2} and stage II_A, chemo–radiotherapy would now normally be advised. The reason for this is that even if radical surgery was to be successful, the likelihood of an unsatisfactory margin or positive nodes is sufficiently great to make adjuvant treatment likely.

For patients with small stage I_{B1} lesions that have been assessed in detail with MRI/CT imaging, and in whom future fertility is important, there is the possibility of radical local treatment. This is called radical trachelectomy and lymphadenectomy. The cervix is removed along with the paracervical tissues but the uterus is left in situ with a special suture left to maintain 'cervical competence'. The lymph nodes are also removed. This approach is still being evaluated – although it offers the patient the potential of future pregnancy, it is not without significant problems.

Stage II_B–IV

The treatment of advanced-stage disease usually involves radical radiotherapy in combination with cisplatin chemotherapy. Failure to cure inoperable cervical cancer may result from suboptimal treatment of the central disease or the existence of lymph node metastases. With large lesions, the sensitivity of adjacent structures to radiation may prevent the use of curative radiation doses at the tumour periphery and, furthermore, some tumours may be radio-resistant.

Recurrent disease

Those patients with recurrence have a 1-year survival of around 10–15%. Most recurrences are suitable for palliative care only. If the patient has not been previously treated with radiotherapy, this may be a treatment option, but the majority of patients will have already had radical radiotherapy. Patients with a central pelvic recurrence may be cured by pelvic exenteration (excision of vagina/uterus with the bladder or

rectum or both). With careful selection, up to 60% of these cases may survive 5 years, but the operation is associated with major morbidity.

The remaining patients may benefit from chemotherapy to palliate symptomatic recurrence or radiotherapy to palliate recurrence involving bone or nerve roots. The most active chemotherapy agent is cisplatin, and combinations based on these drugs cause initial tumour shrinkage in up to 70% of cases. The main benefit from chemotherapy is the relief of disease-related symptoms, such as pelvic pain, but chemotherapy itself can cause considerable toxicity and does not improve survival in these women.

Key points

- Cervical cancer is the most common cancer among women in many developing countries. There are over 450 000 cases worldwide each year. It is relatively uncommon in the UK.
- The risk of cervical cancer is related to sexual behaviour. Early age of first intercourse and a high number of sexual partners are risk factors. Smoking may also increase the risk.
- The important causative agent appears to be HPV, particularly serotypes 16 and 18. In the UK, teenage girls are being inoculated with a vaccine to protect against these two serotypes.
- Screening is possible because of a relatively long precancerous phase and involves a programme of regular cervical smears. Cytological abnormalities on smears (dyskaryosis) correlate to some degree with histologically abnormal CIN. In the UK, screening is now using HPV testing to help triage patients.
- When cervical smears demonstrate dyskaryosis, colposcopy allows identification of abnormal epithelium suggestive of CIN to be located, biopsied and treated.
- Although cervical cancers are mainly of squamous type, around 10–25% are adenocarcinomas.
- FIGO staging of cancer is from stage I–IV. Stage I can be treated by surgery or radiotherapy. More advanced cancer can be treated by radiotherapy ± chemotherapy.

Additional information

www.gov.uk/guidance/cervical-screening-programme-overview
http://www.sign.ac.uk/sign-99-management-of-cervical-cancer.html
www.cancerresearchuk.org/

Gestational trophoblastic disease

Introduction

Gestational trophoblastic disease (GTD) comprises a group of diagnoses, each characterized by the abnormal proliferation of trophoblast cells with constitutive human chorionic gonadotrophin (hCG) production. GTD can be divided into premalignant and malignant forms, with the premalignant diagnoses of complete and partial molar pregnancies, and the malignant forms including invasive moles, choriocarcinoma and placental site trophoblastic tumours (PSTT) (Table 15.1). The malignant forms of GTD have a number of important differences from other more common types of cancer in terms of aetiology, genetic structure, pathophysiology and responsiveness to treatment. Fortunately, the malignant forms of trophoblastic disease are extremely sensitive to chemotherapy, and chemotherapy treatment routinely results in cure, even in patients presenting with advanced metastatic disease.

Overall GTD are rare; molar pregnancies, which are the most common form of GTD, have an estimated incidence of around 1–3 cases for every 1000 live births. The incidence has previously been thought to vary significantly across different geographical regions and racial groups, with historical estimates showing a near 10-fold higher incidence in Korea, the Philippines and China compared with Europe and the USA. However, more recent data indicates that similar rates of 1–3 cases per 1000 are reported in nearly every modern series worldwide.

The incidence of molar pregnancies is significantly higher at the extremes of reproductive age, at approximately 1 in 30 in those aged under 15 and as high as 1 in 5 in those for women in their late 40s or early 50s. As these extremes of the reproductive age group make up only a very small proportion of the women who become pregnant, over 90% of molar pregnancies occur in women aged 18–40 years.

Choriocarcinoma and PSTT are even rarer, occurring in approximately 1 in 50 000 and 1 in 200 000 pregnancies respectively. In view of the rarity of the diagnoses and the complexity of care, the management of trophoblast disease after the initial uterine evacuation is best provided by a specialist centre.

Trophoblast cells in health and disease

In a healthy pregnancy, the trophoblast cells make up a key component of the placental tissue. Their role is to promote invasion of the conceptus into the lining of the uterus, promote angiogenesis and produce hCG.

The malignant forms of GTD, both those arising from molar pregnancies and those arising from malignant transformation of cells in healthy placentae, share many of these characteristics. In addition to the ability to invade into the lining of the uterus and stimulate new blood vessels, the malignant cells are also able to spread to other organs of the body and grow at a very fast rate, without any control on their division. Fortunately, despite these changes, the production of hCG is always retained and this is extremely helpful in establishing a diagnosis and in monitoring the response to treatment.

Premalignant gestational trophoblastic disease

Premalignant GTD (Table 15.1) is divided into partial and complete molar pregnancies. The original derivation of the historical term hydatidiform mole, from the Greek *hydatis* meaning a watery vesicle and the Latin *mola* meaning a shapeless mass, is an accurate description of the appearance of a complete molar pregnancy evacuated after the first trimester. With the near-universal use of first-trimester ultrasound, however, this florid appearance is now rarely seen.

Partial molar pregnancy

Molar pregnancies occur as the result of an error, either in the production of the oocyte or at the time of fertilization. Normally, fertilization combines a 23,X set of haploid chromosomes from the ovum with either a 23,X or 23,Y haploid set from the sperm, the result being a diploid 46,XX or 46,XY zygote, which has the correct balance of maternal and paternal genes. In contrast, a partial molar pregnancy has 69 chromosomes, 23 from the mother and the other

Table 15.1	Classification of GTD		
Classification	**Pathology**	**Usual karyotype**	**Clinical features**
Premalignant			
Partial hydatidiform mole	Focal hyperplasia of villi Benign	69,XXY: two paternal haploid sets and one maternal haploid set	Difficult to diagnose on ultrasound as a fetus can be present during the first 8–10 weeks. Most present as failed pregnancies. Less than 1% require additional treatment after evacuation
Complete hydatidiform mole	Generalized hyperplasia Benign	46,XX: two haploid sets, both paternal ('androgenically diploid')	Uterine cavity filled with vesicular mole tissue on ultrasound without an embryo. Approximately 10–15% become malignant and require additional therapy
Malignant			
Invasive mole	Features of invasion	Virtually all are androgenically diploid	Molar tissue invading the myometrium and may cause uterine rupture if not treated
Choriocarcinoma	Columns and sheets of malignant trophoblast cells containing syncytiotrophoblast and cytotrophoblast cells, frequent haemorrhage and an absence of villi	Contains maternal and paternal chromosomes (unlike choriocarcinoma of ovarian origin)	Most follow a live birth, stillbirth, miscarriage or ectopic pregnancy, but can arise from a hydatidiform mole. There is frequently metastatic spread. Highly curable with chemotherapy
PSTT	Malignant intermediate trophoblast cells infiltrating muscle. No cytotrophoblast cells and no villi. Positive stain for human placental lactogen (hPL)	Contains maternal and paternal chromosomes	Slow-growing malignancy invading the myometrium and potentially metastasizing to the lung. hCG levels are less elevated than in choriocarcinoma. Usually treated with surgery and chemotherapy

46 paternally derived, usually from the entry of two separate sperm into the ovum (Fig. 15.1).

In a partial molar pregnancy, there is usually an embryo which may be seen on an early ultrasound. The ultrasound may have been 'routine' or have been carried out because of vaginal bleeding, vaginal discharge, abdominal pain or excessive morning sickness. Although structurally abnormal, there may be no obvious ultrasound features of this in the early first trimester and the diagnosis may therefore not become apparent until histological tissue examination is carried out after a failed pregnancy. The features are of focal hyperplasia and swelling of the villi, though many areas do not have these obvious changes and pathologically distinguishing a partial mole from a hydropic miscarriage can be difficult. Fortunately, the risk of malignant change after a partial molar pregnancy is less than 1%, and so very few partial mole patients require chemotherapy treatment.

Complete molar pregnancies

In contrast to partial molar pregnancies, complete molar pregnancies have the correct number of chromosomes, with the majority having a 46,XX karyotype. In complete molar pregnancies, however, all the genetic material is from the father and they are therefore termed androgenetic in origin.

There appears to be two mechanisms by which this genetic combination arises:

- the maternal 23,X haploid set of chromosomes in the ovum may be lost at the time of fertilization and the 23,X haploid paternal chromosomes from the fertilizing sperm may duplicate themselves, giving rise to the 46,XX cell

- alternatively, an 'empty' ovum may be fertilized by two separate spermatozoa (dispermy), which also leads to a paternally derived karyotype.

In a complete molar pregnancy, there is no fetal material and the placental tissue has marked hyperplasia and gross vesicular swelling of the villi. The classical macroscopic 'bunch of small grapes' appearance of a complete molar pregnancy generally occurs later in the second trimester; thus, as most molar pregnancies are now diagnosed in the first trimester, this appearance is less often seen (Fig. 15.2). In areas without routine ultrasound, the presentation may be later, with abnormal clinical findings including: a large-for-dates uterus (from the bulk of the tumour), hyperemesis or, more rarely, thyrotoxicosis resulting from the supraphysiological levels of hCG, which mimics the action of thyroid-stimulating hormone on the thyroid gland.

Approximately 10–15% of complete molar pregnancies become malignant and will require chemotherapy after their surgical evacuation.

Malignant gestational trophoblastic disease (Table 15.1)

Invasive mole

Invasive molar pregnancy is rare in areas with routine first-trimester ultrasound but occurs when the molar tissue invades predominantly into the myometrium. The clinical presentation is with a uterine mass and an elevated hCG level. As a result

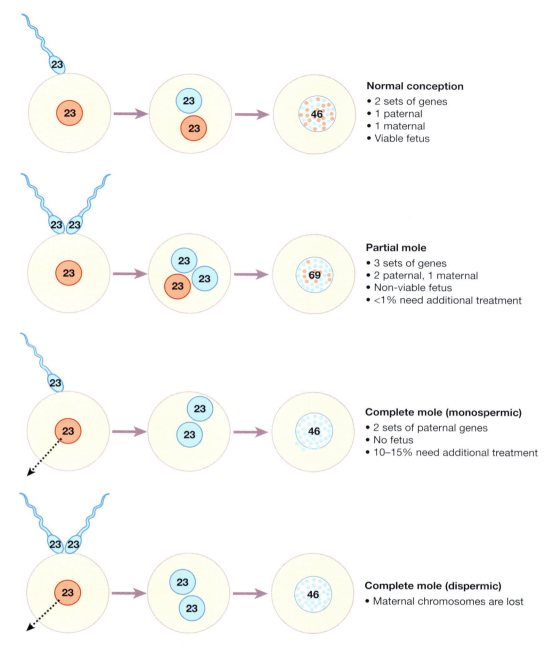

Normal conception
- 2 sets of genes
- 1 paternal
- 1 maternal
- Viable fetus

Partial mole
- 3 sets of genes
- 2 paternal, 1 maternal
- Non-viable fetus
- <1% need additional treatment

Complete mole (monospermic)
- 2 sets of paternal genes
- No fetus
- 10–15% need additional treatment

Complete mole (dispermic)
- Maternal chromosomes are lost

Fig. 15.1 Genetic make-up of normal pregnancy and partial and complete molar pregnancies.

of the myometrial invasion, the tumour can lead to uterine rupture and present with abdominal pain and bleeding. Histologically, invasive mole has a similar appearance to a complete molar pregnancy and is routinely curable with chemotherapy.

Choriocarcinoma

Choriocarcinoma is a highly malignant tumour arising from malignant transformation of the placental trophoblast cells,

and histologically is characterized by haemorrhage, necrosis and intravascular growth. Choriocarcinoma lacks the villous structure of the normal trophoblast or molar pregnancy and is very rare, with approximately 1 case per 50 000 live births. Choriocarcinoma may become apparent shortly after a pregnancy or can present after an interval of up to 20 years after the causative pregnancy.

Presentation is usually with persistent vaginal bleeding and a markedly raised hCG (the serum hCG level, which is usually <100 000 IU/L at the time of delivery, should fall to

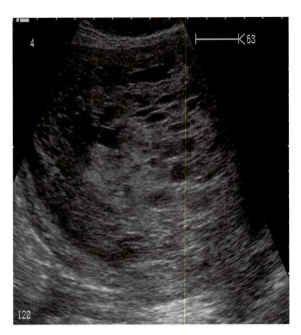

Fig. 15.2 Ultrasound appearance of a complete hydatidiform mole.

normal within 3 weeks postpartum). Diagnosis can also follow presentation of a metastasis in:

- the lung, causing haemoptysis or dyspnoea
- the brain, leading to neurological abnormalities
- the gastrointestinal tract, causing chronic blood loss or melaena
- the liver, leading to jaundice
- the kidney, causing haematuria.

The finding of an elevated hCG level in a woman with advanced cancer is highly suggestive of choriocarcinoma.

In contrast to molar pregnancies, there do not appear to be any specific risk factors or higher-risk groups for the development of choriocarcinoma.

Placental site trophoblastic tumour

PSTT is the least frequent type of gestational tumour, with approximately 1 case for every 200 000 live births. In contrast to choriocarcinoma, PSTT is believed to arise from the intermediate trophoblastic cells that develop slightly later in pregnancy. These cells have a lower capacity to invade and also make relatively less hCG than the syncytiotrophoblast cells that give rise to choriocarcinoma.

The presentation of PSTT is similar to that of choriocarcinoma, though interestingly, it occurs predominantly after the delivery of a female infant and is more likely to be associated with hCG-induced amenorrhoea. PSTT usually presents rather later than choriocarcinoma, tends to grow more slowly and is less chemosensitive.

Management of molar pregnancies

Following an ultrasound scan suggestive of a molar pregnancy, the first step is to arrange a uterine evacuation. In a complete molar pregnancy, where there are no fetal parts, the evacuation should be performed by a suction procedure. The risks of bleeding and perforation during surgical evacuation are significant. The procedure should be performed by a senior surgeon and with cross-matched blood available. Medical evacuation may be appropriate for a partial mole, particularly if larger fetal parts are present, but this should be followed with a surgical evacuation of any retained products of conception. It is recommended that oxytocin is avoided until after the uterine evacuation is completed to minimize the risk of distant spread by uterine contractions.

Following the evacuation, the diagnosis is confirmed on histological examination and supported, if needed, by cytogenetic studies of the trophoblast cells.

Follow-up after a molar pregnancy

Following the evacuation of a complete molar pregnancy, there is an approximately 10–15% chance of persistent disease and the development of malignancy, while after a partial molar pregnancy the risk is only 1%. There is no effective prospective method of determining which patients will develop persistent disease and will therefore require further treatment, but hCG follow-up after the evacuation allows this group to be identified.

To ensure that this is meticulously carried out, in the UK follow-up of molar pregnancies is organized through three central trophoblast centres (in London, Sheffield and Dundee). Each case of molar pregnancy is registered with the nearest laboratory, which will then organize the hCG follow-up directly. This system has been a major factor in producing the extremely high cure rates now seen for the disease, and the clinical experience in these centres has led to most of the major therapeutic developments in these rare tumours.

For the majority of patients with molar pregnancies, the hCG values fall to normal levels within 2 months and relapse after this point is very rare. The standard advice is that follow-up is needed for only 6 months from the time of the evacuation or for 6 months from the first normal hCG level in those where the rate of fall is slower. It is also recommended that women postpone a further pregnancy during the follow-up period, as the hCG from the new pregnancy could mask the hCG from relapsed disease, and this would delay diagnosis and treatment.

There is an increased risk of a further molar pregnancy in subsequent pregnancies, with the risk estimated at approximately 1:70. For women unfortunate enough to have two molar pregnancies, the risk of a third in a later pregnancy is in the order of 1:10.

Indications for treatment after a molar pregnancy
- hCG plateau of 4 values ± 10% over a 3-week period
- hCG increase of >10% of three values over a 2-week period
- Persistence of hCG for more than 6 months after molar evacuation

Management of malignant gestational trophoblastic disease

Following evacuation of a molar pregnancy, there are a number of indications for further treatment (Box 15.1). The most frequent of these is a rise or a plateau in the hCG levels after the evacuation. The majority of patients receive treatment with simple single-agent chemotherapy, which has a high cure rate and is generally well tolerated (Fig. 15.3). A few women who have completed their families and have no evidence of disease spread may opt instead for a hysterectomy, but they still require careful follow-up, as occult extrauterine disease may exist and chemotherapy could still be required.

In contrast, all patients with choriocarcinoma occurring after a pregnancy require chemotherapy treatment and surgery in this group is rarely useful. As GTD is so exquisitely sensitive to chemotherapy, the majority of patients with GTD occurring after a molar pregnancy can be treated with low-toxicity single-agent chemotherapy using methotrexate. This is well tolerated, has minimal side-effects, does not cause hair loss or significant sickness, and there is only a minimal risk of neutropenia.

In contrast, GTD patients with choriocarcinoma after a normal pregnancy require treatment with a more toxic combination chemotherapy regimen, usually etoposide, methotrexate, actinomycin D, cyclophosphamide and vincristine (EMA-CO).

To help determine which type of treatment is required, the International Federation of Gynecology and Obstetrics (FIGO) scoring system can be used (Table 15.2). This allows the calculation of a score based on eight variables. Patients scoring ≤6 points initially receive methotrexate chemotherapy, while those scoring ≥7 start with the EMA-CO combination chemotherapy. In the UK, overall cure rates of 100% for those in the low-risk treatment group and approximately 90% for those in the high-risk group, including those patients presenting with advanced disease (Fig. 15.4), can be expected. The small number of patients who are difficult to

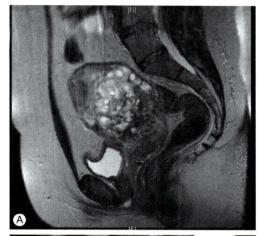
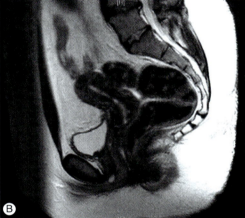

Fig. 15.3 Invasive complete molar pregnancy.
(A) Magnetic resonance imaging appearance prior to chemotherapy treatment. **(B)** Follow-up scan performed 3 months after chemotherapy completion.

cure usually present unwell with choriocarcinoma and a long interval from their causative pregnancy, and may die before treatment can be commenced or from drug-resistant disease.

After the completion of chemotherapy, most patients recover fairly rapidly, and in nearly all cases fertility is retained. An interval of 12 months from the completion of chemotherapy to the next pregnancy is usually recommended, and the majority of women are able to have further children. There is thought to be little or no excess risk of fetal abnormalities in this post-chemotherapy group.

Table 15.2	FIGO prognostic score system for GTD			
	Score			
	0	1	2	4
Age	<40	≥40	–	–
Antecedent pregnancy	Mole	Miscarriage	Term	–
Interval	<4 months	4–6 months	7–13 months	≥14 months
Pre-treatment hCG (IU/L)	<1000	1000–10 000	10 000–100 000	>100 000
Largest tumour size	<3 cm	3–5 cm	>5 cm	–
Site of metastases	Lung	Spleen, kidney	Gastrointestinal tract	Brain, liver
Number of metastases	0	1–4	5–8	>8
Previous chemotherapy	–	–	Single agent	Two or more drugs

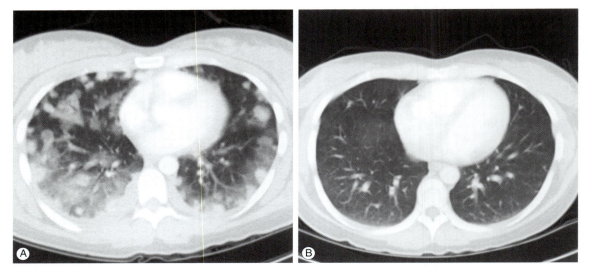

Fig. 15.4 **Choriocarcinoma. (A)** Computed tomography (CT) scan of the chest, demonstrating extensive pulmonary metastases and haemorrhage, in a patient with choriocarcinoma presenting 1 month after a normal delivery. **(B)** A CT scan performed 6 months later shows the complete resolution of the disease in response to chemotherapy.

Key points

- Gestational trophoblastic disorders represent an abnormal proliferation of trophoblastic tissue and may be benign (molar pregnancy) or malignant (invasive mole, a choriocarcinoma or a PSTT).
- Trophoblastic tumours always produce hCG, and this acts as an excellent marker for diagnosis, assessing response to treatment and for follow-up.
- A hydatidiform mole may be complete or partial. A complete mole is diploid (but all the chromosomes are paternally derived) and there is no fetal tissue (only trophoblast). A partial mole is usually triploid (with 46 of the 69 chromosomes being paternally derived) and there may be a fetus.
- The diagnosis of a molar pregnancy is often suggested by ultrasound, in which there is homogeneous solid tissue with a vesicular appearance. The diagnosis is confirmed by histopathological examination of tissue.

- The initial management of a molar pregnancy is to carry out an evacuation of the uterus, and follow-up is required to ensure that the hCG level is falling. Further treatment, usually chemotherapy, is required if the hCG rises progressively following the uterine evacuation, or if the pathology is reported as choriocarcinoma.
- Choriocarcinoma is rare but can occur after any type of conception, including a normal pregnancy, miscarriage or hydatidiform mole.
- All the malignant forms of GTD, including choriocarcinoma, are exquisitely sensitive to chemotherapy and the cure rate is high.
- Following a molar pregnancy, there is a modest increase in risk of further molar pregnancy in any subsequent pregnancies.

16

Disorders of the vulva

Introduction

The vulva consists of the mons pubis, labia majora, labia minora, clitoris and the vestibule (Fig. 2.1). It is covered with keratinizing squamous epithelium, unlike the vaginal mucosa, which is covered with non-keratinizing squamous epithelium. The labia majora are hair-bearing and contain sweat and sebaceous glands: from an embryological viewpoint, they are analogous to the scrotum. Bartholin's glands are situated in the posterior part of the labia, one on each side of the vestibule. The lymphatics of the vulva drain to the inguinal nodes and then to the external iliac nodes. The area is richly supplied with blood vessels.

Examination of the vulva

Before direct examination of the vulva, a general dermatological examination may be useful, particularly:

- the nail beds for signs of pitting (found in psoriasis)
- the extensor surfaces (elbows and knees) also for features of psoriasis
- the flexor surfaces for lichen planus and dermatitis
- the mouth for other features of lichen planus.

The vulva may then be inspected under a good light, as described on page 17. If necessary, closer inspection is possible using a colposcope.

Simple vulval conditions

Urethral caruncle

A urethral caruncle is a polypoidal outgrowth from the edge of the urethra, which is most commonly seen after the menopause. The tissue is soft, red and smooth and appears as an eversion of the urethral mucosa. Most women are asymptomatic, but others experience dysuria, frequency, urgency and focal tenderness. If there are any suspicious features, an excision and biopsy may be required to exclude the very rare possibility of a urethral carcinoma.

Bartholin's cysts

The greater vestibular, or Bartholin's, glands lie in the subcutaneous tissue below the lower third of the labium majus and open via ducts to the vestibule between the hymenal orifice and the labia minora. They secrete mucus, particularly at the time of intercourse. If the duct becomes blocked a tense retention cyst forms, and if there is super-added infection, a painful abscess develops. The abscess can be incised and drained, usually under general anaesthesia, with the incision on the inner aspect of the labium so that secretions bathe the introitus rather than the outside of the vulva. To prevent the cyst reforming, the fistula is kept open by suturing its edges to the surrounding skin, a procedure known as marsupialization (Fig. 16.1). Insertion of a balloon catheter is a non-surgical alternative to incision and drainage or marsupialization. Bartholin's gland carcinoma is rare.

Small cysts

The commonest small vulval cysts are usually either inclusion cysts or sebaceous cysts. Inclusion cysts form because epithelium is trapped in the epidermis, usually following obstetric trauma or episiotomy. They are usually asymptomatic and need no treatment. Sebaceous cysts are usually multiple, mobile, non-tender, white or yellow, filled with a cottage cheese-like substance and more common in the anterior half of the vulva. Excision may be requested by the patient.

Cysts in an episiotomy scar can be tender and need excision. Infected cysts need to be excised and drained, and recurrent infections should be treated by excision in their non-acute phase.

Moles

Vulval moles are usually asymptomatic but become more pigmented at puberty. Any other change in a vulval naevus is an indication for removal. There is a good case to be made for removing all vulval moles, as approximately 2% of malignant melanomas in women arise from the vulva.

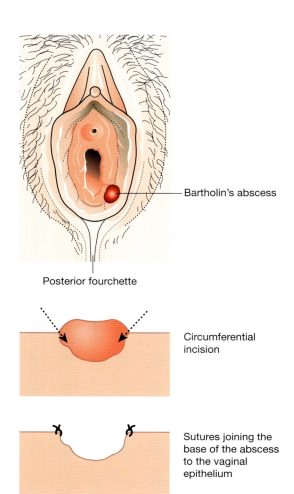

Bartholin's abscess

Posterior fourchette

Circumferential incision

Sutures joining the base of the abscess to the vaginal epithelium

Fig. 16.1   Marsupialization of a Bartholin's abscess. The lower part of the abscess cavity granulates and heals during the subsequent weeks. (From Pitkin J, Peattie A, Magowan BA. Obstetrics and Gynaecology. An Illustrated Colour Text. Churchill Livingstone, Edinburgh, 2003.)

Fibroma, lipoma, hidradenoma

Fibromas and lipomas are benign, mobile tumours of fibrous tissue and fat, respectively. Hidradenomas are rare tumours of sweat glands near the surface of the labia. All are benign, but the diagnosis is usually only made once they have been excised.

Haematoma

The commonest cause of a vulval haematoma is vaginal delivery. It may also occur following any vulval operation, or by 'falling astride' accidents, particularly in children. The possibility of sexual assault should be borne in mind in this situation. Vulval haematomas usually present with severe pain, and evacuation under general anaesthesia is often required.

Simple atrophy

Elderly women develop vaginal, vulval and clitoral atrophy as part of the normal ageing process of skin. In severe cases, the thin vulval skin, terminal urethra and fourchette cause dysuria and superficial dyspareunia, and the labia minora may fuse and bury the clitoris. Introital stenoses can make coitus impossible. A simple effective moisturizer rubbed into the vulva is effective, although some advocate topical oestrogen replacement. There is a small amount of systemic absorption with topical oestrogen therapy, and if this route is chosen, treatment should be for no more than 2 or 3 months without either a break or a short course of progesterone to prevent endometrial stimulation.

Ulcers

These may be:

- aphthous (yellow base)
- herpetic (exquisitely painful multiple ulceration, pp. 163, 165)
- syphilitic (indurated and painless, p. 165)
- associated with Crohn disease ('like knife cuts in skin')
- a feature of Behçet syndrome (a chronic painful condition with aphthous genital and ocular ulceration)
- malignant (see later)
- associated with lichen planus (see later) or Stevens-Johnson syndrome
- tropical (lymphogranuloma venereum, chancroid, granuloma inguinale).

Treatment depends on the cause. The management of Behçet syndrome is difficult, but the combined oral contraceptive or topical steroids may be tried.

Infection

Candida, vulval warts, herpes, lymphogranuloma venereum, scabies, granuloma inguinale, tinea, chancroid and syphilis are discussed in Chapter 18.

Hidradenitis suppurativa is a chronic unrelenting infection of the sweat glands. The glands become obstructed and chronic inflammation follows. Long-term antibiotics reduce further attacks, but the only cure is local excision.

Dermatoses

Vulval 'dystrophy' is an abnormality of vulval epithelium. Epithelial growth may be hypoplastic, hyperplastic or abnormal in some other way.

Lichen sclerosus

This chronic and recurrent condition can present at any age, but is more common in the older patient and usually

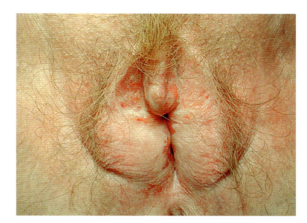

Fig. 16.2   Lichen sclerosus. The skin is white, with some reddened areas, and adhesions have significantly narrowed the introitus.

presents with pruritus. Less commonly, presentation is with dyspareunia or pain. It is an autoimmune condition and there is an association with other autoimmune disorders, including pernicious anaemia, thyroid disease, diabetes mellitus, systemic lupus erythematosus (SLE), primary biliary cirrhosis and bullous pemphigoid. Histologically, the epidermis appears thin, with loss of rete ridges. The superficial dermis is hyalinized and a band of chronic inflammatory cells is seen beneath it.

Clinically, the skin appears white, thin and crinkly, but may be thickened and keratotic if there is coexistent squamous cell hyperplasia (Fig. 16.2). There may also be clitoral or labial atrophy, with loss of the normal vulval features, such as recession of the clitoral hood and shrinkage of the labia minora. Diagnosis is usually made on clinical examination but can be confirmed by biopsy. Lichen sclerosus is nonneoplastic but may coexist with vulval intraepithelial neoplasia (VIN) and there is an association with subsequent development of vulval squamous cell carcinoma in 2–5% of cases. Initial follow-up is required to ensure that the patient is managing her symptoms and there are no suspicious skin changes. Once symptoms are controlled, then clinical review should be prompted by a change in symptom, a failure for routine management to control symptoms or a concern regarding the skin features.

Treatment is required, particularly if the condition is symptomatic, and initially is usually with a potent topical steroid cream (e.g. Dermovate), reducing gradually over a few months to a milder preparation (e.g. 1% hydrocortisone) as symptoms require. An emollient such as Oilatum or Diprobase is symptomatically beneficial. The patient should also cut her nails to try to break the itch–scratch–itch cycle. Avoidance of soaps, perfumed products and baby wipes is recommended. A non-fragranced, non-biological washing powder should be used. Vulvectomy has no role, the recurrence rate after surgery being around 50%.

Squamous cell hyperplasia

Squamous epithelial hyperplasia is characterized by thickened hyperkeratotic skin with white, itchy plaques. Pruritus is usually severe. Diagnosis is again by biopsy, and treatment is as for lichen sclerosus.

Other dermatoses

Allergic/irritant dermatosis

The vulval skin, especially the introitus, is not uncommonly affected by dermatitis. The dermatitis is either due to an irritant (non-immunological) or a true allergy (immunological aetiology). The chemicals causing hypersensitivity of the vulval skin include cosmetics, perfumes, contraceptive lubricants, sprays and douches. Detergents, dyes, softeners, bleaches, soaps and chlorine used to clean undergarments can also cause irritation. In severe cases, hypersensitivity may develop to local anaesthetic creams and even steroid preparations.

Women with contact dermatitis have a red inflamed vulva with features of eczema, and patch-testing may identify local irritants. Temporary relief may be obtained with vulval moisturizers (e.g. Dermol 500 in a daily bath), emollients (e.g. Epaderm) and topical corticosteroids (e.g. a month's course of topical Dermovate). As before, lesions that do not respond should be biopsied to confirm the diagnosis.

Psoriasis

Psoriasis manifests as a well-circumscribed, erythematous eruption with superficial scaling and it may often have a plaque that may extend to the thigh. The diagnosis is easier to make if there is evidence of extra-genital psoriasis or there are nail changes. Because the vulva is often moist, it is often difficult to distinguish psoriasis from candidal infection or dermatitis. *Candida* should be excluded. The lesions may be treated with topical preparations, ultraviolet light, steroid creams or other suitable formulations.

Intertrigo with *Candida*

Intertrigo refers to a moist inflammatory dermatitis, which can occur in any body-fold because of apposition and chafing of skin surfaces. Skin-folds are more likely to rub together in those who are overweight and in those who use occlusive clothing.

The skin is sore, macerated and often red, inflamed and cracked. Weight loss, local hygiene and ventilation should be encouraged, for example the use of stockings and cotton underclothes rather than tights and nylon pants.

Candida often complicates intertrigo and should be treated as on page 160. Providing there is no candidal infection, steroid creams may be used to relieve inflammation.

Lichen planus

Lichen planus is a chronic pruritic, purple, papular rash involving the vulva and flexor surfaces. It can affect other

Box 16.1

Causes of pruritus vulvae
- Infection (*Candida*, pediculosis, thread worms)
- Eczema
- Dermatitis (consider patch testing)
- Irritation from a vaginal discharge
- Lichen sclerosus
- Lichen planus
- VIN
- Vulval carcinoma
- Medical problems, e.g. diabetes mellitus, uraemia or liver failure
- Psychogenic

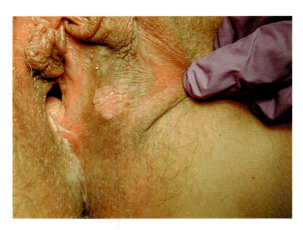

Fig. 16.3 High-grade VIN of the left labia majora. In this case, the lesion is rough surfaced, not unlike the appearance of wart virus infection, but lesions are also commonly macular with indistinct borders.

flexor surfaces and oral mucous membranes, and the diagnosis may be supported by the finding of other lesions, such as Wickham striae, in the buccal mucosa. It is usually idiopathic, but can be drug-related. Treatment is with potent topical steroids or ultraviolet light, and it tends to resolve within 2 years. Surgery should be avoided.

Pruritus

Pruritus describes an intense itching with a desire to scratch. It is commoner in those aged over 40 years, and symptoms are often most severe under times of stress or depression. There are numerous aetiologies (Box 16.1).

A biopsy may be necessary to establish the diagnosis, and patch testing may be of help. It is important to break the itch–scratch–itch cycle and strong short-term topical steroids will reduce the local inflammation caused by scratching. Application of a strong steroid cream twice daily for 3 weeks, followed by hydrocortisone cream 1% daily as maintenance, is useful, as is the use of soap substitutes (e.g. Oilatum). Irritants and bath-water additives should be avoided, soap substitutes used, the area dried gently (e.g. with a hairdryer), loose cotton clothing worn and nylon tights avoided. Antihistamines may also be of help. Coexisting depression may also warrant treatment.

Vulvodynia

This is chronic vulvar discomfort characterized by the complaints of burning, stinging, irritation or rawness with no diagnosis having been identified. There may also be pruritus. The condition may be localized, vestibulodynia, with erythema, severe pain on entry or to vestibular touch, and tenderness to pressure localized within the vestibule. The condition may also be generalized, dysaesthetic vulvodynia. No one factor can be identified as the specific cause. It may also occasionally be associated with previous sexual abuse.

There may be a response to low-dose tricyclic antidepressants (e.g. amitriptyline). Symptomatic relief can also be gained by the use of topical local anaesthetics. Due to the complex nature of this symptom, management can often

be difficult and refractory cases should be reviewed in specialist multidisciplinary clinics where physiotherapy, psychological counselling, pain management and behavioural modification can be explored.

Vulval intraepithelial neoplasia

VIN refers to the presence of neoplastic cells within the confines of the vulval epithelium. In 2004, the International Society for the Study of Vulvovaginal Diseases reclassified VIN. They now recommend that the term VIN be used for what was previously described as high-grade VIN (VIN 2 or 3). VIN is further described as usual type (or undifferentiated type) or the less common differentiated type.

Usual type (or undifferentiated type) is associated with human papilloma virus (HPV). The less common differentiated type is often encountered along with lichen sclerosis, especially where invasive squamous cancers are identified. Many are asymptomatic, although pruritus is present in up to two-thirds of cases and pain is an occasional feature. Lesions may be papular and rough surfaced, resembling warts (Fig. 16.3), or macular with indistinct borders. White lesions represent hyperkeratosis and pigmentation can also be seen. The lesions can be multifocal or unifocal. There is also an association in HPV-related cases with intraepithelial neoplasia of the cervix, vagina and perianal areas.

Diagnosis is by biopsy, which may be taken at vulvoscopy, using 5% acetic acid as at colposcopy, under either local or general anaesthesia. The opportunity should be taken to look at the cervix at the same time, as there is an association with cervical intraepithelial neoplasia (CIN). As the natural history is so uncertain, treatment is controversial. Regression has been observed but progression of high-grade VIN to invasion may occur in approximately 5% of cases, and up to 15% of those with high-grade VIN may have superficial invading vulval cancer.

Treatment of VIN includes surgical excision to obtain clear margins with plastic surgical reconstruction for extensive areas; immunomodulators such as imiquimod cream (Aldara) or laser ablation, which has been employed where there is no concern regarding malignancy. Close follow-up is required as the disease can recur. Smoking is a potent cofactor for the development of high-grade VIN and help with respect to smoking cessation should be offered.

Paget disease (extra-mammary Paget disease)

In this uncommon condition there is a poorly demarcated, often multifocal, eczematoid lesion, associated in 10% of cases with adenocarcinoma either in the pelvis or at a distant site. The development of symptoms may precede the development of cancer by 10–15 years. Treatment is by wide local excision, but due to the indistinct nature of the margins it can be difficult to obtain clearance. Recurrences are common.

Vulval carcinoma

Vulval cancer is relatively uncommon. Squamous cell carcinoma accounts for 90% of vulval cancers. Approximately 5% of vulval malignancies are malignant melanomas and the others include Bartholin's gland ca ncer, basal cell carcinomas and sarcomas. It is usually a disease of older women (60+ years) and, like cervical cancer, is commoner in cigarette smokers and women who are immunocompromised. Many squamous vulval cancers also share a common aetiology with cervical cancer in that high-risk HPV is a common cause.

Clinical presentation

Most women will present with a history of long-standing vulval irritation or pruritus, and some will have had a previous history of lichen sclerosus. A lump or ulcer is common (Fig. 16.4). As the disease advances, the tumour grows and focal necrosis may cause discharge and pain. The diagnosis is confirmed by histological examination of a biopsy.

Pathophysiology

Squamous cell carcinoma spreads to the inguinal nodes and, from there, to the external iliac nodes in the pelvis (Table 16.1). Unless the lesion has only penetrated the basement membrane by <1 mm, node involvement can occur and may include both the superficial and deep inguinal lymph node systems.

Surgical management

The treatment of vulval carcinoma is surgical excision, either a wide local excision or vulvectomy, where this can be achieved without compromising bladder or bowel function.

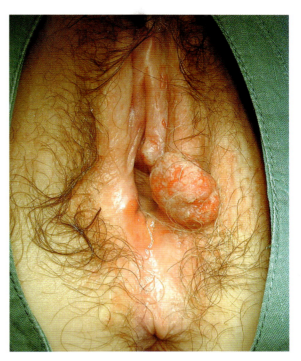

Fig. 16.4 **A stage II left-sided squamous vulval carcinoma.**

Table 16.1	International Federation of Gynecology and Obstetrics (FIGO) staging of vulval carcinoma		
Stage	**Definition**		
I$_A$	Tumour <2.0 cm in dimension and <1 mm of stromal invasion. No lymph vascular space invasion and no nodal disease		
I$_B$	Tumour <2.0 cm in dimension but with >1 mm of stromal invasion		
II	Tumour of any dimension invading the lower one-third urethra/vagina or lower one-third anus with negative nodes		
III	Tumour of any size with or without extension to adjacent perineal structures (lower one-third urethra, lower one-third vagina, anus) with positive inguinofemoral lymph nodes		
	IIIA	(i)	With 1 lymph node metastasis (≥5 mm) or
		(ii)	1–2 lymph node metastasis(es) (<5 mm)
	IIIB	(i)	With ≥2 lymph node metastases (≥5 mm) or
		(ii)	≥3 lymph node metastases (<5 mm)
	IIIC		With positive nodes with extracapsular spread
IV$_A$	(i)		Upper urethral and/or vaginal mucosa, bladder mucosa, rectal mucosa, or fixed to pelvic bone or
	(ii)		Fixed or ulcerated inguinofemoral lymph node
IV$_B$	Any distant metastases including pelvic nodes		

The addition of groin node lymphadenectomy should be performed where the depth of invasion is >1 mm. It is appropriate to carry out only a unilateral exploration if the lesion is well lateralized >1 cm from a midline structure such as the clitoris or posterior fourchette. In all other cases, a bilateral groin node dissection is required. Distant metastases are not a contraindication to radical vulval surgery, as death from a large fungating genital neoplasm or erosion of the femoral artery or vein by metastatic groin nodes is very unpleasant.

The groin explorations are carried out through separate incisions, and the wound will often be drained for around 7–10 days under suction, as lymph fluid accumulates and breakdown is common. To reduce the associated morbidity from groin node dissection, the technique of sentinel node biopsy has been explored and there is growing evidence from large-scale observational studies that this is an acceptable technique with reduced morbidity and false negative rates of 1%. If there is significant groin node involvement, it may be necessary to give adjuvant pelvic node radiotherapy as well.

The commonest complication of a radical vulvectomy is breakdown of the wound, which may take weeks to heal. To reduce the morbidity plastic surgical reconstruction can be offered. In addition, these women are often elderly, immobile and have had surgery on their pelvic vessels close to the femoral vein, leaving them at a high risk of venous thromboembolic disease. Long-term sequelae of surgery include vulval mutilation, if plastic surgical reconstruction is not offered, and lymphoedema. The 5-year survival is around 80% if groin nodes are negative and 40% if positive.

Recurrence

Recurrence of the excised tumour at the primary site is reduced where a 10-mm margin has been achieved. The epithelium is likely to be unstable and there may be multifocal pre-invasive lesions from which new vulval tumours may arise. Treatment of recurrence is surgical, although interstitial radiotherapy may be appropriate. A check should be made at follow-up for signs of tumour spread to nodes.

Key points

- A swollen symptomatic Bartholin's gland or abscess should be marsupialized and not simply incised.
- Lichen sclerosus is associated with squamous carcinoma of the vulva in around 2–5% of women.
- VIN is analogous to intraepithelial neoplasia in the cervix (CIN). Treatment of VIN is local excision of severely dysplastic lesions with careful follow-up.
- Vulval carcinoma is usually of squamous cell type and tends to occur in the more elderly population. The treatment is excision ± unilateral or bilateral inguinal lymphadenectomy. Pelvic radiotherapy may also be indicated if there is a significant chance of nodal spread.

17

Gynaecological surgery

Introduction

The majority of gynaecological surgical procedures are performed electively and, for most patients, preoperative assessment and preparation for surgery can be comprehensive. Although rare, life-threatening complications can arise after minor operations. Counselling and obtaining informed consent should be undertaken by someone capable of performing the proposed procedure, or at least capable of weighing up its risks and benefits. This chapter will address the issues surrounding good surgical practice in patients undergoing gynaecological procedures.

Preoperative counselling

Gynaecological patients require support and assistance when dealing with decisions about surgery. Careful preoperative counselling, competently performed surgery and continuity of care maximize the chance of a successful outcome and a favourable patient experience. Most patients will first be seen in the outpatient clinic where a preliminary assessment and provisional diagnosis will be made. The surgeon must be prepared to spend time discussing and explaining any proposed surgical procedure. This important process is frequently aided by the use of literature and drawings, copies of which should be included in the medical records. It is good practice to provide the patient with written information and invite her to address any uncertainty by direct contact with the clinical team. It is important to keep good records of any communication and meeting with the patient.

Obtaining consent as part of the outpatient clinic visit is viewed as enabling the patient to take this important step away from the stress of admission to hospital on the day of the operation. However, this is to be balanced with the fact that at the time of the clinic visit there may be a lot of information to be considered, possibly affecting the patient's decision-making. It is good practice to reconfirm the wishes of the patient and validity of the consent at the time of their admission for surgery. Standardized, procedure-specific consent forms facilitate good practice.

Patients must give consent for surgery in light of full knowledge of the procedure; what is called 'informed consent'. Risk can be a difficult concept to communicate with a patient, and sensitivity is required when presenting potential adverse outcomes related to a specific operation. Table 17.1 gives an example of how to communicate risk in terms of frequency. It is important to always use accurate terminology with appropriate explanation.

If surgery and general anaesthesia are contemplated for patients with comorbidities, these should be communicated to the anaesthetist to allow satisfactory preparation and to avoid anaesthetic complications. Liaison with other specialties may be necessary to ensure the postoperative course runs smoothly.

Smoking continues to be prevalent in society, especially among younger women. The visit to the hospital is a good opportunity to impress on the patient the importance of stopping smoking. It not necessary to stop the oral contraceptive pill before minor surgery and only those patients at higher risk should have the pill stopped and alternative contraception introduced. Obese patients often have poor exercise tolerance and recover less quickly from the physiological stress of surgery. Unfortunately, the practice of sending the patient away for some time to lose weight is often counter-productive. Sometimes it is impractical to delay treatment (such as in cancer treatment). Prophylaxis for venous thromboembolism (VTE) must be considered for all major procedures.

In most modern centres, preoperative assessment clinics, run by nursing staff, enable the majority of preoperative investigations and admission procedures to be performed on an outpatient basis. Early admission (not on the same day as surgery) may be necessary on occasion for patients who have specific problems which may need optimization prior to surgery, such as infections of the operative field, control of diabetes, nutritional improvement or preoperative physiotherapy.

Gynaecological operations

Gynaecological surgery generally involves removal or repair of the tissues of the female genital tract. In oncological surgery, this will also extend to removal of sites where gynaecological cancer may have spread, for example draining lymph nodes and omentum. Many of the procedures will be discussed in other chapters and, therefore, only an overview will be given here. More common gynaecological procedures are listed in Table 17.2.

Safer surgery principles

Unfortunately, avoidable surgical complications account for a substantial number of preventable injuries and deaths.

Table 17.1	Presenting information on risk (adapted from the Royal College of Obstetricians and Gynaecologists [RCOG] clinical governance advice, presenting information on risk)	
Term	**Equivalent numerical ratio**	**Colloquial equivalent**
Very common	1/1 to 1/10	A person in family
Common	1/10 to 1/100	A person in street
Uncommon	1/100 to 1/1000	A person in village
Rare	1/1000 to 1/10 000	A person in small town
Very rare	Less than 1/10 000	A person in large town

The World Health Organization produced a surgical safety guidance which identified a core set of safety checks for improving performance at critical time points within the patient's care pathway. The checklist provides structure and guidance for surgical teams, allowing them to work together in a safe and effective manner. This guidance has been widely adopted in the UK, with one of the key features being the introduction of safety checks (briefing, sign in, time out, surgical pause, sign out and debriefing) for all surgical procedures (Fig. 17.1). All healthcare professionals are responsible for ensuring that the safer surgery principles are adopted and utilized. All healthcare team members have a responsibility for ensuring that the correct procedure is performed on the correct patient, at the correct site and on the correct side.

A *briefing*, involving all the key team members, must be performed at the start of all procedure sessions. All required members of the procedural team must attend the briefing, including the operator and anaesthetist, their trainee(s)/assistant(s), and the scrub and circulating practitioners. For each patient the discussion should include: the diagnosis and planned procedure, site and side of procedure, its expected duration, infection risk, e.g. methicillin-resistant *Staphylococcus aureus* status, allergies, relevant comorbidities or complications, need for antibiotic prophylaxis, likely need for blood or blood products, patient positioning,

Table 17.2	Gynaecological operations	
Site	**Procedure**	**Indication**
Vulva	Radical vulvectomy	Advanced vulval cancer
	Wide local excision	Early vulval cancer
	Excision biopsy	VIN/suspicious vulval lesion
	Incisional/punch biopsy	Diagnosis of vulval disease
Vagina	Anterior colporrhaphy (anterior repair)	Cystocele
	Posterior colporrhaphy (posterior repair)	Rectocele
	Manchester repair (amputation of cervix and anterior colporrhaphy)	Vaginal prolapse
	Sacrospinous fixation	Prolapse of the vaginal vault
Cervix	Radical trachelectomy	Early-stage cervical cancer
Endometrium	Endometrial ablation	Heavy menstrual bleeding (HMB)
	Hysteroscopic resection	Symptomatic fibroids, endometrial polyps
Uterus	Abdominal total hysterectomy (removal of body of uterus and cervix. Subtotal hysterectomy is when the cervix is conserved)	HMB Endometrial/ovarian cancer (total hysterectomy is one component of treatment)
	Total laparoscopic hysterectomy	HMB/early cervical cancer/endometrial cancer
	Laparoscopic-assisted vaginal hysterectomy	HMB/early cervical cancer/endometrial cancer
	Radical hysterectomy	Stage IB1 cervical cancer
	Vaginal hysterectomy (often with a colporrhaphy)	Uterine prolapse
	Myomectomy (open or laparoscopic)	Fibroids
Fallopian tube	Salpingectomy (open or laparoscopic)	Ectopic pregnancy/hydrosalpinx
	Salpingostomy	Ectopic pregnancy to retain tube
	Laparoscopic tubal ligation	Contraception
Ovary	Oophorectomy (open or laparoscopic)	Removal of normal or diseased ovary
	Ovarian cystectomy (open or laparoscopic)	Removal of ovarian cyst(s)

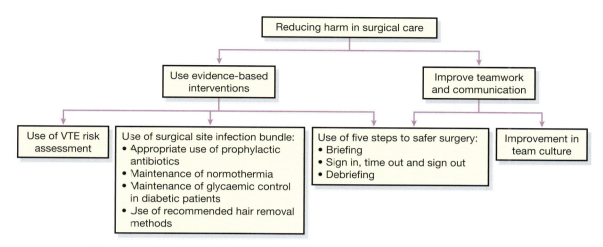

Fig. 17.1 **Safer surgery principles.**

equipment requirements and availability, and the postoperative destination for the patient, e.g. ward or critical care unit.

The checks performed during the *sign in* should include: the patient's name checked against the identity band, consent form, surgical site marking if applicable, operating list, anaesthetic safety checks, allergies, aspiration risk, potential airway problems, arrangements in case of blood loss and the result of the pregnancy test.

The *time out* should be performed before any procedure is commenced and prior to skin preparation and incision, and should include checks of: the patient's name and identity band against the consent form, the procedure to be performed and verification of surgical site marking, the anticipated blood loss, any specific equipment requirements or special investigations, any critical or unexpected steps, any patient-specific concerns, any anaesthetic concerns, any equipment issues or concerns, antibiotic prophylaxis, patient warming, glycaemic control, hair removal, VTE prophylaxis and patient allergies.

Immediately prior to the skin incision, a *surgical pause* must be conducted and must be led by the surgeon. All team members must participate in the surgical pause, which includes verification of the patient identity, procedure and correct site verification.

Sign out checks should be conducted at the end of the procedure and before the patient leaves the operating room. These checks should include: confirmation of the procedure performed (to include site and side if appropriate), confirmation that instruments, sharps and swab counts are complete, confirmation that any specimens have been labelled correctly and discussion of post-procedural care, to include any patient-specific concerns or equipment problems.

A *debriefing* should be performed at the end of all elective procedure sessions. The discussion should include: things that went well, any problems with equipment or other issues that occurred and any areas for improvements.

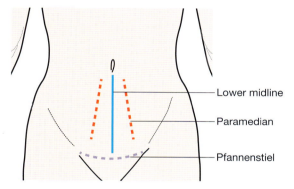

Fig. 17.2 **Skin incisions.**

Surgical anatomy

Normal anatomy is shown in Chapter 1. Underlying disease processes may disrupt normal anatomy by destroying normal tissue planes (e.g. in endometriosis and malignancy), and make identification of anatomical structures challenging for even the experienced surgeon.

Hysterectomy is one operation where the main gynaecological structures are often clearly visible and the principal steps in this procedure will be outlined later. Dissection usually involves a combination of scalpel, scissors and diathermy, but there is increasing use of sealing/cutting devices generated by high-frequency oscillation of the instrument's blade or bipolar diathermy.

Abdominal wall incision

Options for type of skin incision are as shown in Fig. 17.2. The length and position of the abdominal incision will depend on the purpose of the operation and on the body habitus of the patient. The incision must allow the surgeon to carry out the procedure with ease and enable full access to the operative field. The choice of the incision should be determined by the following considerations: simplicity of the incision, the need for exposure, the potential need for enlarging the incision, the cosmesis of the healed incision and the location of previous surgical scars. Most gynaecological procedures are best performed through one of two incisions – the subumbilical midline incision or the low transverse suprapubic incision (Pfannenstiel); the latter is often preferred for cosmetic reasons, as the incision follows the natural skin crease (Langer's lines), hence the alternative term 'bikini-line incision'. The incision has the disadvantage of being more vascular than a midline incision and, if extended too far laterally, can be associated with nerve damage. It also offers only a limited access to the pelvis and a midline or paramedian is preferred when there is a large pelvic mass such as a large ovarian cyst or fibroid uterus. The Pfannenstiel incision has a low incidence of wound herniation due to the criss-crossing nature of the vertical rectus abdominis muscles and the horizontal fibres of the rectus sheath.

Once through the skin and subcutaneous layers of Camper and Scarpa fascia, the rectus sheath is revealed. This is then opened and the rectus abdominis muscle lies beneath. The bellies of this muscle are separated in the midline and the extraperitoneal fat displaced to reveal the peritoneum. This is elevated between two clamps and inspected to ensure no bowel lies below before entry. Care must be taken to identify the inferior epigastric vessels, which bleed heavily if injured.

After entering the peritoneal cavity, the abdomen and pelvis are explored systematically. Following inspection of the pelvis, the bowel is packed away with large gauze swabs and a self-retaining retractor inserted. A variety of retractors have been designed for pelvic and abdominal surgery to allow adequate exposure.

Round and infundibulopelvic ligaments

The uterus is held between two straight forceps and elevated. This delineates the round ligaments, which are then divided. The soft areolar tissue of the broad ligament, which lies between the anterior and posterior leaves of peritoneum, are dissected to reveal the ureter and ensure it is clear of the clamps to be placed on the ovarian vessels running in the infundibulopelvic ligament. This is the most common site for inadvertent ureteric injury. When the ovaries are to be retained the clamp is placed on the medial side of the tubo-ovarian complex and the pedicle divided here instead. With increasing evidence of the tube being the source of high-grade serous cancers of the ovary and peritoneum, it is usual to remove the fallopian tubes but retain the ovaries in patients wishing to retain their ovaries.

Bladder reflection

The uterus is pulled cranially to help identify the uterovesical peritoneum. The peritoneum is then divided and the areolar tissue around the bladder divided, allowing the plane between bladder and anterior uterus and cervix to be developed. This displaces the bladder downwards, reducing the risk of bladder damage later in the dissection.

Division of the uterine vessels

The uterine artery is readily identifiable due to its spiral and tortuous appearance. The vaginal angles are then divided but the vagina not opened.

Opening the vagina

A knife is used to enter the anterior fornix, and when the incision is widened the uterosacral ligaments are clamped and the remaining vaginal tissue divided to permit removal of the uterus from the pelvis.

The vaginal skin edges are grasped and the vaginal cuff oversewn either circumferentially or opposed to either side. It is not necessary to close the peritoneum, which heals whether sutured or not.

Wound closure

Following closure of the vagina and confirmation of haemostasis, the tissues of the abdomen are closed in the reverse order to opening. It is important to appose the tissues and avoid over-enthusiastic tension in the sutures, as this will have a detrimental effect on tissue perfusion and increase the likelihood of wound dehiscence.

Radical (Wertheim) hysterectomy for cervical malignancy differs from the simple hysterectomy by formally dissecting the ureter along its length in the pelvis, dividing the uterine vessels at their source as they leave the anterior division of the internal iliac vessels allowing adequate dissection of the parametrial tissues. A 'cuff' of vagina is removed to achieve adequate margins around the tumour.

Laparoscopic surgery

Nearly all gynaecological operations that are carried out through an open incision can technically be undertaken with laparoscopic surgery. Although gynaecologists have been performing simple laparoscopic surgery for decades, the range of operations is now developing rapidly. There are constant improvements in optics and digital camera equipment that enhance the surgeon's vision. In addition, the evolution of instruments specifically for laparoscopic surgery has meant that procedures have become easier to perform and operating times have reduced. This has considerable benefits for patients who gain by avoiding an open procedure (Box 17.1).

Technique

Patient position

The patient is placed flat in a Lloyds-Davies position with the hips flexed at 45° rather than the near 90° used for many other gynaecological procedures. The use of moveable padded stirrups/boots allows the position of the legs to be altered intraoperatively. The flat position prevents bowel being displaced toward the umbilicus. The bladder should be emptied to reduce risk of injury and, if required, a uterine manipulator can be introduced transvaginally to allow mobilization of the uterus.

Pneumoperitoneum

There is wide variation in the techniques used by surgeons to gain primary entry (first trocar) into the peritoneal cavity with subsequent creation of a pneumoperitoneum. Gynae-cologists have tended to favour the transumbilical **Veress needle (closed) entry** technique, whereby the abdominal cavity is insufflated with CO_2 gas prior to introduction of the primary trocar and cannula. General surgeons have often preferred the **open/cut-down (Hasson) approach**. This method uses a small periumbilical incision to enter the peritoneal cavity under direct vision. **Direct trocar insertion** is a third, acceptable method, which, in experienced hands, is the most rapid method of entry and can be safely used if the cases are carefully selected. It is not widely used within gynaecological practice.

Alternative sites for primary entry have been described, most notably Palmer's point, which is 3 cm below the left costal margin in the midclavicular line. A small incision is made and a Veress needle is inserted vertically. After pneumoperitoneum is established, a 2–5 mm endoscope is used to inspect the undersurface of the umbilical region. If this is free of adhesions, the trocar and cannulae can be inserted under direct laparoscopic vision. If there are many adhesions present, it is possible to dissect these free via secondary ports.

In women who have had previous laparotomies, the intra-abdominal anatomy may be altered by adhesions. In patients who have had complicated abdominal operations, the bowel may be attached under, very close to, or occasion-ally above the umbilicus. Open laparoscopic entry or Palmer's point entry are preferred in women with a history of previous surgery and in women where intra-abdominal adhesions are anticipated.

Once the pneumoperitoneum has been created, subse-quent ports may be introduced, always under direct vision. The inferior epigastric vessels can often be identified to avoid injury prior to any lateral port insertion. Any instruments being inserted into or removed from the peritoneum must be visualized to avoid inadvertent injury. At the end of the procedure, any trocar site with a diameter >10 mm should have the underlying sheath closed to avoid a Richter hernia. Gas should be expelled to reduce referred shoulder-tip pain and trocars removed under direct vision.

Postoperative management

Immediate postoperative care is geared to identify potential complications arising from the surgery or new-onset medical complications secondary to the physiological stresses of surgery and anaesthesia. Regular recording of temperature, pulse, blood pressure, respiratory rate and urine output help early recognition of an adverse event. These physiological parameters can be recorded as a combined score that helps provide an early warning of a patient's deteriorating condition and mandates early medical review.

The use of T.E.D anti-embolism stockings and low-molecular-weight heparin help minimize VTE. Early mobiliza-tion and maintenance of hydration also help to minimize the risk of VTE. Rather than traditional bed rest and fasting post-surgery, emphasis is now placed on 'enhanced recovery', where the patient is allowed oral fluids and diet early in the postoperative period and the use of intra-abdominal drains, naso-gastric tubes and urinary catheters is kept to a minimum. Attention is also focused on good pain relief and prevention of postoperative nausea and vomiting.

Postoperative complications

Postoperative complications can be classified with regard to their timing related to the surgery, i.e. intraoperative, immediate postoperative period and delayed postoperative period. Complications arising from surgery may include bowel, bladder or ureter injury; the management of these are beyond the scope of this chapter but may require the assistance of a general surgeon or urologist. Intraoperative bleeding can be profuse and difficult to arrest if the vessels retract into the pelvic sidewall. In the presence of such bleeding, care must be taken to identify the bowel, bladder and ureter, as frantically placed sutures can lead to their injury and complicate surgery further. Clear communication with the anaesthetist is essential to enable circulatory support and the issue of blood products.

Immediate postoperative complications can also include bleeding and this is often masked in the younger patient by their ability to compensate physiologically for blood loss. However, the combination of abdominal pain, developing tachycardia and oliguria should raise suspicions of post-operative bleeding. It may not be until the patient is *in extremis* before she becomes hypotensive. Postoperative pyrexia is common and has multiple causes. Basal atelectasis of the lungs, bacteraemia and VTE should be considered and managed accordingly. Unrecognized bowel injury may reveal itself within the first 24 h, but iatrogenic ureteric obstruction may not become symptomatic until day 4 postoperatively. The incidence of wound infections is reduced by a strict hand hygiene policy and administration of intraoperative antibiotics. These may be continued further in those at high risk of wound infection, i.e. the obese, patients with diabetes or those on steroid medication.

Voiding of urine can be affected by many gynaecological procedures – pain in itself can result in urinary retention, so close attention to fluid balance should be given in the immediate hours following surgery in those without a urinary catheter. Following removal of the catheter, complete emptying of the bladder should be demonstrated, as residual volumes of urine can predispose to ascending urinary tract infection and longer term voiding difficulties.

Delayed complications may involve delayed wound healing, VTE, bladder dysfunction, chronic pain, lymphoedema, or lymphocyst formation and genital tract fistulae.

Key points

- The decision to proceed with a surgical procedure ideally should be taken by the gynaecologist who will be performing the surgery.
- Alternatives to surgery should be explored thoroughly and discussion documented in the notes.
- Informed consent should be clearly documented and written information provided where possible.
- Familiarity with pelvic anatomy is essential to understand gynaecological surgery and minimize surgical complications.
- Use of a surgical early-warning scoring system can assist in identifying immediate postoperative complications.

18

Pelvic infection and STIs

Introduction

Symptoms commonly associated with genital infection in women include vaginal discharge, abnormal vaginal bleeding, pelvic pain, genital lumps and ulceration. Bacterial vaginosis (BV) and *Candida albicans* are common and do not usually have serious sequelae, but sexually transmitted infections (STIs) such as *Chlamydia trachomatis*, gonorrhoea, syphilis and genital herpes can cause acute and long-term morbidity.

Symptoms of genital infection in women are common and in the majority of cases are not due to STIs. Conversely, most STIs are asymptomatic: about 70% of women with chlamydia, 50% with gonorrhoea, 30% with human papillomavirus (HPV) and 50% with genital herpes have no symptoms. In women, untreated infections can lead to chronic pain or infertility, may significantly increase susceptibility to sexual transmission of human immunodeficiency virus (HIV), and can lead to genital cancers such as cervical carcinoma. STIs in pregnant women can cause serious complications including stillbirth, neonatal death, prematurity, neonatal sepsis, low birth weight and congenital abnormalities.

The World Health Organization estimates that there are over 357 million cases of the four major curable STIs (syphilis, gonorrhoea, chlamydia and trichomoniasis) in adults aged 15–49 throughout the world each year, with 90% in developing countries. Sexually transmissible blood-borne viruses (BBVs), including hepatitis B and HIV, are transmitted horizontally (through sex) and vertically (from mother to child). Hepatitis B is a highly infectious virus affecting 240 million people worldwide, with the main route of acquisition being by neonates at birth or in the first year of life. Of these, 90% will develop chronic infection, with a 15–40% chance of cirrhosis and hepatocellular carcinoma. A total of 37 million people worldwide were living with HIV at the end of 2015, of whom 18 million were taking antiretroviral therapy (ART) – resulting in a 45% reduction in acquired immunodeficiency syndrome (AIDS)-related deaths worldwide since the peak in 2005, when only 2 million accessed therapy. Of pregnant women worldwide in 2015, 77% accessed antiretrovirals to prevent mother-to-child transmission, with a 50% reduction in new HIV infections in children since 2010. Despite these improvements, there have been no overall decline in new HIV infections among adults since 2010. Rates of all STIs can vary dramatically geographically and over time, affected by social disruption such as war, economic decline or mass migration, the availability of tests and services, treatment and vaccination programmes, and social mores and sexual behaviour. For example, rates of gonorrhoea and syphilis fell dramatically in the UK and elsewhere following the widespread availability of effective antibiotics following the end of the Second World War, whereas infections increased substantially in much of Eastern Europe in the 1990s following the collapse of the former Soviet Union. Cases of genital warts in women fell by half in Australia following the introduction of a quadrivalent vaccine against HPV in 2006, and signs of similar changes are beginning to be noted in the UK after the introduction of the same vaccine in 2012. However, the prevailing trend for most STIs in the UK in this century has been upwards, with sustained rises in gonorrhoea, chlamydial and herpes infections in women since 2006. Unsafe sex was identified in 2016 as the fastest growing risk factor for ill health in young women (and men) worldwide between1990 and 2013. Contributory factors include changes in sexual behaviour, ways of sexual mixing (such as the use of mobile phone apps), early sexual debut, increased geographical mobility within and between countries, the emergence of drug-resistant strains, asymptomatic infections, and barriers to accessing testing and treatment services, often affecting those most at risk of infection.

The risk of STI acquisition is increased with younger age (under 25), prior STI diagnosis, frequent partner change or concurrent partners, non-use of condoms and high rates of condom errors. However, for many women, particularly in developing countries, it is the social and demographic risk factors affecting the community from which she chooses a regular partner, rather than her own individual risk factors, that determine her STI risk.

Principles of STI management

To minimize the harms from STI in women the aim is to maximize early diagnosis, appropriate testing, early treatment and partner notification to break the chain of infection. Performing STI testing solely in all women who present with genital symptoms will result in large numbers of tests being performed on women at very low risk of STI, but miss or delay a diagnosis in women at risk both of serious complications and of onward horizontal and vertical transmission of infection. STI syndromic management involves treating the most likely causal organism(s) of a syndrome to ensure prompt treatment. Syndromic management can be applied to both resource-rich and resource-limited settings as part of a public health approach which includes the following components:

- syndromic management *without diagnostic testing* in women at low risk of STI: many women presenting for the first time with vaginal discharge can be treated empirically following a clinical diagnosis
- syndromic management *with diagnostic testing* and early treatment before test results are available in women at higher risk of STI: women who are diagnosed with clinical genital herpes or pelvic inflammatory disease (PID) are treated before STI test results are available
- diagnostic testing for STI according to individual or population-based risk assessment, clinical setting and local and national resources
- partner notification (identifying, tracing, treating and/or testing the partners of women diagnosed with possible STI) to prevent reinfection and/or onward transmission
- routine population-based screening for infections which are common and/or have serious sequelae in particular subpopulations (e.g. antenatal syphilis, HIV and hepatitis B testing, chlamydia screening in under 25s)
- prophylactic treatment in women undergoing procedures associated with the risk of ascending infection (e.g. termination of pregnancy)
- vaccination – highly effective vaccines against hepatitis B and HPV are widely available, vaccines against HIV, herpes simplex virus (HSV) and other STIs are in development.

In most countries, these elements are clearly defined in local, national and international guidelines and policies. In routine clinical practice, the risk of missing a serious STI diagnosis is reduced by maintaining a low threshold for performing tests in both symptomatic and asymptomatic women, a high level of awareness of the genital and non-genital manifestations of STI and, above all, routinely including an STI risk assessment in clinical history-taking.

Once an STI has been diagnosed, partner notification (contact tracing) is essential in the management of bacterial STIs, HIV and hepatitis B, both to prevent reinfection in those that are curable and to avoid further onward transmission. Partner notification strategies include: patient referral, where the patient informs recent partner(s); provider referral, where details are passed to a healthcare professional who then contacts the partners; and conditional referral, where provider referral is initiated if patient referral has not occurred after an agreed period has elapsed. In provider referral, it is usual to protect the identity of the index patient. Enhanced partner notification strategies include providing the patient with antibiotic treatment for the partner or with a pharmacy voucher for treatment, and the use of innovative web applications or mobile apps to allow patients to inform partners, while preserving anonymity, is increasing. Patients are advised to abstain from sex until they and their partner(s) have completed treatment.

Sexual history

A syndromic approach to STI management in individual women depends on an accurate assessment of risk factors for particular STIs. This in turn makes a comprehensive understanding of symptoms, current and past sexual partners, and other risk activities a crucial part of STI management.

A woman presenting with genital symptoms may or may not have considered the possibility of an STI and women attending for other reasons, such as termination of pregnancy, may be unaware of STI risk. Time, sensitivity and privacy must be ensured: interviews should take place in a sound-proof setting. Accurate answers to a risk assessment may not be possible with a partner or relative present. Questioning should be sensitive, inclusive and appropriate, but direct, avoiding euphemisms. As with all history-taking, choice of words and appropriate facial expressions and body language in the questioner are important. Use open language to avoid conveying any impression of being judgmental; examples are the use of inclusive words such as 'partner' rather than 'boyfriend'.

After eliciting a history of any presenting symptoms, medication, contraception and a gynaecological history, the sexual history should be taken. 'When did you last have sex?' is the ideal opening question if the woman has been put at ease, but asking 'Do you have a (sexual) partner?' can be a gentler introduction if she is not expecting questions about sexual contacts. For recent contact(s) the important factors affecting the risk and site of infection include the partner status (one-off, regular or other), partner gender, the types of sex that took place, use of condoms, the partner's place of origin and consent to sex. The same questions should be asked about other partners in the last 3 months. See Box 18.1 for further suggestions on sexual history taking for STIs. If universal testing for HIV and hepatitis is not local policy, an assessment of lifetime risk is useful in deciding on whether testing for BBVs is indicated:

- Was the woman born and brought up in an area with higher HIV or hepatitis prevalence (e.g. sub-Saharan Africa)?
- Has she had any sexual partners from these areas?
- Has she had any male partners she knows to have been bisexual?
- Has she or any partner used intravenous recreational drugs?

Examination for genital infections

The history can provide some indication of both the type and site of infection, but syndromic management requires

Box 18.1

Sexual history taking for STIs

A model for sexual history taking for STI with examples.
1. Open questions should be used at the start. 'Tell me…, Tell me about that …, So tell me the story …'.
2. More open questions are employed to establish detail. 'Tell me more about how this pain developed …, What is the discharge like …?'
3. Straightforward anatomical terms should be used (vagina is OK, vulva often is not). 'So, you mean on the lips of your vagina?'
4. One simple framing statement before taking the sexual history avoids any sense of apology or embarrassment. 'So, thinking about your sex life …, Some questions about your sex life …'.
5. Focussing on events helps to avoid labels and generalizations. 'When did you last have sex, any sort of sex …?'
6. Permission-giving can be included in the question (explicit permission for a range of answers). 'Was that a one-off thing, with a regular partner, or something else? Have your partners been men, women or both? Was that oral sex, vaginal sex, anal sex … or all of them?'
7. The 'non-acceptable' or non-sanctioned answer should be invited. 'So that was without a condom …? Do you ever use condoms? When did you last have sober sex?'
8. Remember that partners' place of origin is a major determinant of STI risk. 'So, was he/she from (this town/city) … or elsewhere? Any partners from outside the UK?'
9. Gentleness should be balanced with directness. 'So, did everything happen with your consent or perhaps not?'
10. Display innocent inquisitiveness to understand social issues. 'I really don't know much about which dating apps people use to meet up … can you tell me more?'
11. Make every question permissive of a full range of possible answers. 'When did you last have sex with anyone else/any other partner?'
12. Understand and mitigate the ways in which your own values might affect your questioning. 'When was your last previous partner?' (which assumes serial monogamy – so avoid).

the use of all available information for clinical diagnosis. Examination should be performed in all women with symptoms. This should be in a private room and the woman should be provided with a gown to cover the areas not being examined. She should give informed consent, understanding what the examination and any samples taken will involve and be offered a chaperone for both the history and examination, regardless of the practitioner's gender. Male clinicians must have a chaperone when examining a woman's genital tract. The woman should be in the lithotomy position, and there should be a good light source behind the examiner. Genital examination is directed by the presenting symptoms and the clinician should:

- inspect the pubic hair and surrounding skin for pubic lice and any skin rashes
- palpate the inguinal region for lymphadenopathy
- inspect the labia majora and minora, clitoris, introitus, perineum and perianal area for warts, ulcers, erythema or excoriation
- inspect the urethral meatus and Skene's and Bartholin's glands for any discharge or swelling

- insert a bivalve speculum into the vagina
- inspect the vaginal walls for erythema, discharge, warts, ulcers
- inspect the cervix for discharge, erythema, contact bleeding, ulcers or raised lesions. Mucopurulent discharge from the cervix should be noted, but is not a reliable indicator of infection
- perform a bimanual pelvic examination to assess size and any tenderness of the uterus, cervical motion tenderness (cervical excitation) and adnexal tenderness or masses.

Taking samples for genital infections

Syndromic management alone, based on a combination of clinical symptoms and signs, is appropriate for women at low risk of STI who present with genital warts or a first episode of uncomplicated vaginal discharge. In most other situations, samples for microbiological testing are indicated to support the clinical diagnosis. Nucleic acid amplification testing (NAAT) is widely available for the diagnosis of chlamydia, gonorrhoea and herpes simplex, and increasingly commonly for trichomoniasis and symptomatic early syphilis (ulcers). When samples for culture or microscopy are required, or during the examination of a symptomatic woman, the swabs required will depend on the laboratory facilities available locally and the presenting symptoms. The following tests are routinely offered to symptomatic and asymptomatic women at risk of STI in non-specialist settings:

- a lower vaginal swab (obtained by the clinician or by the patient) for NAAT for both chlamydia and gonorrhoea
- a blood sample for syphilis and HIV serology
- hepatitis B testing* of the same sample if the woman or any of her sexual partners are from areas of high hepatitis B prevalence (e.g. sub-Saharan Africa or Asia)
- hepatitis B* and C testing, if the woman or any of her sexual partners have ever injected drugs.
- Additional samples may be indicated depending on presentation:
  - samples for NAAT testing for herpes simplex and syphilis may be taken if ulcers or fissures are seen
  - additional samples for NAAT testing for chlamydia and gonorrhoea may be taken from other sites of potential exposure (throat and/or rectum)
  - samples of vaginal discharge may be taken for microscopy in cases of recurrent, complicated or atypical discharge. NAAT and enzyme tests to detect the organisms of BV are available but not widely used

*hepatitis B immunization should be offered if the hepatitis B test is negative and she is at continued risk

❑ if a woman is to be treated for suspected gonorrhoea, in addition to NAAT tests as described above, swabs for culture for gonorrhoea placed in Amies, Stuart's or similar transport medium, or directly inoculating a culture plate, may be taken from the urethra and endocervix, for antibiotic sensitivity testing.

Syndromes associated with genital infections

Asymptomatic

Many infections are completely asymptomatic, so testing should be considered on the basis of risk factors. In many areas, all women attending for healthcare will be offered HIV testing, or those under the age of 25 will be routinely offered testing for chlamydial infection.

Vaginal discharge

An increase in vaginal discharge may be due to a number of infective and non-infective conditions (Table 18.1). Even in areas of high STI prevalence, most women presenting with vaginal discharge alone will not have an STI, so syndromic management of first presentation of vaginal discharge without microbiological testing is often appropriate in women with no recent change of sexual partner.

Symptoms can help to distinguish the causes and anatomical origin of a vaginal discharge including:

■ an increase in vaginal discharge without any itch or irritation accompanied by an unpleasant or fishy odour, which may be worse after sexual intercourse and during menstruation, indicates the possibility of BV)
■ vulval itching accompanied by a thick, white vaginal discharge, vulval burning, external dysuria and superficial dyspareunia may indicate candidiasis
■ a purulent or mucopurulent discharge, with bloodstaining and/or post-coital or intermenstrual bleeding indicates the possibility of a discharge originating from an inflamed cervix, more commonly associated with STI including chlamydia and gonorrhoea

■ abdominal, pelvic or back pain, deep dyspareunia or systemic symptoms may suggest infection that has ascended to the uterus, ovaries and or fallopian tubes, or is systemic.

Signs elicited on examination may assist with the diagnosis:

■ an absence of any inflammation of the vulva or vagina and a discharge with a homogeneous, white appearance which is adherent to the vaginal walls and may be malodourous is typical of BV (Fig. 18.1)
■ vulval erythema, sometimes with satellite lesions, fissuring, excoriation and oedema may indicate vulvovaginal candidiasis. Discharge may be thick or curdy, occasionally with typical white candidal plaques on the vaginal walls (Fig. 18.2)
■ a purulent malodorous yellow or grey vaginal discharge with vulval erythema and excoriation and inflammation of the vaginal walls raises the possibility of trichomoniasis
■ a purulent or bloodstained cervical discharge may increase the suspicion of chlamydial or gonococcal infection, indicating that tests for these infections should be undertaken.

Additional tests can be performed:

■ narrow-range pH paper can be used to test the pH of the vaginal discharge either by pressing a strip of pH against the lateral vaginal walls, or using a swab to transfer a small sample of discharge onto the paper. It is important to avoid sampling cervical secretions, as cervical mucus has a pH of 7 and any contamination will give a falsely high reading. A pH of >4.9 suggests the presence of anaerobic organisms (which metabolize nitrogen into amine compounds) and supports a diagnosis of BV or less commonly trichomoniasis. The pH of the vagina with normal flora, or with candidal infection is below 4.5
■ a swab of vaginal secretions is taken from the lateral vaginal walls and the pool of discharge in the

Table 18.1	Causes of vaginal discharge
Vaginal infections	Bacterial vaginosis
	Candida albicans
	Trichomonas vaginalis
Cervical infections	*Chlamydia trachomatis*
	Neisseria gonorrhoeae
Physiological discharge	Cervical ectopy
Other causes	Retained tampon
	Retained products of conception

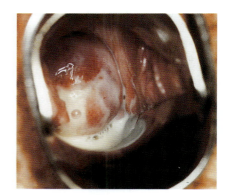

Fig. 18.1   Bacterial vaginosis. BV is due to an overgrowth of anaerobic bacteria, genital mycoplasmas and *Gardnerella vaginalis*. The discharge is milky white, adherent to the vaginal walls, and may be frothy.

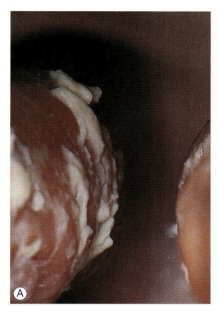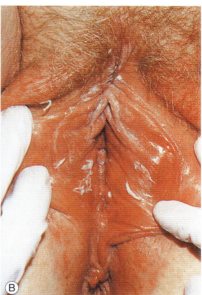

Fig. 18.2   Candidal infection. (A,B) Although *Candida* may present with these 'typical' white plaques, the discharge is sometimes minimal. (**A**, From McMillan A, Young H, Ogilvie MM, Scott GR (eds), Clinical Practice in Sexually Transmissible Infections, Saunders 2003. **B**, From Clutterbuck D, Specialist Training in Sexually Transmitted Infections and HIV, Mosby 2005.)

posterior fornix. Samples can be inoculated onto glass slides for immediate Gram staining and wet-mount direct microscopy – routinely used in many specialist sexual health clinics. In other settings, the swab is sent to the laboratory in a transport medium (e.g. Amies) for examination

- microscopy of a Gram-stained sample may reveal depletion of normal lactobacilli and the presence of mixed organisms – diagnostic of BV. Pseudohyphae and spores of candidal infection may be seen
- examination of a wet mount (suspending the discharge in a drop of saline) may reveal Clue cells (epithelial cells covered with bacteria that are 'clues' to the diagnosis of BV) or the motile flagellate trichomonads of *Trichomonas vaginalis* (TV)
- culture of vaginal samples is not routinely indicated and is rarely helpful.

Infections of the vagina

Bacterial vaginosis

Background information

BV is the most common cause of vaginal discharge in women of reproductive age, found in around 9% of women in general practice, 12% of pregnant women and 30% of women undergoing termination of pregnancy. BV is due to an overgrowth of anaerobic bacteria, genital mycoplasmas and *Gardnerella vaginalis* (all of which can normally be present in small numbers in the vagina). Risk of BV is associated with multiple male or female partners, having a new sexual partner and non-use of condoms. Treating male partners of women with BV, however, does not affect recurrence and is not recommended.

About 50% of women with BV are asymptomatic. A total of 30–50% of women are colonized with *G. vaginalis*, anaerobes and mycoplasmas, as part of their normal vaginal flora, so culture is not helpful in the diagnosis of BV.

Treatment and management

Asymptomatic non-pregnant women do not need treatment. Treatment is recommended in all women with symptoms and those undergoing gynaecological surgery (including termination of pregnancy).

Treatments include:

- metronidazole 400 mg twice daily for 7 days
- intravaginal clindamycin cream 2% once daily for 7 days.

Complications

BV increases vaginal vault infection following hysterectomy, postpartum endometritis following caesarean section and post-abortal PID after surgical termination of pregnancy.

It increases a woman's risk of acquiring HIV infection two- to three-fold, and may also increase the risk of transmission of HIV to a male partner.

Candidal infections

Background information

Some 75% of all women experience at least one episode of symptomatic *Candida* in their lifetime. About 20% of asymptomatic women have vaginal colonization with *Candida*. Increased rates of colonization (30–40%) are found in pregnancy and uncontrolled diabetes. Factors associated with symptomatic *Candida* are pregnancy, diabetes, immunosuppression, antimicrobial therapy and vulval irritation/trauma. It is not sexually acquired, so sexual partners do not need to be treated.

Diagnosis

Microscopy and culture is the most sensitive method of diagnosis, but in many cases syndromic management without testing is appropriate. The sensitivity of clinical diagnosis increases with the number of symptoms and signs present. Up to half of women who self-diagnose candidal infection have another condition.

Treatment and management

Azole antifungals are widely used for treatment:
- oral fluconazole 150 mg single dose (oral azoles are contraindicated in pregnancy)
- clotrimazole pessaries for 1, 3 or 6 nights.

Complications

There are no known long-term complications from candidal infections.

Trichomonas vaginalis

Background information

TV is uncommon in the UK but in other parts of the world, e.g. Africa and Asia, it remains a major cause of vaginal discharge. It is sexually transmitted and only infects the urogenital tract. It may be asymptomatic in 10–50% of women, but can cause significant vulval and vaginal inflammation.

Treatment and management

The recommended treatment is:
- metronidazole 2 g single oral dose, or
- metronidazole 400 mg orally twice daily for 5–7 days.

Of women with TV, 30% have gonorrhoea and/or chlamydia, so they should be tested for other STIs. Patients should abstain from sex until they and their partner(s) have completed treatment.

Complications

TV increases a woman's risk of acquiring HIV infection, and in pregnancy is associated with low birth weight and pre-term delivery.

Infections of the cervix

Chlamydia trachomatis

Background information

C. trachomatis is the most frequently seen bacterial STI, affecting 1–2% of all women aged 16–44 who have ever had a sexual partner in the UK and around 14% of those aged 20–24 years attending sexual health clinics. The natural history of infection is not fully understood and in more than 50% of cases the infection resolves spontaneously without complications. It can, however, cause PID, chronic pain and tubal infertility. Screening for, and treating, asymptomatic chlamydia may reduce the rate of PID. England has a screening programme.

Symptoms and signs

- The cervix is the primary site of infection, but the urethra is also infected in about 50% of cases. Chlamydia can also infect the pharynx and rectum.
- Approximately 70% of women with chlamydia are asymptomatic.
- If symptoms are present, they are usually non-specific, such as increased vaginal discharge, dysuria and post-coital bleeding.
- Lower abdominal pain, dyspareunia and intermenstrual bleeding may be present if the infection has spread beyond the cervix.
- On examination, there may be mucopurulent cervicitis (Fig. 18.3) and/or contact bleeding (Fig. 18.4) but the cervix may also look normal.

Diagnosis

NAAT such as Polymerase Chain Reaction (PCR) have a sensitivity of over 90% for chlamydia and can be performed on vulvovaginal, cervical, pharyngeal, rectal or urine samples. Self-taken vulvovaginal swabs are at least as sensitive as physician-taken cervical swabs and may be used for home-based testing or in the clinic, if examination is not otherwise indicated.

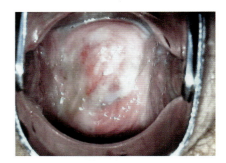

Fig. 18.3   Mucopurulent cervicitis. This may be a feature of infection with *C. trachomatis* or *N. gonorrhoeae*. The cervix, however, can look normal.

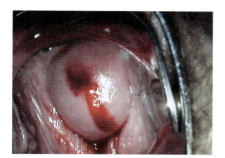

Fig. 18.4 Contact bleeding. This can occur for a number of reasons, one of which is *C. trachomatis* infection.

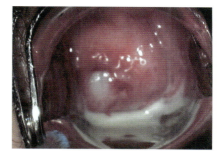

Fig. 18.5 Purulent cervicitis. The cervix is the primary site of infection in 90% of cases of gonococcal infection, and a purulent discharge may be seen.

Treatment and management

Uncomplicated chlamydial infection can be treated with:

- azithromycin 1 g single dose
- doxycycline 100 mg twice daily for 1 week.

Azithromycin is extensively used for the treatment of chlamydia in pregnancy, although this is an unlicensed indication. Patients should abstain from sex until they and their partner(s) have completed treatment. A test of cure is not necessary except after treatment in pregnancy. However, reinfection rates are 10–30%, so re-testing after 6–12 months is often advised.

Complications

C. trachomatis can spread beyond the lower genital tract, causing Skene's and Bartholin's gland abscesses, endometritis, salpingitis and perihepatitis. Around 3–10% of women with untreated chlamydia develop symptomatic ascending infection (PID), which may lead to tubal damage, predisposing to tubal pregnancies and tubal infertility, as well as causing chronic pain. Although asymptomatic upper genital tract infection also leads to tubal damage, the proportion of women who develop infertility following asymptomatic chlamydial infection is thought to be low (<1%). Chlamydial infection during pregnancy can cause miscarriage, pre-term birth, postpartum infection and neonatal ocular and respiratory infection. In genetically susceptible people, sexually acquired reactive arthritis can occur (Reiter syndrome).

Neisseria gonorrhoeae

Background information

Gonococcal infection rates are around five-fold lower than those of chlamydia in the UK, but have increased dramatically in recent years. There has been a 60% rise in the number of cases of gonorrhoea in women in England since 2006. *N. gonorrhoeae* is a highly adaptive organism and gonococcal antibiotic resistance is an increasing global health concern.

Symptoms and signs

- The cervix is the primary site of infection, but the urethra is also infected in 70–90% of cases. Gonorrhoea also commonly affects the pharynx and rectum.
- About 50% of women with gonorrhoea have no symptoms.
- The most common symptoms are increased vaginal discharge, dysuria and post-coital bleeding.
- Lower abdominal pain and intermenstrual bleeding may also be present if the infection has spread beyond the cervix.
- On examination, there may be purulent (Fig. 18.5) or mucopurulent cervicitis and/or contact bleeding, but again the cervix may look normal.

Diagnosis

NAAT for *N. gonorrhoeae* are widely used and offer increased sensitivity and convenience over culture. Confirmation of NAAT-positive results by culture is recommended and has the advantage of allowing antibiotic sensitivity testing. If gonorrhoea is detected in a genital site (e.g. cervix or vulvo-vaginal swab), non-genital sites (throat, rectum) should also be tested and a test of cure from these sites performed. Treatment failure, leading to the emergence of resistance, is more likely in non-genital sites.

Treatment and management

Uncomplicated gonorrhoea in all women, including pregnant and lactating women, can be treated with:

- ceftriaxone 500 mg intramuscular (IM) single dose *plus* azithromycin 1 g orally single dose.

Oral cephalosporins are no longer recommended for treatment of gonorrhoea due to worldwide concerns about the emergence of resistance. About 40% of females with gonorrhoea also have *C. trachomatis* infection, so they should be tested and treated for chlamydia. Patients should abstain from sex until they and their partner(s) have completed treatment.

Table 18.2	Causes of lower abdominal pain
Uterus	Endometritis (PID)
	Endometriosis
Fallopian tubes	Salpingitis (PID)
	Ectopic pregnancy
Ovary	Torsion of, or haemorrhage into, an ovarian cyst
Urinary tract	Cystitis
Bowel	Acute appendicitis
	Irritable bowel syndrome

Complications

N. gonorrhoeae can spread locally beyond the lower genital tract, causing Skene's and Bartholin's gland abscesses, endometritis, salpingitis and perihepatitis. About 10–20% of women with acute gonococcal infection will develop ascending infection (PID), the resulting damage predisposing to tubal pregnancies and tubal infertility. Infection in pregnancy can cause miscarriage, pre-term birth, postpartum infection and neonatal infection. Rarely, gonococcal septicaemia can occur and present as an acute arthritis/dermatitis syndrome (disseminated gonococcal infection). Gonorrhoea increases a woman's risk of acquiring HIV infection four- to five-fold.

Lower abdominal and pelvic pain

Lower abdominal and pelvic pain can be caused by a number of differing conditions (Table 18.2). PID is particularly common in young (under 25 years), sexually active women.

Pelvic inflammatory disease

PID results when infections ascend from the cervix or vagina into the upper genital tract. It includes endometritis, salpingitis, tubo-ovarian abscess and pelvic peritonitis. No specific symptoms, signs or laboratory tests are diagnostic of PID and the diagnosis is often made on clinical findings (presence of lower abdominal pain, increased vaginal discharge, cervical motion tenderness and adnexal tenderness on bimanual examination), which together have a Positive Predictive Value (PPV) of 65–90% compared with laparoscopy.

The history can help to distinguish PID from lower abdominal and pelvic pain of other cause and anatomical origin:

- clinical symptoms of PID vary from none to very severe
- the onset of symptoms often occurs in the first part of the menstrual cycle
- lower abdominal pain (usually bilateral) is the most common symptom. Pain affecting the pelvis with deep dyspareunia suggests involvement of the reproductive tract
- increased vaginal discharge, irregular or intermenstrual bleeding and post-coital bleeding may indicate cervical or vaginal infection

- consider differential diagnoses, including urinary tract infection, appendicitis and ectopic pregnancy
  - When was her last menstrual period; what contraception has she been using and is there any possibility of her being pregnant?
  - Has she any dysuria, urinary frequency, nocturia or haematuria?
  - Has she any nausea, vomiting, diarrhoea or constipation?

Examination findings support the diagnosis:

- the cervix may have a mucopurulent discharge with contact bleeding, indicative of cervicitis
- uterine tenderness or adnexal tenderness or cervical motion tenderness on bimanual examination along with lower abdominal or pelvic pain is sufficient for a diagnosis of PID. Pyrexia and a palpable adnexal mass may also be present.

Diagnosis

- Tests for STI including chlamydia and gonorrhoea should always be performed. Positive results are supportive evidence. Negative results do not exclude the diagnosis.
- Non-specific tests of inflammation such as the Erythrocyte Sedimentation Rate (ESR), white cell count and C-reactive protein may be raised. The absence of pus cells on a slide taken from the cervix or vaginal wall is a sensitive marker of the absence of PID. Laparoscopy, with microbiological specimens from the upper and lower genital tract, is considered the 'gold standard' for diagnosis, but this is not always available or appropriate, particularly for those with mild symptoms. Clinical symptoms and signs do not accurately predict the extent of tubal disease found at laparoscopy.

Background information

C. trachomatis and *N. gonorrhoeae* are important sexually transmitted causes of PID, but *G. vaginalis* and anaerobes associated with BV are also implicated. *Mycoplasma genitalium* may be associated with PID but testing for this organism is not routine. PID is commonly and increasingly seen in women without STI. Sometimes in women with laparoscopically proven PID, no bacterial cause is found. The true incidence of PID is unknown because about two-thirds of cases are asymptomatic.

Treatment and management

Treatment should not be delayed while waiting for bacteriological test results, as early antibiotic therapy improves outcomes. Outpatient therapy with oral antibiotics is appropriate for clinically mild-to-moderate disease, but hospitalization is required if there is diagnostic uncertainty, severe symptoms or signs, or failure to respond to oral therapy. Intravenous therapy for the first few days is recommended in women with severe clinical disease. Therapy requires broad-spectrum antibiotics including cover for gonorrhoea and anaerobes.

Recommended regimens for outpatient therapy include:

- ceftriaxone 500 mg IM single dose plus azithromycin 1 g single dose plus doxycycline 100 mg (oral) twice daily plus metronidazole 400 mg (oral) twice daily for 14 days.

For parenteral therapy, second-generation cephalosporins including cefotetan or cefoxitin plus doxycycline are preferred.

Appropriate analgesia should be given. Patients should abstain from sex until they and their partner(s) have completed treatment. Women with moderate or severe clinical findings should be reviewed after 2–3 days to ensure they are improving. Lack of response to treatment requires further investigation, intravenous therapy and/or surgical intervention. All patients should be seen after treatment to check their clinical response, and that medication has been completed.

Complications

The main complications from PID are due to tubal damage, with the risk of all complications increasing with severity of infection. Tubal infertility occurs in 10–12% of women after one episode of symptomatic PID, 20–30% after two episodes, and 50–60% after three or more episodes. The risk of ectopic pregnancy is increased 6- to 10-fold, with higher rates in women with several episodes. Abdominal or pelvic pain for longer than 6 months occurs in 18% of women. Women with a past history of PID are 5–10 times more likely to need hospital admission and undergo hysterectomy.

About one-third of women have repeated infections. This may be due to relapse of infection because of inadequate treatment, reinfection from an untreated partner, postinfection tubal damage or further acquisition of STIs. In 5–15% of women with salpingitis, the infection spreads from the pelvis to the liver capsule, causing perihepatitis (Fitz-Hugh–Curtis syndrome).

Dysuria

Dysuria is usually due to acute bacterial cystitis, urethritis or vulvitis (Table 18.3). STIs occasionally present with dysuria. External dysuria, particularly in the absence of frequency or abdominal pain, indicates irritation at the urethral meatus.

Questions that help distinguish between the causes are:

- Is the dysuria external, i.e. is it as the urine comes into contact with the vulval mucosa?
- Is there any urinary frequency, nocturia or haematuria?
- Is there any vaginal discharge, post-coital or intermenstrual bleeding or abdominal pain?

Vulval ulcers

Infective lesions are the most common cause of vulval ulcers, with genital herpes the commonest cause of genital ulcers in the UK (Table 18.4).

Table 18.3	Causes of dysuria
Acute bacterial cystitis	Coliform bacteria
	Staphylococcus saprophyticus
Urethritis	*Chlamydia trachomatis*
	Neisseria gonorrhoeae
Vulvitis	Genital herpes
	Candidal infection
	Trichomonas vaginalis
	Vulval dermatological conditions

Table 18.4	Vulval ulcers – types
Infective	Genital herpes
	Syphilis
Non-infective	Aphthous ulcers
	Behçet syndrome

Genital herpes

Genital herpes can be caused by HSV type 1 or 2. The two viral types are clinically similar: symptoms range from none (asymptomatic); mild irritation and soreness; multiple painful ulcers or a severe systemic illness with extensive, confluent anogenital ulceration. After an initial episode (often the most severe), HSV ascends the peripheral sensory nerves into the dorsal root ganglion, where latent infection develops. This can reactivate, resulting in recurrent episodes which may or may not be symptomatic but are potentially infectious. Around 75% of first-episode infections are acquired from an asymptomatic partner. Some 90% of people with HSV-2 infection and 60% with HSV-1 will develop recurrences within the first year. The median number of recurrences in year 1 is one in HSV-1 infection and four in HSV-2. Long-term studies show that symptomatic recurrences gradually decrease with time.

Initial episode

This may be primary infection – the first-ever exposure to either HSV-1 or -2. Over 50% of first-episode genital herpes in the UK is due to HSV-1: oral-to-genital transmission is common. Non-primary, initial-episode genital herpes occurs in people with previous orolabial HSV-1 who then acquire genital HSV-2 infection. There is some cross-protection from this prior infection, resulting in a milder illness than in primary infection. These non-primary infections are more likely to be asymptomatic than are primary infections.

Recurrent herpes

These episodes may be asymptomatic (subclinical shedding). If symptoms are present they are usually milder than in first infections.

The history can help to determine whether genital ulcers are caused by HSV and establish the stage of infection:

- multiple, painful herpetic ulcers may be preceded by a prodrome of tingling, itching or pain in the area

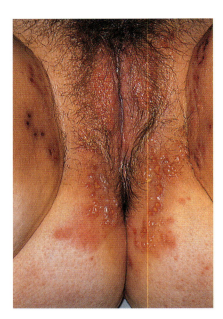

Fig. 18.6   Primary herpes. Multiple painful superficial ulcers are present. (From Clutterbuck D, Specialist Training in Sexually Transmitted Infections and HIV, Mosby 2005.)

- soreness, itch and external dysuria may initially be mistaken for (and treated as) candidiasis
- one or more previous similar episodes may be reported in those presenting with recurrence
- the presence of orolabial or genital sores in a partner supports the diagnosis
- a history of sex with bisexual males or non-UK partners increases the likelihood of other diagnoses including infectious early syphilis.

On examination:
- multiple painful superficial ulcers with evidence of lesions at the recognized erythematous, vesicular, ulcerative and resolving stages (Fig. 18.6) confirms the syndromic diagnosis. Tender inguinal lymphadenopathy is present in about 30% of cases
- in recurrences there are usually just a few ulcers confined to a small area, or the lesions may appear or as fissures or splits
- single and/or painless ulcers raise the possibility of other infections (e.g. syphilis) or non-infective ulcers.

Diagnosis

NAAT of swabs from the lesions for HSV-1 and -2 should routinely be performed. In atypical or painless ulcers, syphilis must be excluded by serological testing and PCR for syphilis on the ulcer swab should be requested if available. Type-specific serological tests for HSV-1 and -2 are not routinely used for diagnosis but may be useful in assessing the susceptibility of a partner to primary infection (e.g. during pregnancy).

Treatment and management

Primary and first-episode genital herpes

Antiviral drugs reduce the severity and duration of the symptoms. They do not prevent latency, so have no effect on future recurrences.

Recommended regimens include:
- aciclovir 400 mg three times daily for 5 days
- valaciclovir 500 mg twice daily for 5 days.

Aciclovir can be used in pregnancy and breastfeeding.

Analgesia and saline bathing are recommended. Patients can be advised to pass urine in a bath or under a shower spray of warm water, to ease external dysuria. Topical analgesia (such as lidocaine gel) may be helpful. The natural history of HSV infection should be explained, covering recurrences, subclinical viral shedding, the potential for sexual transmission and treatments that are available.

Recurrent genital herpes

Recurrences are self-limiting and can often be managed with supportive therapy. Infrequent but severe recurrences can be treated with episodic antiviral therapy. If started early, therapy will reduce the severity and sometimes the duration of an attack, but will not reduce the number of recurrences. The patient should initiate treatment at home as soon as a recurrence is noticed.

Episodic treatment regimens include:
- aciclovir 800 mg three times a day for 2 days
- valaciclovir 500 mg twice daily for 3 days.

For frequent recurrences (more than six recurrences in a year) suppressive therapy may be considered. In around 80% of cases, recurrences are stopped altogether. Therapy does not modify the natural history of infection, but after 12 months of treatment about 20% of patients will have fewer recurrences due to the natural decay in episode frequency. It may be restarted if frequent recurrences persist.

Suppressive treatment regimens include:
- aciclovir 400 mg twice daily
- valaciclovir 500 mg once daily.

Patients should be advised to avoid sexual contact with uninfected partners during the prodrome and recurrence, as this is when the risk of transmission is highest. It should be explained that a low risk of transmission remains even when they have no obvious recurrence, because of subclinical viral shedding. Condoms reduce this risk and suppressive therapy has an additional effect.

Complications

Women who acquire primary genital herpes during pregnancy, particularly in the third trimester, may transmit the infection to the baby at the time of delivery. Herpes neonatorum, though rare in the UK, carries a risk of death or serious disability. The risk of perinatal transmission with recurrent HSV is low. Genital herpes increases the acquisition and transmission of HIV two- to three-fold, although providing suppressive antiviral treatment to women with herpes who are at risk of HIV has not been successful in preventing infection.

Many people with recurrent HSV infection fear rejection by sexual partners and a minority develop psychological problems. Aseptic meningitis and autonomic neuropathy can occasionally occur with primary infection, even leading to urinary retention. Rarely, the infection can disseminate, causing a life-threatening condition. This is more likely in the immunocompromised and in pregnancy.

Syphilis

Background information

Syphilis is caused by the spirochaete *Treponema pallidum*. Infectious syphilis in women in the UK was almost eradicated by the mid-1990s, but has returned to significant levels in this century. Between 20 and 30 cases of congenital syphilis are diagnosed annually in the UK. Worldwide, over 900 000 pregnant women were infected with syphilis in 2012, resulting in 350 000 adverse birth outcomes.

Symptoms and signs

Syphilis can be asymptomatic and identified on screening serology, such as in antenatal testing.

There are several stages of symptomatic syphilis infection:

- *primary syphilis*: about 3 weeks after exposure, a chancre appears. This is usually a single, painless ulcer with rolled indurated edges, which usually goes unnoticed in women. Even without treatment, it heals spontaneously. Syphilis serology may still be negative at this stage of infection
- *secondary syphilis:* after several weeks, a generalized illness develops, with fever, malaise, and skin and mucosal rashes. The rash is present on the trunk, limbs, palms and soles. Wart-like moist papules occur on the vulva (condylomata lata). Even if untreated, these symptoms and signs resolve after 3–12 weeks. Syphilis serology is strongly positive at this stage of infection
- *late syphilis:* up to 40% of untreated patients will develop symptomatic late syphilis, with neurosyphilis, cardiovascular syphilis or gummata.

Diagnosis

Syphilis can be diagnosed by serological testing, commonly using an enzyme immunoassay for syphilis antibodies. NAAT for syphilis ulcers is increasingly available.

Treatment and management

Long-acting penicillins remain the treatment of choice. Management and follow-up should be undertaken by a specialist sexual health service.

Complications

Without adequate treatment, complications of late syphilis can occur. Syphilis in pregnancy can cause miscarriage

Table 18.5	Causes of vulval lumps
Viral infections	Genital warts
	Molluscum contagiosum
	Vulval intraepithelial neoplasia and vulval cancer
Bacterial infections	Syphilitic condylomata lata
	Skene's or Bartholin's gland abscesses owing to *Chlamydia trachomatis* or *Neisseria gonorrhoeae*
Anatomical variants	Sebaceous glands
	Vulval papillae
Other	Sebaceous cysts

and stillbirth, and can be transmitted to the infant, causing congenital syphilis.

Vulval lumps

Raised lesions on the vulva can be due to infections or anatomical variants. Genital warts are by far the most common cause of vulval lumps (Table 18.5).

Genital warts

Background information

Genital warts are the commonest viral STI in the UK. The prevalence of infection with HPV types 6 and 11 in women aged 19–23 years in one UK vaccine study was 23%, and the incidence of clinical genital warts is around 0.8% per annum. HPV is highly infectious: two-thirds of sexual partners will develop warts, and HPV infection is also seen in adolescents who have had only non-penetrative sexual contact. Infection causes painless, benign, epithelial tumours caused by HPV types 6 and 11. The incubation period of months to years means that warts may appear some time into an exclusively monogamous relationship. The immunosuppression of pregnancy may cause warts to appear or recur. A national vaccination programme against oncogenic HPV types (16 and 18) was provided to girls aged 13 in the UK from 2008. From 2012 this was replaced by a quadrivalent vaccine, also protecting against HPV 6 and 11. As this cohort becomes sexually active, the number of women presenting to clinics with genital warts is beginning to fall.

Symptoms and signs

- Genital warts are painless, so in women they may be asymptomatic.
- If symptomatic, it is usual that the woman has felt the vulval lumps.
- There may be a slight itch and discomfort as the warts develop, but pain, bleeding or other symptoms suggest an alternative or coexisting diagnosis.
- On examination the flesh-coloured papules can be seen around the introital opening. They can

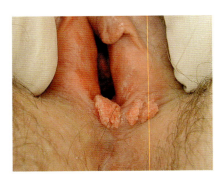

Fig. 18.7 Flesh-coloured papules characteristic of warts. (From Clutterbuck D, Specialist Training in Sexually Transmitted Infections and HIV, Mosby 2005.)

spread onto the labia, perineum and perianal area. They may be single but are usually multiple (Fig. 18.7).

- On the mucous membranes they are usually soft and cauliflower-like (condylomata acuminata).
- On the drier surfaces, they are harder and keratinized.

Diagnosis

They are diagnosed by their clinical appearances. Atypical lesions should be biopsied, particularly in older women, as premalignant and malignant lesions can look similar.

Treatment and management

Warts may resolve spontaneously. No one treatment modality has been shown to be effective in all cases. Fewer (<5) or keratinized warts can be treated with ablative therapy, such as cryotherapy, trichloroacetic acid, curettage or electro-cautery. All of these can be used in pregnancy and a single treatment may be effective. Multiple, soft warts (condylomata acuminata) can be treated with podophyllotoxin solution or cream. It is a cytotoxic agent, so is contraindicated in pregnancy. Imiquimod cream works by stimulating local cell-mediated immunity, resulting in clearance of the warts. It can be used on both soft and keratinized warts, but should also not be used in pregnancy. All treatments can have recurrence rates of up to 25%, because of residual subclinical viral infection. Treatment failure should be followed by change of treatment, and management algorithms improve outcomes. Women with genital warts should be offered testing for other STIs. There is evidence that condoms reduce the spread of HPV, so patients should be advised to use condoms with new partners.

Complications

Genital warts are mainly a cosmetic problem. Psychological morbidity may arise because of their appearance, fears about cervical cancer or concerns about fidelity if they appear in a regular relationship. Physical complications are rare; HPV

6 and 11 are not associated with cervical cancer and vertical transmission is rare.

Systemic presentations of sexually transmitted infections

STIs do not always present with genital symptoms or signs. Syphilis becomes a systemic infection following the primary phase, and herpes, gonorrhoea and chlamydia can all cause disseminated infections, producing symptoms and signs in other systems. HIV is a systemic viral infection which may present with direct effects of viral infection or opportunistic infections and malignancies in any body system.

HIV infection

Background information

HIV infection can be transmitted by contact with body fluids (either sexually or through needles or blood transfusion) and by vertical transmission from mother to baby. It was estimated that 36 000 women were living with HIV in the UK in 2015. The rate of undiagnosed infection in women is significantly lower than men in the UK, demonstrating the effectiveness of the antenatal screening programme introduced in the 1990s. The uptake of testing among pregnant women is 96%. ART allows a near-normal life expectancy for people diagnosed with HIV at an early stage, but deaths from AIDS still occur in people diagnosed too late for therapy to allow immune recovery. The universal provision of antiretroviral treatment, condom use and the use of oral pre-exposure prophylaxis are effective prevention methods currently used in the UK. Topical vaginal microbicides, male circumcision and an HIV vaccine have also been shown to reduce HIV transmission and have great potential to slow the spread of the epidemic worldwide.

Symptoms and signs

- Most people with HIV infection have no symptoms in the first few years of infection.
- There may be a systemic illness with fever, malaise and rash at the time of seroconversion, 6–12 weeks after infection. This is rarely recognized as being HIV related.
- As the immune function is starting to deteriorate, infections such as oral candidiasis and herpes zoster may occur.
- Women with HIV infection get more frequent episodes of vaginal candidiasis and recurrent HSV, and higher rates of HPV-related abnormalities such as cervical intraepithelial neoplasia.
- Opportunistic infections and HIV-related malignancies can present in many different ways. Common early presentations are shown in Fig. 18.8.

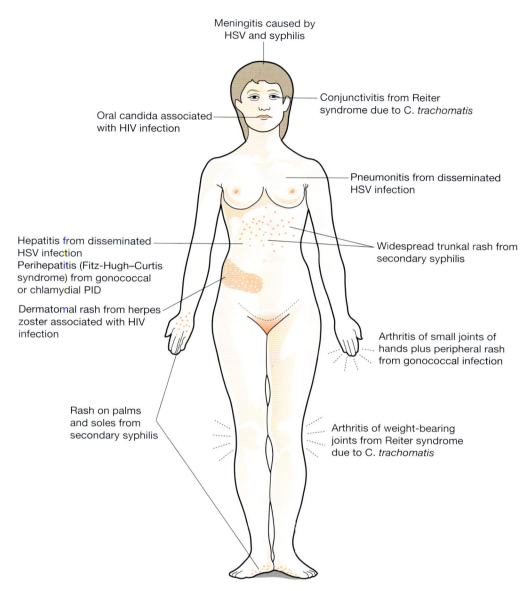

Meningitis caused by
HSV and syphilis

Conjunctivitis from Reiter
syndrome due to C. *trachomatis*

Oral candida associated
with HIV infection

Pneumonitis from disseminated
HSV infection

Hepatitis from disseminated
HSV infection
Perihepatitis (Fitz-Hugh–Curtis
syndrome) from gonococcal
or chlamydial PID

Widespread trunkal rash from
secondary syphilis

Dermatomal rash from herpes
zoster associated with HIV
infection

Arthritis of small joints of
hands plus peripheral rash
from gonococcal infection

Rash on palms
and soles from
secondary syphilis

Arthritis of weight-bearing
joints from Reiter syndrome
due to C. *trachomatis*

Fig. 18.8 Systemic presentations of STIs.

Diagnosis

A fourth-generation serological test for antibodies to HIV and HIV antigen is the preferred method of diagnosis. Point-of-care tests for HIV are widely available and used for routine testing, providing a result in as little as 1 min. They can be particularly helpful in the obstetric setting; for example, when a woman from an area of high HIV prevalence presents in labour. HIV testing should always be a routine part of antenatal care and STI screening, and should be recommended when a patient presents with any HIV clinical indicator condition. Clinical indicator conditions seen in gynaecology include cervical cancer, cervical intraepithelial neoplasia (Grade 2 and above) and vulval and vaginal intraepithelial neoplasia. Testing requires informed consent but not specialist counselling, and can be performed by any clinician.

Treatment and management

Patients should have their CD4 count (this measures cell-mediated immune function) and HIV viral load (this measures the level of viral replication) performed about every 6 months. ART, usually with three drugs in combination, is recommended for all HIV-infected individuals at any stage of infection and almost eradicates the risk of horizontal transmission through sex.

Complications

Without treatment, there is increasing damage to the cell-mediated immunity, leading to susceptibility to opportunistic infections and eventually death, a median of 9–12 years after infection. Treating the pregnant woman with triple ART and avoiding breastfeeding reduces vertical transmission. Rates of transmission are now as low as 1%. Delivery by caesarean section reduces vertical transmission in women who are not taking ART, but is not thought to offer additional benefit in those on effective treatment.

Key points

- STIs in females are often asymptomatic. Detection depends on risk assessment and testing in all women presenting for care.
- High rates of STIs are found in sexually active women aged less than 25 years.
- Testing for HIV infection is routine in women attending for antenatal care and termination of pregnancy, and should also be done in any woman presenting with an indicator condition.
- Syndromic management, with or without the support of diagnostic testing for STIs, can help to ensure early treatment.
- The management of STIs, particularly chlamydia, gonorrhoea and PID, includes treatment of the sexual partner(s) and advice about abstinence from sex until the patient and partner(s) have completed treatment, in order to prevent reinfection.

19

Sexual problems

Introduction

It is important for any doctor to be able to take a sexual history and to have some idea of how sexual problems are managed. Understanding the physiology of the normal sexual response will allow the doctor to better understand many of the uncomplicated sexual problems.

Scientific investigation of the normal sexual response is necessary to our understanding, but, because of conservative attitudes, few scientists have chosen to work in this area until fairly recently. Early workers were:

- Sigmund Freud (1856–1939), an Austrian doctor, was the founder of psychoanalysis and the first to recognize the importance of childhood influences on sexuality. His studies were on patients rather than normal subjects.
- Havelock Ellis (1859–1939) studied medicine at St Thomas's Hospital, London. His seven-volume *Studies in the Psychology of Sex* (1897–1928) caused controversy but was the first detached treatment of the subject.
- Alfred Kinsey (1894–1956), an American zoologist, became director of Indiana University's Institute for Sex Research in 1942. To investigate 'normal' sexual experience, 18 500 Americans were interviewed. *Sexual Behaviour in the Human Male* was published in 1948, and *Sexual Behaviour in the Human Female* in 1953.
- Masters and Johnson: William Masters (1915–2001), a doctor, and Virginia Johnson (1925–2013), a psychologist, working at Washington University, St Louis, carried out the first direct observations on sexual activity under laboratory conditions. *Human Sexual Response* appeared in 1966, and *Human Sexual Inadequacy* in 1970.
- The field of sexual medicine or sexology has developed significantly since the early work of these pioneers and is now a flourishing specialty in itself. There are numerous societies, conferences and journals devoted to the field. Despite this, it is still a niche specialism and not everyone has access to services for sexual problems.

Normal sexual response

The normal human sexual response can be regarded as having five phases: desire, arousal, orgasm, resolution and the refractory phase (Fig. 19.1). This is the most widely accepted model first published by Masters and Johnson. There are criticisms of this model and others have developed slightly different models but this version serves as a useful introduction to the topic.

Desire

Sexual desire refers to the general level of interest in sexuality. It is modulated by hormones – hence the change in sexual interest at puberty. The main hormonal modulator in both sexes is testosterone. Desire is also dependant on contextual factors such as mood, environment and levels of sexual attraction.

Arousal

This phase has three components: central arousal, genital response and peripheral arousal.

Central arousal

This refers to the response to sexual stimuli, which may be visual or tactile or may result from internal imagery or from a relationship. These stimuli act through the cerebral cortex (Fig. 19.2). The areas of the brain involved in sexual arousal are thought to be in the limbic system. There are thought to be excitatory centres with endorphins as the neurotransmitter, and inhibitory centres, linked to the centres for pain and fear.

Genital response

The spinal pathways leading to the genitalia are not precisely known but appear to be near the spinothalamic pathways for pain and temperature. Genital responses are due to vaso-congestion and neuromuscular changes. Arteriolar dilatation is probably controlled by the parasympathetic sacral outflow at S2, 3 and 4 via the nervi erigentes. Thoracic sympathetic outflow also plays a part. The local neurotransmitters involved

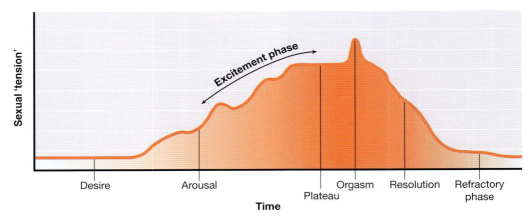

Fig. 19.1   The normal sexual response.

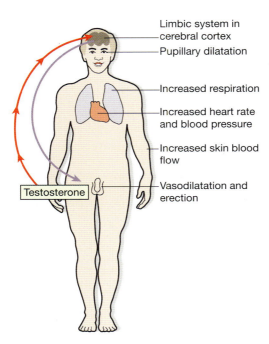

Fig. 19.2   Control of sexual activity.

include vasoactive intestinal polypeptide, a potent vasodilator found in the penis and vagina.

In the male, engorgement of the corpora cavernosa is due mainly to arteriolar dilatation and probably a reduction in the venous outflow which results in penile erection (Fig. 19.3). The scrotum tightens due to contraction of the dartos muscle and the testes are elevated due to contraction of the cremaster muscle.

In the female, there is engorgement of the venous plexus surrounding the lower part of the vagina, and of the erectile bulbs of the vestibule on either side of the introitus (Fig. 19.4). There is reddening and pouting of the labia minora. The clitoris becomes erect and later is said to retract against the symphysis pubis.

The vagina becomes lubricated by a transudate as the blood supply to the vaginal wall increases. This fluid is not the product of mucous glands. Mucus secretion from the cervix makes relatively little contribution to vaginal lubrication (which is therefore usually unaffected by hysterectomy). Secretion from Bartholin's glands, formerly thought to be mainly responsible for lubrication, is only moderate in amount and occurs relatively late during arousal.

Relaxation of the woman's pelvic floor muscles occurs after vaginal lubrication has started. In the later stages of arousal, the uterus becomes engorged, increases in size and rises in the pelvis. The upper part of the vagina 'balloons' and there may be slow irregular contractions of the lower third of the vagina.

In both sexes, but particularly in the male, the genital response interacts with the central response, so that arousal becomes self-amplifying.

Peripheral arousal

Sexual arousal causes:

- a rise in systolic and diastolic blood pressure (which may only be transient)
- general flushing of the skin
- change in heart rate (either an increase or a decrease)
- respiratory changes
- pupillary dilatation.

Plateau phase

When arousal is heightened, there may be a 'plateau' phase during which the couple prolong the pleasure of intercourse before orgasm.

Orgasm

Orgasm involves genital, muscular and sensory changes, as well as cardiovascular and respiratory responses.

In the male

First, there is smooth muscle contraction of the epididymis, vas deferens, seminal vesicle, prostate and ampulla,

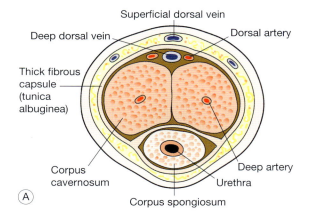

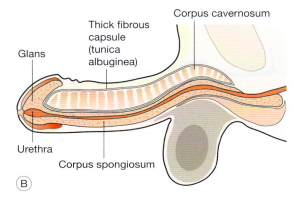

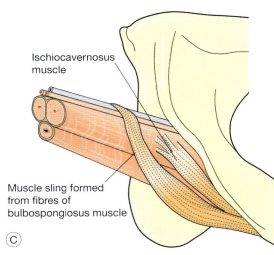

Fig. 19.3   The penis. (A) Cross-section showing erectile spaces and principal blood vessels. **(B)** Erectile tissues. Each crus of the corpora cavernosa is inserted into the pubic bone. **(C)** Muscles.

propelling seminal and prostatic fluid into the urethral bulb. Then, the male becomes aware that orgasm is imminent and ejaculation usually follows within a few seconds. The internal bladder sphincter remains shut but the external sphincter relaxes and semen is propelled along the urethra by rhythmic contractions of the bulbospongiosus and ischiocavernosus muscles.

In the female

A few seconds after the onset of the subjective experience of orgasm, there is a spasm of the muscles surrounding the lower third of the vagina (the 'orgasmic platform') followed by a series of rhythmic contractions. Uterine contractions may also occur.

In both sexes

There is contraction of rectus abdominis, pelvic thrusting, contraction of the anal sphincter and sometimes carpopedal spasm. Systolic and diastolic blood pressure rises by at least 25 mmHg, and hyperventilation occurs. There is a feeling of intense pleasure and an alteration of consciousness to a variable degree.

Resolution

The events of arousal are gradually reversed. In men, there is a moderate immediate loss of erection, followed by a slower complete reversal. In women, if no orgasm has occurred, pelvic congestion may take hours to resolve and can be uncomfortable. In both sexes, there is a subjective feeling of relaxation, though its duration may differ between the man and the woman.

Refractory phase

There follows an interval during which further stimulation does not produce a response. In men, this varies from minutes in young men to many hours in older men. Some women do not experience a refractory period, only a minority of women (14% according to Kinsey) can have multiple orgasms.

The effect of age

Normal sexual behaviour differs from couple to couple. It also alters with age and with the evolution of a sexual relationship. Patients may present with problems due to difficulties in adjusting to the change from one phase to the next of a relationship.

Adolescence

An adolescent usually has a higher capacity for sexual arousal and a need to explore the bounds of their sexuality. However, coupled with the need to learn about sexual behaviour there is an emotional vulnerability. This can lead to high-risk sexual behaviour. Unsatisfactory sexual experience at this time

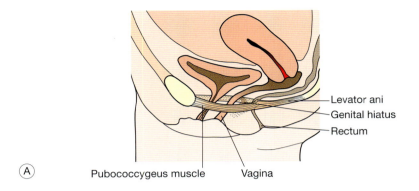

(A)

Levator ani
Genital hiatus
Rectum

Pubococcygeus muscle   Vagina

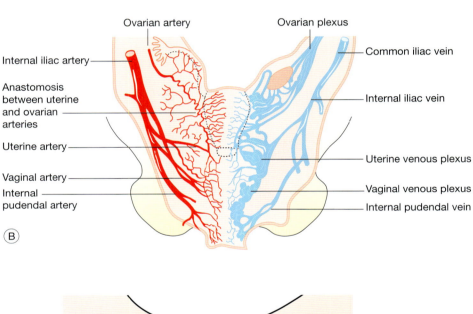

Ovarian artery   Ovarian plexus

Internal iliac artery

Anastomosis
between uterine
and ovarian
arteries

Uterine artery

Vaginal artery
Internal
pudendal artery

Common iliac vein

Internal iliac vein

Uterine venous plexus

Vaginal venous plexus
Internal pudendal vein

(B)

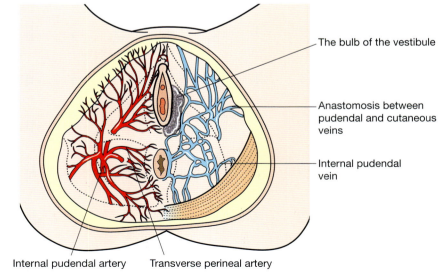

The bulb of the vestibule

Anastomosis between
pudendal and cutaneous
veins

Internal pudendal
vein

(C)   Internal pudendal artery   Transverse perineal artery

Fig. 19.4 Female reproductive organs. (A) The muscular supports of the vagina. This shows the sling of muscle fibres that surround the urethra, vagina and rectum, running from the pubic bone to the coccyx. The levator plate formed by these fibres supports the rectum and vagina in its non-aroused horizontal position. **(B)** Arteries and veins supplying the female reproductive organs. **(C)** Blood vessels of the pelvic floor, showing the rich arterial and venous networks surrounding the vaginal opening.

can result in sexual problems in later life. Young women in their teens are at a higher risk of unwanted pregnancy due to uncertainty about contraceptive needs. In addition, awareness of sexually transmitted diseases can be limited at this age.

The couple

The early months of a relationship may be characterized by frequent sex, but couples need to learn quickly how to establish good communication and to adjust their sexual behaviour to suit each other's needs, as desire usually wanes as a relationship progresses. Should this communication not occur, dysfunctional patterns may develop potentially resulting in sexual problems and relationship difficulties.

Early parenthood

The time taken for sexual interest to return after childbirth is variable and in some women, can be a year or more. Problems can result from a difficult birthing experience or postnatal depression but more commonly are due to tiredness and the difficulties of coping with the demands of the new baby.

Middle age

When the novelty of a sexual relationship has worn off, sexual activity usually becomes less frequent and this may cause anxieties for both genders. Couples may feel they 'ought' to be having sex more often resulting in guilt or anger. Stresses at work for both partners in combination with social commitments can make it difficult for them to find time to relax together. In the years before the menopause, women often have menstrual problems. After the menopause, there may be a reduction in sexual interest or a problem with vaginal dryness; these can usually be corrected by hormone replacement therapy.

Old age

There is a decline in erectile function with age, which can be a manifestation of physical disease (Fig. 19.5). Post-menopausal women may experience low libido and vaginal dryness or atrophy. These factors can impact on the couple's sexual relationship.

The functions of sex

It is important to remember how much people differ from one another and how wide the range of normality may be. Sex can fulfill a multitude of functions including some of the elements described here.

Reproduction

Reproductive sex is often limited to a short interval in a couple's relationship once conception has occurred. Couples

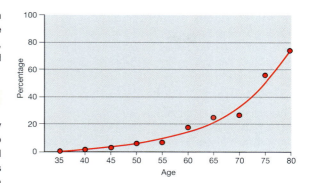

Fig. 19.5 **Erectile dysfunction increases with age.** (From Bancroft 1989, with permission. Data from Kinsey et al. 1948.)

who have fertility problems may find that this causes difficulty with their sex life, or, conversely, may find that after they achieve pregnancy it is difficult to have sex for pleasure only.

Physical exercise

Sexual activity is a form of physical exercise, which improves self-esteem and feelings of well-being but is also something to be mindful of in people with physical problems, such as angina.

Pleasure

Though sex is readily associated with pleasure, there are in some cultures taboos that prevent some people from enjoying sex.

Pair-bonding

Enjoying sex means lowering one's defences, and sharing this experience strengthens the bond between partners. People who have had to build particularly strong defences, for example after emotional abuse in childhood, may have difficulty in relinquishing them.

Asserting masculinity or femininity

People may use sexual activity to reassure themselves about their sexuality.

Bolstering self-esteem

Satisfactory sex can improve one's self-esteem however, for some, promiscuous behaviour to accomplish this can have negative consequences.

Achieving power

Some people see the sexual relationship in terms of dominance and submission. This can apply to coitus itself, or to the power to allow or deny access to sex. Rape can be seen as an example of this.

Reducing anxiety or tension

This can be helpful for most people but, in some cases, can cause relationship or personal problems through risk-taking, for example, promiscuity or use of internet pornography.

Material gain

Prostitution is the most obvious form of sex for gain, and is often the result of poverty. Marriage, even nowadays, may also be a way of using sex to ensure financial security.

History-taking

Some sexual problems may present as another symptom such as pelvic pain, or are discovered fortuitously, for example, when a routine enquiry is made about contraception. It is not possible to take a detailed sexual history from every patient whatever their complaint, but it is reasonable, particularly in a gynaecological clinic, to ask one or two questions about sex as a routine; for example, 'Do you have any trouble with intercourse?' or, if appropriate, 'Is this symptom worse after intercourse?' An evasive reply may suggest that all is not well, which may require some further sensitive questioning.

Elucidating a sexual problem relies mainly on the history, although useful information may be obtained from examination or investigation. The interviewer should be comfortable with the subject, as the patient is likely to be embarrassed by talking about a sexual problem. A sympathetic but matter-of-fact approach may help to reduce this embarrassment. The vocabulary used must also be appropriate, using words that avoid, on the one hand, being too technical and, on the other hand, appearing too crude.

It is usually helpful to see both partners, but not necessarily together on the first occasion. A patient may be more open if interviewed alone, but the partner may give quite a different version of the history. When treatment is planned, however, both partners should ideally be involved.

The history needs to be thorough, but, if too intrusive, it may be off-putting. If a topic seems painful, the subject can be changed and then returned to later. Sometimes more than one interview is necessary; with sensitive topics being explored on the second occasion after a rapport has been established. A detailed account of a specific instance may be more helpful than asking general questions. For example, if the patient is asked 'How often do you have intercourse?' the reply is likely to depend partly on what the patient thinks is expected (e.g. 'About twice a week'). It may be better to ask, 'When did you last have intercourse?', and then, if the couple's last attempt was unsatisfactory, to ask in detail about what went wrong. Open questions should also be used, for example, 'How did you feel when that happened?'

Many patients, especially if talking about their sexual problem for the first time, find it difficult to put their feelings into words. It may be helpful to offer the occasional summary: 'What I think you're saying is that …'. The patient will usually give a clearly positive response if the doctor has summed up the situation correctly. If the patient's response is more guarded, the doctor should be cautious about the conclusions drawn.

Human sexuality

There are several variations of human sexuality which should not be seen as problems unless they are presented as such by the patient. Most people are heterosexual or straight in that they are attracted to a sexual partner of the opposite gender. Some of the more common variations are detailed below.

Homosexuality

This refers to being attracted to a partner of the same gender. Homosexuality or being 'gay' is widely accepted in most societies but in some cultures, there remains a degree of stigma which can be difficult for the homosexual person to cope with. This can result in mental health problems in some cases.

Fetishistic transvestitism

A transvestite is someone who enjoys dressing in the clothes of the opposite gender. This is usually associated with sexual excitement and is not associated with a desire to change their gender. Transgender people may wish to change aspects of their gender but this is not seen as a sexual problem. The vast majority of transvestites are male and rarely present to services unless their behaviour causes relationship difficulties.

Sadomasochism

This is a spectrum of sexual behaviours encompassed in the term, 'BDSM' (bondage, discipline, sadism and masochism), which involve mild to extreme pain being inflicted or received for sexual pleasure. It is unusual for these people to present to services unless they are traumatized either physically or psychologically by their practices or their behaviour results in injury to another person and possibly legal action.

Fetishism

Particular parts of the body, articles of clothing (e.g. shoes) or materials (e.g. rubber or plastic) can become objects of sexual gratification.

Paedophilia

This term refers to a sexual preference for children usually of pre-pubertal age. This is an illegal practice and adults engaging in this behaviour should be reported if it is apparent that they are engaging in this behaviour. This is an instance when medical confidentiality can be breached.

Sexual dysfunction

Sexual dysfunction may be due to psychological or relationship problems or may have an underlying medical or surgical cause. Sexual dysfunction is common, with 43% of women and 31% of men experiencing some form of sexual dysfunction during their lifetime.

The common disorders of sexual function can be classified according to the physiological stages described early in this chapter:

- impaired desire
- disorders of arousal
- disorders of orgasm
- dyspareunia.

The causes of sexual dysfunction can be classified into physiological or psychological factors but it is hard to make a distinction between the two as they often coexist. For example, painful intercourse due to a physical cause such as a herpetic lesion may lead to secondary anxiety in both partners. However, anxiety due to sexual abuse in childhood may lead to spasm of the pelvic floor muscles. Treatment often needs to be directed towards physical and psychological causes at the same time.

A list of pathological causes of sexual dysfunction is given in Box 19.1. These causes are more common in an ageing population. Psychological causes of sexual dysfunction are given in Box 19.2.

Box 19.1

Pathological causes of sexual dysfunction
Medical disorders
- Acute and chronic illness
- Psychiatric illness
- Cancer – especially gynaecological
- Neurological problems, e.g. spinal cord injuries, multiple sclerosis, neuropathy
- Endocrine, e.g. diabetes
- Cardiovascular, e.g. myocardial infarction
- Respiratory
- Arthritic
- Renal, e.g. dialysis
- Gynaecological, e.g. vaginitis

Surgical procedures
- Mastectomy
- Colostomy
- Gynaecological – oophorectomy, episiotomy, vaginal repair
- Amputation

Drug effects
- Anticholinergics
- Anticonvulsants
- Antihypertensives
- Antiinflammatories
- Hormones
- Hypnotics and sedatives
- Major tranquillizers, e.g. antipsychotics
- Alcohol
- Opiates
- Antidepressants

Female sexual dysfunction

Impaired arousal/desire

This is a common presentation to specialist sexual medicine clinics, although it is not such a frequent symptom in routine gynaecology clinics. The woman complains that she is just not interested in sex. Such 'loss of libido' may be primary or secondary.

Primary

Some women have never felt interested in sex and in these cases; there is usually impairment of arousal and orgasm as well. In fact, the new *Diagnostic and Statistical Manual of Mental Disorders,* fifth edition (DSM 5) has not separated disorders of arousal and desire as it is difficult to distinguish between these interrelated concepts. The underlying cause is often psychological. Sometimes woman may try to choose a partner who also has an apparently low sex drive to match her desire.

Secondary

More commonly, loss of libido follows an interval of apparently normal sex drive, during the woman's teens or early 20s, or early in the relationship with her partner. Loss of interest in sex may occur after childbirth, when both parents devote all their attention to the baby, often combining motherhood with a return to paid employment. If there has been postnatal depression, this will exacerbate the problem.

Other causes include:

- depression
- bereavement
- the menopause
- medical causes or drugs (Box 19.1)
- gynaecological investigation, e.g. for an abnormal cervical smear
- loss of self-esteem, e.g. problems at work.

Box 19.2

Psychological factors in sexual dysfunction
Predisposing
- Repressed family attitudes to sex
- Poor sex education
- Sexual or physical trauma

Precipitating
- Psychiatric illness
- Childbirth
- Infidelity
- Partner's sexual dysfunction
- Relationship problem – may be cause or effect

Maintaining
- Anxiety
- Poor communication
- Lack of foreplay
- Depression
- Poor information

Sometimes, the secondary loss of libido has no obvious specific cause. A woman who has suffered sexual or physical abuse in childhood, or who has had a sexually repressed upbringing, may go through a phase of normal or increased sexual activity in her teens and 20s and then present with loss of libido due to the long-term effects of her childhood experiences.

Often, a man reacts to the woman's loss of interest by making persistent sexual demands and then, after some years, gives up approaching her for sex. Loss of desire can be due to, or cause, relationship difficulties, and counselling will be directed towards improving communication between the partners. A specific cause, such as childhood abuse, may require specialist referral. Hormone therapy is appropriate for postmenopausal women but not for those who still have a normal menstrual cycle.

Orgasmic dysfunction

Inability to achieve orgasm is usually associated with lack of interest in sex, but sometimes can be an isolated symptom in a woman who has an otherwise satisfactory sex drive and is able to experience normal arousal. However orgasmic dysfunction may result in extreme frustration and distress.

Primary

This refers to a woman who has never been orgasmic. Inability to achieve orgasm, despite adequate arousal may be due to inexperience of the woman or her partner, or unrealistic expectations, e.g. reading erotic fiction may have led the couple to believe that orgasm occurs automatically on penetration. Often education and reassurance about normal sexual behaviour is all that is required in these circumstances. Sometimes, the cause is more deep-seated; possibly because of childhood/cultural repression resulting in the woman not being able to let go of her defences. Psychological counselling may be helpful in these cases.

Secondary

Secondary orgasmic dysfunction follows an interval of adequate sexual functioning. It is usually associated with reduced desire or arousal, as discussed in the previous section and has similar causes.

Situational orgasmic dysfunction

Some women can achieve orgasm through masturbation but not coitus, or with one partner but not with another. This is usually a pointer towards relationship difficulties.

Vaginismus and dyspareunia

Vaginismus is involuntary spasm of the pelvic floor muscles and perineal muscles, provoked by attempted penetration. It is also provoked by vaginal examination or by attempts to insert a tampon or the woman's own finger into the vagina. When severe, the conditioned reflex includes spasm of the

---

> **Box 19.3**
>
> ### Causes of dyspareunia
>
> **Superficial dyspareunia**
> - Infection, e.g. candida, herpes
> - Atrophic change, particularly after the menopause
> - Vulval dystrophy
> - Vaginismus
>
> **Deep dyspareunia**
> - Endometriosis
> - Pelvic inflammatory disease
> - Bowel dysfunction
> - Pelvic mass
> - 'Unexplained' pelvic pain

adductor muscles of the thighs. The spasm results in intense pain and inability to have penetrative intercourse.

Dyspareunia is the experience of pain on intercourse and is the commonest sexual problem presenting to the routine gynaecology clinic. It is usually classified into superficial and deep dyspareunia, but it is not always possible to make a clear distinction between the two (Box 19.3). With superficial dyspareunia, there is pain at the vaginal introitus or vestibule (vestibulodynia) on attempted penetration, often making full intercourse impossible. In deep dyspareunia, there is pain in the pelvis on deep penetration.

The separation between vaginismus and dyspareunia is increasingly seen as unfounded as the conditions are closely interrelated; with vaginismus being seen as a response to pain but also a cause of pain. The DSM 5 has developed category merging both conditions into 'genito-pelvic pain/penetration disorder' illustrating this overlap.

Primary

Primary vaginismus/dyspareunia is discovered during the first attempt at intercourse and persists thereafter. It may be due to apprehension that intercourse will be painful or due simply to failure to control the pelvic musculature. Persistent attempts at penetration cause more pain and a 'vicious cycle' is set up, reinforcing the vaginismus/pain cycle. There may also be deep-seated psychological problems, such as an inability to accept sexual maturity, sexual repression in childhood, childhood sexual abuse or fear of pregnancy.

Secondary

Symptoms may also follow a physically painful experience, such as a sexual assault, an obstetric problem at delivery or an insensitive vaginal examination. It can sometimes also result from painful infections or other conditions, e.g. lichen sclerosus, therefore an examination is essential in all patients with vaginismus/dyspareunia to exclude organic causes.

Examination of the vulva may reveal the inflammatory appearance of candidal infection, the lesions of herpes, or the presence of atrophy or dystrophy. Careful examination may be necessary to reveal the localized inflammation of vestibulitis. Vulval and vaginal swabs should be taken for microbiological examination and treatment given if appropriate. The Q-tip test elicits intense pain on light touch in the vestibular area and is indicative of vestibulodynia. If no cause is found for what appears to be superficial dyspareunia, it may be necessary to consider the causes of deep dyspareunia.

Bimanual examination may reveal a specific area of tenderness, e.g. the cervix or on palpating the posterior fornix, the rectum, or one or other lateral fornix. Sometimes, however, the tenderness is more general and a specific site cannot be identified. Deep dyspareunia is often associated with other symptoms such as dysmenorrhoea or persistent pelvic pain. The history should include questions about bowel habit. Bowel dysfunction is not uncommon and can be treated with a high-fibre diet. The timing of the pain in relation to the cycle should also be noted – it may occur just before ovulation or menstruation. Bimanual examination may reveal a pelvic mass.

The finding of a retroverted uterus is unlikely to be significant, as uterine retroversion is common. Occasionally, however, a sharply retroverted uterus can be the only site of tenderness. High vaginal and cervical swabs should be taken if there is any suspicion of pelvic infection. In most cases, laparoscopy is necessary to diagnose or exclude endometriosis or pelvic inflammatory disease.

When a specific cause is identified, the appropriate treatment is given. If laparoscopy is negative, a high-fibre diet may help even in the absence of obvious bowel symptoms. If no cause is found and the deep dyspareunia is not associated with other symptoms, the problem may be due to limited foreplay, leading to inadequate arousal and insufficient relaxation of the upper vagina. The couple should try allowing more time for arousal, and may be advised to avoid positions (such as the woman sitting on top of the man) in which penetration is particularly deep. Lubricants can be helpful and are worth trying.

If deep dyspareunia is associated with 'unexplained pelvic pain', treatment can be difficult and may require a combination of endocrine manipulation and psychological support.

Management

Treatment of any underlying condition is important, e.g. steroids for lichen sclerosus or topical oestrogens for postmenopausal atrophy. Where no underlying cause is identified, most cases respond well to simple treatment involving training in relaxation and the use of vaginal dilators/trainers. The woman should be helped to relax completely: she should let her head rest on the pillow and vaginal examination should not be attempted until the adductor muscles of the thighs have fully relaxed. In severe cases, physiotherapy can be helpful. The woman is then taught to insert a small vaginal dilator. Once she is comfortable about inserting the small dilator regularly, she can progress to gradually larger sizes. During treatment, she is also taught pelvic floor exercises, which help her to gain control of the muscles. It may take several weeks or months before full control is achieved.

Attempts at intercourse should be discouraged until she is able to insert the larger-sized vaginal dilators. In most instances, satisfactory intercourse follows. An alternative to vaginal dilators is for the woman to use her own finger and then for the partner to insert one and then two fingers into the vagina. In most instances that present to the clinic, however, the couple is reluctant to do this and prefer the dilators. If primary vaginismus is due to more deep-seated problems, treatment may take many months and the prognosis not as promising. Psychosexual counselling may be appropriate in these cases. In cases of vulvodynia, techniques such as mindfulness have proven to be effective.

For treatment of resistant cases, botulinum toxin (Botox) injected into the pelvic muscles can be very effective to prevent vaginal muscle spasm. The use of topical anaesthetic agents can help to relieve the pain of vestibulodynia.

Male sexual dysfunction

Male sexual dysfunction can be classified as impairment of desire, arousal (erection) or ejaculation.

Impaired desire

In the male, libido is dependent on normal testosterone levels, and serum testosterone should be checked in men complaining of lack of libido. If the level is normal, testosterone supplements are unlikely to help. Further enquiry may then elicit contextual factors, e.g. work stress, relationship difficulties, etc., which may impact on desire. This condition is a lot less common than in females.

Erectile dysfunction

Inability to achieve or maintain a satisfactory erection ('impotence') is the commonest sexual problem among men. It may be associated with impaired desire, but desire usually is normal.

Erectile dysfunction can be due to psychological factors but it is important to exclude organic causes. Erectile dysfunction is often the first sign of cardiovascular disease and all patients who present with this symptom should have their cardiovascular risk status assessed. If a physical cause is found, treatment and modification of risk factors may resolve the problem. The patient may also not accept a diagnosis of a psychological cause until all possible physical causes have been excluded (Box 19.4).

In addition to a full sexual history, the man should be asked about the duration of the problem, whether it is primary or secondary, and whether it is situational (i.e. does he get 'early morning' erections, or can he get an erection by masturbation but not with his partner). Situational erectile dysfunction is usually indicative of psychological causation. Enquiry should be made about symptoms of general disease, including those listed above. Smoking history is also important.

Physical causes of erectile failure

Endocrine disorders

- Hypogonadism. Disorders causing reduced plasma testosterone may cause erectile failure, but these usually cause loss of libido as well
- Diabetes may cause impotence. The incidence of erectile failure at age 50 is 40% among diabetic men, and only 5% among non-diabetic men. The mechanism may be either diabetic neuropathy or vascular disease

Neurological disorders

- Multiple sclerosis
- Spinal injury causes erectile failure but, after the initial phase of 'spinal shock', reflex erectile ability may return if the sacral segments of the spinal cord are intact

Vascular disorders

- There is a decline in sexual activity after myocardial infarction and, interestingly, before a heart attack. Erectile dysfunction is an important warning of likely cardiovascular disease and is often the first sign
- Hypertension is associated with erectile dysfunction

Drugs

- Antihypertensives
- Antipsychotics

Psychiatric illness

- Severe depression causes loss of sexual interest in over 60% of cases
- Severe anxiety

Surgery

- Prostatectomy need not cause impotence, particularly if it is by the transurethral or retropubic route. Radical prostatectomy usually causes erectile failure

Physiological

- Ageing reduces the frequency of erections. Some men may also fail to understand the refractory period, and may have unrealistic expectations of how soon erection can recur after orgasm

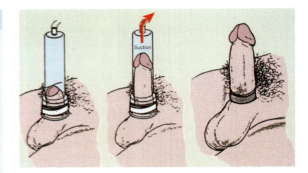

Fig. 19.6   The use of a vacuum device to manage erectile dysfunction.

Clinical examination should include a check for signs of systemic disease. The genitalia should be examined for abnormalities of the penis (such as hypospadias, peyronies disease) or abnormally small testes. Serum testosterone, glucose and lipids should be checked as a matter of routine. Therapeutic options include:

- phosphodiesterase inhibitors (PDE5 inhibitors), e.g. sildenafil (Viagra). Penile erection is due to relaxation of the smooth muscle around the cavernosal vascular spaces, allowing them to fill with blood. This is under the control of the autonomic nervous system, mediated by cyclic guanosine monophosphate (cGMP). These drugs are taken orally and enhance erection by blocking breakdown of cGMP. Alternatives to sildenafil are vardenafil (Levitra), which acts more quickly, and tadalafil (Cialis), which has a longer duration of action. Their success rate in treating erectile dysfunction is about 85%. Side-effects are mild and transient and include flushing, dyspepsia, headache and disturbance of colour vision. These

drugs must not be used by men who use nitrates or have severe cardiac disease, as they may lead to a life-threatening profound drop in blood pressure
- alprostadil (prostaglandin E_1 [PGE_1]). This drug also relaxes cavernosal smooth muscle but has to be injected directly into the corpora cavernosa. It is more effective than sildenafil in severe erectile failure. It is also available as a urethral pellet, but this is less effective
- other treatments used include vacuum devices (Fig. 19.6) and penile implants, the latter only where no other treatment has been effective.

Ejaculatory dysfunction

The most common type of ejaculatory dysfunction is premature ejaculation, affecting around one-third of men. Retarded ejaculation is much less common and may be associated with deep-seated psychological issues. Painful ejaculation is relatively rare and is most commonly a symptom of prostatitis.

Premature ejaculation is normal in early sexual experiences. There are various definitions and the best guide is if the man feels he has insufficient control to satisfy his urge to ejaculate following penetration (usually within 2 min of penetration). Sometimes, ejaculation occurs before penetration or within a few seconds of penetration. The cause of premature ejaculation is unknown but when it occurs it leads to anxiety and a vicious cycle.

Treatment requires the cooperation of the partner and it can be difficult to help a man who presents for treatment without his partner's knowledge. If the couple have a good relationship, they can be instructed in the 'stop–start' technique. This is when the couple have sex until just before the point of orgasm then 'stop' moving or withdraw the penis until the sensation passes then 'start' again and repeating this. Practice with this technique helps to build a feeling of control. This can also be adopted during masturbation. The 'squeeze' technique – firm pressure at the level of the frenulum when an orgasm is imminent – may also help to retard ejaculation. Antidepressant drugs (selective serotonin reuptake inhibitors [SSRIs], e.g. sertraline) are used off license to delay orgasm and are very effective. More recently, an SSRI-like drug, dapoxetine, has been given a license for treatment of premature ejaculation. A small amount of local anaesthetic applied to the frenulum before sex can also be helpful in some cases.

Treatment of sexual problems

The treatment of sexual problems can be divided into two categories:

- counselling, which should be within the scope of any healthcare worker
- sex therapy, which requires specialist training.

Counselling

Some problems can be helped by a single consultation or a few consultations. Simple counselling may include the items below.

Permission giving

Patients can be embarrassed or nervous about discussing sexual problems. Therefore, if the clinician can open the discussion about sexual activity, e.g. 'How is your sex life?' or 'Have these medications affected your sex life?'. These kinds of questions enable patients and let them know that it is OK to talk about sexual activity.

Limited information

An explanation of normal anatomy or physiology may also be helpful. He or she may be reassured by an examination, which shows that the genitalia are normal. The clinician may also recommend a book or website which explains sexual matters.

Specific suggestions

Common-sense advice on sexual techniques may be helpful. Examples of this, would be advice about foreplay, spending time with your partner, using sex aids, e.g. vibrators, suggesting different sexual positions, use of vaginal dilators/trainers or the 'stop–start' technique. The use of specific medication would also be appropriate e.g. PDE5 inhibitors for erectile dysfunction.

Sex therapy

Some problems are more complex and require specialist referral. Specialist treatment usually involves an average of about 12 sessions. Sexual therapy consists of behavioural elements and counselling. Both methods allow exploration of the sexual history in a nonthreatening and supportive environment. A behavioural approach offers practical solutions to sexual dysfunction supported by the counsellor, e.g. the 'stop–start' technique, and also includes elements of education about sexual functioning. Counselling allows exploration of the reasons behind the sexual dysfunction so the patient can develop a greater understanding of their difficulties in order to solve or accept them.

Conclusion

Sexual problems can be very distressing and may present to any clinician. Some problems can be treated easily with simple advice or prescribed medication; whilst others need more prolonged specialist treatment. A few may never respond to treatment. The main aim for a young doctor is to be able to discuss the subject comfortably. This is not easy, as both parties need to overcome their embarrassment. With sexual problems, more than with many aspects of medicine, there are many sensitivities, but with experience and some knowledge, any doctor can develop their skills in this area. Sexual medicine is a diverse and interesting area of work and can be very rewarding for both the doctor and the patient.

> **Key points**
> - Sexual problems are important and history-taking requires considerable skill. The problems may present directly or in the guise of another condition, or may be discovered coincidentally.
> - Normal sexual response has five phases: desire, arousal, orgasm, resolution and a refractory phase, during which further arousal does not occur.
> - Sexual response varies with age and with different phases of a relationship.
> - Sex has several functions in addition to reproduction, e.g. the strengthening of the pair bond.
> - The commonest male problems include erectile dysfunction and premature ejaculation.
> - The commonest female problems include loss of libido, orgasmic dysfunction and sexual pain.
> - Causes of sexual dysfunction may be medical or psychological. Psychological factors include predisposing factors (e.g. poor sex education or childhood abuse). Dysfunction is also more likely after childbirth, or if there has been infidelity, anxiety or poor communication.
> - Treatment involves counselling and education, hormonal therapy and relaxation exercises. Sometimes couple, group or psychotherapy is required.

20

Abortion

Introduction

Therapeutic abortion or termination of pregnancy has been carried out for thousands of years. The provision of abortion in a legal, medically supervised and safe framework remains one of the most contentious issues in modern-day medicine. Many people have strongly held and often divergent opinions about abortion. Those who are pro-abortion maintain that they are 'pro-choice' and support the right of individuals to make their own decisions. They are sensitive to the difficulties of bringing an unwanted baby into the world, and are aware of the impact on both the woman concerned and society more broadly. Those who are anti-abortion, or 'pro-life', argue that the fetus is more than just part of the mother; it is a life in itself and should be protected, even if that means limiting the mother's choices regarding her body.

There are many factors leading to unplanned pregnancy: contraception may have failed, or perhaps was not used at all; occasionally, intercourse without the woman's consent has resulted in pregnancy. Of course, a woman may have an unplanned pregnancy but be pleased to be pregnant and continue the pregnancy. Another may have planned to be pregnant but then her circumstances may change and she feels unable to continue. Among women attending antenatal clinics, research demonstrates that only two-thirds of women had an intended pregnancy, with the rest either ambivalent or having an unplanned pregnancy. Although abortion should not be considered as a method of contraception, contraceptive failures do occur, and access to abortion allows women complete fertility regulation.

Abortion care forms a large part of the gynaecology workload in the UK, and therapeutic abortion is one of the commonest gynaecological procedures. Although doctors may have differing degrees of involvement in abortion services, most will come into contact with women who are seeking abortion at some point in their career, so need to be familiar with the legal framework and options open to the women.

Worldwide perspectives

There are over 100 million acts of sexual intercourse every day across the world, resulting in over 900 000 pregnancies. It is estimated that about 50% of these pregnancies are unplanned, and about 25% are actually unwanted. Many women with an unwanted pregnancy will seek an abortion, and, as a result, about 150 000 pregnancies are terminated by induced abortion every day. There are over 50 million abortions worldwide every year and around one-third of these abortions are carried out in unsafe conditions. Illegal abortions are often performed in unclean conditions by unqualified people, causing considerable morbidity and mortality. Between 100 000 and 200 000 women die each year from unsafe abortion. In contrast, abortion performed in appropriate conditions with trained staff is a very safe procedure, with extremely low morbidity and mortality.

UK perspectives

The Abortion Act was passed in 1967, and after this, there was a rapid rise in the number of abortions carried out in England, Wales and Scotland. Currently, almost 190 000 abortions are carried out each year in England and Wales, with a further 12 000 in Scotland. Women of all reproductive ages have abortions, although the highest rate is among women aged 18–24 years. About 80% of women having abortions are unmarried, although many of these will have a regular partner. Just over half of women have already had a child and over one-third have had an abortion previously. Most terminations (80%) are carried out before 10 weeks of pregnancy, with only 8% performed above 13 weeks of gestation.

Legal and ethical aspects

Abortion is not available 'on demand' in the UK, and can only be carried out if certain criteria are met. The 1967

Circumstances in which an abortion may be carried out under the Abortion Act 1967 (amended 1991)

A. The continuance of the pregnancy would involve risk to the life of the pregnant woman greater than if the pregnancy were terminated
B. The termination is necessary to prevent grave permanent injury to the physical or mental health of the pregnant woman
C. The pregnancy has *not* exceeded its 24th week and continuance of the pregnancy would involve risk, greater than if the pregnancy were terminated, of injury to the physical or mental health of the pregnant woman
D. The pregnancy has *not* exceeded its 24th week and continuance of the pregnancy would involve risk, greater than if the pregnancy were terminated, of injury to the physical or mental health of the existing child(ren) of the family of the pregnant woman
E. There is a substantial risk that if the child were born it would suffer from such physical or mental abnormalities as to be seriously handicapped

Factors associated with coping problems and distress after abortion

- Women with a history of mental health problems
- Younger women
- Women from cultural or religious group who do not believe in abortion
- Women with low self-esteem
- Women without a close supportive person to talk to
- Women undergoing later abortions
- Women in whom the pregnancy was initially planned
- Women who feel there is no choice, e.g. due to financial pressures

Abortion Act, as amended in 1991, states that abortion can be performed if two doctors agree that the pregnancy should be terminated on one or more grounds (Box 20.1).

Most abortions (98%) are carried out under clause C of the Abortion Act, where two doctors agree that continuing the pregnancy would carry greater risk to the physical or mental health of the woman than abortion. A smaller number of abortions (1%) are carried out to protect the health of existing children. Clauses C and D carry an upper gestational limit of 24 weeks. The 1967 Abortion Act does not apply to Northern Ireland, where abortion is only legal under exceptional circumstances, e.g. to save the life of the mother.

Current methods of inducing abortion are now so safe that it is safer for the woman to have an early abortion than to continue to term and have a delivery. Of course, that does not mean that abortion should be recommended for all women, but a clinician may positively consider a request for abortion when a woman feels that her health or well-being (or that of her children) will be adversely affected by continuing the pregnancy.

Although uncommonly used, the Abortion Act also allows abortion to be performed in an emergency situation upon the single signature of the doctor performing the abortion. Such an emergency abortion can be carried out either to save the life of the pregnant woman, or to prevent grave permanent injury to the physical or mental health of the pregnant woman.

Recent opinion polls have shown that most of the public support the right to abortion, with 65% agreeing that if a woman wants an abortion she should not have to continue with her pregnancy. Women requesting abortion need the agreement of two doctors, and will often rely on the support of their general practitioner for referral. Over 80% of British general practitioners described themselves as 'broadly pro-choice', and 18% as 'broadly anti-abortion'. No doctor has to be involved in referring women for abortion, but the General Medical Council guidance advises that if a doctor is unable to make a referral for termination, then a timely referral of the woman to a colleague who does not hold similar views is obligatory; every doctor has an obligation to treat in an emergency situation.

Consultation and counselling before abortion

When a woman is considering abortion, it is important that she is able to weigh up the practical and emotional aspects of her decision, to ensure that the best choice is made in the circumstances. The Royal College of Obstetricians and Gynaecologists's (RCOG) guidance recommends that the initial consultation appointment should be available within 5 days of referral, to avoid any unnecessary delays. She will require sympathetic but non-directional support so that she is able to explore her own feelings and to make her own informed decision. Many women with an unplanned pregnancy will make their decision within a few days of knowing that they are pregnant. Other women may remain undecided for some time. It is important that the decision to abort or continue the pregnancy is made freely by the woman, and that she is not coerced by another party, for example a parent or partner. For this reason, it is imperative to speak to the woman alone at some point during the consultation.

Psychological problems and rates of depression are not increased after abortion when compared with background population risk, but some women may experience coping problems and distress. The counselling process can help to identify these women, and ensure that appropriate support is offered both before and after the abortion. Box 20.2 outlines risk factors for emotional problems.

Women who blame themselves for the pregnancy and subsequent abortion can struggle to come to terms with their decision. It can help to identify what went wrong that led to the pregnancy. Jointly agreeing a contraceptive plan with the woman can return a sense of control to her, and give her something positive for the future to take from the experience.

We are used to taking a structured gynaecological and sexual history, collecting factual information, such as date of last menstrual period, but we can help the woman to express her emotional needs by using some basic counselling techniques:

- ask open-ended questions, e.g. 'How did you feel about the pregnancy?' rather than 'Were you upset when you found out?'
- actively listen to the patient, e.g. show interest in her views, and show understanding
- reassure her that her feelings are normal, e.g. saying 'I understand that you are finding this difficult to talk about'
- encourage questions, e.g. say 'What would you like to ask me about your choices?', rather than 'Any questions?'

Some women need practical information to make their choice, such as details about maternity leave, housing rights, etc. or information about adoption. Timely referral to a social worker should be available.

Pre-abortion investigations

Once the woman has decided to proceed to abortion, there are a number of investigations which are usually performed to ensure that the abortion is as safe as possible:

- *blood tests*: haemoglobin is measured and a sample is sent for blood grouping. Women who are rhesus negative will require anti-D immunoglobulin after the abortion (250 IU if <20 weeks and 500 IU if >20 weeks). Human immunodeficiency virus testing should be offered to all women. Other blood-borne virus testing and haemoglobinopathy screening can be performed if indicated
- *estimation of gestation*: this can be performed by either clinical examination or ultrasound. Most abortion clinics in the UK use ultrasound to confirm gestation before abortion. Ultrasound is essential if there is a possibility of ectopic pregnancy, or where gestation is unclear. Some women will not make the decision until they know the gestation of the pregnancy, i.e. they may decide to abort an early pregnancy, but would not wish to undergo a later abortion. Occasionally, women may request a scan photograph, as a memento of the pregnancy. Ultrasound will sometimes show a non-viable pregnancy, which will then relieve the woman of a decision around abortion, and may avoid an unnecessary procedure
- *prevention of infection*: infection can occur in about 10% of women after abortion, but is reduced with the use of antibiotics. RCOG guidance advises that all women undergoing abortion should be screened for *Chlamydia trachomatis* and receive prophylactic antibiotics on the day of abortion. Screening gives the opportunity to carry out partner notification (contact

tracing) when there is a positive test, thus preventing reinfection of the woman and onward transmission. Some clinics treat everyone having an abortion with prophylactic antibiotics (commonly metronidazole and azithromycin), whereas others have opted to screen women for sexually transmitted infections (STIs), including chlamydia, and only treat positive women and their partners

- *cervical cytology*: if a woman is due cervical cytology within the national screening programme, then this should be offered at the time of the clinic visit
- *provision of information*: information given verbally should be supported with written information for the woman to take away, available in a range of languages. This should include information about the types of abortion available, the risks and complications of abortion and who to contact if there are any problems after the procedure.

Methods of abortion

Historically, a wide range of surgical and medical techniques have been used to cause therapeutic abortion. In the past three decades, advances in abortion techniques mean that safe and effective methods are now available at all stages of gestation. Medical methods have been increasingly used since the licensing of mifepristone in 1991. Both medical and surgical abortion can be offered up to 24 weeks, but availability varies in different geographical areas. In England and Wales, around 55% of abortions are performed using medical methods, whereas in Scotland 80% are medical. The most appropriate method depends on gestation, medical history and the woman's preference (Box 20.3).

Medical abortion

Mifepristone is a synthetic steroid that blocks the biological action of progesterone by binding to its receptor in the uterus and other organs. It is given orally under supervision of a doctor or nurse, in a premises licensed to carry out abortion. The woman is then allowed home. She returns to the unit 24–48 h later (usually 48 h) for administration of a prostaglandin, which can be given vaginally, buccally or sublingually. Bleeding usually starts within a few hours, followed by uterine contractions which expel the fetus and placenta. Most women experience period-like pains but there is much variation, with some women needing no pain relief while others (about 10–20%) require opiates. Bleeding usually continues for about 10 days after medical abortion.

Early medical abortion (up to 9 weeks' gestation)

When a woman is less than 7 weeks' pregnant, medical abortion is the most effective type of termination, with a lower failure rate than early surgical abortion. It is

Abortion options depend on gestation. Providing a choice of abortion method increases satisfaction with method chosen

Medical abortion

- ■ 'Early' medical abortion
  - – under 9 weeks
  - – mifepristone plus single-dose misoprostol
- ■ 'Late' first-trimester medical abortion
  - – between 9 and 12 weeks
  - – mifepristone plus misoprostol (more than one dose of misoprostol may be required)
- ■ Mid-trimester medical abortion
  - – 13–24 weeks
  - – mifepristone plus repeated doses of misoprostol (need to perform feticide intervention if over 22 weeks)

Surgical abortion

- ■ Manual vacuum aspiration
  - – below 7 weeks
  - – under local anaesthesia
  - – higher failure rate
  - – careful follow-up required
- ■ Suction abortion
  - – between 7 and 14 weeks
  - – cervical preparation recommended
  - – local or general anaesthesia
- ■ Dilatation and evacuation
  - – between 14 and 24 weeks
  - – requires specially trained surgeon
  - – not available in all areas

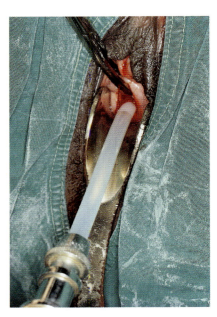

Fig. 20.1 **Surgical termination of pregnancy at 10 weeks' gestation.**

also a good choice between 7 and 9 weeks' (63 days') gestation.

The usual regimen is:

- ■ mifepristone 200 mg orally, followed by misoprostol 800 μg vaginally 24–48 h later. Women can remain in the abortion unit until the abortion is complete, or can go home to complete the abortion.

Medical abortion in the later first trimester (9–12 weeks)

In the past, surgical termination alone has been offered to women in the late first trimester. However, it is now recognized that medical abortion is an effective alternative to surgical termination in the late first trimester.

The usual regimen is:

- ■ mifepristone 200 mg orally, followed by misoprostol 800 μg vaginally 36–48 h later. Up to a further four doses of misoprostol 400 μg, either vaginally or orally, can be given until abortion occurs.

Medical abortion in the second trimester (13–24 weeks)

Traditionally, mid-trimester medical abortion was carried out using prostaglandin alone, or in combination with an oxytocin infusion. Not uncommonly, it would take several days for the abortion to be completed. Giving mifepristone prior to prostaglandin significantly reduces the length of time taken for the abortion to occur.

The usual regimen is:

- ■ mifepristone 200 mg orally, followed by misoprostol 800 μg vaginally 36–48 h later. Up to a further four doses of misoprostol 400 μg orally can be given until abortion occurs.

Surgical abortion

Surgical abortion below 7 weeks' gestation

Surgical abortion below 7 weeks' gestation has a higher failure rate than later surgical procedures and than medical abortion at this gestation. However, abortion by manual vacuum aspiration can be performed at this early gestation, with appropriate measures to ensure the abortion is complete. A narrow suction curette of 4 or 5 mm diameter is inserted into the uterus under local paracervical block. The early pregnancy is aspirated using a 5-mL syringe. It is very important to ensure that the abortion is complete, either by identifying the products of conception or by human chorionic gonadotrophin follow-up.

Surgical abortion at 7–14 weeks

Surgical abortion at this gestation is performed by suction or vacuum aspiration using a flexible suction curette, and a mechanical or electrical pump. The suction curette is inserted into the uterine cavity, after cervical dilatation, and the contents aspirated (Figs 20.1 and 20.2). The procedure can be carried out under general anaesthesia, local anaesthesia or conscious sedation depending on patient choice.

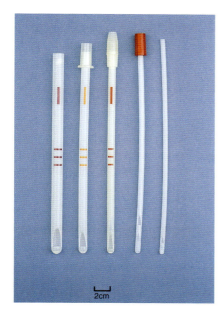

Fig. 20.2 A selection of suction curettes for surgical pregnancy termination.

Cervical treatment with prostaglandin before surgical abortion reduces the risk of cervical trauma and uterine perforation, and is recommended for all cases.

The recommended regimen is:

- misoprostol 400 µg vaginally or sublingually 2–3 h prior to surgery.

Later surgical abortion (14–24 weeks)

Cervical preparation followed by dilatation and evacuation (D&E) can be offered in the second trimester. It is the method of choice in the USA, but in the UK is offered by a limited number of doctors experienced in the technique. It may be necessary to dilate the cervix up to a diameter of 20 mm before the fetal parts can be extracted using special instruments. D&E has the advantage that the woman is under anaesthesia so is unaware of the procedure. There is evidence from the USA that women prefer D&E to medical methods, although some nurses and doctors can find the procedure disturbing.

Complications of abortion

Women should be advised that the risk of complications is low. Indeed, a termination is safer than continuing the pregnancy to term. Complications do occasionally occur, however, and women should be given information about where to seek help if there are problems.

Retained products of conception

Retained products of conception occurs in less than 5% of women. It is more common after medical abortion, and when surgical abortion is carried out at either very early or later gestations. Some women with retained products will require (further) surgical evacuation of the uterus, particularly if there is heavy or prolonged bleeding. However, many women will pass the retained tissue spontaneously, without the need for further intervention. Antibiotics can be given to reduce the risk of secondary infection until the tissue is passed.

Failure of abortion

Ongoing pregnancy after an abortion procedure is unusual, occurring in less than 1% of cases. Women should be advised of the importance of returning for follow-up, if there was any doubt over completion at the time of the procedure, or if there are continuing symptoms of pregnancy.

Post-abortion infection

Pelvic infection can occur in up to 10% of women after termination, but this can be at least halved with pre-abortion STI screening and use of antibiotics at the time of termination. Women should be advised about signs of infection such as pyrexia, pelvic pain and offensive vaginal discharge, and should return if concerned.

Haemorrhage

Significant haemorrhage of over 500 mL at the time of termination occurs in less than 1 in 1000 early abortion cases, rising to 4 in 1000 when over 20 weeks.

Trauma to the genital tract

Perforation of the uterus happens in about 1 in 1000 surgical cases, and is more common with later-gestation abortions and with less experienced surgeons. Cervical trauma is also uncommon (<1 in 100) and is reduced by cervical preparation with prostaglandin. Uterine rupture has been described very occasionally with mid-trimester medical abortion.

Future fertility

Women often ask about the chance of an abortion affecting their future fertility. There is no established positive association between previous termination of pregnancy and future infertility, ectopic pregnancy or placenta praevia. There may be a slight increase in risk of subsequent miscarriage and pre-term delivery with later abortion, although the evidence is unclear.

Psychological sequelae

There is no evidence of lasting psychological harm to women undergoing abortion and indeed there is no difference in psychological sequelae if women abort or continue the pregnancy. Some women may be at higher risk of distress after the abortion, and can be identified at the time of pre-abortion consultation and offered greater support.

Abortion aftercare

Women should be provided with appropriate information of symptoms and signs of complications, and should be given a contact telephone number if she has concerns after the procedure. There is no need for routine follow-up when the completion of the abortion was confirmed at the time.

Post-abortion contraception

Over one-third of terminations are carried out on women who have had a termination in the past, and ensuring that there is adequate contraception available can reduce the chance of a further abortion. All methods of hormonal contraception (combined pill, progestogen pill, implant, injection, patch, ring) can be started on the day of surgical abortion, or on the prostaglandin treatment day of medical abortion, with immediate contraceptive cover. Intrauterine contraception can be fitted immediately following termination. This can be done at the end of the surgical procedure, or following expulsion of the pregnancy with medical termination. Condoms can be used immediately after termination. Women are usually advised not to use a diaphragm within 6 weeks of mid-trimester abortion, in case refitting is required. Female sterilization is not usually performed at the same time as abortion. This is because simultaneous sterilization is associated with a higher sterilization failure rate, and increased subsequent regret about being sterilized. Women who wish to be sterilized can be offered an interval sterilization, with provision of a bridging method of contraception in the interim.

Conclusion

Over 200 000 women undergo therapeutic abortion each year in the UK. Women need to be well informed about pregnancy and abortion options, and supported to make an informed choice. A choice between medical and surgical abortion should be offered. A range of contraceptive options should be made available to women at the time of termination.

Key *points*

- Unsafe abortion is a great threat to women's health worldwide and causes many maternal mortalities.
- Therapeutic abortion is a common, safe and effective procedure in the UK, and is carried out under the terms of the Abortion Act.
- Women considering termination need information about options to guide their choice, and non-directive support to ensure they reach the most appropriate decision.
- A choice between medical and surgical abortion should be offered.
- A contraceptive plan should be agreed and in place immediately after the abortion.

21 Contraception

Introduction

Currently, the World Health Organization (WHO) recommends a 24-month inter-pregnancy interval after childbirth. It has been estimated that worldwide effective family planning could prevent 1 in 10 deaths among babies by helping women to space births at least 2 years apart because a short inter-pregnancy interval of less than 12 months increases the risk of complications such as low birth weight, pre-term birth, stillbirth and neonatal death. The Faculty of Sexual and Reproductive Healthcare (FSRH) has developed the UK Medical Eligibility Criteria (UKMEC), which provide evidence-based recommendations to facilitate the safe use of contraception without imposing unnecessary medical restrictions, and the categories used to define risk are summarized in Table 21.1.

Defining 'contraceptive failure' is not easy, as it depends on the population studied. Studies on a young population will suggest a higher failure rate than in an older group, as fertility is higher in younger people. Caution is therefore required when interpreting relevant figures. The 'method' failure includes the inherent risk of failure providing the method is used correctly. It is quantified in the units per 100 woman-years (HWY), the number of women who would become pregnant if 100 of them used that method of contraception for 1 year. 'User' failure is the failure rate when the method is not used correctly (e.g. missed pills, late injections, drug interactions). If used consistently and correctly, hormonal contraceptives (combined hormonal method, progestogen-only pills [POPs], injectable, implant and intrauterine system) and the non-hormonal methods (copper intrauterine device [Cu-IUD], male and female sterilization) are more than 99% effective in preventing pregnancy. These methods, as well as emergency contraception (EC), barrier methods and natural family planning methods, are described in this chapter.

Methods of contraception

Contraception can be considered as either hormonal (pills, patch, intravaginal ring, injectable, subdermal and the levonorgestrel-releasing intrauterine system [LNG-IUS]) or non-hormonal (Cu-IUD, barrier methods, sterilization, lactational amenorrhoea method [LAM] and natural family planning). In the UK, oral contraception remains the most popular method, with a third of women on contraception using this as their primary method. Increasingly popular are the so-called long-acting reversible contraceptive (LARC) methods, which include subdermal implants and both the Cu-IUD and LNG-IUS. LARCs are cost effective in the prevention of pregnancy and there is no delay in return to fertility after removal of these methods.

Combined hormonal contraception (CHC)

CHC (pills, patch and intravaginal ring) work primarily by inhibiting ovulation via the hypothalamo–pituitary–ovarian axis to reduce luteinizing hormone (LH) and follicle-stimulating hormone. In addition, cervical mucus is less favourable to sperm penetration and the endometrium is thinned. Most data on the use and safety of CHC relates specifically to the combined oral contraceptive (COC) pill. This evidence is extrapolated to the transdermal patch and intravaginal ring, as they also contain oestrogen and progestogen.

Most currently available COC pills contain ethinylestradiol (EE) and a progestogen (synthetic progesterone), which can be norethisterone (first generation), levonorgestrel (LNG) (second generation), desogestrel, norgestimate and gestodene (third generation), and drospirenone, dienogest and nomegestrol acetate (fourth generation).

Contraindications to combined hormonal contraception

Most evidence available relates to the COC, but this evidence can also be applied to the use of the combined patch and intravaginal ring. Women considering the CHC should be informed of the potential risks and benefits associated with use. However, it is safe for most women, most of the time Table 21.2. Oestrogen-containing COCs increase the risk of venous thromboembolism (VTE) above the background risk of 2 per 10 000 woman-years among women not using a COC. The COCs containing LNG, norethisterone or norgestimate have the lowest risk (5–7 per 10 000 women) and those containing drospirenone, desogestrel or gestodene have the highest risk (9–12 per 10 000 women). The risk is greatest in the first few months after initiating the COC and the risk falls to that of non-users within weeks of discontinuation. Nevertheless, when prescribed appropriately, the

Table 21.1	UKMEC categories	
UKMEC category	**Definition**	
UKMEC 1	A condition for which there is *no restriction* for the use of the contraceptive method	
UKMEC 2	A condition for which the *advantages of using the method generally outweigh the theoretical or proven risks*	
UKMEC 3	A condition where the *theoretical or proven risks usually outweigh the advantages* of using the method[a]	
UKMEC 4	A condition which represents an *unacceptable health risk* if the contraceptive method is used	

[a]The provision of a method to a woman with a condition given a UKMEC category 3 requires expert clinical judgement and/or referral to a specialist contraceptive provider, since use of the method is not usually recommended unless other methods are not available or not acceptable.

Table 21.3	Risk of VTE associated with COC use
Absolute risk of VTE per 10 000 woman-years	**Circumstance**
4–5	For women not using COC and not pregnant
9–10	For women using a COC
29	For women who are pregnant
300–400	For women who are immediately postpartum

Table 21.2	Risks and benefits associated with COC use
Disease	**Relative risk with COC use in non-smokers**
Potential harms (risks)	
Coronary artery disease	Very small increase
Ischaemic stroke	Two-fold increase
VTE	Two-fold increase
Breast cancer	Any increased risk likely to be small and will vary with age
	No increased risk above background risk 10 years after stopping COC
Cervical cancer	Small increase after 5 years and a two-fold increase after 10 years
Benefits	
Ovarian cancer	Halving of risk, lasting for >15 years
Endometrial cancer	Halving of risk, lasting for >15 years
Colorectal cancer	Reduction

How to take the combined oral contraceptive

The majority of COCs are usually a fixed dose (monophasic) pill containing 20–35 µg of EE and a progestogen. There are no proven benefits of biphasic or triphasic COCs (where doses of the constituent hormones are varied week to week) over a monophasic pill. The following advice on how to take COC applies to monophasic regimens.

A monophasic COC can be started up to and including day 5 of the menstrual cycle to provide immediate contraceptive protection. If started after this time, condoms or abstinence is advised for the next 7 days (or until 7 consecutive pills have been taken). Most COC packages contain 21 active tablets: one tablet is taken daily for 21 consecutive days, followed by a 7-day pill-free interval (PFI) or placebo pill week. For pills with placebo, 21 active pills are followed by 7 inactive pills with no pill-free week. A withdrawal bleed usually occurs in the PFI due to the withdrawal of hormones, which induces endometrial shedding. Women should be encouraged to take COCs around the same time every day to support compliance. In general, one pill can be missed without requiring any further action as long as all other pills have been taken and are continued to be taken consistently and correctly. Continuous dosing or extended regimens of COC pills are becoming increasingly common modes of administration. The potential advantages of continuous or extended regimens are that they enable women to eliminate or reduce the frequency of their withdrawal bleed and any menstruation-related symptoms. The most common extended regimen is three cycles of active pills taken without a break, followed by a 4- or 7-day break. Giving women more choice in their pill taking regimens may improve compliance and satisfaction.

Drug interactions

Enzyme-inducing drugs increase the metabolism of oestrogens and progestogens, which may in turn reduce

benefits of CHC use generally outweigh the risk of venous thrombosis, which is low overall and is lower than the VTE risk associated with pregnancy and the postpartum period (Table 21.3). A clinical history should identify any risk factors for VTE that fall within the UKMEC categories 3 or 4 for use of hormonal contraception. A personal history of VTE, current VTE, a family history of VTE in a first-degree relative under the age of 45 years, major surgery with prolonged immobilization, immobility and known thrombogenic mutations fall under these UKMEC categories. Non-smokers may safely continue to use CHC, including COC, to age 50 years if they have no contraindications for use. Deaths in COC users over 35 years of age are eight times more common in smokers than non-smokers. For women who continue to smoke (<15 cigarettes/day) at the age of 35 years COC use is given a UKMEC category 3 (risks outweigh benefits); and if smoking ≥15 cigarettes/day a UKMEC category 4 is given (unacceptable health risk). The use of CHC may pose an unacceptable health risk (UKMEC 4) in women with current and/or history of ischaemic heart disease, stroke, vascular disease, hypertension, liver disease (severe cirrhosis, active viral hepatitis, tumours) or migraine with aura at any age or for women within 6 weeks postpartum and breastfeeding. Notably, however, women who are not breastfeeding, are between 3 and 6 weeks postpartum and have no risk factors for VTE can safely start CHC.

the contraceptive efficacy of CHC. Women using enzyme-inducing drugs should ideally switch to a method that is unaffected by their use (such as the Cu-IUD, the LNG-IUS or the progestogen-only injectable). Liver enzyme-inducing drugs include some antiepileptics (such as carbamazepine), some antiretrovirals, certain antibiotics (such as rifabutin and rifampicin) and the over-the-counter herbal medicine St John's Wort. These liver enzyme-inducing drugs can accelerate the hepatic breakdown of contraceptive steroids, thus potentially reducing the efficacy of the COC. Women using COC while on liver enzyme-inducing drugs short-term may continue to use this method if they consider a minimum 50 µg EE pill (such as a 30 µg pill plus a 20 µg EE monophasic) as a tricyling regimen with a PFI of 4 days. This should be used during treatment and continued for a further 28 days after treatment has stopped. The use of two patches or two rings is not recommended. For women using the very potent enzyme inducers rifampicin and rifabutin, an alternative method is always advised. Additional contraceptive precautions are not required when non-liver enzyme-inducing antibiotics are used. Conversely, some medications may themselves be affected by hormonal contraceptive use. Women on lamotrigine (except in combination with sodium valproate), for example, should be advised that there is a risk of reduced seizure control whilst on CHC along with the potential for toxicity in the CHC-free week; therefore, the risks of using CHC may outweigh the benefits in these women.

Follow-up

A 12-month supply of COC can be provided at the first visit, but for some women a follow-up at 3 months may be appropriate to assess any problems and provide re-instruction if necessary. Blood pressure should be assessed annually. Women should be encouraged to attend at any time if problems arise. The pill should be discontinued if any potentially serious side-effects occur (e.g. chest pain, leg pain or swelling). Follow-up visits are also an opportunity to carry out other well-woman screening (e.g. blood pressure, cervical cytology, new risk of sexually transmitted infections [STIs]).

The COC should be stopped and an alternative method used at least 4 weeks before any planned major surgery where immobilization is expected. The COC may be recommenced at least 2 weeks after full mobilization.

Combined hormonal contraceptive patch

The risks and benefits associated with transdermal patch use are as described for the COC (Table 21.2). A patch can be applied to the abdomen, buttock or thigh on the same day each week for 3 consecutive weeks. This is followed by a patch-free week, during which time there is endometrial shedding and a withdrawal bleed. The transdermal patch should be changed every 7 days, although a single patch will provide effective contraceptive protection for up to 9 days. As for the COC, the transdermal patch can be started up to and including day 5 of the menstrual cycle to

provide immediate contraceptive protection. If started after this time, condoms or abstinence are advised for the next 7 days.

Combined hormonal intravaginal contraceptive ring

The risks and benefits associated with intravaginal ring use are as described for the COC (Table 21.2). The intravaginal ring is associated with low and stable serum concentrations of EE of only 15 µg. The ring is inserted into the vagina on the same day each month and is retained for 3 weeks. This is followed by a ring-free week, during which time the endometrium sheds and there is a withdrawal bleed. Once inserted into the vagina by the woman herself the ring sits above the pelvic floor and should not be felt by her and does not need to be removed during intercourse. As for the COC, the intravaginal ring can be inserted up to and including day 5 of the menstrual cycle to provide immediate contraceptive protection. If started after this time, condoms or abstinence are advised for the next 7 days.

Progestogen-only contraception

Progestogen-only contraception (pills, injectables, subdermal implant and the LNG-IUS) avoids the potential increased risks attributed to oestrogen. Most progestogen-only methods are associated with a disturbance in the bleeding pattern, which is often the main reason for discontinuation of these otherwise very effective methods. Other side-effects have been reported (abdominal bloating, weight changes, acne, headaches and mood changes) but few have been objectively related to progestogen use.

Drug interactions

The effect of liver enzyme-inducing drugs on the metabolism of progestogens is similar to that for oestrogens. This reduces the efficacy of a POP or subdermal implant and alternative methods of contraception are recommended. The progestogen-only injectable depot medroxyprogesterone acetate (DMPA) and the LNG-IUS, however, are not affected by liver enzyme-inducing medication and may be a good option for women in these circumstances.

Progestogen-only pills

POPs containing LNG, norethisterone or desogestrel are currently available in the UK. Although POPs are suitable for most women, they are often used by women for whom a COC is contraindicated. All POPs thicken cervical mucus, thus preventing sperm penetration into the upper reproductive tract, and this is the primary mode of action of POPs. In addition, some POPs also inhibit ovulation, although not in every cycle. POPs containing norethisterone or LNG inhibit ovulation in up to 60% of cycles and the desogestrel POP inhibits ovulation in up to 97% of cycles. A POP should be taken at or around the same time every day **without** a PFI. A POP can be started up to and including day 5 of the menstrual cycle (within 5 days of a termination of pregnancy or up to day 21 postpartum) to provide immediate contraception. If started at other times, additional contraception, such as condoms, is required for the first 48 h. A norethisterone or LNG-POP is late if taken ≥3 h after when it was due to be taken; the desogestrel POP is late if >12 h has elapsed. Contraception from intercourse prior to the missed pill is maintained but barrier methods are recommended until two consecutive pills have been taken, by which time the cervical mucus effect preventing sperm penetration is maximal again.

Progestogen-only injectable contraception

The most widely used progestogen-only injectable in the UK is DMPA, which is licensed to be given as an intramuscular (IM) injection every 12 weeks. The primary mode of action of the progestogen-only injectable is inhibition of ovulation. Unpredictable bleeding is common in the initial months of use but usually settles and up to 70% of women are amenorrhoeic at 1 year of use. Women should be informed that there could be a delay of up to 1 year in the return of fertility after stopping the use of injectable contraceptives. This is possibly due to the serum levels of DMPA, which in some women can still be detected between 6 and 9 months after a single injection and, for some women, in concentrations sufficient to inhibit ovulation. Hormonal investigations should not normally be considered until amenorrhoea continues for up to 12 months after the last injection was given.

A reversible loss of bone mineral density occurs with DMPA use. Most of this bone loss is in the initial 2 years of use and, thereafter, there is no further loss. There is no indication to consider dual-energy X-ray absorptiometry bone scans routinely in women using DMPA, even with long-term use. Serum concentrations of oestrogen in women using DMPA are similar to concentrations seen in the follicular phase of the menstrual cycle and therefore women are not hypo-oestrogenic. There is no apparent increase in risk of fracture, and moreover bone mineral density recovers after cessation of DMPA use. In women aged under 18 years, DMPA may be used as first-line contraception after other options have been discussed and considered unsuitable or unacceptable. Women can use DMPA up to the age of 50 years, at which time an alternative method should be considered. This is because of concerns about the impact on skeletal health and the theoretical risk of osteoporotic fracture in the menopause. However, if a woman prefers to continue or start the method at the age of 50 years or over, this would not be an unacceptable health risk providing the benefits and risks have been assessed. Women using DMPA who wish to continue use should be reviewed every 2 years to assess individual situations, and to discuss the benefits and potential risks.

Weight gain is a recognized effect of DMPA use, particularly in women under 18 years of age with a BMI ≥30.

There is now a subcutaneous DMPA preparation that is licensed for self-administration. It is bioequivalent to IM-DMPA and is administered at intervals of 13 weeks ± 7 days. Like the IM-DMPA, the primary mechanism of action is to prevent ovulation. It may be preferable to IM-DMPA in patients at risk of haematoma due to bleeding disorders or anticoagulation.

Progestogen-only subdermal implants

This is a single subdermal etonogestrel implant or rod made from a non-biodegradable polymer that contains an active slow-release progestogen formulation and is about the size of a matchstick. The implant is licensed to provide contraception for up to 3 years. Changes in bleeding patterns are common: infrequent bleeding is the most common pattern (approximately one-third); around one-fifth of women experience no bleeding; and approximately one-quarter have prolonged or frequent bleeding. These bleeding patterns may not settle with time. Women who experience troublesome bleeding while using the progestogen-only implant, and who are eligible to use CHC, may be offered a COC cyclically or continuously for 3 months (outside the product licence). There is no evidence of a causal association between the use of the implant and weight change, mood change, loss of libido or headache. Healthcare professionals who insert and remove progestogen-only implants should be appropriately trained. Insertion is intended to render the implant palpable beneath the skin. Barium sulphate is added to the implant so that if an implant cannot be palpated, an X-ray of the upper arm enables its identification. The incidence of deep insertion is around 1 in 1000 women and ultrasound scan can be used to facilitate location and removal of deep implants lying above muscle.

Levonorgestrel-releasing intrauterine systems

There are two intrauterine systems that contain different doses of LNG and both offer highly effective and reversible contraception. They are T-shaped devices with an elastomer core containing LNG (Fig. 21.1A). The LNG-IUS works primarily by its progestogenic effect on the endometrium that prevents implantation. In addition, effects on cervical mucus reduce sperm penetration. Ovulation may be inhibited in some women. Systemic side-effects due to absorption of LNG are often mild and usually settle in the first 3 months of use.

The 52 mg LNG-IUS is licensed for 5 years' use as contraception or as a treatment for heavy menstrual bleeding. Failure rates for 5 year use are low (1%). Irregular bleeding with the 52 mg LNG-IUS is common in the first few months after insertion but often settles by 6 months after insertion. Menstrual loss is reduced by an average of 90% at 12 months, with 20% of women experiencing amenorrhoea. For women who have the device inserted after the age of 45 years, the 52 mg LNG-IUS may be continued until the menopause is confirmed or until the age of 55 years, at which time the majority of women are postmenopausal.

The 13.5 mg LNG-IUS is a smaller device with a lower dose of LNG. It is licensed for contraception for a duration of 3 years. The device contains a silver ring, which

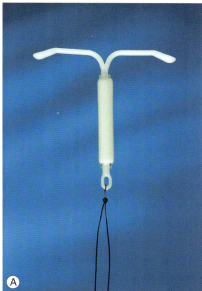

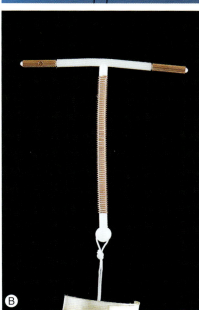

Fig. 21.1 **Intrauterine Contraception (IUC). (A)** LNG-IUS; **(B)** CU-IUD.

Non-hormonal contraception

Copper intrauterine devices

Copper is toxic to ova and sperm, and the Cu-IUD works primarily by inhibiting fertilization. In addition, the endometrial inflammatory reaction generated by the Cu-IUD has an anti-implantation effect and alterations in cervical mucus inhibit sperm penetration. Failure rates for Cu-IUD contraception up to 5 years of use are low (2% with a 380 mm^2 Cu-IUD). Banded Cu-IUDs, which have 380 mm^2 of copper in the vertical stem and copper sleeves on the horizontal arms, are the most effective intrauterine devices available and are recommended to be used as a first-line device (Fig. 21.1B). Some branded devices available in the UK can be used for up to 10 years. Spotting, light bleeding or heavier or prolonged bleeding is common in the first 3–6 months of Cu-IUD use, but this may settle. There are few contraindications to use of IUC (Table 21.4). The management of common problems associated with Cu-IUD and LNG-IUS use is outlined in Table 21.5.

The adverse effects and complications associated with insertion of Intrauterine Contraception (IUC)

The term IUC includes both LNG-IUS and CU-IUD. There are few contraindications to use of IUC (Table 21.4). The management of common problems associated with IUC use is outlined in Table 21.5. Clinicians who insert IUC should be appropriately trained and be able to maintain competency. Discomfort during and/or after insertion of IUC and the need for pain relief during insertion should be discussed with women in advance and administered when appropriate. Emergency equipment must be available in all settings where IUC is being inserted, and local referral protocols must be in place for women who require further medical input.

Expulsion and perforation

The risk of expulsion with IUC is around 1 in 20 and is most common in the first year of use, particularly within 3 months of insertion. The risk of uterine perforation associated with IUC is up to 2 per 1000 insertions, and is approximately six-fold higher in breastfeeding women. Most perforations occur at the time of insertion, but a delayed 'migration' is recognized to occur. Immediate perforation may be detected because of acute pain or it may be detected later, if pregnancy occurs. Most commonly, perforation is identified following the investigation of 'missing threads', although the most common reason for missing threads is that they have curled up in the endocervical canal in the presence of a normally placed device. The management of suspected perforation and lost threads are outlined in Table 21.5. If the device is not in the uterine cavity, an abdominal X-ray will identify IUC if it is lying within the peritoneal cavity (Fig. 21.2). They may cause dense adhesion formation and should be removed by laparoscopy or laparotomy.

distinguishes it from other intrauterine devices on ultrasound scan or X-ray. Women using the 13.5 mg LNG-IUS are less likely to experience amenorrhoea. Higher failure rates and ectopic pregnancy rates have been reported in some trials of the 13.5 mg LNG-IUS, but numbers are currently too small to confirm a significant difference. This is still a highly effective method with low failure rates and low ectopic rates overall.

The adverse effects and complications associated with insertion of the LNG-IUS are as for a Cu-IUD (see later).

Table 21.4	UKMEC categories where risks may outweigh benefits or pose an unacceptable health risk for use of IUC		
UKMEC category 3 (risks outweigh benefits)	**UKMEC category 4 (unacceptable risk)**	**Where Cu-IUD and LNG-IUS are given different UKMEC categories**	
Between 48 h and <4 weeks postpartum	Postpartum sepsis	A UKMEC category 1 is given for a Cu-IUD and a category 3 is given for the LNG-IUS due to the progestogen content for the following medical conditions: • *continuation* of LNG-IUS if a new diagnosis of ischaemic heart disease or stroke is made • having a LNG-IUS if there is a past history of breast cancer • severe decompensated cirrhosis • hepatocellular adenoma • malignant hepatocellular carcinoma	
Initiation following a complicated organ transplant: graft failure (acute/chronic), rejection, cardiac allograft vasculopathy	Post-abortion sepsis	A UKMEC category 1 is given for a Cu-IUD and category 4 is given for the LNG-IUS due to the progestogen content for the following medical conditions: • current breast cancer	
Initiation in long QT syndrome	*Initiation* of the method in women with unexplained vaginal bleeding		
Initiation in women with HIV whose CD4 is <200	Gestational trophoblastic neoplasia when serum human chorionic gonadotrophin (hCG) concentration persistently elevated or malignant disease		
Gestational trophoblastic neoplasia when serum hCG concentrations are decreasing	Initiation of the method in women with cervical cancer awaiting treatment or in women with current endometrial cancer		
Initiation in women with radical trachelectomy	Initiation of intrauterine methods in women with current PID or purulent cervicitis or gonorrhea		
Uterine fibroids or uterine anatomical abnormalities distorting the uterine cavity	Initiation in women with symptomatic chlamydia infection		
Initiation in women with asymptomatic chlamydia infection	Initiation of intrauterine methods in women with known pelvic tuberculosis		
Continuation of intrauterine methods in women with known pelvic tuberculosis			

Note: Liver enzyme-inducing drugs are not thought to reduce the contraceptive efficacy of a Cu-IUD or the LNG-IUS.
https://www.fsrh.org/standards-and-guidance/external/ukmec-2016-digital-version/

Pelvic infection

There is an increased risk of pelvic infection in the 20 days following insertion of IUC; after this, however, the risk is the same as for the non-IUC-using population. The risk of acquiring pelvic inflammatory disease (PID) is related to the insertion procedure and background risk of STIs. A relevant history (including sexual history) should be taken to identify those at higher risk of STIs. Women aged <25 years, or 25 and over with a new sexual partner or more than one partner in the last year, or those with a regular partner who has other partners are at a higher risk of STIs. For these women (or for women who request STI testing), a self-administered low vaginal swab dual test for *Chlamydia trachomatis* and the gonococcus should be taken in advance of insertion. If results are unavailable before insertion, prophylactic antibiotics should be considered for the higher risk group (at least to cover *C. trachomatis*).

Pregnancy

An IUC-failure pregnancy is rare but, if it occurs, the chance of having an ectopic pregnancy is higher than in those without a device (Table 21.5). The overall risk of ectopic pregnancy is reduced with the use of an IUC when compared with using no contraception. If the pregnancy is intrauterine, there is an increase in the risk of spontaneous miscarriage and pre-term labour (Fig. 21.3). Removal of the IUC reduces these risks and should be carried out as soon as is practical, ideally before 12 weeks' gestation, provided the threads are easily seen. If they are not present, no attempt at retrieval should be made (Table 21.5).

Barrier methods

Barrier methods of contraception aim to prevent sperm gaining access to the female upper reproductive tract. Barrier

Table 21.5	Managing common problems associated with IUC
Problems associated with IUC	**Management**
Suspected perforation at the time of insertion	The procedure should be stopped and vital signs (blood pressure and pulse rate) and level of discomfort monitored until stable
	An ultrasound scan and/or plain abdominal X-ray to locate the device if it has been left in situ should be arranged as soon as possible
'Lost threads'	Advise women to use another method (condoms or abstinence) until medical review
	Consider the need for emergency hormonal contraception
	If no threads are seen and uterine placement of the intrauterine method cannot be confirmed clinically, an ultrasound scan should be arranged to locate the device and alternative contraception recommended until this information is available
	If an ultrasound scan cannot locate the intrauterine method and there is no definite evidence of expulsion, a plain abdominal X-ray should be arranged to identify an extrauterine device
	If the intrauterine method is not confirmed on an ultrasound scan, clinicians should not assume it has been expelled until a negative X-ray is obtained (unless the woman has witnessed expulsion)
	Hysteroscopy is not readily available in all settings but can be useful if the ultrasound scan is equivocal. Surgical retrieval of an extrauterine device is advised
Abnormal bleeding	Gynaecological pathology and infections should be excluded if abnormal bleeding persists beyond the first 6 months following insertion of IUC. Women using the LNG-IUS who present with a change in pattern of bleeding should be advised to return for further investigation to exclude infections, pregnancy and gynaecological pathology
	For women using a Cu-IUD, non-steroidal anti-inflammatory drugs can be used to treat spotting, light bleeding, or heavy or prolonged menstruation. In addition, antifibrinolytics (such as tranexamic acid) may be used for heavy or prolonged menstruation
Pregnancy	Most pregnancies in women using IUC will be intrauterine, but an ectopic pregnancy must be excluded
	Women who become pregnant with an intrauterine contraceptive in situ should be informed of the increased risks of second-trimester miscarriage, pre-term delivery and infection if the intrauterine method is left in situ. Removal would reduce adverse outcomes but is associated with a small risk of miscarriage
	If the threads are visible, or can easily be retrieved from the endocervical canal, the intrauterine contraceptive should be removed up to 12 weeks' gestation
	If there is no evidence that the intrauterine method was expelled prior to pregnancy, it should be sought at delivery or termination and, if not identified, a plain abdominal X-ray should be arranged to determine if the intrauterine method is retained
Suspected pelvic infection	For women using IUC with symptoms and signs suggestive of pelvic infection, appropriate antibiotics should be started. There is no need to remove the intrauterine method unless symptoms fail to resolve within the following 72 h or unless the woman wishes removal
	All women with confirmed or suspected PID should be followed up to ensure: resolution of symptoms and signs, their partner has also been treated when appropriate, completion of the course of antibiotics, STI risk assessment, counselling regarding safer sex and partner notification
Presence of Actinomyces-like organisms (ALOs)	IUC users with ALOs detected on a swab who have no symptoms should be advised there is no reason to remove the intrauterine method unless signs or symptoms of infection occur. There is no indication for follow-up screening. If symptoms of pelvic pain occur, women should be advised to seek medical advice. Other causes of infection (in particular, STIs) should be considered and it may be appropriate to remove the intrauterine method

methods offer advantages in terms of safety and reversibility, but their efficacy is critically dependent upon consistency and quality of use. The failure rates can be low when they are used correctly by well-motivated couples.

Male and female condoms

Used consistently and correctly, male condoms are up to 98% effective at preventing pregnancy and female condoms are up to 95% effective. Failure rates with 'real life' use can be much higher at 18%, and often failures are not recognized at the time. In general, evidence supports the use of condoms to reduce the risk of STI transmission but, even with correct and consistent use, transmission may occur. The consistent and correct use of male and female condoms is recommended to reduce the risk of transmission of genital human papillomavirus.

Men and women with latex sensitivity or allergy can use polyurethane or deproteinized latex condoms. Condom users should be made aware of the risk of pregnancy, emergency contraceptive use and risk of STIs should a condom fail.

Condoms lubricated with non-spermicidal lubricant are recommended for use. Non-oil-based lubricants are recommended, as they can be used safely with latex and non-latex condoms. The female condom is a polyurethane

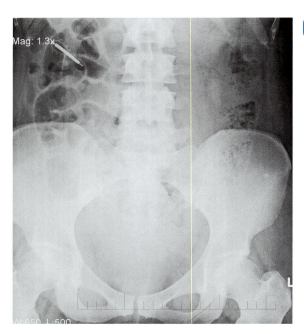

Fig. 21.2 The IUD has perforated the uterus and attached itself to the omentum.

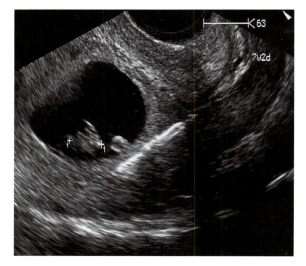

Fig. 21.3 Ultrasound scan of a 7-week fetus with an IUD visible low in the uterine cavity.

sheath, its open end attached to a flexible polyurethane ring, which sits at the vaginal entrance, and is available in one size.

Female diaphragms and caps

When used consistently, correctly and with spermicide, diaphragms and cervical caps are estimated to be between 92% and 96% effective at preventing pregnancy. These methods require a relatively high degree of user motivation,

---

Box 21.1

Instructions for women using a diaphragm or cervical cap

- Initial assessment of diaphragm and cervical caps should be done by a suitably trained healthcare professional
  - Before the woman relies on the method for contraception she should be asked to return to wearing the diaphragm/cap
- All methods can be inserted any time before intercourse
- The use of spermicide is recommended when using diaphragms and cervical caps
- If intercourse is repeated or occurs ≥3 h after insertion, more spermicide is required and should be inserted with an applicator or as a pessary without removing the diaphragm or cervical cap
- The diaphragm or cervical cap must be left in situ for at least 6 h after the last episode of intercourse. Sperm in the lower reproductive tract are unlikely to be alive after 6 h
- Oil-based lubricants can damage latex, and women should be advised to avoid use when using latex diaphragms or cervical caps
  - Water- or silicone-based lubricants are recommended when using latex condoms
- Women should be advised to check the diaphragm or cervical cap regularly for tears, holes or cracks
- There is no evidence that a colour change or change in shape of the outer ring of a diaphragm reduces efficacy
- Women should be advised on the use of EC should female barrier methods be used incorrectly
- Women should be advised to attend for a review of contraception if they have
  - any problems with the method
  - had a pregnancy

---

and failure rates are comparable with those observed with the male condom. There is the diaphragm and a cervical cap. The diaphragm is a soft dome, the edge of which contains a supporting metal spring to exert a slight pressure on the vaginal walls. It is inserted to lie diagonally across the vagina between the back of the symphysis pubis and the posterior fornix. Diaphragms are available in different diameters ranging from 55 to 5 mm, in 5 mm increments. It is important that the diaphragm covers the cervix after fitting and a vaginal examination by a competent healthcare professional is essential to ensure the correct diaphragm size is used. However, women may purchase a silicon diaphragm in a single size designed to fit most women (approximately 80%) where no fitting is required by a healthcare professional. Cervical caps depend on suction to hold the cap over the cervix and only one type is currently available in the UK and it also does not require a healthcare professional for fitting.

There is limited evidence on the use of diaphragms and cervical caps for reducing the risk of STIs or the development of cervical intraepithelial neoplasia. Women with sensitivity to latex proteins can use silicone diaphragms or cervical caps. For women with a history of toxic shock syndrome, the use of diaphragms and cervical caps is not recommended. Guidance on the correct use of diaphragms and caps is outlined in Box 21.1. It is usually recommended that diaphragms and caps are used with a spermicide. The use of spermicide alone is not considered to provide effective contraception. Nonoxinol-9 (N-9) is the main spermicide commercially available in the UK. N-9 is a surfactant, which disrupts cell membranes. Epithelial disruption in the vagina and rectum has been identified in association with N-9 use in human and animal models. Repeated and high-dose use of N-9 is associated with an increased risk of genital lesions, which may increase the risk of human immunodeficiency virus (HIV) acquisition, and the WHO recommends that women at high risk of HIV infection should not use N-9. The risks of using a diaphragm or cervical cap (with N-9) in women with a high risk of HIV or those with HIV or acquired immune deficiency syndrome generally outweigh the benefits (UKMEC 3).

Natural family planning

Women who choose to use fertility-awareness methods should be made aware of the different fertility indicators and the failure rate of different combinations in order to decide on the most appropriate method for them. The use of single fertility indicators is not recommended, as the typical pregnancy rate at 1 year is approximately 24%. Combining fertility indicators is considered more effective than using single fertility indicators alone. The symptothermal method (uses a combination of monitoring cervical secretions and basal body temperature with a calendar calculation to identify the fertile window) has been shown to be an effective method of contraception when used consistently and correctly, with fewer than 1 in 100 women expected to experience a pregnancy with perfect use of the method over 1 year. There are several commercially available fertility-monitoring devices that are designed to identify the period of fertility, usually by measuring urinary LH. However, because these methods are primarily designed to identify the most fertile window, they may underestimate the time of risk for women who do not wish to become pregnant. There are also fertility-awareness applications for mobile phones that require women to enter information such as body temperatures, ovulation test results and date of menstruation prior to informing them of their fertile period that month. More rigorous research is required before conclusions can be drawn regarding the effectiveness of these devices and applications.

The LAM can provide very effective contraception (98%) if the woman is fully breastfeeding (day and night on demand) with no supplementary feeds, she is less than 6 months postpartum and she is amenorrhoeic. Women using LAM should be advised that the risk of pregnancy is increased if the frequency of breastfeeding decreases (stopping night feeds, supplementary feeding, use of pacifiers/dummies), when their period returns or when >6 months postpartum. They should be supported to commence another method of contraception ideally prior to this occurring (Fig. 21.4).

Emergency contraception

EC can be used:

- after unprotected sexual intercourse (UPSI)
- after 'accidents' with a barrier method (e.g. burst condom or diaphragm removed too early)
- if pills are missed, injectable methods are late or an intrauterine method is expelled.

It can be difficult to accurately assess an individual woman's risk of pregnancy. A woman who has a single act of UPSI mid-cycle has an approximately 20–30% chance of pregnancy. The risk reduces to 2–3% before day 10 and after day 17 (in a regular 28-day cycle). Other factors have an effect on pregnancy risk, such as the age of the woman. Three methods of EC are currently available; the Cu-IUD, oral levonorgestrel emergency contraception (LNG-EC) and oral ulipristal acetate emergency contraception (UPA-EC).

The most effective emergency method of contraception is the Cu-IUD and all women should be offered this option. Unlike the Cu-IUD, oral EC does not provide contraception for the remainder of the cycle and effective contraception or abstinence is advised after it is taken. The Cu-IUD is the only method of EC that is known to be effective after ovulation has occurred. Women who experience vomiting within 3 h of administration of the oral methods (LNG-EC and UPA-EC) will require a repeat dose or may wish to consider a Cu-IUD.

The Cu-IUD

EC providers should be aware that a Cu-IUD can be inserted up to 5 days after the first UPSI in a natural menstrual cycle, or up to 5 days after the earliest likely date of ovulation, i.e. up to day 19 in a woman with a regular 28-day cycle. Almost 99% of expected pregnancies can be prevented. It is for this reason that women of any age may opt for this method of EC. The copper is immediately toxic to ovum and sperm, thus making it effective immediately after insertion. The LNG-IUS is not effective as EC and should not be used for this indication.

Ulipristal acetate

The progesterone receptor modulator UPA (30 mg) is licensed to be used up to 5 days (120 h) after UPSI. The primary mode of action of UPA is to inhibit or delay ovulation. UPA-EC is significantly more effective than LNG-EC at preventing pregnancy when taken up to 5 days after UPSI. This is likely to be due to UPA-EC's ability to delay ovulation even after the start of the LH surge, a time when LNG-EC is no longer effective. Therefore, UPA-EC should be the first-line oral EC for a woman who has had UPSI within the last 5 days, if the UPSI is likely to have taken place during the 5 days prior to the estimated day of ovulation. Studies estimate that UPA-EC can reduce the risk of pregnancy by 60–80%.

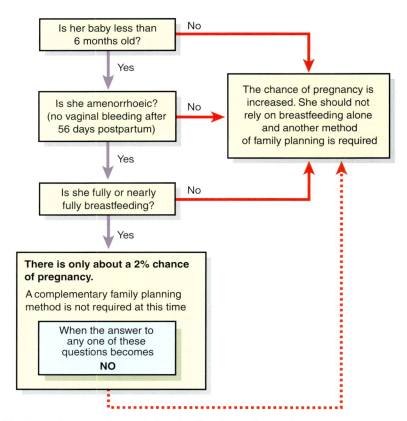

Fig. 21.4 **Use of lactational amenorrhoea during the first 6 months postpartum.**

Use of UPA can cause delay in the onset of menstruation and menstrual irregularities (similar to LNG-EC). For women using a liver enzyme-inducing drug, UPA is not recommended. Use of UPA is not recommended for women with severe asthma controlled by oral glucocorticoids. Women who are currently breastfeeding should be advised to express and discard breastmilk for 1 week after they have taken UPA-EC.

Following UPA administration, women should be advised to wait 5 days before starting suitable hormonal contraception. This is because hormonal contraception may reduce the efficacy of the UPA-EC. Women should be made aware that they must use condoms reliably or abstain from sex during this 5 days and then until their contraceptive method is effective again (e.g. 2 days for POP and 7 days for other hormonal methods).

If a woman has already taken UPA-EC in a cycle, UPA-EC can be offered again after further UPSI in the same cycle, provided ovulation has not occurred. Evidence suggests that UPA-EC does not disrupt an existing pregnancy and is not associated with fetal abnormality.

Levonorgestrel emergency contraception

LNG-EC is effective up until 72 h after UPSI. The 1.5 mg tablet inhibits ovulation, delaying or preventing follicular rupture and causing luteal dysfunction. If taken prior to the start of the LH surge, LNG-EC inhibits ovulation; however, in the late follicular phase and once ovulation has occurred, LNG-EC becomes ineffective. If taken within 72 h of a single episode of UPSI, LNG-EC is thought to prevent between 60% and 80% of expected pregnancies. For women using liver enzyme-inducing drugs, a single 3 mg tablet of LNG can be considered, but women should be informed that the effectiveness of this approach is unknown.

After taking LNG-EC, women can start hormonal contraception immediately. Women should be made aware that they must use condoms reliably or abstain from sex until their chosen method of contraception becomes effective (2 days for POP and 7 days for other hormonal methods). If a woman has already taken LNG-EC in a cycle, LNG-EC can be used again after further UPSI, provided ovulation has not occurred

Sterilization

Counselling and advice on sterilization procedures should be provided to women and men within the context of a service providing a full range of information and access to other methods of contraception. This should include information on the advantages and disadvantages and relative failure rates. Failures can occur with all methods of sterilization and a pregnancy can occur several years after the procedure. Women should be informed that other female methods of contraception such as IUD and subdermal implants are as, if not more, effective than sterilization and may confer non-contraceptive benefits. Men and women seeking sterilization counselling should be informed of the different methods of sterilization available including laparoscopic tubal occlusion, hysteroscopic tubal occlusion and vasectomy.

Female sterilization

Laparoscopic sterilization is still the most common method of female sterilization in the UK and is usually achieved with a titanium clip, under general anaesthesia. All women must be informed of the risks of laparoscopy, including those of visceral and vascular injury necessitating additional surgery. The lifetime risk of failure is estimated to be 1 in 200 for laparoscopic sterilization. Laparoscopic sterilization is intended to be permanent, however it may be reversed, but this has variable success rates and women should be informed of this. Sterilization involving ligation of the fallopian tubes can be performed at the time of caesarean section, but only if there has been appropriate pre-procedure counselling.

Hysteroscopic female sterilization involves tubal cannulation and occlusion of the fallopian tubes from within the uterine cavity using flexible micro-inserts. The micro-inserts cause fibrosis, resulting in the permanent occlusion of each tube after approximately 3 months. The procedure is designed to be performed under local anaesthetic. Women should be informed that hysteroscopic sterilization is irreversible, that hysteroscopic access or micro-insert placement may be unsuccessful in 4% of women, and that contraception must be continued for at least 3 months until tubal occlusion is confirmed. Hysteroscopic tubal occlusion has a similar failure rate to laparoscopic tubal occlusion. Tubal occlusion can be confirmed by transvaginal scan or hysterosalpingography.

Compared with women using no method of contraception, the overall risk of ectopic pregnancy is not increased after sterilization; however, women should be informed that, if pregnancy occurs, the resulting pregnancy may be ectopic (because tubal anatomy is distorted).

There is no causal effect between female sterilization and the development of heavy menstrual bleeding. However, whilst there is evidence to suggest an association between tubal occlusion and undergoing a subsequent hysterectomy, there is no evidence of causation.

Vasectomy

Vasectomy is ligation of the vasa deferentia for the purpose of excluding spermatozoa from the ejaculate. The procedure is usually performed under local anaesthesia. Vasectomy is intended to be permanent, but men should be given

information on the success rates associated with reversal. Following vasectomy, an effective contraceptive must be used until azoospermia has been confirmed by semen analysis. It can take up to 20 ejaculations to clear any sperm ahead of the now blocked vasa deferentia. Twelve weeks' post-vasectomy is the optimal timing to schedule the first post-vasectomy semen analysis.

There is no increase in the risk of testicular cancer or heart disease associated with vasectomy. The association, in some reports, of an increased risk of being diagnosed with prostate cancer is currently considered not to be causal. Men should be informed about the possibility of chronic testicular pain after vasectomy. Serum testosterone concentrations, libido, and the colour, consistency and volume of the ejaculate are unaffected by undergoing a vasectomy. Vasectomy is highly reliable, with a failure rate of 1 in 2000.

Key points

- Medical eligibility criteria can be used to ensure the safe provision of contraception to women and men without imposing unnecessary medical restrictions.
- Efficacy of contraception is measured by failure rate expressed as pregnancies per HWY.
- Consistent and correct use of contraception is important to maintain efficacy. Methods that reduce the risk of user failure, such as long-acting methods (implant, injectable and intrauterine methods), are more effective than methods that rely on user input (pill taking or patch use).
- The combined hormonal methods (pill, patch, vaginal ring) contain oestrogen and a progestogen. These methods may be unsuitable for some women, such as those with significant cardiovascular disease (e.g. myocardial infarction, stroke, hypertension, VTE), smokers aged ≥35 years, women with migraine with aura and women with breast cancer.
- Progestogen-only contraception consists of pills, injections, implants and the LNG-IUS. They are useful for women with contraindications to oestrogen use and can be used as a first-choice contraceptive.
- The LARC methods, which include intrauterine methods and subdermal implants, can be used by women of any age. They are the most cost-effective contraceptive options with high levels of satisfaction and low discontinuation rates.
- Barrier methods are less effective than other methods. Male and female condoms will provide some protection against STIs.
- EC can reduce the risk of unplanned pregnancy following UPSI or contraceptive method failure.
- Male and female sterilization provide effective permanent contraception. Vasectomy has lower failure rates than female sterilization and can be performed without general anaesthesia. Newer hysteroscopic female sterilization methods offer a technique that avoids the risks associated with laparoscopy and can be performed under local anaesthesia

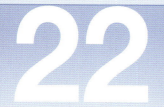

Antenatal and postnatal care

The aim of antenatal care

The aim of antenatal care is to maximize the chance of a positive outcome from a pregnancy: a healthy mother and a healthy baby or babies.

High-quality antenatal care includes regular contact between a pregnant woman and a suitably educated healthcare professional or group of healthcare professionals. At these contacts, risks, complications and emerging problems will be screened for and identified. Where any problems are identified, an appropriate care plan will be implemented to minimize the negative impact on the health and well-being of the mother and infant. High-quality antenatal care will also focus on the promotion of positive health and well-being, using the opportunities provided by regular contact to promote positive health behaviours and provide education and guidance.

Models of antenatal care

Models of antenatal care, and maternity care more generally, vary widely across the world (Fig. 22.1). The model of maternity care is determined by a range of factors including history and tradition, resource level and organization of care. The model of antenatal care includes how often the care is given, who provides the care and where the care is located.

In middle- and high-income countries, the pattern of antenatal appointments is generally around ten appointments for a woman in her first pregnancy and seven for a woman in a subsequent pregnancy. In low-income countries the number of contacts is often much lower.

The providers of antenatal care also vary considerably between countries. In the UK, the great majority of antenatal care is provided by registered midwives working for the state-funded National Health Service (NHS). Healthy women without any significant risk factors or obstetric problems may receive all of their care from midwives. Women with risk factors, health problems, obstetric problems or poor obstetric history will also receive some of their antenatal care from other members of the multidisciplinary maternity team, including obstetricians. Continuity of carer during the antenatal period, that is, when the woman has the majority of her antenatal care by the same person or a small group of healthcare professionals, is associated with improved outcome and satisfaction.

The first trimester

The first contact between a healthcare professional and a pregnant woman occurs after the confirmation of pregnancy. This first contact may take place as early as 6 weeks. In the UK, the great majority of women will have their first 'booking' appointment with their midwife by 10 weeks' gestation.

The aims of this first appointment are to identify risks, screen for abnormalities or illness, develop a rapport and encourage future attendance by ensuring the woman has a positive first experience of maternity care and provide key health-promotion messages.

The first appointment is an opportunity to gain initial observations of the mother, which enable care planning and identification of any later deterioration. The healthcare professional is also able to establish the likely gestation of the pregnancy through establishment of the first day of the last menstrual period and abdominal examination.

There are a range of risk factors that increase the probability that problems or complications may emerge for the mother or fetus in pregnancy, during labour and childbirth, or postnatally. Being under 18 or over 40 years of age represents increased probability of developing some problems during pregnancy, as is having had more than six previous births or having a first pregnancy.

Women may have conditions for which they take medication. The healthcare professional should identify what medication is currently being taken and seek advice on the risks and benefits of the medication in pregnancy and of discontinuing the medication in pregnancy. Risk factors should be recorded and be taken into account when planning care (Table 22.1).

If risk factors are identified, the healthcare professional should follow local referral pathways to ensure that women receive the appropriate surveillance, treatment, advice or support to reduce the impact of the risks identified.

Some family history and previous personal history risks will require additional screening appointments and multidisciplinary care planning: a personal history of postpartum psychosis has a recurrence risk of 1 in 2 to 4 (background risk of 1 in 500); a family history of blood disorders will require relevant counselling and screening. Medical conditions such as diabetes, thyroid conditions and epilepsy will require

multidisciplinary care planning and monitoring throughout the pregnancy. Previous obstetric complications or interventions, such as previous caesarean section, require discussion of choices relating to delivery.

Identifying lifestyle risks may prompt referral for smoking cessation support or dietetic support to promote healthy eating. Identifying mental health risks, such as a personal history of bipolar disorder, will require liaison with mental health services to ensure a coordinated plan of care is in place during pregnancy and immediately after birth. Social difficulties will require liaison with local social care or voluntary sector organizations.

At the first antenatal appointment, the healthcare professional will undertake a general physical examination including calculation of the woman's body mass index (BMI), blood pressure measurement and heart rate. In areas with a high incidence of heart and respiratory conditions, auscultation of heart and lung sounds is recommended. An abdominal examination will be undertaken to identify the uterine size and any abnormal masses or surgical scars.

Urinalysis should be undertaken for the presence of protein and glucose; proteinuria prompts testing for urinary tract infection, persistent glycosuria prompts testing for hyperglycaemia.

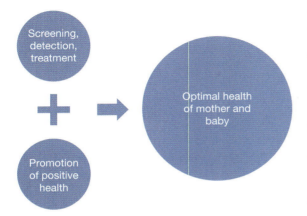

Fig. 22.1 The dual purpose of antenatal care

Table 22.1	Risk factors to be identified at first appointment, through discussion with mother and reference to previous medical or obstetric notes		
Personal history and current health	**Family history**	**Obstetric history previous pregnancies**	**Current pregnancy**
History of subfertility and fertility treatment	Pregnancy related – first-degree relative with a congenital abnormality or genetic abnormality, pre-eclampsia, venous thrombosis	Miscarriage at >14 weeks, stillbirth or neonatal death	Hyperemesis
Medical condition including diabetes, thyroid problems, epilepsy, asthma, heart disease, hypertension, renal disease, cancer	Medical conditions – diabetes, heart disease, inherited conditions, e.g. sickle cell anaemia, cystic fibrosis	Recurrent miscarriage (three consecutive first-trimester losses)	Vaginal bleeding
Surgical history – gynaecological procedures, treatment to the cervix, breast surgery, abdominal surgery	Mental health – first-degree relative with postpartum psychosis, schizophrenia, bipolar disorder, severe postnatal depression or depression	Premature birth or small for gestational age infant	Abdominal pain
Raised BMI or very low BMI		Pregnancy-related hypertension, gestational diabetes, rhesus isoimmunization, antepartum haemorrhage	Findings from pregnancy ultrasound
Mental health – bipolar disorder, postpartum psychosis, schizophrenia, depression, postnatal depression, anxiety disorders, eating disorders		Induction of labour – indication	
Lifestyle – smoking, non-prescription and prescription drug use		Operative birth (caesarean section or instrumental delivery), shoulder dystocia, breech birth	
Social difficulties – domestic abuse, financial difficulties, previous child-protection concerns		Postpartum haemorrhage, retained placenta, OASI	

Further screening should be offered:

- full blood count to screen for maternal anaemia and thrombocytopenia
- blood group to determine the ABO and rhesus status of the mother and to identify any red cell antibodies
- rubella status has traditionally been determined in order to identify those mothers who are not immune, but since 2016 this has been discontinued as part of normal care in the UK due to the high population coverage provided by the measles-mumps-rubella vaccine
- haemoglobin (Hb) electrophoresis to screen for conditions such as thalassaemia and sickle cell anaemia
- hepatitis B status
- syphilis
- human immunodeficiency virus (see p. 166).

A clear process should be in place and shared with the woman about how and when she will receive test results following this first appointment.

Many women experience some discomfort or symptoms that may cause them to be concerned during the early stages of pregnancy. These include nausea and vomiting ('morning sickness'), some lower abdominal discomfort, frequency of micturition, vaginal 'spotting' (small amounts of bleeding per vagina) and breast tingling or discomfort.

The healthcare professional should ask women about symptoms to identify when normal and transient discomforts appear to be more serious.

Discussion about a woman's options for screening for chromosomal and structural fetal abnormalities should be undertaken at this first appointment. Screening approaches vary in different countries but are likely to include blood tests often combined with ultrasound scans, such as screening for Down syndrome with nuchal translucency testing between 11 and 14 weeks, and the routinely offered fetal anomaly scan between 18 and 22 weeks. Women should be advised that initial screening for Down syndrome will not provide them with a conclusive diagnostic answer about the presence or absence of an abnormality, but will present them with a risk factor, enabling them to make a further decision about diagnostic testing (chorionic villus sampling or amniocentesis).

Some women will choose not to undergo screening for fetal abnormality as they would choose not to terminate a pregnancy if an abnormality were found and do not feel they would benefit from knowing about any conditions prior to the birth. Other women may choose to have screening as they may wish to make a decision not to continue with a pregnancy if an abnormality is found or they may wish to have time to prepare for a baby with additional needs.

For a significant proportion of women, pregnancy is the first time that they have regular contact with health services. It is important to ensure that this contact is as positive as possible to ensure that women feel motivated to return for regular appointments and are confident to seek help should any problems arise.

All healthcare professionals undertaking this first appointment should treat the woman with respect:

- introduce yourself by role and name, and ask the woman what she prefers to be called
- call the woman by this name
- ensure that the woman's conversation with you is private and cannot be overheard by other women attending for care
- provide enough time to complete the appointment adequately
- explain the purpose of the appointment and the questions being posed
- ensure that the woman is able to communicate effectively with the healthcare professional. Provide an interpreter where required
- offer the woman evidence-based information to assist her in coming to an informed choice on care options or screening
- ask for verbal consent before undertaking any physical examination or taking a blood sample
- offer the woman, and her partner (if present), the opportunity to ask any questions they have regarding the pregnancy, any problems or the care planned
- explain the plan of care for the remainder of her pregnancy and the importance of attending regularly for antenatal care to monitor her and the baby's health and well-being.

Where a woman is helped to feel relaxed and comfortable during this first appointment she will be more likely to share concerns with her healthcare professional and to attend future appointments.

Motivational interviewing or brief intervention approaches can be helpful in exploring a woman's readiness to make positive health behaviour changes such as giving up smoking, drinking alcohol or using drugs; eating healthily and being more physically active. The healthcare professional can best support women to make positive changes through providing clear information about the impact of particular behaviours on maternal and fetal health, while remaining non-judgemental in approach.

Smoking, alcohol and drug use

The healthcare professional should advise all women that it is best not to smoke, drink any alcohol or take illegal drugs during pregnancy. Smoking in pregnancy is linked to miscarriage, premature birth, small for gestational age babies, stillbirth, sudden unexpected death in infancy (SUDI) and increased hospital admissions in the first year of a baby's life. Alcohol, including 'binge drinking', is related to a spectrum of potential problems categorized as fetal alcohol spectrum disorder (FASD). It is estimated that as many as 1 in a 100 babies are born with effects from alcohol. FASD has a lifelong impact on the affected person, including learning and behavioural difficulties. Illegal substances increase the risk of fetal abnormalities, premature birth, small for gestational age babies and neonatal abstinence syndrome.

Diet

Where relevant, the healthcare professional can provide helpful information about a healthy diet during pregnancy, including eating plenty of fruit and vegetables, good food hygiene and foods to avoid. Vitamin and mineral supplements are a helpful addition to a balanced diet for pregnant women. In the UK, it is recommended that all women take 400 mcg folic acid supplements for the first 12 weeks of pregnancy to reduce the risk of neural tube defects; 5 mcg daily vitamin D supplements are also recommended for all pregnant women. Women should be informed to avoid vitamin A supplements, as they may be teratogenic.

Physical activity and exercise

It is beneficial for women to be physically active during pregnancy. Advice about physical activity in pregnancy is the same as for all adults in the UK, i.e. five periods of moderate physical activity for around 30 min each week. Moderate physical activity includes walking, swimming, gardening, yoga. Physical activity and exercise is helpful in maintaining and improving physical and mental health in pregnancy and may help to relieve some of the discomforts of pregnancy.

The second trimester (12–20 weeks)

Antenatal care during the second trimester includes follow-up of results from initial blood tests, fetal anomaly screening at 18–22 weeks and instigating any treatment or further surveillance indicated by these results.

At each antenatal appointment throughout the second trimester the following should be assessed and recorded:

- maternal blood pressure
- maternal urinalysis
- enquiry about any pain or vaginal loss
- auscultation of the fetal heart from 18 weeks.

The healthcare professional should enquire about the woman's well-being, both physical and emotional, at each appointment. Many women experience symptoms that cause them discomfort or concern during pregnancy. Through discussing the impact of symptoms on a woman's life, the healthcare professional can identify when any problems are of concern and require further investigation and possible follow-up (Table 22.2).

Social and environmental factors

Healthcare professionals should ensure that, on at least one occasion during the pregnancy, they have some time alone with a woman in order to enquire about the woman's

Table 22.2	Common problems or 'minor disorders' of pregnancy
Condition	**Advice, possible treatment**
Nausea and vomiting	Investigate severity through history-taking – if more than occasional, monitor weight, dehydration (urinalysis), consider hospitalization; exclude urinary infection as cause; eat little and often. Antiemetics can be safely prescribed.
Heartburn	Antacids; monitoring of diet to identify which foods worsen or improve symptoms; eat little and often. If persistent and not relieved by common treatments, consider treatment with H_2 antagonists.
Haemorrhoids	Over-the-counter treatments; need to avoid constipation through remaining well hydrated and eating plenty of fruit and vegetables.
Constipation	Over-the-counter treatments; need to avoid constipation through remaining well hydrated and eating plenty of fruit and vegetables; increase fibre in diet.
Pelvic girdle pain, sciatica, back pain	Avoid over abduction of hips; refer for physiotherapy – use of prescribed exercises to relieve pain, improve mobility and strengthen muscles; in more severe cases may require walking aids.
Anaemia	Usually iron deficiency, so prescribe an iron supplement; improve intake of iron rich foods and monitor improvement.
Carpal tunnel syndrome	Monitor severity; exclude pre-eclampsia; refer for physiotherapy; wrist splints may be helpful.
Bleeding gums	Gingivitis or gum disease is more common due to hormonal changes in pregnancy. Careful oral hygiene and dental check up recommended.
Fatigue	Fatigue is common in pregnancy, particularly the first trimester. Screen for anaemia; encourage physical activity to improve sleep quality.
Itching	Itching is quite common in pregnancy due to hormonal changes and stretching of the skin. However, severe itching, particularly after 30 weeks, can indicate obstetric cholestasis, which requires confirmation by biochemical testing.
Rashes	• Polymorphic eruption of pregnancy (1 : 240 pregnancies); presents with abdominal urticaria and vesicles (with no bullae), rarely occurs in the periumbilical area, sometimes extends to the proximal limbs. Treat with antihistamines and topical steroids. • Pemphigoid gestationis (1 : 10 000 pregnancies); pruritic erythematous papules, plaques and wheals spreading from the periumbilical area to the breasts, thighs and palms associated with fetal compromise. Treat with antihistamines, topical steroids and systemic steroids.
Vaginal discharge	A heavier discharge is normal during pregnancy. However, if the discharge is malodorous or accompanied by itching, a vaginal swab for culture is appropriate.

home situation and whether she is experiencing domestic violence or abuse. Research suggests that violence against women in their own homes can begin or escalate in pregnancy. If a woman discloses violence or abuse, the healthcare professional should offer the woman support and appropriate onward referral.

Healthcare professionals have a responsibility to consider the welfare of the woman, her new baby and any other children in the family, by considering issues of concern in the woman's life. These issues include domestic abuse, substance misuse, involvement with the judicial system, homelessness and poverty. Healthcare professionals should talk to the woman about the need to make referral for social support through social services and/or voluntary sector organizations. Healthcare professionals should familiarize themselves with their local safeguarding and child-protection procedures.

The third trimester (20 weeks–term)

All of the aforementioned physical examinations should continue at each antenatal contact through the third trimester of pregnancy and be clearly recorded in her maternity records. In addition, the healthcare professional will undertake the following at each antenatal contact:

Abdominal examination

This examination will include inspection, palpation and auscultation of the fetal heart using a Pinard stethoscope or hand-held Doppler device. If the fetal heart cannot be heard in this way, an ultrasound scan should be undertaken to assess fetal well-being.

Presentation

Examination and palpation of the uterus will identify the presentation, position and descent of the fetus into the pelvis. Further information about malpresentations can be found in Chapter 33, page 312.

Evaluation of fetal growth

At each appointment from 24 weeks onwards the healthcare professional should measure from the symphysis pubis to the fundus of the uterus and plot the measurement (symphysis-fundal height [SFH]) on a size chart. Where the SFH measurement falls outwith the normal range or is static over a few weeks, then an ultrasound examination should be offered (Chapter 26).

Enquiry about fetal movements

Each woman should be encouraged at each appointment to become familiar with the individual pattern of their baby's movements. Movements will generally increase in frequency and strength until 32 weeks and then are likely to remain relatively stable until the birth. There should not be a reduction in movements closer to the birth, though the size of the movements may change. Women should be advised that the baby's movements are a sign of the baby's well-being. If they become aware of any reduction in the baby's normal pattern of movements, they should lie down for an hour to rest and focus on the baby's movements. If the movements continue to be reduced, they should seek advice from a healthcare professional. Reduced fetal movement can be an indicator of fetal hypoxia and is a risk factor for intrauterine death.

A woman's description of reduced fetal movements is important and should be responded to by a face-to-face consultation with fetal heart rate monitoring by cardiotocography (CTG) and the selective use of ultrasound.

Polyhydramnios (increased amniotic fluid volume)

Palpation and measurement may identify polyhydramnios. Where polyhydramnios is suspected during routine antenatal care, the woman should be referred for an ultrasound scan.

Polyhydramnios is diagnosed with ultrasound and may be described by a single pool >8 cm in depth, and/or an amniotic fluid index (AFI) >90th centile for gestational age. The AFI is a measurement of the maximum depth of amniotic fluid in the four quadrants of the uterus.

Polyhydramnios occurs in 0.5–2% of all pregnancies and is associated with maternal diabetes (pre-existing or gestational, ~20%) and congenital fetal anomaly such as oesophageal atresia (~5%).

Polyhydramnios is associated with an increased risk of:

- placental abruption
- malpresentation
- cord prolapse
- a large for gestational age infant (association with diabetes)
- requiring a caesarean section
- postpartum haemorrhage
- premature birth and perinatal death.

When polyhydramnios is confirmed by ultrasound it is necessary to exclude gestational diabetes. It is rarely necessary to aspirate amniotic fluid for maternal comfort, as if amniotic fluid is aspirated, it quickly re-accumulates. Increased antenatal fetal surveillance is important during the remainder of the pregnancy and during labour. Following birth, a paediatrician should examine the baby for congenital anomalies, particularly oesophageal atresia.

Oligohydramnios (reduced amniotic fluid volume)

Abdominal palpation and measurement may suggest oligohydramnios. Oligohydramnios is unlikely to be specifically suspected by clinical palpation but may contribute to a smaller than expected SFH measurement. Where oligohydramnios is suspected, the woman should be referred for ultrasound. Oligohydramnios is diagnosed by ultrasound when the AFI is <5 cm or a single cord-free pool of <2 cm. Oligohydramnios affects 1–3% of pregnancies and is associated with poorer perinatal outcomes. Oligohydramnios usually presents in the third trimester of pregnancy and is associated with prolonged pregnancy, rupture of the membranes, fetal growth restriction and, rarely, fetal renal congenital abnormalities (when oligohydramnios may be present from mid-trimester onwards). Oligohydramnios may indirectly cause fetal hypoxia as a consequence of cord compression.

Identifying other antenatal complications

Regular antenatal contacts facilitate screening for potential or emerging conditions during the third trimester.

Hypertension and pre-eclampsia

At each antenatal contact during the third trimester, blood pressure measurement and urine testing for proteinuria is undertaken. Each appointment will also include enquiry about symptoms that may be indicative of hypertension including headache, visual disturbances, severe upper abdominal quadrant pain and significant facial, hand or ankle oedema (Chapter 36).

Screening for anaemia

Blood should be taken to assess each woman's full blood count in the third trimester to identify anaemia and abnormal platelet numbers. Anaemia in pregnancy is defined as a Hb concentration of less than 105 g/L. As there is a physiological fall in Hb as pregnancy advances, there is often uncertainty about the value of treating mild anaemia (e.g. Hb 90–100 g/L). Iron supplements may lead to gastrointestinal side-effects and have no proven benefits in the absence of demonstrable iron deficiency. Most maternity units will recommend oral iron if the Hb is less than 100 g/L or if the mean corpuscular volume is low (<80 fL), but it is advisable to estimate serum folate, vitamin B_{12} and ferritin before embarking on therapy. Oral iron is well absorbed, and the only indication for parenteral iron is when there are concerns regarding compliance or there are prohibitive side-effects with oral supplements. In addition to screening for anaemia, women are offered further screening for red cell antibodies at 28 weeks.

Impaired glucose tolerance and diabetes

If a woman has risk factors for diabetes or gestational diabetes or is found to have glycosuria during antenatal appointments, a glucose tolerance test should be undertaken (Chapter 23).

Mental health problems

Antenatal care includes screening for pre-existing and emerging mental health problems throughout pregnancy.

Women with pre-existing mental illness should be referred to a mental health team for additional support and care in pregnancy and the postnatal period. The team should advise on the continuance of medication and any contraindicated medications in pregnancy. The risks and benefits of continuing or stopping medications should be weighed up. Women who discontinue medication during pregnancy can be at high risk of relapse in late pregnancy and the postnatal period. Women who have taken mood stabilizers such as lithium and sodium valproate may be at higher risk of fetal abnormalities.

Some women develop mental health problems for the first time in pregnancy including depression, anxiety disorders such as obsessive-compulsive disorder (OCD) and panic attacks. Healthcare professionals should ask women about their emotional well-being at each antenatal contact. Healthcare professionals should ask open questions to encourage women to be honest if they are feeling low or hopeless or very anxious. Mental health problems including depression and anxiety that develop during pregnancy should be monitored and women should be offered additional support. Women with mental health problems during pregnancy are at higher risk of developing significant mental health conditions including postnatal depression. Suicide is one of the leading causes of maternal death in the UK – effective screening and multidisciplinary care is vital to reduce the impact of mental health problems.

Prolonged pregnancy

Prolonged pregnancy is defined as a pregnancy beyond 42 weeks' gestation. By this definition, around 10% of pregnancies are prolonged. The risk of intrauterine death and intrapartum hypoxia increase significantly beyond 42 weeks. To reduce these risks, induction is generally offered between 41 and 42 weeks' gestation. Prior to formal induction of labour, women should be offered a vaginal examination for membrane sweeping.

Some women may not wish to be induced as they are concerned about the medical interventions involved and the resulting restrictions on their choices during labour and birth. From 42 weeks, women who decline induction of labour should be offered increased antenatal monitoring typically consisting of a twice-weekly CTG and the ultrasound estimation of amniotic fluid volume.

Antenatal summary

For healthy women without significant risks or complications, antenatal care is provided by midwives. For women with health problems or increased risk of complications, antenatal care is generally provided by a multidisciplinary team including midwives, general practitioners, obstetricians and other specialists.

Antenatal contacts should be planned to provide women with regular appointments that are accessible to them, as near as possible to where they live. Antenatal care systems should be designed to maximize the opportunity for women to get to know the healthcare professionals caring for them.

All antenatal contacts should aim to identify risks and needs for the woman and the baby through history-taking, physical examination and offering screening tests. Each contact is an opportunity for the healthcare professional to encourage women to ask questions and to provide education and information. Each contact is an opportunity to promote positive physical and mental health. Care should take into account woman's physical, emotional and social context, and should be responsive to changing need.

Postnatal care

The aim of postnatal care is to monitor and promote the health and well-being of the mother and baby during the first 6 weeks after birth

Postnatal care aims to:

- monitor the well-being of the mother and newborn(s)
- identify any emerging problems and initiate appropriate review or treatment if problems are detected
- support parents in the early days of parenting through the provision of advice and guidance.

Models of postnatal care

Approaches to postnatal care vary considerably between different countries. In the UK, the majority of postnatal care is provided by midwives in maternity units and the woman's home for between 10 and 28 days after the birth. Increasingly, the postnatal care of healthy women with healthy newborns when they have returned home is shared with maternity support workers. After 10–28 days, the health visitor takes over as the lead healthcare professional for continuing postnatal care. Obstetricians provide elements of care in the immediate postnatal period, particularly if there have been complications during the birth.

Immediate post-birth care

Immediately following the birth, if the baby does not require resuscitation, the mother and baby should be supported to have uninterrupted 'skin-to-skin' contact. Placing the newborn onto the mother's chest next to her skin supports the physiological transition of the newborn from intrauterine life and provides an important opportunity for 'bonding'.

'Skin-to-skin' contact supports neonatal thermoregulation, respiratory regulation and increases the rate of successful breastfeeding. Babies are often very alert during the first hour after birth. Being held close with the familiar voice of their mother can calm the baby and allows the mother to spend time to get to know and feel close to her baby. Close physical contact with the baby stimulates the production

of the hormone oxytocin, which increases uterine contractions, milk production and a feeling of love and protectiveness towards the baby.

Care should be taken to ensure that the baby is kept warm during this time. The room should be at a comfortable temperature; the baby should be gently dried and covered with a towel or blanket on the mother's chest.

Routine oral suction of the baby should not be undertaken, as this may stimulate the vagal nerve and negatively impact the establishment of normal respirations.

If the mother is rhesus negative, blood should be taken from the umbilical cord to identify the baby's blood group. If the baby is rhesus positive, the mother should receive anti-D via injection to prevent sensitization to the rhesus gene (rhesus isoimmunization).

Following birth by caesarean section, the care outlined in Table 22.3 is appropriate but, in addition, the mother requires a period of observation in the recovery area of the delivery suite, maintenance of intravenous hydration and observation of urine output from her urethral catheter.

If the woman and baby are well with normal observations following a normal vaginal birth, it is possible for them to return home within 6 h of birth in a hospital or birth centre. Prior to returning home, it is advisable that both the baby and mother have passed urine and that the baby has fed.

Table 22.3	Care in the first hours after vaginal birth	
Neonate	**Mother**
Assessment of condition (represented by the Apgar score) at 1, 5 and 10 min – resuscitation only if indicated	Observation of vaginal blood loss, palpation of uterine fundus to identify if contracted
'Skin-to-skin' contact	Examine for perineal, labial and vaginal trauma, with repair as required. Offer analgesia
Clamp and cut the umbilical cord – once the cord has finished pulsating or after approximately 60 seconds	Support mother to hold baby skin-to-skin and, where she wishes, offer the breast to the baby
Measurement and recording of birth weight, length, head circumference, temperature	Observations – general well-being, colour, respirations, pulse, blood pressure, temperature
Initial physical examination of the neonate to identify any abnormalities – this should include examination of the head and facial features, the palate, limbs, digits, spine and external genitalia	Offer something to eat and drink
A record should be made of the neonate's first micturition and first feed	A record should be made of the mother's first micturition after the birth
Discussion with parents about administration of vitamin K and administer with consent	Categorization of the mother's risk of venous thrombosis and commencement of prophylactic measures as appropriate

Carers should ensure that parents feel informed about feeding the baby, care including changing clothing, nappies and washing, and safe sleeping arrangements.

Before discharging a woman and her baby home, caregivers should identify whether there are any risks or concerns including a raised risk of postpartum psychosis or severe depression, potential child-protection issues or significant social concerns. Where such concerns are present, a care plan should normally be devised before the birth. If no such plan has been devised, a consultation with the appropriate multidisciplinary team including mental health specialists and social workers should be undertaken before the mother and baby leave the hospital or birth centre.

Postnatal follow-up in the first 10 days

In the UK, women are visited on at least three occasions by a community midwife in their own home during the first 10 days after the birth. The aims of these visits are to identify physical or emotional problems and support the mother with feeding and parenting.

During these visits, the mother and birth partner should be given the opportunity to discuss their baby's birth with the midwife caring for them. A proportion of women (and birth partners) experience birth as 'traumatic' and may develop symptoms of post-traumatic stress disorder (PTSD). It is important to enable parents to be open about their feelings about the birth and identify when further support may be required.

At each visit, the midwife should ask the mother about her emotional well-being. Suicide is a leading cause of maternal death, with the first 6 weeks after the birth the period of highest risk. All healthcare professionals caring for women in the postnatal period should be aware of the signs and symptoms of postpartum depression and/or psychosis.

A physical examination should be undertaken at each visit:

- pulse, blood pressure and temperature as indications of haemorrhage, anaemia or sepsis
- abdominal examination is undertaken to establish that the uterus is involuting and non-tender. On the first day after birth, the uterine fundus should be palpable at the umbilicus and it gradually reduces in size until, by the 10–14th day, it is no longer palpable above the symphysis pubis
- perineal examination seeking indications of wound breakdown in women who have experienced perineal trauma and/or required suturing. Cool gel packs may be applied intermittently, although ice packs are not recommended. Simple analgesia can be prescribed and local anaesthetic gels or sprays may alleviate discomfort.

Contraception should be discussed (see Chapter 21).

A physical examination of the baby should be undertaken (Chapter 2). The parents should feel enabled to raise any concerns and for the midwife to provide advice.

Caregivers should ensure that parents are confident with parenting skills including feeding, winding, changing clothes and nappies, and washing the baby.

It is important to discuss safe sleeping with all new parents. Premature babies, low birth weight babies, bottle-fed babies and babies with parents who smoke are at higher risk of SUDI or 'cot death'. All babies should be laid down to sleep on their backs. They should sleep in a flat, clear space. Bed sharing should be discouraged, especially where parents smoke, drink alcohol or take sedative drugs.

Late postnatal examination

This usually takes place around 6 weeks after the birth and is an opportunity for the healthcare professional to spend time with the mother to review the birth, address any questions and place these in context for possible future births. This is likely to be particularly important where a mother has required medical intervention during the birth.

The healthcare professional should ask the mother about physical symptoms including perineal pain, pain during sexual intercourse (if resumed), faecal or urinary incontinence, vaginal bleeding or breast pain. The maternal Hb concentration may be determined and cervical cytology performed, as appropriate. Contraceptive requirements and preferences are revisited.

Postnatal problems

Physical problems

Anaemia

The incidence of postnatal anaemia is 25–30%. It is reasonably simple to treat non-symptomatic anaemia with oral iron supplements, reserving blood transfusion for those with significant symptoms and usually with a Hb concentration <70 g/L.

Bowel problems

Constipation is reported by up to 20% of women in the puerperium and is due to a number of factors, including fear of defaecation in the presence of perineal trauma, reduced mobility, oral medications such as iron or codeine, or narcotic analgesia received in labour. Haemorrhoids commonly affect pregnant women and these often persist after birth.

Breast problems

Two-thirds of women will have a problem relating to their breasts, including nipple pain, nipple cracks, bleeding from the nipple, breast engorgement, mastitis and breast abscesses. For women who are not breastfeeding, breast engorgement generating symptoms of discomfort is common. For breastfeeding women, problems can largely be prevented by proper advice regarding positioning of the baby's mouth.

If mastitis occurs, it is usually the result of a blocked mammary duct and frequently requires antibiotic treatment, principally aimed at *Staphylococcus aureus*.

Perineal breakdown

This is not uncommon, but long-term problems are fortunately uncommon. If the wound is clean, perineal resuturing may be considered. If there is any suggestion of infection, which is usually the case, it is advisable to allow healing by secondary intention and antibiotics are usually only considered when cultures from the lower genital tract are positive.

Incontinence

Following a vaginal birth, at least 20% of women suffer from urinary incontinence if assessed 3 months after birth. This is mostly from neurapraxia (impaired pudendal nerve function due to compression at the time of delivery) and commonly resolves spontaneously. However, a small percentage of women will not fully regain urinary continence and will require additional help from a physiotherapist or gynaecologist.

Inability to control flatus or faeces occurs in around 5% of women after birth but, as it is embarrassing, women may be reluctant to mention it. According to endo-anal ultrasound studies, up to 35% of primiparae undergoing a vaginal birth have damage to the anal sphincters (obstetric anal sphincter injury [OASI]), although such damage may be asymptomatic (Fig. 22.2). Both OASI and nerve damage following spontaneous or instrumental delivery contribute to the problem. Investigation and treatment of symptoms is warranted, particularly if they persist beyond the initial postnatal weeks.

Puerperal pyrexia

This is defined as a temperature of >38°C on any occasion in the first 14 days after birth. Pyrexia is usually due to urinary or genital infections (including endometritis, the 'classical' cause of puerperal sepsis) but may also be related to infection in the chest or breast. Deep venous thrombosis (DVT) and pulmonary thromboembolism should be considered as a cause of pyrexia. After a clinical examination including breasts, legs, perineum, chest and abdominal palpation of the uterus, a mid-stream specimen of urine, endocervical/vaginal and wound swabs, as appropriate, and blood cultures are sent for microbiological analysis. A chest infection necessitates physiotherapy and sputum should also be sent for culture.

Sepsis represents a major cause of maternal morbidity and mortality, and it is important to be vigilant to the possibility of infection in the postnatal period. Risk factors for puerperal sepsis include maternal obesity and delivery by caesarean section. If the mother is unwell (pyrexia, tachycardia, hypotension, occasionally hypothermia, confusion), treatment should be started with broad-spectrum antibiotics and fluid resuscitation without delay, with further investigation as necessary, in conjunction with advice from specialists in microbiology. Mastitis and breast abscess are particularly common in the puerperium and may be overlooked. Antibiotic therapy may be required for breast infections but breastfeeding or hand expression should continue where possible. A breast abscess may require surgical incision and drainage.

Secondary postpartum haemorrhage

See page 243.

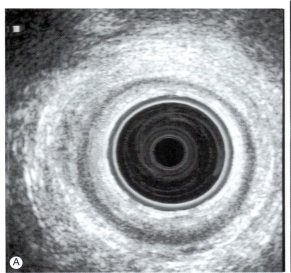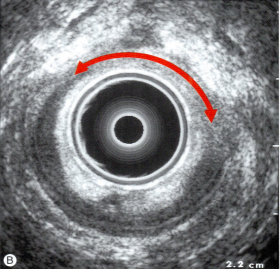

Fig. 22.2 **Anal sphincter damage on endo-anal ultrasound.** (A) Normal anal sphincter scan. (B) Anterior anal sphincter defect between the 10 o'clock and 3 o'clock position.

Venous thromboembolism (VTE)

The puerperium is the period in which women are at the highest risk of developing VTE. Women with risk factors, such as raised BMI or those who are post-caesarean section, are at particular risk, and thromboprophylaxis with graduated compression stockings and low-molecular-weight heparin (LMWH) are widely prescribed after appropriate categorization of risk of VTE. It is important to encourage early mobilization and avoid dehydration. VTE can present as a DVT or pulmonary embolus (PE). Signs and symptoms of DVT include swelling, redness and pain in the leg or calf but may be asymptomatic, whereas a PE is typically accompanied by dyspnoea, chest pain and, sometimes, cardiorespiratory collapse. Prompt diagnosis and treatment, usually with LMWH, is essential.

Superficial thrombophlebitis affects about 1% of women. There is a painful, erythematous and tender (usually varicose) vein. Treatment is with support stockings and anti-inflammatory drugs.

Mental health problems

Around 50% of women will experience transient feelings of tearfulness and emotional lability in the first few days after birth. These are often described as the 'baby blues'. New mothers should be encouraged to talk about their feelings and given support and reassurance.

Talking about the 'baby blues' provides healthcare professionals with an opportunity to discuss the symptoms of a range of more serious mental health problems that may occur postnatally:

- 10% of new mothers are likely to develop a depressive illness. Of these, one-third to a half will be suffering from a severe depressive illness
- 2% of new mothers will be referred to a mental health team
- 2 per 1000 (0.2%) will suffer from postpartum psychosis
- postnatal depression may develop at any time during the first year after the baby's birth, but generally peaks around 3–4 months postnatally
- untreated, postnatal depression can have a significant detrimental impact on the developing mother–infant relationship
- many women do not disclose their true feelings of depression to healthcare professionals after the birth as they are afraid that their baby will be removed from them
- postpartum psychosis generally has an earlier, more acute onset, often within the first few days after the birth
- maternal suicide is one of the leading causes of maternal death.

Signs and symptoms of postnatal depression

Cognitive

- Clouded thinking, difficulty making decisions or choices
- Lack of concentration/poor memory

- Avoidance – physical/psychological
- Fear of rejection by partner
- Worry about welfare of partner/baby
- Thoughts of harming the baby
- Suicidal ideation
- Broken sleep and early-morning awakening
- Feeling hopeless on waking
- Loss of appetite and loss of weight
- Extreme tiredness and lack of vitality
- Loss of pleasure ('not loving her baby' or 'not being a proper mother')

Emotional

- Persistent low mood for up to 10–14 days
- Feelings of inadequacy, failure
- Exhaustion, emptiness, sadness, tearfulness
- Lack of love for the baby/distance from the baby/dislike of the baby
- Guilt, shame, worthlessness
- Confusion, anxiety, panic
- Irritability, anger
- Fear for/of the baby
- Fear of being alone or going out
- Feeling of being on the outside – distanced from those around them

Behavioural

- Lack of interest/pleasure in usual activities
- Sleep disturbances/appetite changes
- Decreased energy/motivation
- Social withdrawal
- Poor self-care/inability to cope with routine tasks

Postpartum psychosis

Many women who develop postpartum psychosis will have previously been well without obvious risk factors, but some women will have particular risk factors:

- a similar illness with a previous child
- non-postpartum bipolar affective disorder, from which they are now recovered
- family history of bipolar illness or postpartum psychosis.

Postpartum psychosis is thought to be caused by biological factors following labour and birth:

- most commonly occurs 3–14 days postpartum
- postpartum psychosis deteriorates rapidly over 48 h whilst the 'baby blues' tends to resolve spontaneously
- commonly thought to be a distinct mental illness but now recognized in many cases to be a variant of bipolar disorder.

Earliest signs are:

- perplexity, fear (even terror), restless agitation, insomnia
- purposeless activity, uncharacteristic behaviours, disinhibition, irritation, fleeting anger, resistive behaviours

- fear for her own or baby's health and safety or identity
- elation and grandiosity, suspiciousness, depression or ideas of horror.

As the condition develops, there is generally a combination of symptoms of mania, depression and psychotic symptoms.

Early recognition and diagnosis is key. A woman's partner or family are likely to be the first to pick up on unusual behaviour. It is important for healthcare professionals to listen to family members' concerns. If treated, postpartum psychosis has a very good recovery rate. Treatment will usually include:

- admission to a 'mother and baby' unit
- antipsychotic or mood-stabilizing drugs initiated to reduce disturbance of the mother–infant relationship. Other medication such as antidepressants may also be indicated
- the psychiatrist will ensure suitable drug therapy if breastfeeding

- community follow-up with the perinatal mental health team
- once recovered, discussion with the woman about risk of future illness and ways of reducing risk following a future pregnancy.

Key points

- The aim of antenatal care is to maximize the chance of a positive outcome from a pregnancy: a healthy mother and a healthy baby or babies.
- Antenatal care involves providing as much support as possible, along with a screening programme to identify maternal and fetal problems at an early stage.
- The puerperium is a time of major physiological change and a time of major personal upheaval.
- Postnatal checks are useful to assess both the mother and baby. The main maternal complications are sepsis, haemorrhage, thromboembolic disease and depression.

23

Maternal medicine

Introduction

Medical disorders are relatively common in pregnancy and often have no implications for the mother or her baby. However, the alteration in maternal physiology, which occurs during pregnancy, may affect the medical condition, or the medical condition itself may affect the pregnancy and the baby. Treatment options for the mother may be limited by concerns for fetal welfare and there is therefore the potential for difficult clinical decision-making.

The following conditions will be considered, but see also hypertension (p. 204) and infection in pregnancy (p. 216):

- diabetes mellitus
- venous thromboembolic disease
- cardiac disease
- connective tissue disease
- epilepsy
- hepatic disorders
- renal disorders
- respiratory disorders
- thrombocytopenia
- thyroid disorders.

Diabetes mellitus

Diabetes mellitus may be diagnosed before pregnancy (pre-existing) or may be discovered for the first time during pregnancy. Discovery during pregnancy is rare for type 1 (insulin-dependent) diabetes but not uncommon for type 2 (non-insulin-dependent) diabetes. In addition to these, a transient, self-limiting state of hyperglycaemia may occur in pregnancy as a result of maternal endocrine changes.

Glucose homeostasis is maintained by the balance between insulin, which reduces glucose levels by increasing cellular uptake, and other hormones such as glucagon and cortisol, which increase glucose production. In pregnancy, the placenta produces multiple hormones and cytokines, such as human placental lactogen and human chorionic somatomammotrophin, which increase insulin resistance and increase production of insulin, respectively. If there is maternal insulin resistance and the pancreatic β islet cells are unable to produce sufficient insulin, the mother may develop a state of hyperglycaemia referred to as gestational diabetes mellitus (GDM).

Pregnant women with pre-existing poorly controlled diabetes mellitus in the first trimester at the time of organogenesis have an increased rate of fetal congenital abnormalities. The abnormalities are principally cardiac defects, neural tube defects and renal anomalies. Although the mechanism of this teratogenesis is unclear, there is evidence that improved pre-pregnancy and early pregnancy blood glucose control reduces the risk of congenital abnormality.

Fetal glucose levels closely reflect those of the mother, with glucose crossing the placenta through facilitated diffusion. Maternal insulin does not cross the placenta and the fetus produces its own insulin from around 10 weeks' gestation. This insulin is recognized to have a significant role in promoting fetal growth. As maternal levels of glucose are higher in mothers with diabetes, fetal levels are also increased and, in turn, there is increased fetal insulin production. This fetal hyperinsulinaemia often results in macrosomia (large babies) and organomegaly, as well as increased erythropoiesis and neonatal polycythaemia.

In addition to the risk of congenital abnormality, there is also a risk of unexplained intrauterine fetal death, possibly because fetal hyperinsulinaemia leads to chronic hypoxia and acidaemia. A macrosomic fetus may be more at risk of these complications because of its increased oxygen demands.

Because babies of women with diabetes are often macrosomic, labour and delivery may be complicated by shoulder dystocia. Neonates may also become hypoglycaemic if the mother is hyperglycaemic during labour and there is an increased incidence of hyaline membrane disease.

Effects of pregnancy on diabetes

Insulin requirements may be static or decrease during the first trimester. It typically increase during the second and third trimesters and may reduce slightly towards term. Improvement in glycaemic control or tight control in pregnant women with pre-existing diabetes may worsen diabetic retinopathy. The optic fundi should be assessed for signs of proliferative retinopathy, with laser treatment advised as necessary.

Effects of diabetes on pregnancy

The incidence of pre-eclampsia is increased. There is also an increased incidence of maternal infection, particularly of the urinary tract. Polyhydramnios, which probably results from fetal polyuria, may result in unstable lie, malpresentation and pre-term labour.

Screening for gestational diabetes

This is a controversial subject. The National Institute for Health and Care Excellence (NICE) UK guidelines recommend offering a 2-h 75 g glucose tolerance test (GTT) at 24–28 weeks to women with risk factors, including a family history of diabetes; a raised body mass index (BMI) (>30); a previous macrosomic baby (>4.5 kg); those with previous GDM; or ethnic minorities with high prevalence of diabetes. For those with previous GDM, early self-monitoring or GTT should also be offered at booking.

NICE UK (2015) diagnostic criteria for gestational diabetes after 2-h 75 g GTT:

- fasting blood glucose level ≥5.6 mmol/L
- 2-h blood glucose level ≥7.8 mmol/L.

Management of gestational diabetes

Treatment with dietary advice and exercise should be the first step. Metformin and subsequently insulin therapy should be instituted if the target levels are not achieved. As per NICE UK guidelines (2015), insulin treatment should aim to keep the fasting glucose <5.5 mmol/L and 1-h postprandial <7.8 mmol/L.

Women with GDM have an increased risk of developing diabetes mellitus in the subsequent 25 years. Recurrence of GDM in subsequent pregnancies is up to 75% (especially if treatment with insulin was required).

Antenatal management of established diabetes

At pre-pregnancy counselling, advice should be given about good diabetic control, diet, smoking cessation, weight loss if BMI >27 kg/m^2 and high-dose (5 mg) folate supplements. Glycosylated haemoglobin should be checked when planning a pregnancy and in early pregnancy, aiming for levels below 48 mmol/L (6.5%).

Pregnancy management should be in a joint diabetic and antenatal clinic, with frequent visits planned as required. Capillary blood glucose should be measured on average four times a day (fasting and 1 h postprandial), aiming for tight control (e.g. with preprandial levels of 4.0–5.5 mmol/L and 1 h postprandial levels of <7.8 mmol/L).

Insulin is commonly given as a short-acting analogue three times a day (with meals), with long-acting background insulin once or twice a day. Ketoacidosis should be avoided, as it is associated with an increased risk of perinatal mortality. All women with type 1 diabetes should be offered ketone testing strips and a ketometer.

Maternal kidney function and optic fundi should be examined in early pregnancy. A detailed anomaly scan including a fetal heart scan should be offered at 18–22 weeks. The maternal abdomen should be examined for polyhydramnios, macrosomia or fetal growth restriction (measurement of symphysis-fundal height), and serial ultrasound fetal biometry is recommended.

Delivery

Delivery between 37 and 38 + 6 weeks by elective birth (induction of labour) is recommended for patients with pre-existing diabetes and by 40 + 6 weeks for patients with gestational diabetes, if there are no complications (NICE UK guidelines 2015). Concern regarding fetal macrosomia and the potential for shoulder dystocia in particular, may necessitate a planned caesarean section.

If pre-term labour occurs, steroids may be given as for the non-diabetic patient, but will lead to deterioration in diabetic control, unless insulin doses are increased appropriately or a variable rate insulin infusion (VRII) employed.

The aim of a VRII is to maintain tight intrapartum glycaemic control, whether during labour or for caesarean section, to reduce the risk of neonatal hypoglycaemia. In the immediate postpartum period, insulin requirements rapidly return to pre-pregnancy levels and the previous subcutaneous (SC) regimen can be re-established. For women with GDM, insulin should be discontinued following delivery.

Venous thromboembolic disease

Antenatal

In pregnancy, the balance of the coagulation system is altered towards thrombus formation. There are increased levels of fibrinogen, prothrombin and other clotting factors, together with reduced levels of endogenous anticoagulants. This tendency to clot formation is only in part offset by an increase in fibrinolysis. In addition to the clotting system changes, the gravid uterus causes a degree of mechanical obstruction to the venous system and leads to peripheral venous stasis in the lower limbs.

Venous thromboembolic disease appears to be very rare in Africa and the Far East but is the commonest direct cause of maternal mortality in the UK. In the UK, over 50% of maternal deaths from thromboembolism occur antenatally.

Over 80% of deep venous thromboses (DVTs) in pregnancy are left-sided, in contrast to only 55% in the non-pregnant woman. This difference may reflect compression of the left common iliac vein by the right common iliac artery and the ovarian artery, which cross the vein on the left side only. The gravid uterus lies over the right common iliac artery. Furthermore, over 70% of DVTs in pregnancy are iliofemoral rather than femoral popliteal compared with the non-pregnant rate of around 9%, and are therefore more likely than lower calf vein thromboses to give rise to pulmonary embolism.

Thromboembolism may be asymptomatic but usually presents with the traditional symptoms and signs, such as calf tenderness, breathlessness and chest pain. It may also present with lower abdominal or groin pain. It is essential to make a definitive diagnosis, not just for management of the current pregnancy but because there are major implications with regard to the need for thromboprophylaxis in subsequent pregnancies.

Haematological testing for D-dimers is not helpful in pregnancy. Radiological investigations are required if there is clinical suspicion. Duplex Doppler ultrasound is particularly useful for identifying femoral vein thromboses, although iliac veins are less easily seen (Fig. 23.1). It is safe and should be the first-line investigation. X-ray venography is more specific, but has the disadvantage of radiation exposure. Venography or magnetic resonance venography is appropriate if Doppler studies give equivocal results, or negative results, despite strong clinical suspicion. Pregnancy is not a contraindication to carrying out a chest X-ray and/or a ventilation-perfusion ($\dot{V}/\dot{Q}$) scan – any radiation risks are outweighed by the benefits of accurate diagnosis (Fig. 23.2). A normal scan virtually excludes the diagnosis of pulmonary embolism. A computerized tomography pulmonary arteriogram (CTPA) may also be appropriate, especially if the chest X-ray is abnormal or an alternative diagnosis is suspected. CTPA, despite involving less radiation to the fetus than ($\dot{V}/\dot{Q}$) scanning, is associated with significant radiation to the maternal breasts.

Treatment of DVT or pulmonary embolism in pregnancy is with SC low-molecular-weight heparin (LMWH). Intravenous (IV) unfractionated heparin is appropriate in cases of massive pulmonary embolus. LMWH therapy is interrupted for delivery to allow for regional analgesia and anaesthesia, and to minimize the risk of haemorrhage. After delivery, the woman may choose to continue with SC LMWH or commence warfarin, continuing anticoagulation for 6–12 weeks, as decided by timing of onset and clinical severity of the thrombosis. Direct oral anticoagulants are not advisable in lactating women.

Women with a previous history of venous thromboembolism (VTE) – except women who have experienced a single episode of VTE provoked by major trauma, who in the absence of other risk factors such as thrombophilia may not require thromboprophylaxis – (Box 23.1) should be offered antenatal and postnatal (for 6 weeks) prophylaxis with LMWH.

Antenatal and postnatal risk assessment

The risks of thromboembolism should be assessed in all women at booking, at the time of any antenatal hospital admission and after delivery (see Box 23.2), and those at risk (previous thrombosis, thrombophilia, emergency caesarean section, or any two [postnatal] or three [antenatal >28 weeks] or four [antenatal throughout pregnancy] of the other risk factors) offered thromboprophylaxis with LMWH (e.g. enoxaparin 40 mg once daily). Admission to hospital is also a risk factor and pregnant women admitted to hospital should usually be offered LMWH unless they have active bleeding or delivery is imminent.

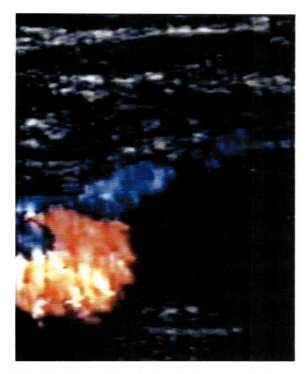

Fig. 23.1 **Normal Doppler flow in the femoral artery (red, left) with no flow through the occluded femoral vein (black, right).**

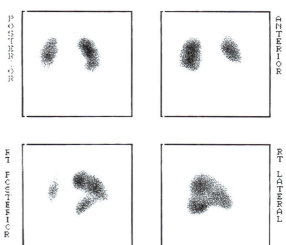

Fig. 23.2 **Positive Q̇ scan.** Note the lack of perfusion in the right lower lobe. The ventilation scan was normal. (From Pitkin J, Peattie A, Magowan BA. Obstetrics and Gynecology. An Illustrated Colour Text. Churchill Livingstone, Edinburgh, 2003.)

Box 23.1

Heritable thrombophilias
- Antithrombin deficiency
- Protein C deficiency
- Protein S deficiency
- Factor V Leiden mutation
- Prothrombin gene variant

Acquired thrombophilias
- Lupus anticoagulant and anticardiolipin antibodies

Box 23.2

Thromboembolic risk factors in pregnancy and postpartum
- Age >35 years
- Obesity (BMI >30)
- Para 3 or more
- Gross varicose veins
- Current infection
- Pre-eclampsia
- Immobility (>4 days)
- Major current illness, e.g. heart or lung disease; cancer; inflammatory bowel disease; nephrotic syndrome
- Caesarean section, particularly emergency caesarean section in labour
- Extended major pelvic or abdominal surgery, e.g. caesarean hysterectomy
- Women with a personal or family history of deep vein thrombosis, pulmonary embolism or heritable thrombophilia
- Women with antiphospholipid antibody (cardiolipin antibody or lupus anticoagulant)
- Paralysis of lower limbs
- Smoking, multiple pregnancy and assisted conception (in vitro fertilization)

Cardiac disease

Heart disease complicates less than 1% of all pregnancies but accounts for around 20% of maternal deaths in the UK. Rheumatic heart disease remains a significant problem in the developing world and it is also encountered with increasing frequency in western countries, as a result of migration. There are increasing numbers of fertile women who have had surgery as children for congenital heart disease. Maternal mortality is highest in conditions where pulmonary blood flow cannot be increased to compensate for the increased demand during pregnancy – particularly Eisenmenger syndrome, where maternal mortality rates reach 20–40%.

Unfortunately, many symptoms and signs similar to those of heart disease occur commonly in normal pregnancy, making a clinical diagnosis difficult. Breathlessness and syncopal episodes are present in 90% of normal pregnancies, atrial ectopic beats are common, and up to 96% of normal women may have an audible ejection systolic murmur. Further investigation should be considered if the murmur is loud (>2/6), diastolic, if a precordial thrill is present or if there are any other suspicious features, especially in migrant women.

If problems are discovered, a cardiologist with expertise in pregnancy cardiology should be involved during the antenatal period. If there is no haemodynamic compromise

Box 23.3

Severe cardiac disease and delivery
- Labour should be conducted in a high-dependency or intensive care unit, possibly with central venous catheter and arterial line monitoring, aiming for a vaginal delivery. Hypotension, hypoxia and fluid overload should be avoided
- Epidural analgesia may be used in most circumstances
- For the third stage, Syntocinon should be given slowly – rather than Syntometrine, because ergometrine can cause hypertension and bolus syntocinon can cause vasodilation
- Particular care is required in the immediate postpartum period, as the increased circulating volume following delivery of the placenta may lead to fluid overload and congestive failure

(e.g. congenital mitral valve prolapse), the prognosis is good and there is often no requirement for cardiac follow-up. If there are potential haemodynamic problems, very close follow-up by a multidisciplinary team is mandatory and a careful plan should be made for delivery. Serious consideration of pregnancy termination is advisable in women with Eisenmenger syndrome, any cause of pulmonary hypertension, pulmonary veno-occlusive disease, in those with aortopathy with significant aortic dilatation and in those with severely impaired left ventricular function. With atrial fibrillation, anticoagulation is required to prevent atrial clot forming and subsequent embolic problems. If the maternal partial pressure of oxygen (PO_2) is decreased, the fetus is at risk from hypoxia and fetal growth restriction, and should be monitored closely.

Severe cardiac disease can cause problems at delivery, particularly in those with prosthetic valves, aortic stenosis, mitral stenosis, left ventricular dysfunction or pulmonary hypertension (Box 23.3).

Myocardial infarction is rare in pregnancy but is a common cardiac cause of maternal mortality. Peripartum cardiomyopathy is also rare (<1:5000), but carries a 5% mortality and is associated with hypertension in pregnancy, multiple pregnancy, high multiparity and increased maternal age. It presents with sudden onset of heart failure and, on chest radiology or echocardiography, there is usually a grossly dilated heart (Fig. 23.3).

Connective tissue disease

These diseases are not uncommon and, as they often affect women during their childbearing years, they are not infrequently found in association with pregnancy. See also antiphospholipid syndrome (p. 63).

Systemic lupus erythematosus (SLE)

There is an increased chance of an exacerbation of SLE (flare-up) occurring in pregnancy and during the postnatal period. Women should be discouraged from becoming pregnant when their disease is active, to minimize problems. Active lupus nephritis during pregnancy is associated with significant maternal and perinatal mortality and morbidity, and in particular with a risk of pre-eclampsia.

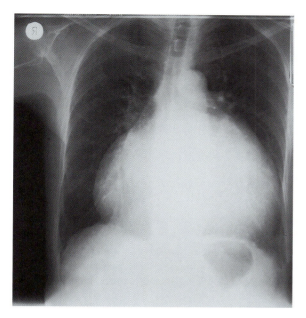

Fig. 23.3 **Postpartum cardiomyopathy after twin delivery in a mother aged 42 years.**

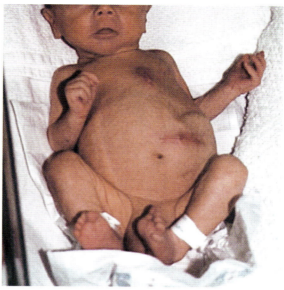

Fig. 23.4 **Pacemaker in a baby with congenital heart block in association with anti-Ro antibodies.**

SLE nephritis is associated with increased fetal loss rates from spontaneous miscarriages and pre-term delivery. This is particularly so in those with antiphospholipid antibodies. There is an increased incidence of pre-eclampsia and this may be difficult to differentiate from a disease flare, as both are associated with hypertension and proteinuria. There is no increase in the rate of fetal abnormalities, although there is a risk of fetal congenital heart block associated with the presence of anti-Ro and anti-La antibodies (Fig. 23.4). Neonatal lupus may rarely occur and is characterized by haemolytic anaemia, leucopenia, thrombocytopenia, discoid skin lesions, pericarditis and congenital heart block.

If lupus anticoagulant or anticardiolipin antibodies (antiphospholipid antibodies) are present, low-dose aspirin should be given and in women with a previous history of thromboembolic disease or adverse pregnancy outcome, LMWH is indicated. Careful monitoring of renal function is appropriate. Disease flares should be managed where possible with oral prednisolone and there should be regular ultrasound fetal biometry owing to the increased risk of fetal growth restriction.

Epilepsy

A first seizure in the second half of pregnancy should be assumed to be eclampsia until proven otherwise. Around a third of pregnant women with epilepsy have an increase in seizure frequency independent of the effects of medication. For women with epilepsy on treatment, the fall in antiepileptic drug (AED) levels due to dilution, reduced absorption, reduced compliance and increased drug metabolism is partially compensated for by reduced protein binding (and therefore an increase in the level of free drug) for phenytoin, but for most AEDs the free drug levels fall in pregnancy. This is particularly the case for lamotrigine. There is an increased incidence of fetal anomalies in association with the older AEDs (phenytoin, carbamazepine) (6% vs 3% in the general population) (Fig. 23.5). Single-drug regimens are less teratogenic than multidrug therapy (Table 23.1) and sodium valproate carries the highest risk of teratogenesis (10%), as well as being associated with an increased risk of neurocognitive impairment, autism spectrum disorders and attention deficit disorder. The risk of congenital malformations appears lower with lamotrigine and leveteracetam.

Hepatic disorders

There are a large number of potential causes of liver dysfunction in pregnancy (Tables 23.2 and 23.3). A history of a prodromal illness, overseas travel or high-risk group for blood-borne illness may suggest viral hepatitis. Itch is suggestive of cholestasis. Abdominal pain is associated with gallstones, HELLP (haemolysis, elevated liver enzymes and low platelets) syndrome (p. 260) or acute fatty liver. Urea and electrolytes (U&Es), liver function tests (LFTs), blood glucose, platelets and coagulation screen should be performed and blood sent for hepatitis serology. Liver autoantibodies may suggest pre-existing liver disease; anti-smooth muscle antibodies are a marker for autoimmune chronic active hepatitis and antimitochondrial antibodies are a marker for primary biliary cirrhosis. A mild transaminitis is common in non-alcoholic steatohepatitis, which may be diagnosed for the first time in pregnancy. Abdominal ultrasound of the liver and gall bladder may show obstruction or gallstones.

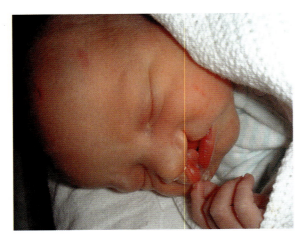

Fig. 23.5 AEDs are associated with neural tube, cardiac and craniofacial defects (with permission).

It is normal for the alkaline phosphatase level to increase in pregnancy (1.5–2 times normal).

Renal disorders

In pregnancy, there is a physiological increase in the size of both kidneys as well as dilatation of the ureter and renal pelvis. This dilatation is greater on the right than on the left because of dextrorotation of the uterus. There is also an increase in creatinine clearance owing to the increased glomerular filtration rate (maximal in the second trimester). In pregnancy, the normal serum urea is <4.5 mmol/L and creatinine <75 μmol/L.

Infection

Urinary tract infections (UTIs) occur in 3–7% of pregnancies and, if untreated, may lead to septicaemia and pre-term labour. Asymptomatic bacteriuria should be treated, since

Table 23.1	Management of epilepsy in pregnancy
Pre-pregnancy counselling	Monotherapy with AED ideal. Folate supplementation (5 mg/day) should be continued until at least 12 weeks
AED dosage	AED doses adjusted on clinical grounds. There are fetal risks from AEDs as well as from not taking the drugs (from increased fit frequency). Increased doses recommended for lamotrigine therapy
Detailed ultrasound scan at 18–22 weeks	Neural tube, cardiac and craniofacial abnormalities, as well as diaphragmatic herniae, are more common
Vitamin K for women on enzyme-inducing anticonvulsants	Oral vitamin K should be given daily from 36 weeks in women receiving enzyme-inducing AEDs to reduce the risk of haemorrhagic disease of the newborn. The baby should be given intramuscular vitamin K stat. at birth
Seizures	Most seizures in pregnancy will be self-limiting; if prolonged, however, rectal or IV diazepam or IV lorazepam, with or without ventilation, may be required
Postnatal	The mother may breastfeed safely (drugs pass into the milk but neonatal levels are low for most AEDs). Advice should be given about safe and suitable settings for feeding, bathing, etc. Carbamazepine, phenytoin, primidone and phenobarbitone induce liver enzymes, reducing the effectiveness of the standard-dose combined oral contraceptives, and a higher-dose oestrogen preparation or alternative form of contraception is therefore required

Table 23.2	Liver disorders specific to pregnancy
Hyperemesis gravidarum	This may occasionally be associated with abnormal LFTs
Intrahepatic cholestasis of pregnancy	Usually presents after 30 weeks' gestation, possibly due to a genetic predisposition to the cholestatic effect of oestrogens. Pruritus affects the limbs and trunk, and it is often severe. There may be a positive family history in up to 35% of cases. Serum total bile acid concentration is increased early in the disease and is the optimum marker for the condition. Transaminases may be increased (<3-fold). Bilirubin is usually <100 μmol/L, and there may be pale stools and dark urine. There are no serious long-term maternal risks but there is a risk of pre-term labour, fetal distress and intrauterine fetal death. Delivery at 37–38 weeks is appropriate, if bile acids >40 μmol/L, in an effort to prevent fetal death
HELLP syndrome	See page 260
Acute fatty liver of pregnancy	This is very rare, is associated with increased maternal and fetal mortality, and may progress rapidly to hepatic failure. It usually presents with vomiting in the third trimester associated with malaise and abdominal pain, jaundice, thirst and polyuria, and may cause hepatic encephalopathy. LFTs are elevated, urate is very high and there is often profound hypoglycaemia. There may be hypertension and proteinuria. Coagulopathy, hypoglycaemia and fluid imbalance should be corrected and the fetus delivered. N-acetylcysteine should be administered. Following delivery, there is a risk of postpartum haemorrhage and liver dysfunction may be prolonged. Hepatic encephalopathy may develop and liver transplant is occasionally necessary. If the patient recovers, there is no long-term liver impairment

Table 23.3	Liver disorders coincidental to pregnancy
Viral hepatitis	Serology should be performed for hepatitis A, B and C, as well as for cytomegalovirus, Epstein-Barr virus and toxoplasmosis (see p. 230)
Gallstones	Asymptomatic gallstones do not require treatment. Cholecystitis should be managed conservatively if possible
Cirrhosis	In severe cirrhosis, there is usually amenorrhoea. If pregnancy occurs, and the disease is well compensated, there is usually no long-term effect on hepatic function. The main risk is bleeding from oesophageal varices
Autoimmune chronic active hepatitis	Pregnancy does not usually have any long-term effect on liver function. Immunosuppressant therapy with prednisolone and azathioprine should be continued in those with autoimmune disease
Primary biliary cirrhosis	This is variable in severity. The prognosis for mother and fetus is good in mild disease. It may present during pregnancy for the first time in a similar way to obstetric cholestasis

there is a 30–40% risk of developing a symptomatic UTI. Pyelonephritis should be treated aggressively.

Obstruction

Acute hydronephrosis is characterized by loin pain, ureteric colic, sterile urine and a renal ultrasound scan showing dilatation of the renal tract greater than normal for pregnancy (Fig. 23.6). If the symptoms are not settling and the ultrasound scan does not demonstrate the cause of the obstruction, a limited IV urogram or magnetic resonance imaging should be considered. Treatment is with ureteric stenting or nephrostomy. There may be no obvious cause of obstruction and complete resolution may occur following delivery. Renal tract calculi are associated with an increased incidence of UTIs but otherwise do not usually affect pregnancy (unless obstruction is severe).

Chronic kidney disease (CKD)

With CKD in pregnancy, the fetal prognosis is best if maternal renal function and blood pressure are optimized. If the plasma creatinine is <125 μmol/L, the maternal and perinatal outcome is usually good. If pregnancy occurs with a creatinine >250 μmol/L, there is a high risk of deterioration in renal function as well as a lower chance of a successful pregnancy outcome. Between these levels, women should be advised that pregnancy may cause their renal function to deteriorate and that there are also risks to the fetus (mainly fetal growth restriction and pre-term delivery). Some renal diseases carry a poorer prognosis than others and specialist advice is required.

Women with CKD should receive pre-pregnancy counselling. The woman should be seen frequently antenatally, particularly in the third trimester. Hypertension should be treated aggressively, U&Es, plasma albumin, urinalysis and mid-stream urine samples checked at each visit, and a protein–creatinine ratio sent each month to quantify proteinuria. Close fetal monitoring is important. It is difficult to distinguish pre-eclampsia from increasing renal compromise, as both may present with hypertension, rising serum creatinine and proteinuria.

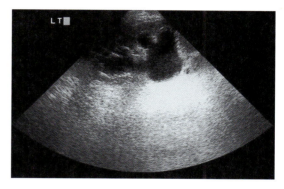

Fig. 23.6   Ultrasound of left kidney with ureteric obstruction and calyceal clubbing. There was a calculus in the lower-third of the ureter.

Pregnancy should be discouraged in women with CKD 4–5 (estimated glomerular filtration rate <30) or on dialysis, as the fetal prognosis is poor. Pregnancy in women who have had a renal transplant is increasingly common and usually successful with good allograft function. As with other causes of CKD, pregnancy and renal outcome is dependent on the baseline renal function.

Respiratory disorders

Breathlessness due to the physiological increase in minute ventilation is a common symptom in pregnancy. Although there is an increased tidal volume from early pregnancy, the exact cause of the feeling of breathlessness is unclear. Investigation should be considered if the breathlessness is of sudden onset, associated with chest pain or if there are clinical signs. It should be remembered that breathlessness can also be a feature of pulmonary thromboembolic disease and heart failure.

Asthma is a common condition. In most women, the disease is unchanged in pregnancy. Treatment is the same that outside pregnancy and women already established on treatment should continue. Inhaled beta-sympathomimetics and inhaled steroids are considered safe. Oral steroids should be given if clinically indicated.

Thrombocytopenia

Maternal thrombocytopenia in pregnancy

In the second half of normal pregnancies there is a mild thrombocytopenia (platelet count $100–150 \times 10^9/L$) in 8% of women, which is not associated with any additional risk to the mother or fetus. The platelet count may also be reduced in pre-eclampsia.

Autoimmune thrombocytopenic purpura is the commonest cause of thrombocytopenia in early pregnancy (but can also arise in later pregnancy) and may be acute or chronic. Antiplatelet antibodies may cross the placenta and, rarely, cause fetal thrombocytopenia, although this seldom is associated with long-term morbidity (cf. alloimmune thrombocytopenia below). No treatment is required in the absence of bleeding, providing the platelet count remains above $50 \times 10^9/L$. If the platelet count falls below this level, steroids and/or immunoglobulin can be given. Specialist haematological advice is appropriate before considering treatment. Treatment may be warranted towards term to ensure the platelet count is $>70–80 \times 10^9/L$ to permit regional analgesia/anaesthesia.

Fetal (alloimmune) thrombocytopenia

This is a rare disorder, in which there are maternal antibodies to fetal platelets. This has some similarities with rhesus disease, in which there are maternal antibodies to the fetal red cells. The maternal platelet count is normal but there may be profound fetal thrombocytopenia and antenatal or intrapartum fetal intracranial haemorrhage. The diagnosis should be suspected when a previous child has experienced neonatal thrombocytopenia and maternal antiplatelet antibodies have been identified (often to the HPA-1a antigen). Antenatal therapy is usually with fetal platelet transfusion.

Thyroid disorders

In total, 1% of pregnant women in the western world are affected by thyroid disease, with *hypo*thyroidism being commoner than *hyper*thyroidism. The fetal thyroid gland secretes thyroid hormones from the 12th week and is independent of maternal control.

Hypothyroidism

This may present with fatigue, hair loss, dry skin, abnormal weight gain, poor appetite, cold intolerance, bradycardia and delayed tendon reflexes. If untreated, there is an increase in the rate of spontaneous miscarriages and stillbirths compared with the euthyroid population, as well as a risk of fetal neurological impairment. There is fetal risk if the mother is treated and is euthyroid. Thyroid function should be regularly monitored, aiming to keep thyroid-stimulating hormone (TSH) and free thyroxine (T_4) within the normal range for pregnancy. If the woman is already on treatment and euthyroid at booking, the dose need not be increased. There is no evidence that treating subclinical hypothyroidism (normal free T_4 with TSH 4.6–1) either before or during pregnancy benefits pregnancy outcome.

Hyperthyroidism

Thyrotoxicosis presents with weight loss, exophthalmos, tachycardia and restlessness. It is usually due to Graves disease but may be secondary to a toxic thyroid adenoma or multinodular goitre. Untreated thyrotoxicosis is associated with high fetal mortality and a risk of maternal thyroid crisis at delivery. Well-controlled hyperthyroidism is not associated with an increase in fetal anomalies, but there is a tendency for babies to be small for gestational age. Graves disease usually improves during pregnancy.

Carbimazole and propylthiouracil cross the placenta but are safe in pregnancy and potentially cause fetal thyroid suppression only in high doses. Radioactive iodine is contraindicated in pregnancy and surgery is indicated only for those with a very large goitre or poor compliance with oral therapy.

Postpartum thyroiditis

This occurs following 5–10% of all pregnancies, usually with initial hyperthyroidism followed by hypothyroidism and then recovery. Because the hypothyroidism occurs at around 1–3 months, the condition may be confused with postnatal depression. Symptoms of hyperthyroidism may be treated with propranolol (antithyroid drugs). Hypothyroidism should be treated with thyroxine as above, withdrawing around 6 months after delivery. Affected women may require long-term treatment or may develop subsequent hypothyroidism.

Key points

- Diabetes carries increased risks of congenital abnormality, macrosomia and intrauterine death for the fetus. Good periconception and antenatal glycaemic control is the cornerstone of management.
- Pregnancy-related venous thromboembolic disease is the commonest direct cause of maternal mortality in many western countries. Relevant symptoms should be appropriately investigated. Thromboembolic prophylaxis is important in both obstetrics and gynaecological practice.
- AED, particularly sodium valproate and polytherapy, increase the risk of fetal abnormality.
- Abnormal LFTs may be related to the pregnancy or incidental viral infections or pre-existing liver disease.
- Asymptomatic UTIs should be treated.
- Well-controlled thyroid disease poses little serious risk to the mother or fetus.

24 Fetal medicine

Introduction

In the UK, approximately 2.5% of fetuses have congenital malformations, the most common of which are listed in Box 24.1 The identification of a 'congenital abnormality' in pregnancy transforms what is usually a joyful and exciting experience into one that is fraught with anxiety and distress. Providing couples with accurate information in an understanding and tactful way is essential and often requires input from senior obstetric staff, ideally those with fetal-medicine experience, as well as paediatricians, surgeons, clinical geneticists and radiologists.

The aims of prenatal diagnosis are four-fold:

- to identify at an early gestation, congenital abnormalities incompatible with life or that are likely to result in significant handicap so as to prepare the parents, involve other specialist clinicians and offer the option of termination of pregnancy (TOP) if appropriate
- to identify conditions which may influence the timing, site or mode of delivery
- to identify fetuses who may benefit from early neonatal paediatric intervention
- to identify fetuses who may benefit from in utero treatment.

Detailed discussion and non-directional counselling are essential. It should not be assumed that all couples will request TOP, even in the presence of lethal abnormalities. It is important to remain completely neutral and avoid using expressions such as 'high risk' or 'severe handicap', which imply a judgement. The sentence 'the risk of handicap is 5%' sounds worse than 'the baby has a 95% chance of being unaffected' and these aspects of counselling should be carefully considered when talking couples through the diagnosis and their options.

Many couples opt to continue pregnancies in the face of severe defects which have resulted in either intrauterine or early neonatal death, subsequently expressing the view that they found it easier to cope with their grief having held their child. Other parents make the difficult decision not to carry on with the pregnancy. More controversial still is the identification of conditions likely to cause long-term handicap and suffering for both the child and their parents. In this situation the parents must decide what is acceptable to them; we can only advise, guide and respect their final wishes, irrespective of our own personal opinions.

All discussions should be complemented with written information. Parents need time to absorb information and it is important that they are given time to reflect on the facts and to consider all options carefully. It can be extremely useful to arrange a follow-up appointment a few days after the initial visit and indeed sometimes it takes several appointments before they have come to a decision.

Assessing the chance of abnormalities

The likelihood of an autosomal trisomy, especially trisomy 21 (Down syndrome) increases with advancing maternal age. In some cases, however, there may be a family history of an inherited condition, for example Duchenne muscular dystrophy, cystic fibrosis and sickle cell disease. Consanguinity increases the chance of single gene abnormalities, especially relating to autosomal recessive conditions. Structural abnormalities are also slightly more likely to occur in those with a family history of the condition and, in some instances, the chance may be higher still if the parents have had a previously affected child. A mother who has a child with spina bifida, for example, has an approximately 2% chance of recurrence compared with a background chance of about 0.2%. Mothers with pre-existing diabetes have a higher chance of cardiac and neural tube defects, whilst women with epilepsy are at increased chance of structural abnormalities, especially if taking potentially teratogenic antiepileptic drugs. Despite this, however, the majority of structural and chromosomal anomalies occur de novo in women with no predisposing risk factors, hence screening tests are offered to all women in pregnancy.

Whilst screening for fetal abnormality is offered to all couples in pregnancy, it is important to appreciate that it may not be appropriate for everyone. When counselling couples for screening, it should be made clear that most tests (particularly those for chromosomal problems) will only

Selected congenital abnormalities

Genetic disorders

- Down syndrome (trisomy 21)
- Edwards syndrome (trisomy 18)
- Patau syndrome (trisomy 13)
- Triploidy
- Sex chromosome abnormalities
- XO (Turner syndrome)
- XXY (Klinefelter syndrome)
- XYY
- XXX
- Apparently balanced rearrangements (translocations or inversions)
- Unbalanced chromosomal structural abnormalities
- Gene disorders (e.g. fragile X syndrome, Huntington chorea, Tay-Sachs disease)

Structural disorders

- Congenital heart disease
- Neural tube defects (e.g. anencephaly, encephalocele, spina bifida)
- Abdominal wall defects (e.g. exomphalos, gastroschisis)
- Genitourinary abnormalities (e.g. renal dysplasia, polycystic kidney disease, pyelectasis, posterior urethral valves, Potter syndrome)
- Lung disorders (e.g. pulmonary hypoplasia, diaphragmatic herniae, cystic fibrosis)

Congenital infection

- Toxoplasmosis
- Rubella
- Cytomegalovirus (CMV)
- Herpes simplex virus (HSV)
- Chickenpox
- *Erythrovirus*
- Human immunodeficiency virus (HIV)
- Zika
- Hepatitis
- *Listeria monocytogenes*
- Syphilis
- Beta-haemolytic streptococci – group B

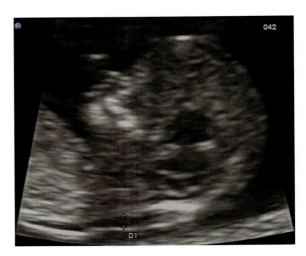

Fig. 24.1 This is the view required to measure the nuchal translucency (between the on-screen calipers).

trisomy 21 when using a 'cut off' of 1 in 150 as 'high risk.' In dichorionic twin pregnancies, each twin is given an 'individualized' risk; however, in monochorionic twins the risk is calculated as an average of that allocated to both twins. As previously discussed, these screening tests can only identify fetuses at increased risk of problems; for absolute certainty a diagnostic test is required (see amniocentesis and chorionic villous sampling [CVS] later).

Serological screening

For those in whom it is not possible to obtain a first trimester screening test (poor fetal position or a pregnancy already beyond 14 weeks' gestation), serological testing may be offered. Alpha-fetoprotein (AFP) is lower than expected in Down syndrome and levels can be combined with β-HCG, oestriol and inhibin A in what is referred to as the 'quadruple test'. A raised AFP should prompt an ultrasound scan looking for a neural tube defect or gastroschisis (see later).

Non-invasive prenatal screening test (NIPT)

NIPT is based on the analysis of cell-free fetal DNA (cffDNA) extracted from maternal blood and is used to screen for various chromosomal disorders, as well as to identify fetal rhesus blood type if required. Although not yet widely available, is it much more sensitive and specific than conventional tests and is currently recommended as an option to women who have been identified as 'high risk' by the screening methods mentioned previously but who wish to try to avoid invasive diagnostic procedures. Mothers who are deemed 'high risk' by this test are still advised to undergo invasive testing as detailed later. The accuracy of NIPT is reduced in multiple pregnancy, obesity and in women at less than 10 weeks' gestation.

identify those at 'high or low risk' for a condition, rather than whether that condition is actually present. Couples must understand that if they were placed in the 'high risk' group, further tests would then be offered and they should be aware of what that would involve. They should ideally also have given thought to what they would do should the pregnancy be affected.

Screening for chromosomal abnormalities

First trimester combined screening test

Screening for chromosomal abnormalities (principally trisomy 21) is possible by measuring the thickness of nuchal fluid behind the fetal neck (nuchal translucency [NT]) on first trimester scan and combining it with the first trimester biochemistry (free β-HCG and PAPP-A) to provide an estimate of the risk of Down syndrome (Fig. 24.1). This combination of tests has a sensitivity of up to 90% for the detection of

Ultrasound scanning

Many structural abnormalities may be reliably diagnosed on ultrasound scan and it is recommended that all women should be offered a detailed ultrasound between 18 and 21 weeks' gestation (see structural abnormalities later). The timing is such that it maximizes the likelihood of obtaining satisfactory images, whilst allowing those in whom major or lethal abnormalities have been detected to consider TOP. Despite highly skilled operators and optimal machinery, ultrasound scanning has its limitations. Some abnormalities may not be evident at this gestation and so cannot be identified on routine scanning, and maternal obesity reduces the quality of images obtained. It is therefore essential to explain that, whilst a normal detailed scan is reassuring, it cannot completely exclude structural abnormalities.

Other problems associated with the routine anomaly scan include the identification of minor abnormalities or 'soft markers' that are often associated with, but not diagnostic of, other problems, especially chromosomal abnormalities. These markers are found in approximately 5% of detailed scans and include choroid plexus cysts (Fig. 24.2), mild renal pelvic dilatation, echogenic cardiac foci (Fig. 24.3) and mild cerebral ventricular dilatation. If the soft marker is noted in isolation, the chance of chromosomal problems is low; if more than one is seen, however, or it is seen in conjunction with a structural defect, the chance of a chromosomal problem is likely to be increased.

Unlike structural abnormalities, chromosomal abnormalities can be much harder to identify on ultrasound scan. Around two-thirds of fetuses with Down syndrome (trisomy 21) will have a normal detailed scan, with the remaining third only demonstrating minor defects not diagnostic for the condition. Most fetuses with the less common trisomies, for example Edwards syndrome (trisomy 18) or Patau syndrome (trisomy 13), usually do show some anomaly; however, again this is usually non-specific and not diagnostic. These latter conditions are usually fatal in the perinatal period and do not pose the same lifelong implications as for trisomy 21. It is for that reason that much of the emphasis in screening has been focused on identifying women at high risk for Down syndrome.

Diagnosis of chromosomal abnormalities

If screening tests have identified a mother at 'high risk' of carrying a baby with a chromosomal abnormality, then she will be offered a diagnostic test, either amniocentesis or CVS, which aims to sample fetal cells. Both of these carry a small risk of miscarriage. Given the possibility of rhesus sensitization, rhesus-negative women require 250 IU of anti-immunoglobulin D. More recently, it has been possible to extract fetal DNA from maternal circulation to identify specific conditions; however, this is not yet widely available.

Amniocentesis

Diagnostic amniocentesis may be performed after 15 weeks' gestation and involves passing a thin needle transabdominally into the amniotic cavity, under continuous ultrasound guidance, to extract 10–15 mL of amniotic fluid (Fig. 24.4). The risk of miscarriage is around 1%. Traditionally, amniocyte culture was previously used to obtain karyotype results, but this was replaced with quantitative fluorescence polymerase chain reaction (QFPCR) to exclude the more common aneuploidies. Most recently, developments in microarray analysis allows examination of many more segments of the genome, and can detect very small changes that may not have been identified on conventional testing.

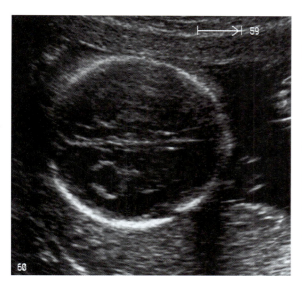

Fig. 24.2 Although there are bilateral choroid plexus cysts, the baby was karyotypically normal.

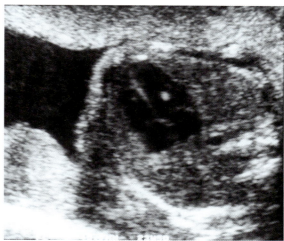

Fig. 24.3 Echogenic focus in the left ventricle of a four-chamber cardiac view.

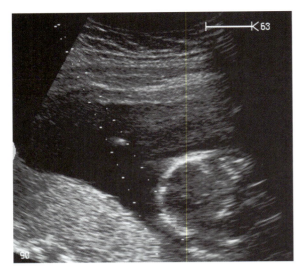

Fig. 24.4 **Amniocentesis is carried out under direct ultrasound guidance.** The tip of the needle can be seen between the dotted guidelines 2 cm above the fetal head.

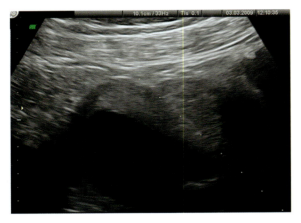

Fig. 24.5 **Chorionic villus sampling is performed under direct, real-time ultrasound imaging.** Here, the needle follows the on-screen needle guide dots. (Courtesy of Dr M Ledingham, Glasgow.)

Chorionic villus sampling

CVS or placental biopsy may be performed after 10 weeks' gestation and involves passing a needle transabdominally, or occasionally transvaginally, under ultrasound guidance to take a sample of placental tissue (Fig. 24.5). The risk of miscarriage is slightly higher than with amniocentesis at 1.5–2%.

Chromosomal abnormalities

Down syndrome (trisomy 21)

The overall incidence is approximately 1:1000 live births; however, this is known to increase with advancing maternal age:

- 20 years, 1:1500
- 30 years, 1:800
- 35 years, 1:270
- 40 years, 1:100
- 45 years, 1:50.

All children born with Down syndrome have some degree of neurodevelopmental delay; however, this is extremely variable. Likewise, the physical characteristics commonly associated with the condition including hypotonia, short stature, small facial features with flat nasal bridge and protruding tongue, upward slanting eyes, broad hands and single palmar crease, manifest to differing degrees. Around 50% of those born with Down syndrome will also have a congenital heart defect, most commonly a septal defect. Down syndrome is also associated with gut mobility problems, hypothyroidism and an increased risk of early-onset dementia. Life expectancy for those affected with Down syndrome has increased dramatically in the last 50 years, from 25 in the 1980s to 60 today. Of all cases, 95% are due to chromosomal nondisjunction, with 4% due to translocation and the remaining 1% mosaicism.

Edwards syndrome (trisomy 18)

The incidence is around 1 in 6000 live births, with the majority resulting from nondisjunction of chromosome 18. Clinical presentation is characterized by early-onset growth restriction, specific craniofacial features, including a small strawberry-shaped cranium, small facial features and low-set ears, and skeletal abnormalities including overlapping fingers and prominent calcanei (rocker bottom feet). Major systemic abnormalities are common and include congenital heart disease, complex urogenital anomalies and problems with the gastrointestinal system. Outcome is poor, with a median survival of 2 weeks after birth. 20% will live to 3 months, and only 8% survive past 1 year.

Patau syndrome (trisomy 13)

The incidence is low, ranging from 1 in 5000 to 1 in 29000 live births. It is associated with multiple severe congenital abnormalities which result in significant physical and mental impairment. The majority of babies affected are stillborn, with survivors rarely expected to live longer than a few days. Around 50% will survive to 1 week, with <5% living longer than 1 year.

Triploidy

This describes the presence of an additional set of chromosomes acquired either from the mother (causing severe fetal growth restriction and fetal abnormality) or father (associated with a partial mole, see Chapter 15) during fertilization, resulting in a total of 69 as opposed to the normal 46. Affected fetuses usually miscarry in early pregnancy and survival to birth is rare. There is no expected survival past the immediate neonatal period, with the affected fetus generally severely growth restricted and affected by multiple severe abnormalities.

Turner syndrome (45,XO)

This affects around 1:2500 live-born girls and, in most cases, is due to the loss of the paternal chromosome, although some individuals have a mosaic pattern. Antenatally it is associated with cystic hygroma (Fig. 24.6), cardiac defects and non-immune hydrops, which results in many affected pregnancies miscarrying. If not identified antenatally, the majority of girls affected are diagnosed in infancy or childhood as a result of characteristic physical features. These include short stature, webbed neck, widely spaced nipples and cubitus valgus. Other associated problems include renal dysgenesis, coarctation of the aorta and ovarian failure necessitating long-term hormone replacement therapy (HRT) requirements. Intelligence is largely unaffected, although there may be some impairment of non-verbal skills.

47,XXX

This is the most common female chromosomal abnormality, occurring in 1:1000 live births, although higher in pregnancies to women over 40 years. Those affected are phenotypically normal, with normal development of secondary sexual characteristics and fertility. There is often a delay in motor and speech development and an association with genitourinary problems including premature ovarian insufficiency requiring HRT.

Klinefelter syndrome (47,XXY)

This affects 1:1000 live births and is a frequent cause of male factor infertility. Those affected tend to be tall males with sparse body hair and gynaecomastia. Typically, the

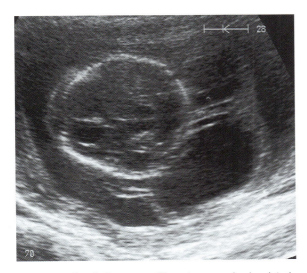

Fig. 24.6 Cystic hygroma. There is a massive loculated cystic swelling behind the fetal neck.

testes remain small and many cases are diagnosed during puberty as a result of this. There is some association with reduced IQ, hypothyroidism, cardiovascular disease and type 2 diabetes.

Jacobs syndrome (47,XYY)

Incidence is around 1:1000 live births. Those affected tend to be very tall males and, whilst intelligence is in the normal range, there may be an association with behavioural problems including impulsivity.

Single gene disorders

Single gene disorders are those caused by a mutation in a single gene. There are over 6500 conditions in this group and they are broadly classified into autosomal, where the mutation is in a gene on a non-sex chromosome, or X-linked, where the mutated gene is found on the X chromosome.

Cystic fibrosis

This is an autosomal recessive condition, with a UK incidence of around 1:2500. It is caused by mutations in the cystic fibrosis transmembrane conductance regulator gene on chromosome 7, which codes for a protein involved in chloride ion channel function. Alterations in this protein can lead to thickened mucous affecting the lungs, resulting in recurrent chest infections, pancreatic insufficiency and malabsorption. Azoospermia in males is common, with subsequent subfertility. Prognosis remains variable but the median predicted survival of sufferers is 41 years. If a couple are known to be carriers, there is a 25% of their baby being affected, and so it is reasonable to offer invasive testing with either amniocentesis or CVS if they felt that they would not continue with an affected pregnancy.

Huntington disease

This is an autosomal dominant condition with a peak age of onset between 40 and 45 years. It is caused by a CAG trinucleotide expansion and can result in chorea, dementia and neuropsychiatric disturbance. Generally, those affected deteriorate over time and life expectancy tends to be about 20 years from the onset of symptoms. Given the lack of treatment and the fact that the disease tends to manifest in later life, issues around testing the children of sufferers are complex. At present, testing is offered to those over 18 who wish to proceed following genetic counselling. There is also the option for invasive prenatal testing, although this becomes even more complex if one-half of the couple is at risk but does not wish to find out if they are affected.

Tay-Sachs disease

This is an autosomal recessive condition characterized by a build-up of gangliosides in the central nervous system resulting in progressive neurodegeneration, seizures and blindness from the age of 3–6 months. The mutation is in the HEXA gene on chromosome 15 and can be tested for by measuring the level of hexosaminidase A in leucocytes. It is common in Ashkenazi Jews but rare in other groups. Sadly, most of those affected die before the age of 4.

Fragile X syndrome

This results from an expansion in the CGG triplet repeat on the X chromosome, causing moderate neurodevelopmental delay. Unaffected individuals typically have 29 repeats; however, they this is increased to up to 200 in those with a pre-mutation. These individuals are phenotypically normal; however are at risk of expansion to a full mutation. Full mutation is defined by over 200 repeats and is characterized by varying degrees of neurodevelopmental delay. The condition affects males more severely than females and is often associated with hyperactive behaviour and impulsiveness. Physical characteristics evolve with age and include a long narrow face with a prominent jaw and forehead and enlarged testicles in males. Prenatal screening is possible and CVS can be used to identify the degree of amplification of the CGG repeats in potential offspring.

Structural abnormalities

Cystic hygroma

Cystic hygromas are fluid-filled swellings at the back of the fetal neck, which are thought to develop as a result of a defect in the formation of lymphatic vessels. It is likely that the lymphatic and venous systems fail to connect, with lymph accumulating in the jugular lymph sacs. They are often associated with cardiac and renal abnormalities, and may manifest alongside oedema, ascites and pleural and pericardial effusions. They are also frequently associated with chromosomal abnormalities, and so prenatal karyotyping should be discussed and offered to parents. 'Isolated cystic hygromas' may be corrected surgically after birth and have a good prognosis; in cases of generalized fetal hydrops, however, the outlook is poor.

Congenital heart disease

This is one of the most common congenital malformations in children, affecting just under 1% of live births. In most cases there is no obvious cause; however, associated risk factors include family history, type 2 diabetes, maternal infection with rubella or cytomegalovirus (CMV), chromosomal abnormalities including the trisomies, and drugs, including some anticonvulsants, alcohol and lithium. Antenatal detection rates vary. Forty to fifty percent of major abnormalities may be identified on the cardiac four-chamber view, including ventriculoseptal defect, ventricular hypoplasia (Fig. 24.7), valvular incompetence and arrhythmias. Scanning to include the outflow tracts will increase detection, identifying problems

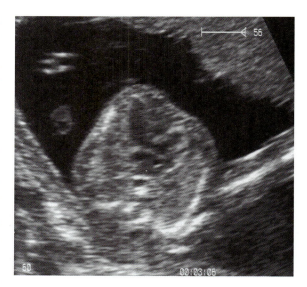

Fig. 24.7   Hypoplastic right heart. The normal four-chamber view is not obtained. The baby died in the early neonatal period.

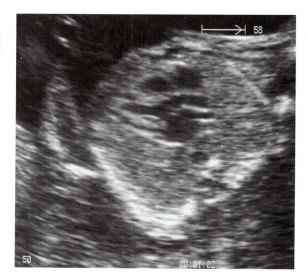

Fig. 24.8   Aorta. The aorta in this normal heart is seen to be arising exclusively from the left ventricle, excluding the diagnosis of tetralogy of Fallot.

such as tetralogy of Fallot and transposition of the great vessels (Fig. 24.8).

Neural tube defects

The neural tube is formed from the closing of the neural folds, with both anterior and posterior neuropores closed by 6 weeks' gestation (Fig. 24.9). Failure of closure of the anterior neuropore results in anencephaly (40%) or encephalocele (5%), with failure of the posterior neuropores to close

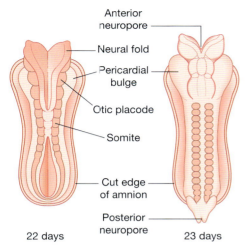

Anterior
neuropore

Neural fold

Pericardial
bulge

Otic placode

Somite

Cut edge
of amnion

Posterior
neuropore

22 days   23 days

**Fig. 24.9   Dorsal view of embryo on days 22 and 23,
demonstrating neural tube closure.**

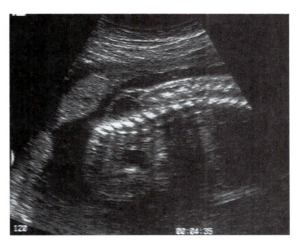

Fig. 24.11   Spina bifida. There is a large lumbosacral
defect, with the sac of the myelomeningocele clearly
visible.

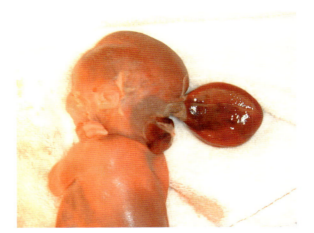

Fig. 24.10   Encephalocele. There is a defect in the
posterior aspect of the skull, allowing brain tissue to
herniate into the sac.

resulting in spina bifida (55%). The overall incidence of all
neural tube defects is around 1:1000.

Anencephaly

This is characterized by the absence of the cerebral hemi-
spheres and cranial vault giving rise to prominent orbits and
a typical 'frog-like' appearance on ultrasound. Most of those
affected will be stillborn, with the remainder dying shortly
after birth.

Encephalocele

This describes the protrusion of the dura mater sac (with
or without brain tissue) through a bony defect in the cranial
vault (Fig. 24.10). The majority are occipital. Prognosis
depends on the presence on brain tissue within the sac and
the degree of resultant herniation.

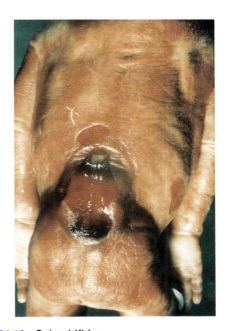

Fig. 24.12   Spina bifida.

Spina bifida

This is the commonest central nervous system malformation,
resulting from the failure of closure of the neural groove.
Lesions may be open or closed, closed defects having a
skin covering, and may take the form of a meningocele or
myelomeningocele. In a meningocele, the meninges of the
neural tissue bulge through a posterior wall defect, whereas in
a myelomeningocele there is additional involvement of neural
tissue (Figs 24.11 and 24.12). Scalloping of the frontal bones
gives rise to the typical 'lemon' sign seen on ultrasound, and
the descent of the cerebellum, pons and medulla through the
foramen magnum results in a 'banana' shape to the cerebellum

also visible on ultrasound. The extent of the associated disability depends on the site and size of the defect and can include abnormalities in lower limb neurology including paralysis, with bladder and bowel dysfunction. Intelligence can be normal, although this is difficult to predict antenatally and depends in part on the degree of ventriculomegaly.

The protective effect of pre-conceptual folic acid is well established, and all women planning pregnancy are advised to take 0.4 mg daily for at least a month prior to conception. Women at increased risk of neural tube defects, for example those with type 2 diabetes, a raised body mass index or on antiepileptic medications are advised to take a higher dose of 5 mg daily.

Ventriculomegaly

In a normal fetus the mean size of the lateral ventricles is 7 mm. Ventriculomegaly refers to an increase in this size over 10 mm and is thought to affect up to 1% of pregnancies. In some cases this is in association with other structural or chromosomal abnormalities and detection should prompt discussion regarding possible karyotyping and serial scanning to look for the development of any structural anomalies which may not have been obvious on previous scans. Normal development is very common, but not necessarily predictable from the degree of dilatation.

Hydrocephalus

This occurs when an accumulation of cerebrospinal fluid (CSF) leads to dilation of the ventricular system. For diagnosis, the lateral ventricles should have a lateral atrial diameter over 15 mm with anterior displacement of the choroid plexus. The three main forms are aqueductal stenosis, communicating hydrocephalus and Dandy-Walker syndrome. Outcome is variable and depends on the severity of the hydrocephalus, as well as the presence of other abnormalities.

Abdominal wall defects

Exomphalos (omphalocele)

This occurs following failure of the bowel to return to the abdominal cavity at 8 weeks' gestation, resulting in a midline defect through which the peritoneal sac protrudes (Fig. 24.13 A,B). In some cases the sac contains small bowel or liver. Exomphalos affects 1:5000 pregnancies and in 30% of cases is associated with chromosomal abnormalities, especially trisomy 18. Ten to fifty percent of cases occur in conjunction with other structural abnormalities, in particular cardiac and renal problems. Management should involve the offer of karyotyping and increased surveillance due to the increased risk of intrauterine death.

Gastroschisis

This occurs in 1:2500–3000 pregnancies and is associated with a young maternal age, smoking and recreational drug

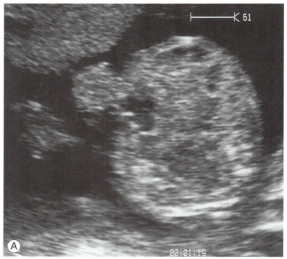

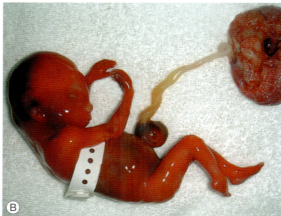

Fig. 24.13 **(A and B) Small exomphalos in a fetus terminated for multiple abnormalities.**

misuse (Fig. 24.14). It is a paraumbilical defect through which the gastrointestinal organs, usually bowel, herniate allowing them to float freely in the amniotic fluid. There is no increased chance of chromosomal abnormality and concurrent structural defects are rare. There is, however, an association with bowel atresia and affected babies tend to be small for gestational age, requiring increased surveillance. With early surgical correction the prognosis is good, although 10% of affected pregnancies will result in stillbirth.

Genitourinary abnormalities

Multicystic dysplastic kidney disease

This may be unilateral, bilateral or may only affect a small segment of kidney. It occurs in 1:1000 pregnancies and is characterized by the presence of multiple non-communicating cysts (Fig. 24.15). If only one kidney is affected and there is adequate liquor then the prognosis is good; if the disease is bilateral, however, and especially if there is associated

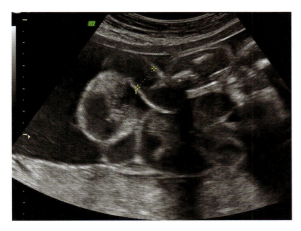

Fig. 24.14 Gastroschisis, with multiple loops of bowel free in the amniotic fluid.

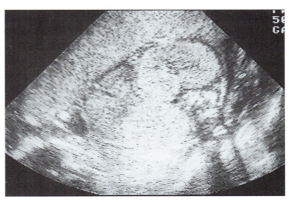

Fig. 24.16 Infantile renal cystic scan. Note anhydramnios and bright renal echoes from the microscopically small cysts.

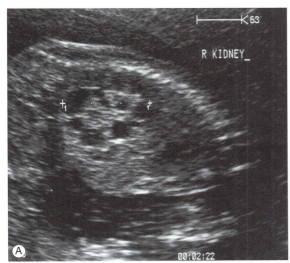

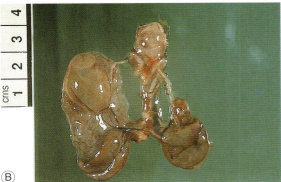

Fig. 24.15 Dysplastic renal scan. Note the enlarged kidney containing fluid-filled cysts: **(A)** ultrasound; **(B)** post-mortem specimen.

oligohydramnios, then the outcome is very poor with a high perinatal mortality.

Polycystic kidney disease

Infantile polycystic kidney disease is characterized by the presence of multiple cysts of various sizes affecting the kidneys bilaterally (Fig. 24.16). The condition has an auto-somal recessive inheritance and expression is variable. Diagnosis is usually made in the antenatal period by the ultrasound findings of bilateral enlarged hyperechoic kidneys, absent bladder and oligohydramnios. Cysts may also be present in the liver and pancreas. Prognosis is poor and long-term survival rare.

Adult polycystic kidney disease is a relatively benign condition which has an autosomal dominant inheritance and is rarely diagnosed until adulthood. Nearly all babies have ultrasonically normal kidneys at birth.

Renal tract dilatation

Dilation of the renal tract may be unilateral or bilateral and can occur at any level of the renal tract (Fig. 24.17). Renal pelvic dilatation or pyelectasis can affect one or both kidneys and is usually due to a neuromuscular defect at the junction of the ureter and renal pelvis. It affects about 2% of pregnancies and presents with increasing pelvic dilatation in the presence of a normal ureter. The majority resolve spontaneously postnatally, although there is an association with postnatal urinary tract infections and reflux nephropathy, and so it is prudent to consider neonatal prophylactic antibiotics in those with marked dilatation and arrange postnatal radiological follow-up.

Hydronephrosis refers to renal pelvic dilation >15 mm and is most commonly caused by ureteric obstruction. It is unilateral in 80–90% and affects males more commonly than females. If the fetal bladder appears normal, the level of obstruction is proximal to the ureterovesical junction.

Bladder dilation is most commonly caused by obstruction from posterior urethral valves, a condition almost exclusively

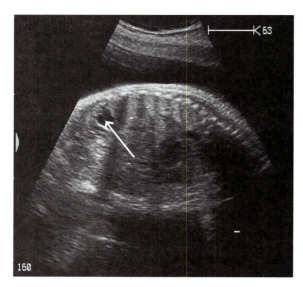

Fig. 24.17   Pyelectasis. The renal pelvis is markedly dilated, although the renal cortex looks well preserved.

affecting males, where folds of mucosa at the bladder neck prevent urine from leaving the bladder. The result is progressive bladder dilatation with hydroureter and hydronephrosis. The kidneys may become dysplastic and the resultant oligohydramnios can lead to problems with lung development. There is the potential for vesicoamniotic shunting, whereby a stent is placed into the fetal bladder to relieve pressure by diverting urine out into the amniotic cavity, although success with this is poor.

Bilateral renal agenesis (Potter syndrome)

Potter syndrome is a lethal condition affecting 1:3000–10000 births. It is characterized by the ultrasound finding of an absent bladder and severe oligohydramnios; confirmation of absent kidneys is often quite challenging due to difficult visualization of the fetal anatomy in the absence of liquor. Without amniotic fluid there is resultant pulmonary hypoplasia and limb deformities.

Lung disorders

Pulmonary hypoplasia

Amniotic fluid is essential for the normal development of the fetal lungs and without it there is a >95% chance of pulmonary hypoplasia, especially with severe oligohydramnios prior to 20 weeks. The causes are variable and include Potter syndrome and pre-term pre-labour rupture of membranes. Pulmonary hypoplasia is also associated with some congenital abnormalities including diaphragmatic hernia and cystic lung lesions.

Diaphragmatic hernia

Congenital diaphragmatic hernia occurs in <1:1000 and is characterized by a defect in the diaphragm, most commonly

on the left, through which the stomach, colon and even the spleen can herniate. The heart is pushed to the right, and the lungs are compressed and may become hypoplastic. The incidence of aneuploidy is 15–30% and there is an association with structural abnormalities including neural tube defects, congenital heart disease and skeletal anomalies. Diagnosis made after 24 weeks and defects occurring on the left side carry a more favourable prognosis; however, polyhydramnios, mediastinal shift and left ventricular compression are associated with a poor outcome. Postnatal surgery is advised soon after delivery to reduce the hernia and correct the defect.

Prenatal congenital infection

Whilst the relative immune suppression of pregnancy affects the maternal response to infection, maternal infections in pregnancy are also important, as some have the potential to affect the fetus. A number of agents are known to be teratogenic, especially if contracted early in pregnancy, whilst others have the potential to cause miscarriage, pre-term labour, severe neonatal sepsis or long-term carrier states. It is worth remembering, however, that infection in itself does not necessarily mean that the baby will be affected.

Infection in general raises the maternal serological level of immunoglobulin G (IgG) and immunoglobulin M (IgM). Maternal IgG crosses the placenta, whilst IgM, a much larger molecule, does not. The fetus does not make IgM until after 20 weeks' gestation and its presence in fetal or early neonatal blood implies infection, although its absence does not always exclude it. In 'high-risk' cases, the detection of pathogenic DNA in fetal blood or amniotic fluid by polymerase chain reaction has revolutionized the specificity of infection detection.

Risk factors

Farm workers are at increased risk of infection with chlamydia and *Listeria*, both of which are associated with miscarriage. Toxoplasma may be acquired from cows, sheep and cats, and certain foods have been implicated in congenital infection, as detailed in Table 24.1

Table 24.1	Foods that carry potential infection risks in pregnancy
Soft cheeses	Unpasteurized milk and its products may contain *Listeria*. Those made from pasteurized milk are safe
Raw eggs	Must be avoided, as there is a risk of salmonella (including puddings)
Meat or pâté	Undercooked meat may transmit toxoplasma or, rarely, *Listeria*
Fruit	This should always be washed before eating as it may be contaminated with salmonella, toxoplasma or one of several intestinal parasites

Specific infections (see also Table 24.2)

Varicella-zoster virus (VZV/chickenpox)

Having usually had chickenpox as a child, the majority of the antenatal population are seropositive for the VZV IgG antibody and so primary infection in pregnancy is rare, affecting around only 1 in 1000. If contracted in pregnancy, the illness tends to be more severe in the mother and may result in pneumonitis. Fetal infection is rare, affecting 1–2%, with no cases documented after 28 weeks. Fetal varicella syndrome is characterized by limb deformity, microcephaly and growth restriction. Maternal infection just prior to delivery may result in neonatal infection, and in some, clinical varicella. If delivery occurs within 5 days of maternal infection, or if the mother develops chickenpox within 2 days of giving birth, the neonate should be given varicella-zoster immunoglobulin and monitored for 2 weeks. If neonatal infection occurs, it should be treated with aciclovir.

Hepatitis

Hepatitis A is not known to cause any significant complication in pregnancy. All women are screened for hepatitis B at booking, with the risk of transmission to the fetus depending on the antigen status. Vertical transmission is most likely to occur with acute infection or in the presence of HBeAg, a marker of high infectivity. Ninety-five percent of cases of transmission occur at delivery. Babies who are considered to be at high risk of acquisition should be given passive hepatitis B immunoglobulin for 24 h after delivery and then immunized. Those at lower risk are simply immunized. There is no routine antenatal screening for hepatitis C, although this should be considered in high-risk women. The risk of vertical transmission is related to viral load, and there is no evidence to suggest that treatment during pregnancy will reduce this risk. Acute infection with hepatitis E in pregnancy is associated with a 15% risk of fulminant liver failure and carries a mortality rate of 5%.

Herpes simplex virus (HSV)

HSV is divided into two subgroups: type 1, which is generally associated with facial lesions and type 2, which predominately affects the genitals. The management of genital herpes in pregnancy is dictated by the gestation at presentation and whether the episode is primary or secondary. Women presenting with primary herpes up to 28 weeks should be treated with aciclovir to limit the duration of symptoms and be reassured that there is no association with congenital abnormalities. Provided that mothers do not labour within 6 weeks of a primary infection, vaginal delivery is advocated and encouraged. The maternal management of primary infection after 28 weeks is unchanged, although women often continue aciclovir until delivery. Delivery, however, should be by elective caesarean section to avoid the potential risk of neonatal transmission. Secondary genital herpes presenting at any gestation is associated with a low risk of neonatal infection and vaginal delivery is encouraged even in the presence of lesions during labour. If recurrent episodes occur during pregnancy, aciclovir suppression from 34 weeks should be considered.

Rubella

As a result of immunization programmes, rubella is rare in the UK, with less than 2% of women susceptible. Infection during pregnancy may result in a collection of abnormalities known as congenital rubella syndrome, with transmission most common in the first trimester. Defects include pulmonary stenosis, patent ductus arteriosus, cataracts, neurodevelopmental delay, microcephaly and sensorineural deafness. If primary infection has occurred in the first 12 weeks of pregnancy, the risk of congenital defects is high and it is reasonable to discuss TOP.

Erythrovirus (parvovirus B19)

Maternal infection is often asymptomatic and diagnosis is made on serological testing, usually following contact with an infected child. Around 50% of the pregnant population will already be immune as a result of past exposure. The risk of transplacental infection increases with gestational age and is associated with miscarriage in the first trimester. After that there is a risk of fetal anaemia, resulting in hydrops (Fig. 24.18) and high-output cardiac failure, although in many cases the consequences may be self-limiting. Middle cerebral artery (MCA) Doppler peak velocity measurements correlate well with the degree of fetal anaemia and can be used to identify those who would benefit from in utero transfusion.

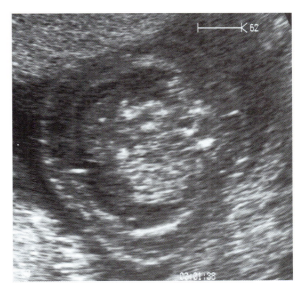

Fig. 24.18 Hydrops fetalis caused by infection with *Erythrovirus*. There are ascites and marked skin oedema in this ultrasound image of a cross-section of the fetal abdomen.

Table 24.2 Infections in pregnancy

Agent	Epidemiology	Maternal features	Fetal, neonatal and infant features	Risk	Treatment/prevention
Rubella	Person-to-person. UK immunity now 97% and congenital infection is rare	Asymptomatic or mild maculopapular rash	Miscarriage, fetal growth restriction, ↓platelets, hepatosplenomegaly, jaundice, deafness, congenital heart disease, mental handicap, cataracts, microphthalmia, microcephaly, cerebral palsy	Risk of affected fetus: <4 weeks 50% 5–8 weeks 25% 9–12 weeks 10% >13 weeks 1%	Consider TOP if <12 weeks Postnatal maternal vaccination if she is not immune
Toxoplasmosis (protozoan-*Toxoplasma gondii*)	From cats, uncooked meats and unwashed fruits	May have fever, rash and lymphadenopathy, but most are asymptomatic	Hydrocephalus, chorioretinitis, intracranial calcification, ↓platelets	<12 weeks: transmission is 10–25%, of which 75% will be severely affected. 12–28 weeks: transmission is 54%, of which 25% will be severely affected. >28 weeks: transmission is 65–90%, of which <10% will be severely affected	Consider TOP only if primary infection <20 weeks
CMV (herpes virus)	Person-to-person	Nearly always asymptomatic	Hepatosplenomegaly, ↓platelets, fetal growth restriction, microcephaly, sensorineural deafness, chorioretinitis, hydrops fetalis, exomphalos, cerebral palsy	40% of fetuses infected. Risk is unaffected by gestation. Of these, 90% are normal at birth, although 20% develop late sequelae. Of the 10% who are symptomatic, 33% die and the rest have long-term problems	Primary infection carries a 10–25% risk of severe abnormality
Erythrovirus	Respiratory transmission	Erythema infectiosum (slapped cheek disease) May be asymptomatic	Aplastic anaemia, hydrops fetalis (Fig. 24.18) and myocarditis ± fetal loss (if <20 weeks). Transmission <20 weeks: ~10%, of which ~10% are lost. If >20 weeks, transmission ~60%, but no adverse effects have been demonstrated	If <20 weeks and the fetus survives the infection (~90%), it is likely to result in a healthy live birth	IUT may be possible to correct hydrops fetalis
Chickenpox (varicella-zoster virus)	Person-to-person	Papules and pustules	Limb hypoplasia, skin scarring, fetal growth restriction, eye abnormalities, neurological abnormalities and hydrops fetalis	25% transmission Probably <1–2% have problems if <20 weeks. No structural problems if >20 weeks See also 'Chickenpox at term' p. 229	Give zoster immunoglobulin to the mother if <10 days from contact or <4 days from onset of rash (although the benefits are not proven)

Listeria monocytogenes

Listeria is a rare bacterial infection transmitted by food, usually soft ripe cheese, paté, cooked–chilled meats and undercooked ready meals. Infection causes a non-specific illness with nausea and vomiting and bacilli cross the placenta, causing amnionitis, pre-term labour or miscarriage. There may be meconium, neonatal jaundice, conjunctivitis or meningoencephalitis. Diagnosis can be made following culture of blood, stool, CSF or placental culture. Treatment is with penicillin.

Beta-haemolytic streptococci – group B

Group B streptococcus is a common vaginal commensal occurring in around 15–20% of pregnant mothers. Colonization with group B streptococci has been linked to pre-term labour, and there is a small chance that the bacteria could be transmitted to the baby during delivery, leading to a serious neonatal infection. Although some countries offer a screening program, the condition does not truly fulfil the recognized criteria for screening, and in the UK intrapartum antibiotics are offered to those known to be colonized, those with risk factors for colonization and those with a previously affected baby.

Syphilis

Whilst congenital syphilis is rare in the UK, it is a significant cause of perinatal morbidity and mortality worldwide. Many of those infected will be unaware of this and testing for syphilis at booking is part of the UK screening programme. The risk of fetal infection increases with gestation and the effects include miscarriage and stillbirth, along with hydrops and growth restriction. There may be deafness and abnormal neurological signs in later life. If diagnosed in pregnancy, syphilis should be treated with penicillin.

Zika

Zika virus disease is a mosquito-borne infection that has gradually spread from a narrow equatorial belt in Africa and Asia across to the Americas, leading to an epidemic in 2015–6. It usually only causes a mild maternal illness but epidemiological and pathological evidence suggests that it may also lead to fetal microcephaly and other fetal neurological problems referred to as congenital Zika syndrome.

The diagnosis of Zika virus infection should be considered among individuals who experience symptoms suggestive of acute Zika virus infection within 2 weeks of leaving an area with active Zika virus transmission or within 2 weeks of sexual contact with a male sexual partner who has recently travelled to such an area. Testing of symptomatic individuals may be possible in some situations, but diagnosis of affected babies can be extremely difficult, especially as microcephaly may only become apparent in the third trimester or even postnatally.

Termination of pregnancy for fetal abnormality

Prenatal diagnoses are often made after 14 weeks of pregnancy and termination is therefore usually medical rather than by surgical means. In the UK, TOP under clause E of the Abortion Act (1967) allows the offer of TOP for fetal anomaly if two registered practitioners agree that a fetal anomaly carries significant risk of serious handicap. Such a consultation requires sensitivity: not all couples will opt for prenatal TOP and it is important that neonatal palliation is discussed as an alternative in such situations. If parents opt for a termination after 22 weeks' gestation, feticide should be offered.

Parents may initially be reluctant to see the baby after delivery but should be strongly encouraged to take the opportunity, and other family members may wish this opportunity too. Photographs and other mementos are extremely important.

Post-mortem examination should be discussed and encouraged, especially if the cause of the anomaly is unknown. If parents decline, they may accept a limited post-mortem investigation with X-rays, clinical photographs and specimens for karyotype studies instead. Follow-up to discuss the results and their implications for subsequent pregnancy is also essential.

Haemolytic disease of the newborn

Haemolytic disease is likely to occur when maternal antibodies develop against fetal red blood cells. Red cells not infrequently cross from the fetus to the mother, either antenatally or at some intrapartum event and, if they are antigenically different from the mother's red cells, there may be a maternal immune response with antibody production. IgG antibodies may cross in the opposite direction, back to the fetus, leading to haemolysis, anaemia, high-output cardiac failure and fetal death. There are numerous known red cell antigens but the rhesus D antigen accounts for approximately 85% of haemolytic disease.

Maternal rhesus alloimmunization exemplifies the achievements of systematic scientific and clinical research. In just 40 years, it has been possible to unravel the pathophysiology, devise useful treatments and introduce an effective means to prevent a condition which had previously caused extensive fetal morbidity and mortality. Among populations with access to an anti-D prophylaxis programme, the fully developed clinical condition of haemolytic disease of the newborn is rare.

The blood group system

Blood groups are determined by antigens on the erythrocyte cell wall. In the ABO system, the letter O is used to refer to those who lack both the A and B antigens. If the mother is group O and the fetus has paternally inherited the A or B antigen, the mother may, if exposed, develop antibodies to these fetal cells. In practice these antibodies rarely cause significant haemolytic disease and no antenatal investigations are warranted.

The next most important system is the rhesus system, which comprises at least 40 antigens, the most important of which are C, D and E. C and E have immunologically distinct isoforms which are designated 'c' and 'e', but it seems unlikely that a 'd' isoform exists. If there is a 'd' antigen, it seems to have little if any immunogenic potential and the notation 'd' is used to indicate the absence of 'D'. A parent contributes one or other antigen (e.g. C or c) to the offspring from each of these three alphabetically designated pairs. An individual can therefore be homozygous or heterozygous for any of the six (e.g. Cde/cDE, cde/cdE). Those who carry the D antigen, which is inherited as autosomal dominant, are referred to as rhesus D positive, whether in the homozygous or heterozygous form.

Any of the rhesus antigens are capable of stimulating antibody formation, but the D antigen is by far the most immunogenic, followed by c and E. If a rhesus-negative mother has a rhesus-positive baby and is at some stage sensitized to the baby's red cells, there is a chance of anti-D antibodies developing against the fetal cells. These antibodies may cross back to the fetus and lead to fetal haemolytic anaemia.

There are other significant antigens in addition to the ABO and rhesus systems. Many of these (e.g. Ce, Fya, Jka, Cw) are poorly developed on the red cell surface and usually stimulate only low levels of antibody production, often of the IgM category (which does not cross the placenta). Some, however, will cause significant haemolytic disease.

One notable exception is the anti-Kell antibody, which has the potential to cause significant fetal anaemia and, along with anti-RhD and anti-Rhc, are the most commonly reported antibodies in cases requiring intrauterine transfusion (IUT). Kell alloimmunization differs from RhD alloimmunization in that the anaemia is not solely due to haemolysis – erythroid suppression has an important role. In addition, past obstetric history cannot be relied on to predict the severity of disease in the current or subsequent pregnancies. Fortunately, the incidence of Kell alloimmunization is low (0.1–0.2%). Since only 9% of the Caucasian population is Kell positive, the majority being heterozygous, the number of cases of haemolytic disease of the newborn is small.

Pathophysiology of haemolytic disease

Exposure to a foreign antigen leads to an antigen-specific antibody response, initially of IgM antibodies, which do not cross the placenta. On subsequent exposure, for example in a second pregnancy, the already primed B cells produce a much larger response, this time of IgG antibodies, which do cross the placenta. In the fetal circulation, an antibody–antigen complex is formed on the red cell membrane, which provokes phagocytosis of the cell by the reticuloendothelial

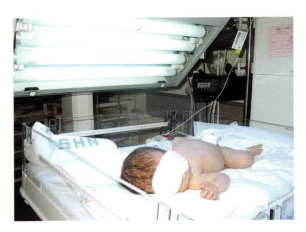

Fig. 24.19 **Baby delivered at 37 weeks because of high anti-D levels.** The bilirubin level rose steeply in the first 24 h but, with phototherapy, exchange transfusion was avoided.

system and results in fetal haemolysis. This will lead to anaemia unless there is sufficient compensatory haemopoiesis from the marrow, spleen and liver.

Increasing anaemia causes progressive fetal hypoxia and acidosis, leading to hepatic and cardiac dysfunction. Generalized oedema of skin develops, as well as ascites, pericardial and pleural effusions. This syndrome is known as 'immune hydrops fetalis' and it is potentially fatal.

Red cell haemolysis results in increased production of bilirubin, most of which passes across the placenta to the mother and is cleared by the maternal system. The fetus therefore does not become jaundiced antenatally, but after delivery its own liver is unable to metabolize bilirubin sufficiently quickly and the neonatal bilirubin level rises (Fig. 24.19). If untreated, the bilirubin can rise to levels which endanger the nervous system, and bilirubin deposition in the basal ganglia leads to a condition known as 'kernicterus'.

Although most fetal bilirubin is readily cleared, some also passes into the fetal urine and then into the amniotic fluid. The level of amniotic bilirubin is therefore an indicator of the severity of the haemolysis.

Incidence

The incidence varies widely. Before the availability of anti-D prophylaxis, rhesus haemolytic disease was common in populations where there was a high prevalence of Rh(D)-negative individuals and where high parity caused an accumulation of alloimmunized women. In the UK, 17% of the population is Rh(D) negative; 55% of Caucasian males are heterozygous for the RhD antigen. Assuming random mating without intervention, around two-thirds of Rh(D)-negative mothers would be expected to carry a rhesus-positive fetus. Approximately 10% of pregnant women are therefore at risk of developing anti-D antibodies.

Since the effective use of prophylactic anti-D, the perinatal mortality from haemolytic disease has fallen from around

46/100 000 to 1.9/100 000. Newly sensitized cases are detected at a rate of approximately 1/1000 maternities.

Aetiology and predisposing factors

Transfer of fetal erythrocytes to the maternal circulation during pregnancy (fetomaternal haemorrhage) may occur without any obvious predisposing event, and about 75% of women may be found to have fetal red cells circulating at some stage during the pregnancy or delivery. Fetomaternal haemorrhage is more likely, however, with disruption of the placental bed, and this may occur with:

- miscarriage and ectopic pregnancy
- invasive intrauterine procedures, e.g. amniocentesis, CVS, fetal shunts
- external cephalic version
- abdominal trauma
- antepartum haemorrhage
- labour and delivery, particularly with delivery of the placenta.

An immune response may, but does not inevitably, follow fetomaternal haemorrhage. The response depends in part on the volume of blood, its antigenic potential, and on the maternal responsiveness. ABO incompatibility between mother and fetus may paradoxically offer some protection, as the transfused cells are likely to be haemolysed by circulating maternal antibodies, reducing the risk of immunization. This observation illustrates the mechanism for the use of prophylactic anti-D immunoglobulin, in that exogenous anti-D is used to bind and lyse any rhesus-positive fetal red cells that reach the maternal circulation.

Prevention of haemolytic disease

The most effective preventive measure is the use of intramuscular anti-D to provide passive immunization of non-sensitized women around the time of exposure. A rhesus-negative mother who has a potentially sensitizing event (see Box 24.2) before 20 weeks' gestation should be given 250 IU of anti-D as soon as possible after the event, and certainly within 72 h if possible. At more than 20 weeks, the dose is 500 IU. At delivery a sample of fetal cord blood should be rhesus grouped and, if positive, a film made of the mother's blood for Kleihauer testing. The Kleihauer test estimates the volume of fetomaternal transfusion and allows an appropriate dose of anti-D to be calculated.

Immunization can occur as a result of silent fetomaternal haemorrhage, therefore, prophylaxis is likely to be more effective if anti-D is given to all non-sensitized rhesus-negative mothers routinely in the third trimester (either 500 IU at 28 and 34 weeks, or a single larger dose early in the third trimester). This is standard practice in most areas.

Surprisingly, there is some evidence of benefit from anti-D prophylaxis even for women already mildly sensitized, in that subsequent children appear less severely affected by haemolytic disease than would otherwise have been expected.

Box 24.2

Indications for anti-D immunoprophylaxis
First trimester
- Ectopic pregnancy
- Surgical or medical TOP
- Miscarriage with heavy loss or requiring surgical evacuation of the uterus
- CVS

Second trimester
- Amniocentesis
- Threatened miscarriage or antepartum haemorrhage
- Abdominal trauma

Third trimester
- Routine prophylaxis
- Antepartum haemorrhage
- External cephalic version
- Delivery
- Abdominal trauma

Table 24.3	Possible screening programme for antibodies in haemolytic disease of the newborn
All pregnant women	Offer ABO and RhD group and antibody screen at booking and again at 28 weeks' gestation
Patients identified with significant alloantibodies (e.g. anti-D, c or Kell related	Consider paternal or fetal genotyping. Frequency of further screening ± antibody titre and quantification depends on antibody and titre

Prediction of at-risk pregnancies

Routine maternal screening

All pregnant women at their first visit have serum sent for ABO and Rh(D) grouping with screening for irregular antibodies. The maternal serum level of any antibody discovered (usually anti-D) is used as an initial screening test for further action. There are regional variations, but an example of when to check for antibody levels is shown in Table 24.3.

Having identified an irregular antibody in the maternal circulation, the next stage is to assess the likely rhesus status of the baby by establishing the genotype of the putative father and remembering that the D antigen is inherited as an autosomal dominant. If the father is found to be d/d, it is likely that anti-D antibodies in a rhesus-negative woman have developed from exposure to some other source of incompatible red cells, for example a previous blood transfusion or the fetus of a previous partner. Assuming confident paternity, the fetus will be unaffected and further specific action is unnecessary. If the father is homozygous for the D antigen, it follows that the fetus will also be rhesus D positive and will be at risk of haemolytic disease. Where the father is believed to be D/d, half of his offspring will be rhesus positive. In this situation it is important to establish the fetal blood group to determine whether or not the pregnancy is at risk. This can be done non-invasively by examining cffDNA present in a maternal blood sample. Accuracies of around 96% are reported for RhD genotyping. DNA amplification of amniotic fluid should only be performed for fetal genotyping if the patient is already undergoing amniocentesis for other indications.

Clinical significance of the antibody

Red cell antigens vary in their likelihood of stimulating an immune response, with the D antigen being the most immunogenic. Apart from c and Kell, most of the other antigens are less likely to lead to significant clinical problems and are not discussed further in this section. The D antibody titre in maternal serum and an actual quantification (level) can be measured. The level is recognized to correlate well with disease severity. Severe disease is rare if the maternal antibody level is <4 IU/mL and additional specific intervention is probably not required. The risk of significant problems is only moderate between 4 and 15 IU/mL, but above 15 IU/mL there is a risk of severe anaemia in 50% of fetuses. These higher levels call for further investigation, described later, and the management of these relatively uncommon cases should be centralized within specialized units. A sudden rise in levels, rather than a particular absolute level, is also likely to be significant.

Fetal assessment and therapy

Clinical symptoms and signs of fetal haemolytic anaemia occur late, are easily missed and are of little help in management. In advanced disease, fetal movements are reduced or even absent, and there may be fetal growth restriction. In severe cases, there may be fetal hydrops with signs of ascites, pericardial and pleural effusions, and oedema of the skin. Polyhydramnios, which is associated with fetal hydrops, may also be detected. Cardiotocography may reveal an unreactive pattern or even decelerations, but again only in advanced disease. A sinusoidal fetal heart pattern is thought to be fairly specific for severe anaemia. All of the above represent the 'end-stage' of the process of progressive fetal anaemia. It is critical in the management of known alloimmunized pregnancies to detect the fetus that will benefit from intrauterine therapy before the fetal condition is seriously compromised. A rise in antibody titre or quantification should prompt non-invasive monitoring, as described next.

Non-invasive testing

Historically, serial amniocentesis and measurement of amniotic fluid bilirubin levels was the method of assessing at-risk pregnancies. However, this has been superseded by non-invasive testing utilizing fetal MCA Doppler studies (Fig. 24.20). A hyperkinetic circulation correlates very well with the degree of fetal anaemia, and can be used to predict the requirement for further therapy. Table 24.4 indicates the level for different antibodies at which there is a moderate or severe risk of anaemia, and once these levels are reached MCA Doppler monitoring should be commenced. The peak

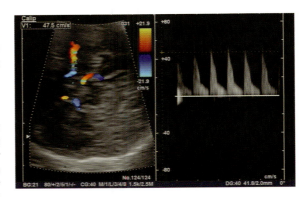

Fig. 24.20 **Measuring the blood velocity in the fetal MCA correlates very well with the level of fetal anaemia.** This non-invasive assessment can be used to determine the need for IUT.

Table 24.4	Risk of fetal anaemia according to antibody quantification/titre		
	Antibody level		
Risk of fetal anaemia	**Anti-D (IU/mL)**	**Anti-c (IU/mL)**	**Anti-K (titre)**
Low	0–4	0–7.5	<1:8
Moderate	4–15	7.5–20	
High	>15	>20	≥1:8

systolic velocity of the MCA is measured and, if >1.5 multiples of the median for gestational age, is predictive of moderate-to-severe fetal anaemia in 100% of cases for a false positive rate of 12%. The test is reliable up to 34 weeks' gestation. Once moderate-to-severe anaemia is predicted, intrauterine therapy should commence. Non-invasive monitoring with MCA Doppler avoids the procedure-related loss rate associated with amniocentesis and exacerbation of the degree of sensitization that results from invasive procedures.

Fetal blood sampling and intrauterine transfusion

Access to the fetal circulation is achieved by inserting a needle into the baby's cord, ideally at its point of placental insertion (Fig. 24.21) or, alternatively, the intrahepatic portion of the umbilical vein. This enables an immediate haemoglobin (or haematocrit) estimation to be made and facilitates simultaneous IUT of blood. Group O rhesus-negative blood is cross-matched to the mother's own serum prior to the procedure and, if the haemoglobin/haematocrit is low, a calculated volume can be transfused during the same sampling procedure. IUT carries the risk of cord haematoma, fetal bradycardia, intrauterine death, and further sensitization of the mother-to-fetal red cell antigens. A procedure-related loss rate in the region of 1% is quoted. It is likely that multiple IUTs will be required owing to the relentlessly progressive anaemia that occurs in alloimmunized pregnancies.

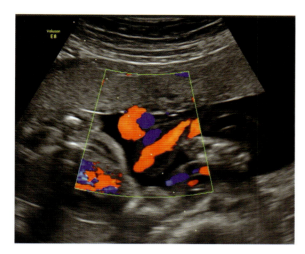

Fig. 24.21   The needle is best inserted into the umbilical vein at the point where the cord is inserted into the placenta.

If an intravascular transfusion is technically too difficult, for example at very early gestations (<18 weeks), it is possible to inject the red cells directly into the peritoneal cavity, from which they are subsequently absorbed by the fetal lymphatic system. This results in a slower increase in fetal haematocrit than direct intravascular transfusion.

Additional measures

In severe early cases, when hydropic change occurs before fetal transfusion is technically possible, repeated maternal plasma exchange may reduce the levels of maternal antibody. The technique requires special equipment to separate red cells from plasma and is both time-consuming and expensive. Maternal immunosuppression has also been tried in very severe cases.

Delivery

All babies with haemolytic disease should be delivered in a specialist unit with full neonatal intensive care facilities. If ultrasound assessment is normal and the antibody level relatively low, a conservative approach with delivery at term is appropriate. If premature delivery is anticipated, maternal corticosteroid therapy is warranted. Babies in whom mild anaemia is suspected, or who have been successfully treated with IUT, can be delivered vaginally, unless there are other obstetric indications for caesarean section. For cases managed with IUT, labour is induced at around 35 weeks' gestation. If a hydropic fetus requires delivery, this should be by caesarean section. Experienced paediatric attendance at delivery is essential and cord blood must be collected for assessment of haemoglobin, platelets, blood grouping, bilirubin and direct Coombs testing. The neonate may require intensive support with measures to control anaemia, hyperbilirubinaemia and any associated cardiorespiratory problems.

Prognosis

For mildly affected fetuses, in whom intrauterine therapy is unnecessary, the outlook, in experienced units, is excellent. Survival rates for non-hydropic fetuses undergoing IUT are ≥90%, compared with approximately 75% if hydrops is present.

Early reports suggested serious neurological impairments, including cerebral palsy, abnormal development and hearing problems, especially in those children who were transfused in utero. Recent experience is very much more reassuring and suggests there are few, if any, additional risks beyond the well-recognized hazards of prematurity.

Key *points*

- Approximately 2% of newborn babies have a serious abnormality detectable at, or soon after, birth. Many of these can be diagnosed antenatally.
- There are a number of different strategies for prenatal screening programmes to detect chromosomal and structural abnormalities. Adequate verbal and written information is essential prior to undertaking screening.
- Parents are often confronted with difficult decisions. Explanations may need to be repeated and often involve experts from several disciplines.
- Isoimmunization occurs when maternal antibodies develop against fetal red blood cells. These antibodies cross to the fetus and may lead to haemolysis, anaemia, high-output cardiac failure and fetal death. There are numerous known red cell antigens, but the rhesus D antigen accounts for more than 85% of haemolytic disease.
- Entry of fetal cells to the maternal circulation is particularly likely with disruption of the placental bed, for example with antepartum haemorrhage. Passive immunization with anti-D IgG prevents sensitization in most cases.
- Appropriately regular serological screening of all pregnant women for irregular antibodies is essential to ensure timely detection of isoimmune fetal haemolytic disease.
- Treatment of severe disease is highly specialized and requires referral to appropriately experienced units. Assessment involves the use of Doppler ultrasound, and when fetal anaemia is suspected, fetal therapy with IUT is possible.

25

Obstetric haemorrhage

Introduction

Obstetric haemorrhage is one of the leading causes of maternal mortality worldwide, and even in the more developed healthcare settings, with ready access to resuscitation, uterotonics, blood transfusion and surgery, deaths still occur. Haemorrhage may be of rapid onset. It is important to recognize its severity promptly, institute effective therapy and keep ahead of the blood loss via intravascular volume replacement.

In mid-trimester, most women will have undergone ultrasound to assess placental site but, despite this, a vaginal examination (PV) should not be performed in the presence of antepartum vaginal bleeding without first excluding placenta praevia (PP) – 'No PV until no PP'. This will usually involve confirming placental site from an earlier ultrasound.

Definitions

Vaginal bleeding associated with intrauterine pregnancy is divided into the following categories:

- threatened miscarriage – up to 24 weeks' gestation
- antepartum haemorrhage (APH) – from 24 weeks' gestation until the onset of labour
- intrapartum haemorrhage – from the onset of labour until the end of the second stage
- postpartum haemorrhage (PPH) – from the third stage of labour until the end of the puerperium (6 weeks after delivery).

Antepartum haemorrhage

APH affects 3–5% of pregnancies. Placental abruption and placenta praevia are the most important causes of APH but are not the commonest. The majority of APH remain unexplained after clinical and ultrasound examination. The magnitude of APH can be usefully classified as follows; minor APH is <50 mL and stopped, major APH is 50–1000 mL and no hypovolaemic shock, massive APH is >1000 mL and/or hypovolaemic shock.

Causes

APH is further classified according to the source of the bleeding.

Local

There may be bleeding from the woman's vulva, vagina or cervix. Bleeding from the cervix is not uncommon in pregnancy and may follow sexual intercourse (post-coital bleeding). A cervical ectropion or benign polyp is often found, and rarely a diagnosis of cervical carcinoma is made. The passing of a blood-stained 'show', mucus along with a small amount of blood, may herald the onset of labour as the cervix becomes effaced.

Placental

Placenta praevia

This is when the placenta encroaches upon the lower segment of the uterus, with the lower segment arbitrarily defined by ultrasound scanning as extending 5 cm from the internal cervical os. Placenta praevia is more common among women with a previous caesarean section, but the majority of women with placenta praevia have no discernible risk factors. Transvaginal ultrasound is a reliable and safe method of determining the distance between the edge of the placenta and the internal os. Placenta praevia is classified as major or minor, or graded I–IV (Table 25.1, Fig. 25.1).

Haemorrhage in labour is inevitable in the presence of a major placenta praevia, but it may be possible to deliver safely vaginally with a minor degree of praevia. In the assessment of suitability for a vaginal birth, engagement of the presenting part is important together with the actual distance of the placenta from the internal os determined by ultrasound (Fig. 25.2). Women with pregnancies where the placental edge is not at least 2 cm from the internal os are not recommended to deliver vaginally. Placental location is routinely determined at the time of the fetal anomaly scan at 18–22 weeks and may be found to be 'low lying' at that stage. As the uterus grows from the lower segment upwards, the placenta appears to move upwards with advancing gestation. Approximately 2% of pregnancies with a low-lying placenta before 24 weeks, 5% of those at 24–29 weeks and 25% of those at >30 weeks will have a placenta praevia at term. This is not a reflection of placental migration, but simply a feature of uterine growth. When a low-lying placenta is detected on ultrasound scanning early in pregnancy, it is necessary to repeat the scan early in the third trimester and then review the management if the placenta praevia is present.

The risk of placenta praevia is of a sudden, unpredictable, major or massive haemorrhage, and some clinicians advocate

Table 25.1		Classification of placenta praevia
Minor	I	Encroaches the lower uterine segment
	II	Reaches internal os of the cervix (marginal)
Major	III	Covers part of internal os (partial)
	IV	Completely covers the internal os (complete)

hospital admission from 30–32 weeks onwards, so that facilities for resuscitation and delivery are immediately available. This can be difficult for the woman and her family. Outpatient management is frequently undertaken, particularly for those who have had no bleeding (placenta praevia, an incidental ultrasound finding) or just light bleeding, and who live close to the hospital with good support and transport availability. Elective delivery is usually planned for 38–39 weeks, but will be earlier if there is a major or massive haemorrhage.

Caesarean section in the presence of placenta praevia should be directly supervised by, or performed by, a senior obstetrician, since a large blood loss is frequently encountered due to the relatively poor capacity of the lower segment of the uterus to contract.

Anterior placenta praevia in the presence of a history of one or more caesarean sections predisposes the woman to a morbidly adherent placenta (abnormally invasive placenta or placenta accreta), where the placenta invades the myometrium and cannot be readily separated from the uterus following delivery. Such abnormal placentation is usually diagnosed with ultrasound antenatally and magnetic resonance imaging is also used to evaluate the presence and degree of invasion. The presence of a morbidly adherent placenta markedly increases the risk of massive PPH and a multidisciplinary approach to delivery is recommended. Stopping the massive PPH may require hysterectomy and women should be warned of this possibility prior to delivery by caesarean section.

Placental abruption

Placental abruption is defined as retroplacental haemorrhage (bleeding between the placenta and the uterus) and usually involves some degree of placental separation. Its management depends on the amount of bleeding, presence or absence of maternal haemodynamic compromise, the maturity of the fetus and its condition. Separation of the placenta results in a reduced area for gas exchange between the fetal and maternal circulations predisposing to fetal hypoxia and acidosis. It is crucial to remember that with placental abruption the amount of 'revealed' blood (bleeding from the vagina) may not reflect the total blood loss and a woman may have considerable retroplacental bleeding without any external loss at all – a 'concealed abruption', the most hazardous type of abruption (Fig. 25.3).

History of a previous pregnancy affected by placental abruption and maternal cigarette smoking are among the risk factors for placental abruption, but the majority of

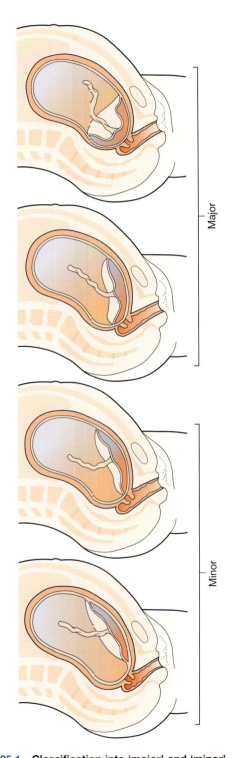

Fig. 25.1   Classification into 'major' and 'minor' placenta praevia depends on the distance of the placenta from the internal os of the cervix. In the presence of a caesarean section scar, an anterior placenta praevia may result in abnormal invasion (morbidly adherent placenta, placenta accreta).

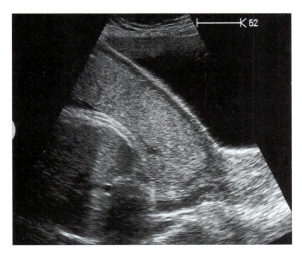

Fig. 25.2 Transabdominal ultrasound scan of an anterior placenta praevia extending to just beyond the internal os.

placental abruptions occur by chance in women without identifiable risk factors.

Light bleeding from the edge of a normally situated placenta does not normally compromise the fetus. A brief episode of inpatient observation and often surveillance of subsequent fetal growth with ultrasound fetal biometry is appropriate. Repeated episodes of placental abruption may lead to a decision to deliver early.

Major revealed haemorrhage is obvious, and urgent delivery is usually required. A major concealed abruption is inferred from the degree of pain, uterine tenderness and evidence of hypovolaemic shock; urgent delivery may be required. The decision between vaginal delivery and caesarean section is influenced by the degree of bleeding, and maternal and fetal conditions.

If intrauterine fetal death is diagnosed, vaginal delivery is to be preferred, if safe to do so, as the mother should not be subjected to an avoidable caesarean section. However, in such a situation it is likely that there will have been a major degree of blood loss. Hypovolaemic shock may develop and may progress to multisystem organ failure if not corrected. In addition, release of thromboplastins from the damaged placenta may lead to disseminated intravascular coagulation (DIC) with depletion of platelets, fibrinogen and other clotting factors. Waiting for vaginal delivery therefore carries risks, and caesarean section may occasionally be indicated to minimize these systemic maternal risks. Deciding on the appropriate mode of delivery is further complicated by the risks of carrying out an operation in the presence of DIC.

Less severe degrees of placental separation can still be associated with fetal compromise. The woman usually describes pain and frequent contractions, the contractions precipitated by irritation of the myometrium from the retro-placental clot. The fetal heart rate will often show a suspicious or pathological pattern which may progress to a fetal

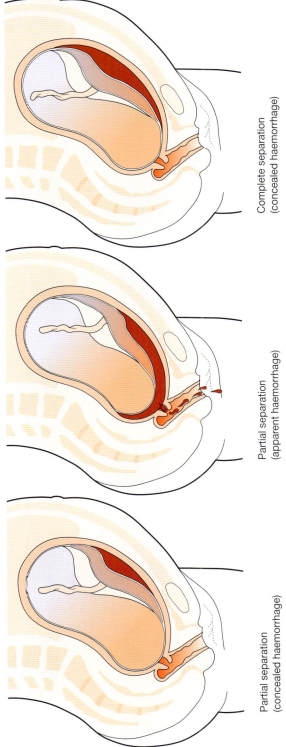

Fig. 25.3 Classification of placental abruption.

bradycardia and fetal death unless delivery is expedited. Placental abruption predisposes the mother to PPH. The adage 'abruption kills the baby but the PPH kills the mother', fortunately, is experienced only rarely in modern obstetric practice, but to remember it serves the obstetrician well.

Unexplained antepartum haemorrhage

In the majority of cases a specific explanation for the APH is not found. Bleeding with no explanation is the commonest clinical scenario and, in the absence of maternal or fetal compromise, is managed expectantly. Unexplained APH, especially if more than one episode (recurrent unexplained APH), is a recognized risk factor for subsequent poor fetal growth and additional ultrasound surveillance is recommended.

Clinical presentations

Bleeding can be spotting (minor staining of underwear or sanitary protection), minor, major or massive, and can occur with or without pain. Other than in circumstances of spotting that has stopped, admission to hospital is advised, as even minor bleeding may herald heavier bleeding.

An attempt should be made to determine the cause of the bleeding. In practice, history and initial examination are carried out simultaneously. It is relevant to ask when the bleeding started, how much blood has been lost, and when the baby was last felt to move. Observation will tell if the mother is in pain, which suggests abruption or labour, and there may be visible blood on the bed, her legs or the floor. If the mother is pale, with low blood pressure and rapid pulse, there is probably hypovolaemic shock. With an abruption, the uterus is typically hard and tender ('Couvelaire' uterus) and the fetal heartbeat may be absent. There may be frequent contractions or continuous pain. When the bleeding is from a placenta praevia, the uterus is usually soft, the presenting part will usually be free, and the fetal heartbeat is usually present. Subsequent management depends on the estimated severity of haemorrhage.

Minor haemorrhage with a soft uterus and normal cardiotocography

An ultrasound scan should be arranged to determine the placental site (if not already established by an earlier scan) and, providing the placenta is not praevia, a speculum examination should be performed to look for cervical efface-ment or dilatation, an ectropion or a cervical polyp. If all is normal, it is common practice to admit the woman at least until the bleeding stops. However, most clinicians will not admit the woman if the bleeding is minor and clearly seen to be coming from an ectropion. Women who are rhesus negative are advised to receive prophylactic anti-D.

If there is a placenta praevia and the pregnancy is at more than 37–38 weeks' gestation, it is reasonable to arrange for delivery by caesarean section. If less than this gestation, a conservative approach is usually appropriate.

Minor or major haemorrhage, but with a hard, tender uterus

The diagnosis is probably a placental abruption (concealed and revealed) and management revolves around maternal resuscitation, correction of hypovolaemia, coagulation defects, and evaluation of the fetal condition by cardio-tocography. Prompt delivery is highly likely to be appropriate; the route of delivery will be influenced by a number of factors, including evidence of fetal compromise and the presence or absence of maternal coagulopathy.

Antepartum haemorrhage requiring maternal resuscitation

Whether the diagnosis is placenta praevia or an abruption, such a massive APH is highly likely to prompt delivery almost irrespective of gestational age.

Intrapartum haemorrhage

Abnormal bleeding during labour should be distinguished from a 'show' that may occur during cervical dilatation. In a previously low-risk pregnancy, intrapartum bleeding is considered to be an indication for continuous electronic fetal monitoring.

Causes

Placental abruption

Placental abruption (see earlier) can occur during labour and should be particularly considered if the uterus does not relax between contractions.

Placenta praevia

As the cervix dilates, so the placenta separates from the uterine wall and typically painless bleeding occurs.

Uterine rupture

Uterine rupture is relatively rare, and is discussed on page 334.

Vasa praevia

This is relatively rare, and occurs when the umbilical cord vessels run in the fetal membranes and cross the internal os of the cervix. These vessels may rupture spontaneously in early labour or be ruptured at the time of amniotomy and this may lead to fetal exsanguination. It may be that the cord is inserted into the membranes rather than directly into the placenta (type 1 vasa praevia, Fig. 25.4), or that the vessels are running from the placenta to a separate succenturiate placental lobe (type 2 vasa praevia). The condition typically presents as a pathological cardiotocography (CTG) or fetal death following a minor intrapartum haemorrhage. In the presence of an APH, diagnostic tests to differentiate fetal from maternal blood are seldom reliable and the baby is usually delivered urgently by caesarean section because of

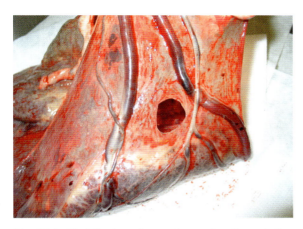

Fig. 25.4 Umbilical cord vessels running through the membranes. If these vessels overlie the internal cervical os, it is termed 'vasa praevia'.

the fetal compromise. The diagnosis of vasa praevia is often only made retrospectively, by examination of the placenta and membranes. Although it is possible to diagnose the condition antenatally with colour flow Doppler ultrasound, routine screening for vasa praevia is not established practice.

Postpartum haemorrhage

It is not possible to predict which women will have a PPH, and it is important to appreciate that a major haemorrhage can very rapidly lead to maternal death. Anticipation of PPH and an awareness of the relevant interventions is essential.

Definitions

There is inevitably some bleeding during the third stage of a labour, usually around 200–300 mL following a vaginal birth.

- A primary PPH is defined as a blood loss of 500 mL or more within 24 h of delivery. The PPH is 'minor' if blood loss is 500–1000 mL with no hypovolaemic shock, 'major' if >1000 mL and continuing or associated with hypovolaemic shock.
- A secondary PPH is any significant loss between 24 h and 12 weeks after the birth.

Primary postpartum haemorrhage

This occurs in around 5% of all deliveries. It is more common in grand multiparity (four deliveries or more); women over 35 years of age; women with a body mass index of over 35; multiple pregnancy; women with fibroids; placenta praevia; and in those who have had a long labour or an instrumental delivery. It may also follow an APH and is more likely in women with a past history of primary PPH. Women with risk factors for PPH are advised to give birth in a consultant-led unit.

Prevention

It is important to treat anaemia in the antenatal period (haematinic supplements), particularly if the woman has risk factors for PPH. It is recommended practice to give a uterotonic (typically Syntocinon 10 IU IM) with delivery of the baby's anterior shoulder; such 'active management' of the third stage of labour is associated with a lower incidence of primary PPH.

Causes

The causes of primary PPH are often recalled as the 'four Ts': i.e. 'Tone' (poor uterine contractility or atony); 'Trauma', e.g. perineal tears; 'Thrombin' (coagulopathy) and 'Tissue', e.g. retained placental tissue inhibiting uterine contractility.

- *Atony*: this is the most common cause of primary PPH (90%). Normally, contraction of the uterus in the third stage of labour causes compression of intramyometrial blood vessels, and bleeding from the placental site stops promptly (Fig. 25.5). If there is uterine atony, this compression does not occur. Atony can occur following delivery of the entire placenta (the myometrium simply does not contract sufficiently well) or when part or all of the placenta is retained. The physical presence of placental tissue prevents effective uterine contraction and the partial placental separation results in bleeding from the placental bed.
- *Trauma*: bleeding may be from an episiotomy, a vaginal tear, cervical laceration (Fig. 25.6) or a rupture of the uterine wall. Lacerations of the genital tract are more common after an instrumental delivery.
- *Coagulation problems*: usually DIC. DIC can occur in association with a number of different causes including maternal sepsis, placental abruption and PPH, where the blood loss causes the DIC and the DIC exacerbates the blood loss.
- *Multiple causes*: may be present, necessitating a systematic approach to the woman experiencing a primary PPH, e.g. uterine atony in association with retained placental tissue.

Clinical presentation

The bleeding is usually obvious, but, occasionally, an atonic uterus can fill up without obvious external loss and the first sign of the PPH is hypovolaemic shock. A less dramatic, prolonged trickling of blood may go unnoticed, the significance of which may not be initially appreciated. With blood-soaked pads and bedding, it is common to underestimate the loss.

The key questions are:

1. Has the placenta been delivered and is it complete?
2. Is the uterus firmly contracted?
3. If so, is the bleeding due to trauma?

Management

A reassuring presence is important. PPH is a common obstetric emergency but it is stressful to the mother and

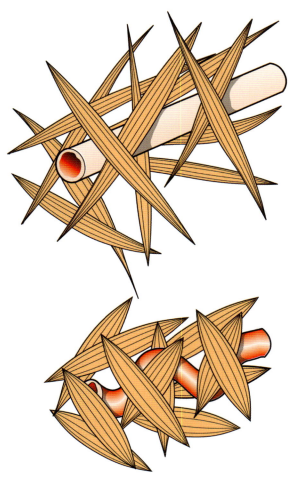

Fig. 25.5   Postpartum haemostasis is principally achieved by the contracting myometrial fibres constricting the blood vessels within the uterine wall.

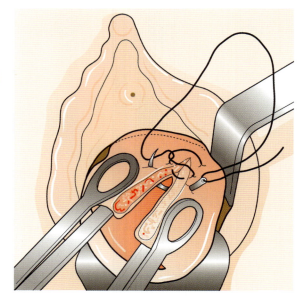

Fig. 25.6   Cervical lacerations may cause a primary PPH.

her birth partner. Ensure appropriate numbers, skill mix and expertise of staff are in attendance or are *en route*.

Assessment

- Make an estimate of the loss.
- Determine the pulse and blood pressure.
- Palpate the abdomen to assess the size and tone of the uterus.

Treatment

- If the uterus is atonic, a contraction can be 'rubbed up' by abdominal massage. Bimanual compression may also be performed (Fig. 25.7).
- Intravenous (IV) access should be established with two wide-bore cannulae and blood taken for haemoglobin concentration, platelet count, blood clotting and a red cell cross-match (the number of units depends on volume lost).

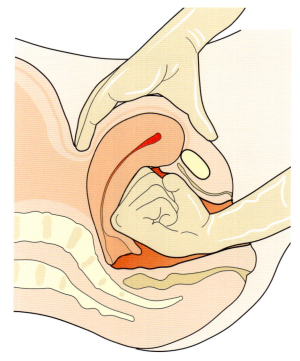

Fig. 25.7   Bimanual compression is often effective in the initial management of primary PPH.

- An IV bolus of Syntocinon 5–10 IU should be given to further contract the uterus, followed by a Syntocinon infusion.
- Crystalloid and/or colloid up to 3.5 L should be rapidly infused to maintain the circulating volume. With

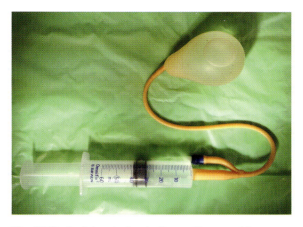

Fig. 25.8 **An intrauterine balloon often provides effective uterine tamponade in atonic PPH.**

rapid blood loss, O rhesus-negative blood may need to be given. A urinary catheter should be inserted to measure urine output and avoid a full bladder becoming an obstacle to uterine contraction.

- If the placenta has not been delivered, a gentle attempt at umbilical cord traction should be tried. If still retained, a regional block or general anaesthetic will be required for a manual removal of the placenta.
- Further oxytocics can be given, e.g. further boluses of IV Syntocinon, IM ergometrine, IM carboprost and/or rectal misoprostol (carboprost and misoprostol are synthetic prostaglandin analogues).
- Bleeding from genital tract lacerations should be diagnosed promptly by examination (often under regional block or general anaesthesia) and bleeding arrested by application of clamps and suturing.

If the haemorrhage continues an arterial line should be considered and inserted by the anaesthetist, and a blood transfusion commenced. The coagulation defects of DIC should be corrected with fresh frozen plasma or cryoprecipitate, depending on advice obtained by the duty haematologist. Tranexamic acid 1 g IV will assist in achieving haemostasis. Additional techniques to stop haemorrhage due to atony are aimed at either maintaining compression of the uterus or applying pressure directly to the placental bed. A 'brace' suture involves an additional laparotomy (unless the haemorrhage is following a caesarean section) and the placing and tying of sutures around the uterine body in order to maintain compression. Placement of an intrauterine balloon does not require a laparotomy and works by applying pressure directly to the placental bed (Fig. 25.8); balloon insertion is effective in the majority of cases where it is considered appropriate. Hysterectomy may be indicated, especially if there is an abnormally invasive placenta. Internal iliac artery ligation is occasionally performed but requires a high degree of surgical skill. Radiologically directed arterial embolization is an option in the management of PPH, provided the woman is stable for transfer to the radiology theatre suite. This procedure is highly specialized and is performed by interventional radiologists. Embolization often enables haemorrhage to be controlled without resorting to hysterectomy.

Secondary postpartum haemorrhage

This is usually due to infection of the uterine cavity (endometritis), retained products of conception or both; exceptionally, it is due to trophoblastic disease. Pulse rate, blood pressure and temperature are measured and the uterus palpated for tenderness. Endocervical and vaginal swabs are sent for culture. An ultrasound scan is often helpful in ruling out retained tissue.

The management decision is usually between conservative management with antibiotics, or arranging for an evacuation of retained products under regional or general anaesthesia. In the first week, the evacuation can often be carried out digitally without the need to instrument the uterus. Clinical judgement is important, often giving broad-spectrum antibiotics in the first instance if the bleeding is not severe, and arranging an evacuation if the bleeding does not settle. Care is required to avoid perforating the postpartum uterus and many clinicians perform the evacuation with real-time ultrasound to ensure the instrument remains within the uterine cavity.

> ### Key *points*
> - Obstetric haemorrhage is one of the leading causes of maternal mortality. APH and PPH are unpredictable. Delivery suite staff are trained and prepared to deal with this obstetric emergency.
> - It can be rapidly fatal, and it is important to establish adequate IV access, initiate resuscitation and identify the cause of the bleeding.
> - Early involvement of senior obstetric, anaesthetic and midwifery staff is important.
> - Providing an explanation to the woman and her birth partner ensures that the anxiety generated by experiencing the haemorrhage is reduced.

Introduction

The focus of this chapter is on fetuses who appear to be small for their gestational age. These babies may simply be small, in other words they are normal babies who just happen to be at the lower end of a normal range (constitutionally or genetically small), or they may be small for a pathological reason. These latter fetuses are referred to as being affected by fetal growth restriction (FGR, previously called intrauterine growth restriction). As a group, small for gestational age (SGA) fetuses are at increased risk of perinatal mortality but most adverse outcomes are within the group affected by FGR.

The key issues are how to screen a low-risk population in order to identify these small fetuses and, once identified, how best to identify those that are risk of developing problems in utero or in labour.

Accuracy of dating

The reliable diagnosis of SGA and FGR requires knowledge of gestational age. The estimated date of delivery is calculated as 40 weeks after the date of the start of the last menstrual period (LMP), providing the cycle length is 28 days. A correction may be made for those with regular longer or shorter cycles; for example, if the cycle is 35 days long, then 7 days should be added to the date of the LMP. Menstrual dating has significant inherent inaccuracies. The dates may be inaccurately recalled, the cycle may be irregular and bleeding in early pregnancy may be mistaken for menses. Abdominal palpation is an inaccurate way of establishing gestational age, as is the date that fetal movements were first noted. Gestational age is most accurately determined by an ultrasound scan undertaken before 20 weeks' gestation, as it is reasonable to assume that all fetuses of a given gestational age are of a similar size up until this point. The natural variation in size after this stage makes pregnancy dating less accurate. The most reliable fetal measurements for dating are the crown–rump length between the 10th and 14th weeks, and the head circumference between the 15th and 20th weeks.

The rest of this chapter will assume that gestational age is reliably established.

Small for gestational age

SGA describes the fetus or baby whose estimated fetal weight or birth weight is below the 10th centile. As the centile reduces, for example to the 5th or 3rd, then so the risk of adverse outcome increases.

Fetal growth restriction

The term FGR indicates 'a fetus which fails to reach its genetic growth potential'. FGR presents as a fetus whose growth on serial ultrasound scanning falls below a certain threshold. This threshold is poorly defined and is often implied as the crossing of centiles on a chart of fetal biometry (see later).

Babies with FGR appear thin, as measured by the ponderal index (the ratio of body weight to length), and their skin-fold thickness, a measure of subcutaneous fat, is reduced. There is clearly an overlap in the categorization of small and/or growth-restricted fetuses; a proportion of SGA fetuses will be growth restricted but the majority will be constitutionally small, i.e. genetically determined to be small. Some growth-restricted fetuses will not be SGA, i.e. their growth is failing but they do not have a size below the 10th centile.

Aetiology

Fetal growth is determined by the baby's intrinsic genetic potential, which is then modified by various fetal, maternal and placental factors (Box 26.1).

Fetal factors affecting fetal growth

The genetic make-up of the fetus is the main determinant of its growth and is related to a number of factors, including ethnicity. Asian mothers, for example, have smaller babies than their European counterparts.

This intrinsic genetic drive to grow is more related to the maternal genome than the genome of the father, and involves 'genomic imprinting'. It is well recognized that while large women often have correspondingly large babies, the correlation between large men and the size of their baby is poor.

Factors affecting fetal growth
Fetal factors

- Genetic – depends on ethnic background and personal characteristics. Maternal genes are more relevant than paternal genes
- Chromosomal – decreased growth in association with fetal aneuploidy
- Fetal anomaly

Maternal factors

- Pre-pregnancy maternal disease, e.g. renal disease, essential hypertension
- Drugs/cigarette smoking
- Maternal disease in pregnancy, e.g. pre-eclampsia

Placental factors

- Adequate/inadequate invasion of maternal spiral arteries
- Adequate/inadequate vascular function

Many developmentally abnormal fetuses are small, presumably as a result of a decreased intrinsic drive. This is particularly seen with chromosomal abnormalities, for instance trisomies 18, 13, 21 and triploidy. Small babies are also found in association with structural abnormalities of all the major organ systems, as well as with fetal infection. These infections include toxoplasmosis, cytomegalovirus and rubella but, worldwide, the main association is with malaria.

Maternal factors affecting fetal growth

Small variations in diet do not have a measurable effect on fetal growth, but extreme starvation does cause significant growth impairment. This was observed in the Dutch winter famine of 1944. There is no evidence, however, that food supplementation above a normal diet can improve growth in utero.

Oxygen supply is important. Babies born at high altitude are smaller, presumably as a result of the decreased oxygen content found in the rarefied atmosphere. This is also true of babies born to mothers with chronic hypoxia secondary to congenital heart disease. The fetus is able to partly compensate through placental hypertrophy, but this compensation is incomplete.

Drugs such as tobacco, heroin, cocaine and alcohol may decrease fetal growth. It has been estimated that smoking, for example, will decrease neonatal weight by an average of approximately 150 g. Maternal chronic disease also has an adverse effect on fetal growth, particularly if there is renal impairment.

Placental factors affecting fetal growth

Adequate placental function depends on adequate trophoblastic invasion. In the first trimester, trophoblast cells invade the maternal spiral arteries in the decidua. In the second trimester, a secondary wave of trophoblast extends this invasion along the spiral arteries and into the myometrium.

This results in the conversion of thick-walled muscular vessels with a relatively high vascular resistance to flaccid thin-walled vessels with a low resistance to flow. In certain conditions, such as pre-eclampsia, it would appear that there has been failure of this secondary trophoblastic invasion, the consequences being subsequent placental ischaemia, atheromatous changes and secondary placental insufficiency. Why this failure should occur is unclear, but it may be related to the immunological interface between the fetal and maternal cells. Impaired trophoblast invasion can be inferred from Doppler studies of the maternal uterine arteries; impaired blood flow is associated with an increased risk of delivering an SGA baby and is an indication for serial ultrasound surveillance of fetal growth (see later).

The overall effect of uteroplacental insufficiency, whatever the cause, is a decrease in the nutrient supply to the fetus. It is not surprising, therefore, that these fetuses are often found to be hypoxic, hypoglycaemic and sometimes acidotic. To compensate for this hypoxia, the fetus increases erythropoiesis in order to increase its oxygen-carrying capacity, and redistributes blood away from the peripheral circulation, gut and liver towards the brain, heart and adrenal glands.

The result is a baby with normal growth in length and brain development, but who is thin and has little or no subcutaneous fat. Glycogen stores are minimal. As these babies have relatively large heads compared with their bodies, their growth has previously been described as 'asymmetrical', although the terms 'symmetrical' and 'asymmetrical' are no longer used to describe patterns of fetal growth or neonatal nutritional status.

Screening and diagnosis

A number of risk factors for delivery of an SGA baby have been identified. Some of these are identifiable at the first visit, whereas others only feature during the course of the pregnancy (Box 26.2). The presence of such a risk factor justifies undertaking serial ultrasound fetal biometry from 26–28 weeks onwards in order to diagnose poor fetal growth. Often, however, small babies are identified following routine clinical examination.

Clinical examination

Estimation of fetal weight from clinical examination is unreliable. The fundus reaches the umbilicus by around 20–24 weeks and the xiphisternum by approximately 36 weeks. The height of the uterine fundus should be measured with a tape measure at each antenatal clinic visit from 26 weeks onwards; the height of the uterus, measured from the pubic symphysis, is approximately equal to the gestation in weeks. Symphysis-fundal height (SFH) charts facilitate the interpretation of these measurements. An SFH less than the 10th centile or serial SFH measurements suggestive of poor growth is an indication for ultrasound fetal biometry.

Risk factors for delivery of an SGA baby
Available from maternal history

- Age >40 years
- Smoker >10/day
- Cocaine use
- Previous SGA baby
- Previous stillborn baby
- Chronic hypertension
- Diabetes with vascular disease
- Renal impairment
- Antiphospholipid syndrome

Current pregnancy complications or results

- Threatened miscarriage (heavy bleeding = menstruation)
- Pre-eclampsia
- Placental abruption
- Unexplained antepartum haemorrhage (especially if recurrent)
- Abnormal uterine artery Doppler waveform
- Low level of maternal Plasma Associated Placenta Protein-A (PAPP-A) (a component of Down syndrome screening)
- Hyperechogenic fetal bowel (usually at the time of fetal anomaly scan)

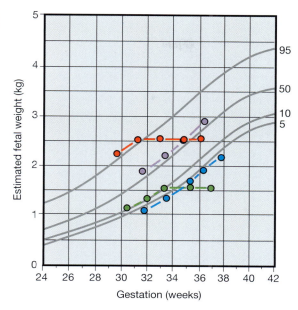

Fig. 26.1 Fetal growth charts. ◐ The fetus is growing along the 50th centile. ● The fetus is SGA but does not have FGR. ● The fetus becomes SGA and has FGR. ● The fetus is growth restricted but is not SGA.

Ultrasound examination

Ultrasound is used to establish or refute the diagnosis of fetal SGA or FGR. Certain diagnosis of SGA or FGR can only be made postnatally, but this is of little value to the obstetrician and midwife in planning antenatal care/surveillance. Measurements can be made of the fetal head (circumference or biparietal diameter), the abdominal circumference and the femur length, and various equations can be used to estimate fetal weight. For practical purposes, it is reasonable to consider the abdominal circumference alone, as measurements below the 10th centile have an approximately 80% sensitivity in the prediction of SGA neonates in high-risk pregnancies. There is no evidence that routine ultrasound screening is of value in low-risk women.

Small for gestational age or fetal growth restriction?

This is a key question and one that is not always possible to answer. Those fetuses less than the 10th centile include those who are simply constitutionally small (around 50–70%) and those who have FGR. The increased risks of stillbirth, birth hypoxia, neonatal complications and impaired neuro-development are principally in the FGR group, and it would be of great value to be able to reliably differentiate between the two groups. The diagnosis of SGA is straightforward, but the diagnosis of FGR less so. Current clinical practice is to plot two or more fetal measurements on a chart of estimated fetal weight (or abdominal circumference) against gestational age. Examples of such plots in four fetuses are presented in Fig. 26.1. Charts of fetal size are not specifically designed for interpretation of serial measurements and the

use of specifically constructed charts of fetal growth rates or velocity can improve diagnosis. An alternative strategy is to employ charts of fetal size, which have been customized or individualized to a specific pregnancy. By calculating a 'term optimal fetal weight' based upon a number of easily obtained maternal and pregnancy physiological variables that have an influence upon fetal size – e.g. maternal weight, parity, ethnic origin – a customized 'growth' curve with centiles can be produced. This chart will be different for each pregnancy. A fetus with an estimated weight below the 10th centile of a customized chart is more likely to be genuinely growth restricted than a fetus that is small based on a population chart. The use of customized charts to improve the identification of growth restriction is recommended.

Once SGA or FGR is diagnosed, it is then necessary to evaluate other parameters of fetal well-being, which are considered later. In practice, most fetuses less than the 10th centile require close observation, and whether they have FGR or are SGA only becomes apparent in retrospect.

Management

The main principle is to monitor the fetus and deliver at the appropriate time (Box 26.3). No antenatal therapy is of proven benefit. The options for fetal monitoring include fetal movement charts, fetal cardiotocography (CTG), biophysical scoring and Doppler blood flow studies. Of these, Doppler flow studies are the most valuable.

Box 26.3

Clinical management of FGR

- Screening by serial ultrasound prompted by risk factors and/or SFH measurements
- Ultrasound confirmation that the baby is small or growth restricted
- Exclude fetal abnormality (unless already done at 20-week scan)
- Consider whether the fetus is SGA or FGR. Use Doppler studies
- Monitor with Doppler studies and CTG as appropriate
- Consider corticosteroids if <34 weeks and delivery anticipated
- Deliver if fetal demise is anticipated; threshold for delivery is strongly influenced by gestation

Fetal movement monitoring

A poorly nourished fetus will attempt to conserve energy by becoming less active. It is useful to ask the mother about the frequency of perceived fetal movements; any sudden change in the pattern of movements may be of significance and should be brought to the attention of the woman's midwife or obstetrician. However, the utility of routine, self-documented formal fetal movement counting is not supported by scientific evaluation of its efficacy in reducing perinatal deaths.

Fetal cardiotocography

The interpretation of CTGs is discussed on page 294. The CTG gives an indication of fetal well-being at a particular moment but has limited longer term value. The routine use of antenatal CTG is not associated with an improved perinatal outcome and antenatal CTG monitoring should be restricted to specific indications.

Biophysical profile (BPP)

The predictive value of adverse outcomes in cases of FGR is low. The test takes a long time to carry out, sometimes up to an hour. As most fetuses with an abnormal BPP also have abnormal umbilical artery Doppler flow, it is more appropriate to rely on Doppler studies. A BPP may be helpful in certain circumstances, such as when the Doppler waveform is already abnormal, but the BPP is seldom indicated in modern-day practice.

Doppler ultrasound

Doppler ultrasound of the umbilical artery is used as an assessment of 'downstream' placental vascular resistance. A normal waveform (described by semi-quantitative pulsatility or resistance indices) indicates that an SGA fetus is constitutionally small rather than growth restricted because of impaired placental function. Reduction or loss of end-diastolic flow identifies a fetus at high risk of hypoxia, and absent end-diastolic flow (AEDF) has been shown to be a useful discriminator between those growth-restricted fetuses at high risk of perinatal death and those at a lower risk (Fig. 26.2). Studies have shown that the use of umbilical artery studies to monitor high-risk fetuses reduces perinatal morbidity and mortality.

Doppler studies of the fetal cerebral circulation can also provide additional useful information, particularly in the term fetus (Fig. 26.3). As the growth-restricted fetus redistributes its blood flow away from the less vital organs towards the brain in response to hypoxia, it is reasonable to expect an increased cerebral flow. This is indeed observed to happen, with Doppler studies showing a decreased resistance of the middle cerebral artery. As the hypoxia becomes more severe, this resistance increases again, possibly secondary to cerebral oedema. Doppler examination of the fetal venous circulation provides useful information when considering the timing of delivery. Doppler signals from the ductus venosus (a vein within the fetal liver) can be used to indirectly interpret the function of the right side of the fetal heart. Abnormal ductus venosus waveforms herald fetal demise.

In general, the sequence of changes observed with progressive fetal hypoxia is impaired growth, abnormal umbilical artery waveform, increased cerebral blood flow, abnormal ductus venosus flow followed by an abnormal fetal heart rate pattern and fetal demise. The rate of deterioration in fetal condition is unpredictable and this sequence of changes is not always present, but it does permit the development of a strategy for the management of the SGA/FGR fetus.

Overall strategy

Fig. 26.4 illustrates the probable sequence of events in fetal decompensation. As umbilical artery Doppler abnormalities are the first to appear, it is logical to use Doppler as the main screening tool. Thereafter, the optimal surveillance strategy in fetuses with absent or reduced end-diastolic flow involves frequent monitoring with CTG and Doppler studies of fetal vessels. The timing of the delivery will be decided by balancing the risks of keeping the baby in utero against the risks of prematurity, but delivery is appropriate when the CTG becomes abnormal (decelerations or reduced variability), there is AEDF in the umbilical artery with abnormal ductus venosus flow, or there is reversal of end-diastolic flow. If FGR is suspected before 36 weeks and delivery is anticipated, it is appropriate to give corticosteroids to the mother to enhance fetal lung maturation.

One strategy for the outpatient management of women with an SGA pregnancy is presented in Fig. 26.5.

The mode of delivery depends on the individual circumstances, but it must be remembered that the placental reserve of some of these fetuses may be extremely low and careful monitoring in labour is required. Early recourse to caesarean

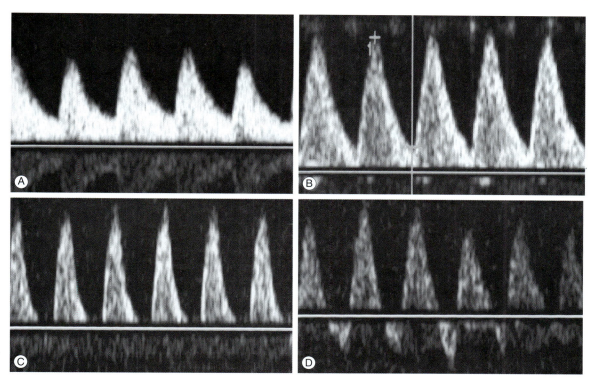

Fig. 26.2 **Doppler ultrasound of the umbilical cord demonstrating (A) normal, (B) reduced, (C) absent and (D) reversed end-diastolic flow.** Absent and reversed end-diastolic flow are associated with fetal compromise of placental origin.

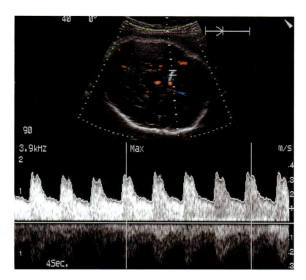

Fig. 26.3 **In FGR, there is an increased flow in the middle cerebral artery.**

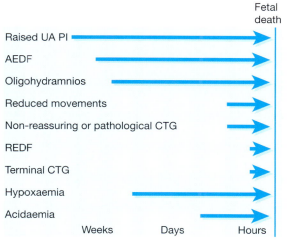

Fig. 26.4 **The 'decompensation cascade' of FGR.** Absent end-diastolic flow (AEDF) is a relatively early sign of hypoxaemia, with reduced fetal movements, cardotocographic abnormalities and reversed end-diastolic flow (REDF) late features. UA PI, Umbilical artery pulsatility index.

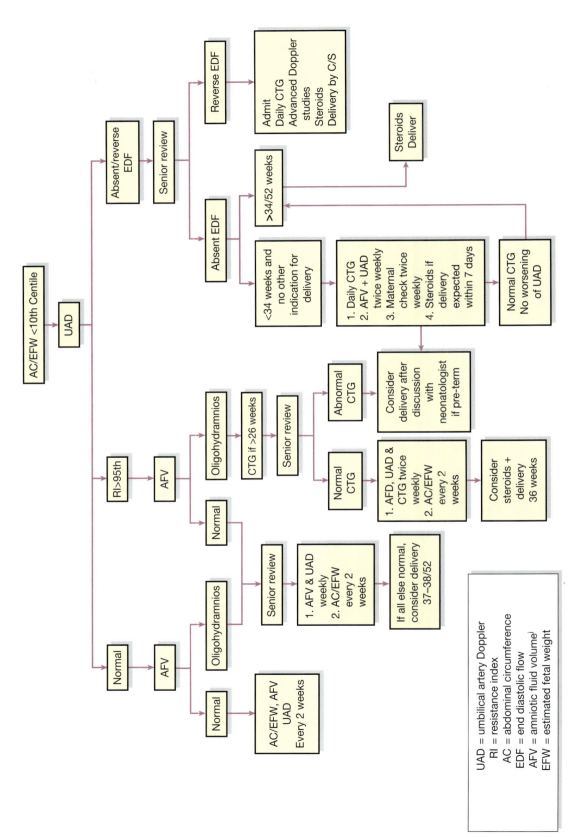

Fig. 26.5   Flowchart for the management of an SGA fetus.

UAD = umbilical artery Doppler
RI = resistance index
AC = abdominal circumference
EDF = end diastolic flow
AFV = amniotic fluid volume
EFW = estimated fetal weight

section is appropriate if the monitoring shows signs of fetal compromise. Pre-labour caesarean section may be appropriate if there are significant pre-labour concerns about fetal well-being, particularly if there is absent or reversed flow in the umbilical artery Doppler waveform.

Long-term implications of fetal growth restriction

Babies exposed to FGR are at increased risk of perinatal mortality including stillbirth (Box 26.4). Antenatal or intrapartum hypoxia may lead to long-term neurological handicap, as may more acute intrapartum hypoxia. Even if there is no overt evidence of handicap, studies of long-term development suggest that growth-restricted fetuses may be more clumsy and that their IQ may be 5–10 points lower than a normally grown sibling.

There is also evidence to suggest that FGR predisposes babies to problems much later in life, particularly non-insulin-dependent diabetes and coronary heart disease. It may be that the fetus alters its metabolism to cope with poor nutrition in utero and is subsequently less able to cope with normal carbohydrate levels in later postnatal life. It is also possible that there are vascular compensatory changes with FGR that predispose to later arterial disease.

Box 26.4

Clinical significance of FGR

Increased risk of: fetal anomaly
- perinatal asphyxia
- operative delivery
- perinatal death including stillbirth
- neonatal hypoglycaemia and hypocalcaemia
- necrotizing enterocolitis
- long-term handicap
- non-insulin-dependent diabetes and coronary artery disease in adult life

---

Key points

- An accurate estimation of gestation is a prerequisite to the accurate diagnosis of fetal growth abnormality.
- SGA refers to those fetuses whose estimated weight is <10th centile for their gestational age. Most SGA fetuses are healthy.
- FGR refers to any fetus failing to achieve its growth potential. Not all SGA fetuses are growth restricted and not all growth-restricted fetuses are SGA. FGR carries an increased risk of intrapartum asphyxia, neonatal hypoglycaemia and possible long-term neurological impairment. There is also an increased risk of perinatal mortality.
- Diagnosis of FGR requires at least two ultrasound scans at least 3 weeks apart. The use of customized or individualized charts of fetal size more reliably differentiates between the SGA and FGR fetus.
- Successful management involves appropriate monitoring, with expedited delivery as necessary.

27

Hypertension in pregnancy

Hypertensive disorders of pregnancy are responsible for over 60 000 maternal deaths worldwide annually. Both maternal and neonatal morbidity and mortality are increased in pregnancies complicated by hypertension, including chronic hypertension and pre-eclampsia. There is significant personal cost to families affected by the disease and economic implications for the health service.

Women who are hypertensive and pregnant may be subdivided into those with chronic hypertension or those with pregnancy-induced hypertension (PIH). Women with PIH (also known as gestational hypertension) can be classified further; the majority have non-proteinuric PIH, a condition associated with less maternal or perinatal sequelae if pre-eclampsia does not develop before delivery, whereas a minority have the major pregnancy complication of pre-eclampsia.

Definitions

Hypertension

National Institute of Health and Care Excellence (NICE) guidelines include threshold values of ≥140 mmHg systolic or 90 mmHg diastolic blood pressure to define hypertension in pregnancy (Fig. 27.1).

Chronic hypertension

Chronic hypertension is defined as:

- The presence of hypertension before 20 weeks' gestation (in the absence of a hydatidiform mole) or
- Persistent hypertension beyond 6 weeks postpartum.

Chronic hypertension may be further subclassified into:

1. Chronic hypertension (without proteinuria)
2. Chronic renal disease (proteinuria with or without hypertension)
3. Chronic hypertension with superimposed pre-eclampsia (new-onset proteinuria).

Gestational hypertension

Gestational hypertension may be classified into:

1. Gestational hypertension (without proteinuria)
2. Gestational proteinuria (without hypertension)
3. Gestational proteinuric hypertension (pre-eclampsia).

Pre-eclampsia

The definition of pre-eclampsia was revised in 2014 to reflect the multisystem nature of the condition and is defined as hypertension developing after 20 weeks' gestation with one or more of: proteinuria, maternal organ dysfunction or fetal growth restriction. This new definition means that proteinuria is no longer essential for diagnosis.

Potential forms of maternal organ dysfunction include:

- Renal insufficiency (creatinine >90 μmol/L)
- Liver involvement (elevated transaminases – at least twice the upper limit of normal ± right upper quadrant or epigastric abdominal pain)
- Neurological complications (examples include eclampsia, altered mental status, blindness, stroke or, more commonly, hyperreflexia when accompanied by clonus, severe headaches when accompanied by hyperreflexia, persistent visual scotomata)
- Haematological complications (thrombocytopenia – platelet count below 150 000/dL, disseminated intravascular coagulation, haemolysis).

Eclampsia

Neurologic involvement in the form of generalized tonic-clonic convulsions in women with pre-eclampsia is termed eclampsia, if the seizures cannot be attributed to any other cause (such as epilepsy, cerebral infection, tumour or ruptured aneurysm).

Pathophysiology

Phase 1: abnormal placentation

Placentation occurs between 6 and 18 weeks' gestation. During normal placental development, major structural alterations of the spiral arteries occur, allowing an increase in blood supply to the placenta. Trophoblast invasion of the maternal spiral arteries causes the diameter of these arteries to increase approximately five-fold, converting a high-resistance, low-flow system to one with a low resistance and high flow. In women who develop pre-eclampsia there is inadequate trophoblast invasion, resulting in inadequate or deranged placental perfusion.

During early pregnancy trophoblast invasion is regulated at the maternal decidual barrier by the action of factors

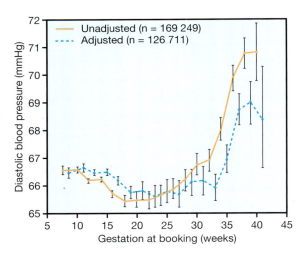

Fig. 27.1 Maternal diastolic blood pressure measurements throughout pregnancy.

expressed within the decidua and on the trophoblast cells. These regulatory factors include cell adhesion molecules and the extracellular matrix, proteinases and their inhibitors, growth factors and cytokines. Underlying genetic and immunological abnormalities may result in abnormalities in any one of these factors.

It has been suggested that the primary factor in the aetiology of pre-eclampsia is immunological in origin. Abnormal placentation may be the result of maternal immune rejection of paternal antigens expressed by the fetus. For example, women who develop pre-eclampsia appear to have an extra-villous trophoblast that does not express human leucocyte antigen-G. The predominance of pre-eclampsia in first pregnancies and the protective effect of parity further support an immunological mechanism for the condition.

Phase 2: endothelial dysfunction

The second phase of pre-eclampsia is characterized by widespread endothelial damage and dysfunction. This is likely to be mediated through oxidative stress originating from the ischaemic placenta. Women with pre-eclampsia have increased circulating levels of markers of endothelial dysfunction. Endothelial damage promotes platelet adhesion and thrombosis, and disturbs the normal physiological modulation of vascular tone, further amplifying the response. This phase of pre-eclampsia is characterized by an exaggerated maternal systemic inflammatory response, with associated activation of leucocytes, platelets and the coagulation system.

There is a relative deficiency of prostacyclin, which is a vasodilator. This occurs either because of reduced prostacyclin synthesis or because of an increased production of thromboxane A_2 (a vasoconstrictor with a tendency to promote platelet aggregation). This imbalance leads to platelet

stimulation and also vasoconstriction and hypertension. Aspirin may reduce risks by redressing this imbalance.

Epidemiology of hypertensive disorders in pregnancy

Hypertension is the commonest medical problem encountered in pregnancy, complicating 10–15% of pregnancies. Pre-existing or chronic hypertension is one of the most common conditions in women of childbearing age, and is becoming more prevalent due to increasing maternal age and increased prevalence of obesity. Chronic hypertension is estimated to affect 1–5% of pregnant women, and is frequently diagnosed for the first time during antenatal care.

The prevalence of pre-eclampsia varies with the definition used and the population studied; however, pre-eclampsia occurs in less than 5% of an average antenatal population. The incidence of non-proteinuric PIH is approximately three times greater.

The incidence of eclampsia was 2.7 cases per 10 000 births in 2005 in the UK, which has been steadily declining. The incidence has decreased by 45% since 1992, and this decrease reflects a continued temporal decline over the past century, with reductions of over 90% observed since the 1920s, related to improved detection and management of hypertensive pregnancies. Risks of serious adverse maternal and perinatal outcomes are high among women with eclampsia. In industrialized countries the case-fatality rate is below 1%, but severe maternal complications (such as coma, stroke and acute respiratory distress) occur in 10–30% of cases, with 5–8% of pregnancies resulting in a perinatal loss.

Chronic hypertension

The cause of primary hypertension is considered to be multifactorial, with both genetic and environmental contributions. Secondary hypertension is identified in less than 5% of the general population, but has been shown to be present in 14% of women of childbearing age. Renal disease is the most common cause of secondary hypertension in pregnancy. Chronic kidney disease affects up to 3% of women aged 20–39 years and pregnancy may be the first time it is identified.

History and examination

The majority of women will be asymptomatic, however, a careful history for end organ damage and potential underlying aetiology should be taken. Questioning about late enuresis and recurrent urinary tract infections in childhood may suggest reflux nephropathy, and a detailed family history may confirm a genetic basis for primary hypertension or identify familial renal disease. Paroxysmal or severe hypertension associated with headache and sweating or palpitations may be indicative of a phaeochromocytoma, which can be fatal in pregnancy if missed.

Examination should include fundoscopy to identify hypertensive retinopathy and assessment for radio-femoral delay (coarctation of the aorta). Other findings may include enlarged kidneys (polycystic kidneys), a renal bruit (renal artery stenosis) and clinical features of endocrine disease (e.g. hyperthyroidism, tachycardia, goitre, proptosis). Some of these conditions may have genetic or endocrine implications for the fetus.

Investigations

Any woman of childbearing age identified to have chronic hypertension should have confirmation with 24-h ambulatory monitoring, and be investigated for end organ damage including an echocardiogram to assess for left ventricular hypertrophy and assessment of renal function and proteinuria. Referral for investigation for secondary causes should be made to an appropriate specialist depending on local expertise and interest (e.g. nephrology, clinical pharmacology, cardiology, endocrinology).

Chronic kidney disease

The most common causes of renal disease in women of childbearing age are reflux nephropathy, lupus nephritis, IgA nephropathy and autosomal dominant polycystic kidney disease (ADPKD), although hypertensive nephropathy and obesity-related focal segmental glomerulosclerosis are becoming increasingly common. Women with reflux nephropathy and ADPKD may have affected family members but both conditions can also occur spontaneously.

Endocrine

Many endocrine disorders are associated with hypertension. The most common being hyperthyroidism in women of childbearing age. A careful clinical history and examination may identify features of other conditions including primary hyperparathyroidism, phaeochromocytoma, carcinoid, and acromegaly.

Management

Pre-pregnancy counselling

Pre-pregnancy counselling is essential for all women with chronic hypertension in order to optimize their hypertensive control, to plan switching from teratogenic medication to alternative agents, and inform women about potential complications in the pregnancy. Women should be advised that statin and fibrate treatment should be stopped before or at conception.

In addition, exacerbating factors can be addressed with lifestyle adaptation such as weight loss, reduced alcohol intake, a low-salt diet and exercise. Smoking cessation should be recommended for all smokers.

Regarding treatment for chronic hypertension, some drugs that are commonly used in the non-pregnant (such as ACE inhibitors) are best avoided as they have adverse fetal effects. The agents commonly used, labetalol and methyldopa, are outlined in Table 27.2. The dose of a single agent should be maximized before introduction of a second agent.

All women with essential hypertension should be advised to take 75 mg aspirin from 12 weeks until delivery in order to reduce the risk of pre-eclampsia.

Maternal complications

The incidence of superimposed pre-eclampsia in women with chronic hypertension is approximately 20%, but can be higher in women with secondary hypertension. Women with chronic hypertension may have undetectable renal damage that is only revealed by pregnancy, therefore a quantitative assessment of proteinuria should be performed at booking for comparison in later pregnancy.

Superimposed pre-eclampsia may be difficult to distinguish from physiological changes, but the following features are suggestive of the condition:

- A rapid rise in hypertension
- New onset or doubling of proteinuria
- Other laboratory parameters, e.g. low platelets, raised liver enzymes or creatinine.

Timing of delivery

Pre-term delivery, often iatrogenic, is more common in women with chronic hypertension compared with the general population. Timing of delivery should be guided by the severity of hypertension, the presence of proteinuria and fetal compromise, and balanced against the risks of prematurity at lower gestations. NICE guidelines suggest that delivery for women with chronic hypertension should be managed the same as for women with gestational hypertension, or if proteinuria is present then as for pre-eclampsia.

Neonatal complications

Neonatal complications are also more commonly reported for women with chronic hypertension than normotensive women including higher rates of perinatal mortality, fetal growth restriction and admission to neonatal special care.

Postpartum management

Peak postpartum blood pressure usually occurs at 3–5 days. It is recommended that women with chronic hypertension should continue to have their blood pressure measured postpartum, and treatment titrated to keep blood pressure lower than 140/90 mmHg.

Women with previously diagnosed chronic hypertension can be discharged when their blood pressure is stable and <140/90 mmHg or <150/100 mmHg with treatment. All women with chronic hypertension should be offered a medical review 6–8 weeks after delivery for future pre-pregnancy counselling.

It is recommended that oestrogen-containing contraceptives be avoided in women with hypertension due to their potential to exacerbate sodium retention and hypertension.

Gestational hypertension and pre-eclampsia

Risk factors

More than a third of pre-eclampsia occurs in women with risk factors, and not recognizing risk accounts for a considerable amount of substandard care in maternal deaths. Distinguishing at-risk patients allows administration of antiplatelet agents (aspirin) prior to 16 weeks' gestation, which appears to reduce the risk of pre-eclampsia, particularly reducing earlier presentations of the syndrome. Recognized risk factors for gestational hypertension and pre-eclampsia are shown in Box 27.1.

One of the strongest risk factors for development of pre-eclampsia is a history of the disease in previous pregnancies, particularly those requiring delivery before 37 weeks, resulting in a 20% chance of developing pre-eclampsia again. A family history in a first-degree relative increases the risk of pre-eclampsia four- to eight-fold, illustrating the strong genetic influence.

A woman has double the risk of pre-eclampsia if pregnant by a partner who had previously fathered an affected pregnancy. This indicates the immunological element to the disease process, where there is an effect of exposure to the paternal antigen, via either the fetus or the partner. Pre-eclampsia occurs more commonly in first pregnancies; miscarriages or terminations of pregnancy provide some reduction in risk in subsequent pregnancies. A new partner increases risk, whereas non-barrier methods of contraception and increased duration of sexual cohabitation reduce risk. It is sustained exposure to a partner's protective 'foreign' antigens that links these risk factors. Teenage mothers and pregnancies conceived by donor insemination have an increased risk of pre-eclampsia, presumably due to the lack of exposure.

Underlying medical disorders, particularly those involving vascular disease such as chronic hypertension, increase the risk of pre-eclampsia (to over 20%). All forms of glucose intolerance, including gestational diabetes, are associated with an increased risk. This may be related to obesity, which is an independent risk factor. Other maternal risk factors include chronic kidney disease and autoimmune disorders. Women with antiphospholipid syndrome and multiple pregnancies are at increased risk. Risk may be related to the size of the placenta; molar pregnancies have been associated with pre-eclampsia, as have pregnancies complicated by hydrops fetalis (mirror syndrome) or trisomy chromosomal complement.

Other moderate risk factors include first pregnancy, age 40 years or more, a pregnancy interval greater than 10 years, body mass index of 35 kg/m^2 or more, polycystic ovarian syndrome, vitamin D deficiency and multiple pregnancy. Low dietary calcium and low serum calcium concentrations are associated with pre-eclampsia, although the role of calcium in preventing pre-eclampsia remains controversial.

Clinical assessment

Patients may have raised blood pressure during their pregnancy or up to 6 weeks postpartum, and full clinical assessment is important to differentiate between the hypertensive disorders of pregnancy and determine severity. There are many non-specific symptoms and signs that are important indicators of widespread multisystem involvement and these symptoms may herald the onset of severe pre-eclampsia (Box 27.2).

When women have the presenting symptom of hypertension, both the gestational age and the previous pregnancy history are important factors in establishing risk of progression to pre-eclampsia; late-onset hypertension after 37 weeks' gestation rarely results in serious morbidity to mother or baby, but prophylactic delivery may be justified and induction of labour does not result in an increased risk of caesarean section. In cases of pre-eclampsia, delivery at 37 weeks'

Box 27.1

Predisposing factors for developing gestational hypertension/pre-eclampsia

- First pregnancy
- Family history – mother/sister
- Extremes of maternal age
- Obesity
- Medical factors:
  - pre-existing hypertension
  - renal disease
  - acquired thrombophilia – antiphospholipid antibodies
  - inherited thrombophilia
  - connective tissue disease (e.g. systemic lupus erythematosus)
  - diabetes mellitus
- Obstetric factors:
  - multiple pregnancy
  - previous pre-eclampsia
  - hydatidiform mole
  - triploidy
  - hydrops fetalis (immune and non-immune)
  - inter-pregnancy interval of >10 years

Box 27.2

Signs and symptoms of pre-eclampsia

Symptoms of pre-eclampsia

Severe headache	Visual disturbances including blurring, flashing or scotoma
Severe right upper quadrant and epigastric abdominal pain	Vomiting
Sudden swelling of the face, hands or feet	Restlessness or agitation

Signs of pre-eclampsia

Hypertension and proteinuria	Clonus
Hyperreflexia	Haemolytic anaemia
Serum creatinine raised	Elevated liver enzymes
Platelet count decreased	Retinal haemorrhages and papilloedema

gestation is routinely recommended. However, in those who develop early-onset gestational hypertension, particularly before 28 weeks, almost half will develop pre-eclampsia.

1. Blood pressure measurement (Fig. 27.2A)

Care in assessing blood pressure will prevent misdiagnosis; blood pressure measurement is poorly performed in clinical practice. The antenatal population within the UK has a significant proportion of obese women. The standard bladder used in sphygmomanometer cuffs (23 × 12 cm) is too small for about a quarter of the antenatal population, resulting in the over diagnosis of hypertension, usually by more than 10 mmHg. Automated 'oscillometric' devices often under-read the true blood pressure in pre-eclampsia, and only those shown to be specifically accurate in pregnancy should be used. Otherwise, Korotkoff sounds by a trained observer should be used for decision-making. Repeating the blood pressure, or obtaining a series of readings in the day unit, will limit the over-diagnosis of hypertension. Uncontrollable blood pressure may indicate need for urgent delivery.

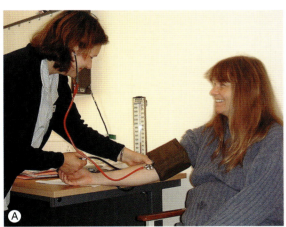

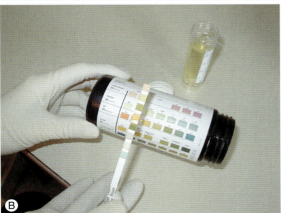

Fig. 27.2 **Early detection of pre-eclampsia is important. (A)** Measurement of blood pressure (reproduced with permission). **(B)** Testing for urinary protein.

2. Urine dipstick (Fig. 27.2B)

Assessing for proteinuria, typically by dipstick of a mid-stream urine sample, is a routine screening tool that should be performed at each clinical interaction with all pregnant women. Urinary protein excretion is considered abnormal in pregnant women when it exceeds 30 mL/dL, a level that usually correlates with 1+ on a urine dipstick. However, errors in the interpretation of proteinuria are common with dipstick urine analysis, as false positives may be caused by dehydration, contamination of samples after ruptured membranes or certain medications. False negatives may occur due to dilutional effects of drinking and overhydration. Therefore 24-h collections of urine are necessary to confirm the diagnosis. More than 300 mg in 24 h is considered abnormal. Newer automated devices that can be used by the bedside relate the proteinuria to creatinine, and closely equate to 24-h collections.

3. Blood tests

In addition to blood pressure and proteinuria, pre-eclampsia has significant effects on other organs (Table 27.1).

Uric acid has in the past been used to detect pre-eclampsia but is not reliable. Spuriously high levels of uric acid are associated with acute fatty liver of pregnancy. Aspartate transaminase (AST) and other transaminases indicate hepatocellular damage and should routinely be checked. It should be remembered that the normal range for transaminases is approximately 20% lower than the non-pregnant range.

When liver involvement is associated with haemolysis and low platelets, this is known as HELLP (haemolysis, elevated liver enzymes and low platelets) syndrome, which is a severe variant of pre-eclampsia and will require urgent delivery. If proteinuria excretion is high (usually >3 g/24 h), circulating albumin may fall, increasing the risk of pulmonary oedema. A raised AST can be associated with either haemolysis or liver involvement; lactate dehydrogenase levels are also elevated in the presence of haemolysis.

If delivery or induction of labour is likely to be imminent, or if the platelet count is low, it is also sensible to screen for clotting abnormalities. Pre-eclampsia can cause disseminated intravascular coagulation, and clotting must be adequate for regional anaesthesia.

Table 27.1	Blood test investigations in pre-eclampsia
Investigation	**Finding in pre-eclampsia**
FBC	Reduced platelets, reduced haemoglobin, haemolysis on blood film
Renal function	Reduced urine output Increased urate, increased urea, increased creatinine
Coagulation system	Prolonged coagulation indices
Hepatic system	Elevated alanine transaminase (ALT) and aspartate transaminase (AST)

FBC, full blood count.

A low albumin, low platelet count or clotting derangement may indicate urgent need for delivery, as the disease of pre-eclampsia is progressive and the only cure is removing the placenta.

4. Fetal assessment

Fetal well-being must be carefully considered in all cases, particularly with early-onset disease. A symphysial–fundal height should be carefully measured in all women who present with pre-eclampsia, in addition to discussing patterns of fetal movements. At early gestations, or in pregnancies with suspected growth restriction, it is usual to confirm fetal growth with ultrasound and to assess the amniotic fluid volume and umbilical artery Doppler waveform. When fetal compromise is detected, urgent delivery is important to prevent fetal demise.

5. Prediction of pre-eclampsia

Doppler velocimetry to assess impedance of uteroplacental flow in pregnancies complicated by pre-eclampsia was described in the 1980s and now forms part of second-trimester screening for women at high risk of developing pre-eclampsia. As the disorder originates in the placenta, blood flow in the uterine artery is abnormal in most women destined to present with the syndrome (Fig. 27.3).

More recently, it has been demonstrated that angiogenic factors such as placental growth factor levels and soluble fms-like tyrosine kinase 1 can be measured in women with suspected disease to accurately determine who will require delivery in the short term.

Prophylaxis

Various preventive strategies have been employed in women considered to be at risk of developing pre-eclampsia (Box 27.3).

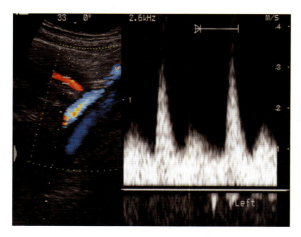

Fig. 27.3 Uterine artery Doppler notching at 24 weeks is predictive of pre-eclampsia and fetal growth restriction in high-risk mothers.

Aspirin inhibits prostaglandin synthesis via cyclooxygenase, and the dose of aspirin required to inhibit thromboxane synthesis is less than that required for prostacyclin inhibition. Low-dose aspirin should reduce the vascular and prothrombotic effects of thromboxane A_2 in women at risk of developing pre-eclampsia. Taking 75 mg aspirin daily from 12 weeks' gestation leads to a 15% reduction in the incidence of pre-eclampsia.

Restriction of salt intake and limiting weight gain during pregnancy are not useful in this regard.

Clinical management of hypertension in pregnancy without proteinuria

If the maternal blood pressure is found to be elevated, measurement should be repeated after 10–20 min. If it settles, and there are no other signs or symptoms of pre-eclampsia, no further action is needed; if still elevated, further assessment is required, ideally at an antenatal day care unit.

In the absence of severe hypertension (blood pressure ≥150/110 mmHg), significant proteinuria or symptoms of pre-eclampsia, and with normal biochemistry and haematology results, the woman can usually be managed as an outpatient. She should be seen at least twice weekly, for blood pressure and urinalysis checks. Serum biochemistry and haematology should also be repeated at least once a week. The woman should be advised to return to hospital if she feels unwell, or if there is any headache, visual disturbance or epigastric pain.

Treatment of the mother with antihypertensive drugs controls the hypertension but does not alter the course of pre-eclampsia. Treatment of hypertension may allow prolongation of the pregnancy and thereby may indirectly improve fetal outcome. Antihypertensive treatment should be commenced with consistent blood pressure recordings of ≥150/100 mmHg.

Clinical management of pre-eclampsia

In a woman with pre-eclampsia, it is important to consider the overall picture, rather than make decisions on the basis of a single parameter. Progression of the disease is not consistent and further management should be tailored to the individual woman. All women with pre-eclampsia should

---

Box 27.3

Prevention of pre-eclampsia

Proven to be of value
- Low-dose aspirin

Possibly of value
- Calcium supplementation

Not of value
- Diet with high protein content
- Restriction of salt in diet
- Restriction of weight gain
- Vitamins C and E

be admitted at initial diagnosis for assessment, as the condition may progress aggressively or follow a longer time course.

The aim should be to prolong the pregnancy in order to reduce the risk to the baby, but this must be balanced against the risks to the mother. The only true 'cure' for pre-eclampsia is delivery of the fetus and placenta.

The decision to deliver and the method of delivery are dependent on many factors. There are usually fetal advantages to conservative management before 34 weeks if the blood pressure, laboratory values and fetal condition are stable.

The principles of management of pre-eclampsia:

- *To control the maternal blood pressure.* Reduce the diastolic blood pressure to <100 mmHg using labetalol, nifedipine, hydralazine or methyldopa (Table 27.2). Effective control of hypertension is essential to prevent cerebrovascular accidents. As intracerebral haemorrhage complicates a significant proportion of deaths, systolic blood pressure should always be <150 mmHg, and treated aggressively if not. Labetalol is now recommended as first-line treatment. Regimens vary, but NICE guidelines now recommend a standard approach to hypertensive management
- *To assess maternal fluid balance.* Pre-eclampsia is associated with an increased vascular permeability and a reduced intravascular compartment. In women with pre-eclampsia, administering too little fluid risks maternal renal failure and giving too much fluid may cause pulmonary oedema. Fluid input and urine output should therefore be monitored. In severe pre-eclampsia, the maternal oxygen saturation (SaO$_2$)

should also be monitored, along with serum urea and electrolytes, liver function tests, haemoglobin, haematocrit, platelets and coagulation. If there is marked oliguria, central venous pressure monitoring may be helpful to differentiate intravascular volume depletion from renal impairment
- *To prevent seizures (eclampsia).* The use of magnesium sulphate (MgSO$_4$) in severe pre-eclampsia halves the risk of subsequent eclampsia, and may reduce the risk of maternal death. MgSO$_4$, given to those who have had an eclamptic seizure, also prevents further seizures
- *To consider delivery.* The timing of this depends on the maternal condition, the fetal condition and the gestational age. Maternal indications for delivery include gestation ≥37 weeks, an inability to control hypertension, deteriorating liver or renal function, progressive fall in platelets or neurological complications. Fetal indications include abnormal fetal heart rate monitoring or a fetal condition that is clearly deteriorating. If pre-term delivery is being considered, corticosteroids should be administered to the mother to reduce the risks associated with prematurity unless there is acute compromise requiring immediate delivery
- *To optimize postnatal care.* Women with pre-eclampsia who remain hypertensive in the initial postpartum period are still at risk of pre-eclampsia-related complications, particularly for the initial 72 h following delivery when the blood pressure often peaks. Continued vigilance is advisable during this period, as an inpatient if necessary.

Complications

Complications of pre-eclampsia involve several organs and also the clotting system (Box 27.4), with the most common complication being compromised placental blood supply leading to fetal growth restriction (Fig. 27.4), fetal hypoxia or intrauterine death. Additionally, since the successful management of pre-eclampsia revolves around delivery,

Table 27.2	Drug treatment of hypertension in pregnancy		
Drug	Action	Side-effects	Comments
Methyldopa (oral)	Central acting	Initial drowsiness	Safe; Slow onset of action. Not suitable if history of depression
Labetalol (oral/intravenous [IV])	Alpha- and beta-antagonist	Postural hypotension, tiredness	Widely used in antenatal setting (oral) and hypertensive crisis (IV)
Hydralazine (oral/IV)	Direct-acting vasodilator	Precipitate precipitates hypotension	Widely used in hypertensive crisis (IV)
Nifedipine (oral/Sub-lingual)	Calcium-channel antagonist	Flushing, headaches	Caution – interacts with MgSO$_4$. Watch for precipitous fall in blood pressure

Box 27.4

Complications of pre-eclampsia

Maternal

Placental rupture
Disseminated intravascular coagulation
HELLP syndrome
Pulmonary oedema
Aspiration

Eclampsia
Liver failure or haemorrhage
Stroke
Death
Long-term cardiovascular morbidity

Neonatal

Pre-term delivery
Intrauterine growth restriction
Hypoxia-neurological injury

Perinatal death
Long-term cardiovascular morbidity (associated with low birth weight)

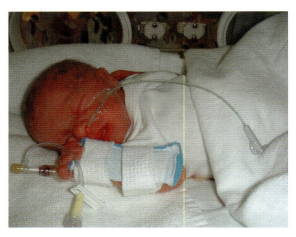

Fig. 27.4   This baby, born at 36 weeks to a mother with severe pre-eclampsia, weighed 1.6 kg. (Usual weight at 36 weeks: 2.2–3.3 kg.)

Treatment of eclampsia

- The patient should be turned onto her left side to avoid aortocaval compression. The airway should be secured and high-flow oxygen should be administered.
- $MgSO_4$ should be administered intravenously to terminate the seizure and then by intravenous (IV) infusion to reduce the chance of further convulsions. The infusion should be continued for at least 24 h following delivery or after the last seizure. $MgSO_4$ can depress neuromuscular transmission and the patient should be monitored for signs of toxicity. The respiratory rate and patellar reflexes should be monitored (reduced patellar reflexes usually precede respiratory depression). If there is significant respiratory depression, calcium gluconate can be used to reverse the effects of $MgSO_4$ and consideration given to ventilation.
- Urgent delivery is necessary if the seizure has occurred antenatally or intrapartum.
- Paralysis and ventilation should be considered if the seizures are prolonged or recurrent.

prematurity and its related problems are more common among babies born to mothers with pre-eclampsia.

HELLP syndrome (which affects 10–20% of eclamptic pregnancies) is defined by the presence of haemolysis, elevated liver enzymes and a low platelet count. Associated morbidity commonly includes disseminated intravascular coagulation, placental abruption and acute renal failure, and it is associated with maternal mortality in between 1.1% and 25% of cases (with the most common causes of mortality being haemorrhage and stroke).

Eclampsia is a less common complication, considered to complicate approximately 1% of pre-eclampsia cases, although this is higher in developing countries. It occurs when tonic-clonic seizures (not attributable to other causes) complicate pre-existing hypertensive disease of pregnancy. The management of eclampsia is outlined in Box 27.5.

A diagnosis of pre-eclampsia usually has no long-term serious sequelae, although may rarely result in a range of complications with significant long-term implications on the mother, such as liver rupture, stroke, pulmonary oedema or kidney failure. Furthermore, the diagnosis may have future implications on the management of the health of the mother, as a history of pre-eclampsia is a risk factor for future cardiac disease and stroke.

Global challenges

The most serious of all complications of pre-eclampsia is maternal death. A triumph of modern obstetrics is illustrated in a recent report showing that maternal deaths in the UK from hypertensive disorders are at the lowest ever rate, with less than one maternal death per million births, which equates to less than one death per year.

The low rate of maternal deaths from pre-eclampsia in the UK is in stark contrast with the global setting, where an estimated 60 000 women die each year from this condition, which equates to about five deaths every hour. Eighty-five percent of this burden lies with sub-Saharan Africa and Southern Asia, where restricted or under-staffed maternity services, particularly in rural areas with poor transport systems, mean that women may present late or infrequently to antenatal care.

Key points

- Pre-eclampsia is an important complication of pregnancy, resulting in effects on multiple organ systems with severe consequences if not detected and managed adequately.
- Clinical assessment involves interrogation of patient symptoms, accurate blood pressure assessment, testing for proteinuria, checking liver and renal function, assessing platelet count, and monitoring of the fetus.
- Complications include maternal stroke, liver failure, pulmonary oedema, seizures and ultimately death, along with fetal effects including growth restriction and stillbirth.
- Appropriate management involves prompt detection of the condition, blood pressure management with antihypertensives, monitoring fluid balance, $MgSO_4$ to reduce seizure risk and timely delivery of the baby.
- In the UK, this has resulted in low maternal death rates, although many global challenges exist which must be overcome to continue the promising improvements that have been made in reducing the mortality from pre-eclampsia and eclampsia over recent years.

28
Prematurity

Introduction

Prematurity is defined as delivery between 24 and 37 weeks' gestation. It occurs in around 10% of births and affects 15 million pregnancies worldwide annually. There is often no apparent cause for pre-term labour (idiopathic), although it is recognized to be more common with multiple pregnancy, antepartum haemorrhage, fetal growth restriction, cervical incompetence, chorioamnionitis, congenital uterine anomaly, polyhydramnios and systemic maternal infection. Almost one-third of pre-term births in the UK are iatrogenic following deliberate medical intervention when the risk of continuing the pregnancy (for either the mother or the fetus) outweighs the risks of prematurity.

Prematurity, especially before 33 weeks' gestation, is the leading cause of perinatal morbidity and mortality. Perinatal mortality rates are proportional to the immaturity of organ systems, especially the lungs, brain and gastro-intestinal tract. It is exceptional to survive if delivered before 24 weeks' gestation, especially without significant disability. Of those infants who survive, 10% overall will suffer some form of long-term disability requiring additional needs, and a greater number may suffer from lesser developmental or behavioural problems; these proportions are higher with delivery at an earlier gestational age.

Research into mechanisms involved in pre-term labour and its prevention has been relatively unsuccessful to date; as a result, prematurity is currently one of the most challenging problems facing obstetricians and neonatologists.

Definitions

Pre-term – a gestation of less than 37 completed weeks.
Very pre-term – a gestation of less than 32 completed weeks.
Pre-term labour – regular uterine contractions accompanied by effacement and dilatation of the cervix after 20 weeks and before 37 completed weeks.
Pre-term pre-labour rupture of the membranes (PPROM) – rupture of the fetal membranes before 37 completed weeks and before the onset of labour.

Low birth weight (LBW) – birth weight of less than 2501 g. It is important to note that LBW infants may be pre-term or growth restricted, or both (see Chapter 26).
Very low birth weight – birth weight of less than 1501 g.
Extremely low birth weight – birth weight of less than 1000 g.
Perinatal mortality rates – see Chapter 36.

Aetiology and predisposing factors

As mentioned earlier, the incidence of pre-term birth is 10% (Table 28.1) and approximately 1.5% will deliver before 32 weeks. Although only 0.5% deliver before 28 weeks, this group accounts for two-thirds of the neonatal deaths.

Two-third of pre-term deliveries are with spontaneous pre-term labour. Obstetric decisions to intentionally bring about delivery result in a quarter of pre-term births, and the rest are associated with Pre-Term Pre-Labour Rupture of Membranes (PPROM).

The aetiological factors that trigger spontaneous pre-term labour are largely unknown and considered to be multifactorial. In some instances it is thought to relate to increased uterine size, or cytokines and prostaglandins. Infection has been implicated in pre-term delivery, and it may be that bacterial toxins initiate an inflammatory process in the chorioamniotic membranes, which in turn release prostaglandins. Bacteria may damage membranes by direct protease action, or generation of cytokines, which stimulates the uterine smooth muscle. None of these mechanisms satisfactorily explains every case of pre-term labour.

Identifying women at increased risk of pre-term birth

A number of techniques or strategies have been proposed to identify pregnancies at increased risk of pre-term birth. These include clinical risk scoring, cervical assessment and the measurement of fetal fibronectin (fFN).

The risk scoring is based on the recognized risk factors available from the maternal obstetric, gynaecological and

Table 28.1	Aetiology of pre-term delivery	
Spontaneous labour, cause unknown		35%
Elective delivery (iatrogenic), e.g. maternal hypertension, fetal growth problems, antepartum haemorrhage		25%
Pre-term premature ruptured membranes		25%
Multiple pregnancy		15%

Box 28.1

Conditions during pregnancy associated with pre-term delivery

Fetal and placental

- Bleeding in the first or second trimester
- Antepartum haemorrhage
- Placenta praevia
- Intrauterine infection
- Pre-labour rupture of the membranes
- Fetal growth restriction
- Congenital fetal anomaly
- Multiple pregnancy
- Polyhydramnios

Maternal

- Congenital uterine anomaly
- Severe systemic maternal disease
- Pre-eclampsia
- Urinary tract infection, including asymptomatic bacteriuria
- Other infections and fevers, including malaria
- Bacterial vaginosis
- Psychological stress and domestic violence

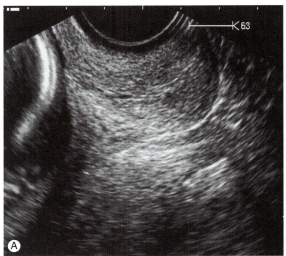

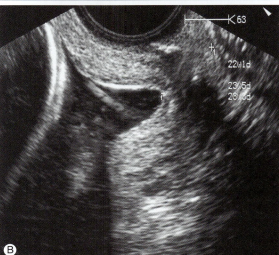

Fig. 28.1 Cervical length as measured by transvaginal scan. (A) Normal. **(B)** There is shortening of the cervix and funnelling at the internal os. Note the transvaginal cervical suture in situ.

medical histories, with smoking status, body weight and socioeconomic status. The strongest of these is a history of previous pre-term birth, but this is clearly not applicable to first-time mothers. Other recognized associations are presented in Box 28.1. Unfortunately, the performance of these scoring systems has been poor, with successful prediction less than 40%. The system at least serves to highlight the potentially avoidable factors such as urinary tract infections, vaginal infections, smoking, drugs and chaotic lifestyles.

A normal cervical length in pregnancy when measured by transvaginal ultrasound is between 34 and 40 mm, and there should be no funnelling at the internal os (Fig. 28.1). Measurement of cervical length in the second trimester can be useful in stratification of the risk of pre-term labour. Women with a cervix less than 25 mm can be considered for other interventions to improve outcome. Even so, around 1 in 5 women with a short cervix will deliver after 34 weeks' gestation without intervention. Conversely, a cervical length over 25 mm can provide reassurance.

fFN is an adhesion molecule involved in maintaining the integrity of the choriodecidual extracellular matrix. It is usually not detectable on a high vaginal swab (HVS) of cervicovaginal secretions after 20 weeks until term or membrane rupture. If it is found to be present, it implies disruption of the matrix or an inflammatory process. The positive predictive value of a positive result is low for pre-term delivery, making it unsuitable for risk stratification in asymptomatic women. On the other hand, a negative fFN result (<10 ng/mL) means the risk of delivery before 34 weeks is under 3% in asymptomatic women. In symptomatic women, a negative fFN gives a similar risk of delivery under 34 weeks, whereas a strongly positive result means up to half will deliver in the next 14 days.

Screening for vaginal infection has been considered as a method to identify those at high risk of pre-term labour. Bacterial vaginosis, which is present in 10–20% of pregnant women, is associated with a doubling of the risk of pre-term delivery if identified in the third trimester and a five-fold increased risk if identified in the first or early second trimester.

Unfortunately, clinical trials have demonstrated that the risk of pre-term labour is unchanged after treating bacterial vaginosis. In those considered to have other risk factors for pre-term labour, it is reasonable to treat bacterial vaginosis if identified rather than screen asymptomatic women.

Accurately predicting women at risk of pre-term delivery would mean interventions could be offered to those likely to benefit most, and avoid unnecessary intervention in others. The available strategies to achieve, outlined previously, are moderately useful in identifying at-risk women and better at helping to avoid unnecessary intervention.

Prevention of the onset of pre-term labour

The aim of the following interventions is to improve the perinatal morbidity and mortality associated with pre-term birth. Research is ongoing to see whether women treated with these interventions to prolong gestation have corresponding improvements in long-term outcomes for their children.

Antibiotics

Evidence suggests that screening for, and treating, asymptomatic bacteriuria can reduce the risk of pre-term labour, presumably by avoidance of progression to maternal infection with pyelonephritis. As noted earlier, evidence does not demonstrate an effect on reducing pre-term delivery with treatment of presumed pathogenic vaginal bacteria. This lack of effect may be because antibiotic treatment is started after the inflammatory cascade from bacterial membrane colonization has already become established.

Cervical cerclage

There is some evidence that elective cervical cerclage (e.g. with a Shirodkar suture or a McDonald suture) performed in early second trimester is of benefit in those with a history of pre-term labour or mid-trimester miscarriage. Under anaesthesia, a non-absorbable high-strength suture (Mersilene or similar) is placed through the tissue of the cervix in a purse-string fashion. It is removed between 36 and 37 weeks' gestation or as an emergency if labour establishes beforehand (see Fig. 28.1).

Transabdominal cerclage is a specialist procedure reserved for those with a poor pregnancy outcome despite previous standard cervical cerclage. It can be performed pre-conception by laparotomy or laparoscopy. Subsequent delivery has to be by caesarean section and the suture is usually left in place for the benefit of any future pregnancies.

'Rescue' cerclage refers to the emergency insertion of a suture in early pre-term labour before or around the limit of viability where cervical factors are suspected. Careful selection criteria are employed, since cerclage in the presence of infection can result in significant maternal morbidity without advantage to the fetus.

Progesterone

Progesterone supplementation reduces the risk of pre-term birth, and selecting the group of women who may benefit from progesterone is key. Potential mechanisms are oxytocin antagonism (leading to relaxation of smooth muscle), maintenance of cervical integrity and anti-inflammatory effects. Progesterone is administered vaginally or rectally, and is usually commenced around 20 weeks. Women with a singleton pregnancy and previous pre-term birth, and women with a singleton pregnancy and a short cervix, will have fewer deliveries before 34 weeks when given progesterone.

Prophylactic tocolytics and bed rest are not effective interventions in the prevention of pre-term labour and delivery. Neither progesterone nor cerclage are of benefit to women with twin pregnancies.

Diagnosis and management of pre-term labour

The definition of pre-term labour is similar to the diagnosis of labour at term: regular painful contractions associated with progressive cervical dilatation. Diagnosis may be difficult in the early stages, because in most cases regular painful contractions may not progress to established labour with normal abdominal and speculum examination. Labour may also be insidious or heralded by a 'show', bleeding or abruption. Objective assessment may be helpful in the presence of normal examination findings; a negative fFN result means that only around 1% of women will deliver within the following week. Similarly, a cervical length of >25 mm is reassuring and a high threshold for intervention can be set.

Maternal well-being is assessed by seeking evidence of infection or haemorrhage. The white cell count may be raised in infection, as may the C-reactive protein. Vaginal swabs and urine should be sent for culture.

The fetus can be assessed with cardiotocography (CTG), and then ideally with ultrasound, to evaluate liquor volume, presentation and estimated fetal weight. If the risk of pre-term labour is high without the start of pre-term labour itself, the neonatologist should be alerted and arrangements made for in utero transfer if local facilities for neonatal care are insufficient for the current gestation.

Inhibition of pre-term labour

In view of the high morbidity and mortality associated with prematurity, an attempt may be made to stop pre-term labour, particularly at gestations less than 33 weeks. Tocolysis is the suppression of uterine activity, and this may delay labour sufficiently for an in-utero transfer to take place, or for a course of corticosteroids to be administered. Whether this delay in itself translates into an improvement for the baby in the long term, remains unproven. As no tocolytic drug has been shown to reduce perinatal mortality or neonatal morbidity, it is also reasonable to use no tocolysis. Contraindications are listed in Box 28.2.

The most commonly used tocolytics are discussed below. If the decision is made to use a tocolytic drug, nifedipine and atosiban appear to have comparable effectiveness in delaying delivery, with fewer maternal adverse effects. Nifedipine is also considerably less expensive. There is little information about the long-term growth and development of the fetus exposed to any of these.

Nifedipine

This calcium-channel blocker inhibits inward calcium flow across cell membranes. The side-effects of dizziness, hypotension, flushing and headache are all related to peripheral dilatation, and serious adverse effects are rare. There seem to be no obvious adverse fetal effects provided there is no precipitous fall in maternal blood pressure resulting in uterine underperfusion.

Oxytocin antagonist

Atosiban is a synthetic competitive inhibitor of oxytocin, which binds to and blocks myometrial oxytocin receptors, inhibits intracellular calcium release and leads to uterine smooth muscle relaxation. It is given as a continuous intravenous infusion and has been shown to be as effective as nifedipine and has minimal maternal or fetal side-effects.

Cyclo-oxygenase inhibitors

Most experience in this class of drugs is with indomethacin. It inhibits cyclo-oxygenase conversion of fatty acids into prostaglandin endoperoxidases and thereby reduces prostaglandin production. Indomethacin may lead to maternal gastrointestinal irritation, headaches and dizziness. The main risks are to the fetus. The ongoing patency of the ductus arteriosus in the fetus is prostaglandin dependent and ductal constriction has been demonstrated in human fetuses in response to these drugs. Significant adverse neonatal effects have not been convincingly demonstrated, however, caution is nonetheless advised.

Beta-sympathomimetics

Salbutamol and terbutaline cause stimulation of β2-adrenergic receptors on myometrial cell membranes, leading to a reduction in intracellular calcium and inhibition of actin–myosin interaction necessary for smooth muscle contraction. Beta-sympathomimetics stimulate the sympathetic nervous system and side-effects are common, including maternal tachycardia, skin flushing and hypokalaemia. Pulmonary oedema and arrhythmias may occur. The main use for beta-sympathomimetics is for short-term uterine relaxation during external cephalic version or in the presence of hyperstimulation of the uterus during induction of labour.

Pre-term pre-labour rupture of the membranes (PPROM)

This occurs in 2–3% of all pregnancies but in 20–50% of all spontaneous pre-term deliveries, and is more likely with polyhydramnios, twins and vaginal infection. If the mother does not establish in labour, the problem is one of balancing the increased risk of developing ascending chorioamnionitis, leading to maternal and fetal morbidity, against the risks of prematurity and induction of labour.

The neonatal prognosis is poorer the earlier the membrane rupture occurs, on account of secondary pulmonary hypoplasia and severe skeletal deformities resulting from the absence of amniotic fluid (Box 28.3). The amniotic fluid normally allows fetal movement and it circulates into the fetal lungs. Pulmonary hypoplasia occurs in 50% of cases with spontaneous membrane rupture before 20 weeks and in 3% after 24 weeks; reliable antenatal prediction of pulmonary hypoplasia remains elusive.

Chorioamnionitis is potentially extremely serious for both mother and baby, as both may develop rapid and overwhelming fatal sepsis. Infection supervenes after the membranes have ruptured in between 0.5% and 25% of cases, depending on criteria employed for diagnosis, and is more likely if vaginal examinations have been performed. Vaginal examinations are therefore contraindicated unless there is high suspicion of pre-term labour. It may be appropriate to carry out a sterile speculum examination to initially confirm the diagnosis, exclude cord prolapse and take a HVS. The

---

Box 28.2

Contraindications to tocolysis
Relative contraindications
- Significant vaginal bleeding
- Pre-eclampsia
- Fetal growth restriction

Absolute contraindications
- Fetal death
- Lethal congenital anomaly
- Chorioamnionitis
- Fetal distress on monitoring
- Maternal condition requiring immediate delivery

Box 28.3

Risks to the infant of pre-term rupture of the membranes
- Pre-Term Delivery
- Intrauterine infection
- Cord prolapse
- Complications caused by ongoing oligohydramnios such as pulmonary hypoplasia and skeletal deformities

membrane rupture may be a secondary process resulting from an already establishing infection, and the HVS may identify the organism and guide treatment.

The diagnosis of chorioamnionitis is suggested by maternal pyrexia, maternal and fetal tachycardia, abdominal pain, uterine tenderness, drainage of offensive liquor and raised blood inflammatory markers. It is more likely if there has been a proven vaginal or urinary infection. It is therefore important to check the maternal temperature, inflammatory markers and urine for infection. It should be noted that the white cell count rises after maternal steroid administration (see later), and C-reactive protein measurements are therefore preferred as a better predictor of infection.

Management of pre-term pre-labour rupture of the membranes

Most mothers will establish in labour, with around 75% of those at 28 weeks' gestation delivering within 7 days. There is again no evidence that tocolysis is beneficial in this group. For those who do not establish in labour, regular fetal monitoring is essential. It is considered acceptable practice to manage these women on an outpatient basis following an initial inpatient stay, and the woman is advised to take her own temperature at home frequently and re-attend if a pyrexia is detected or if she feels unwell. Delivery around 34–36 weeks probably strikes the appropriate balance between fetal maturity and risk of chorioamnionitis, but it is important to individualize management. As there is such As there is such a high risk of pre-term delivery and infection, corticosteroids and antibiotics should be given if PPROM occurs at less than 35 weeks gestation. Prophylactic use of a total of 24 mg of either betamethasone or dexamethasone given as two intramuscular injections 24 hours apart is routinely recommended. Prophylactic oral erythromycin (250 mg x4 daily) for 10 days following PPROM has been shown to be associated with improved neonatal outcome when compared to placebo and is also routinely recommended.

Delivery and optimising neonatal outcome

Despite advances in neonatal medicine, prematurity leads to neonatal morbidity and mortality through a number of mechanisms, and interventions to minimize harm to the immature fetus ex utero have been developed.

Mode of delivery

The mode of delivery needs to be considered. Caesarean section may be indicated for an apparently compromised fetus. Pre-term delivery by caesarean section can lead to significant fetal trauma. Vaginal delivery is preferred on the whole for those with cephalic presentation and the routine advocacy of epidurals, forceps or episiotomy is not required.

In the event that an assisted vaginal delivery is required, forceps are safer than vacuum devices for a fetus less than 34 weeks' gestation to avoid the increased risks of cephalohaematoma, subgaleal haematoma and intraventricular haemorrhage.

There is uncertainty about the most appropriate route of delivery in those with breech presentation, but most babies in breech presentation before 26 weeks are delivered vaginally and many of those after this gestation are delivered by caesarean section.

Corticosteroids

Corticosteroids should be administered to the mother if delivery before term is considered likely; among their many effects they cross the placenta and increase the amount of pulmonary surfactant produced by type II fetal pneumocytes. Intramuscular betamethasone or dexamethasone is given by intramuscular injection in divided doses over 24 h, reducing the incidence of respiratory distress syndrome (hyaline membrane disease) by 44%. Corticosteroids also reduce the incidence of intraventricular cerebral haemorrhage and neonatal death by 46% and 31%, respectively. There are additional reductions in necrotizing enterocolitis and neonatal intensive care admission, and no adverse neurological or cognitive effects following steroid treatment have been demonstrated. There is no identifiable increase in the incidence of maternal or fetal infection, but steroids are contraindicated if there is active maternal sepsis. It is advisable to limit steroid administration to one 'course' during the pregnancy, as there are some concerns regarding the effect repeated doses may have on the developing fetus, and there is no additional benefit to the fetus with repeated courses. Steroids can be used in pregnant women with diabetes if required, but as they can precipitate ketoacidosis, tight control of blood glucose is recommended, with an insulin sliding scale if necessary.

As described earlier, tocolysis can be used to delay delivery temporarily, and allow time for completion of a full steroid course, or an in utero transfer if a higher level of neonatal care is anticipated than is available locally. Centres with advanced facilities for neonatal resuscitation can justifiably avoid tocolysis, and any inherent associated risks.

Prevention of infection

Ten days of oral erythromycin following PPROM has been shown to be of benefit to the fetus and is strongly recommended. Antibiotics for specific culture-proven infections are also known to prevent the development of systemic maternal infection and reduce pre-term delivery, and are also recommended.

In women known to be colonized with group B *Streptococcus* (*Streptococcus agalactiae*) in pre-term labour, intrapartum antibiotic prophylaxis (penicillin or clindamycin) is recommended to reduce infection of the neonate.

Should a woman with PPROM develop clinical signs of chorioamnionitis, broad-spectrum antibiotics should be administered and delivery expedited in both the maternal and fetal interest: the mother to remove the source of infection, and the baby to minimize the risk of sepsis and subsequent cerebral palsy.

Magnesium sulphate

Intravenous magnesium sulphate administered, as used in severe pre-eclampsia and eclampsia, has been noted to reduce the risk of subsequent cerebral palsy in the baby. This neuro-protective effect is more pronounced at earlier gestations, with babies less than 34 weeks' gestation likely to benefit most. Magnesium is beneficial to the baby both in pre-term labour and pre-term caesarean section. The infusion should be started more than 4 hours before delivery to ensure the ideal effect, although even a short exposure to magnesium prior to delivery is likely to be of benefit. Vigilance is required to assess the mother for magnesium toxicity, and once delivery has occurred, the magnesium can be stopped unless also being given to prevent eclampsia in the mother.

Intrapartum monitoring

If pre-term labour or tocolysis is unsuccessful, then close monitoring is important, as a pre-term fetus is more susceptible to intrapartum hypoxia and acidosis than a fetus at term. Women in pre-term labour should be cared for on the labour ward with monitoring of the fetus, usually in the form of a continuous CTG if the fetus is over 26 weeks' gestation. Fetal scalp electrodes are generally avoided, and expediting delivery by forceps or caesarean is preferred to fetal blood sampling in the presence of a persistently abnormal CTG. Intrapartum complications such as abnormal lie, cord prolapse, abruption and intrauterine infection are more common. Good communication with the neonatal team is needed to allow preparation and attendance to deliver care at delivery.

Delayed cord clamping after delivery of the baby should be undertaken, if the condition of the baby permits, to improve circulating blood volume and hence organ perfusion. Very pre-term babies are particularly susceptible to hypothermia and it is often helpful to place these babies quickly into a plastic bag to minimize this (Fig. 28.2).

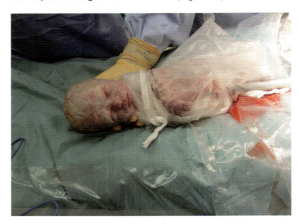

Fig. 28.2   A plastic bag minimizes heat loss in very pre-term babies.

Key points

- Pre-term labour occurs in 10% of pregnancies, and the burden of neonatal mortality and morbidity is high.
- Predicting pre-term labour is difficult, but there are encouraging results from ultrasound cervical assessment.
- Interventions, such as cervical cerclage, may delay labour in carefully selected women, although any benefit to the baby is unproven at present.
- Tocolytics can delay labour in the short term only, and have no proven perinatal benefit alone.
- Antenatal corticosteroids and erythromycin are effective in reducing respiratory distress syndrome and other complications of prematurity in the neonate.
- Magnesium sulphate given prior to delivery can reduce neonatal disability.

29

Multiple pregnancy

Introduction

The natural incidence of twinning has a large geographical variation, ranging from 54/1000 in Nigeria, 12/1000 in the UK, to 4/1000 in Japan. This difference is almost entirely due to variations in the rate of non-identical twins, while the incidence of identical twins remains remarkably constant at around 3/1000. In developed countries, the actual incidence of twin pregnancies is significantly greater than the natural incidence, due to in vitro fertilization and ovulation induction techniques. Around 25% of twin pregnancies, 50–60% of triplet pregnancies and 75% of quadruplet pregnancies are a result of assisted reproduction techniques. One in sixty-four (15.6/1000) pregnancies in the UK is now a twin pregnancy.

Overall, the perinatal mortality in twin pregnancies is four to five times higher than for singleton pregnancies, largely because of pre-term delivery, fetal growth restriction, twin-to-twin transfusion syndrome (TTTS) and a slightly increased incidence of congenital malformations. Perinatal mortality rates rise exponentially with fetal number in higher order pregnancies. The outcome of any multiple pregnancy is also significantly affected by its chorionicity (whether each fetus has its own or shares a placenta) (Fig. 29.1).

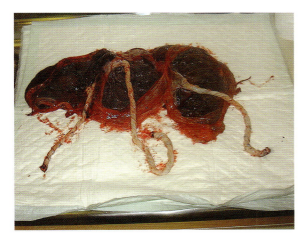

Fig. 29.1 Trichorionic placenta.

The nature of twinning and chorionicity

'Zygosity' refers to whether the twins have developed from a single ovum or from different ova – in other words, whether they are identical or non-identical. 'Chorionicity' refers to the number of placentae (Fig. 29.2).

Dizygotic twinning (non-identical)

Dizygotic twins account for approximately 70% of twins. This process occurs when two ova are fertilized and implant separately into the decidua. Each developing embryo will form its own outer chorion (chorionic membrane and placenta) and its own inner amniotic membrane. Dizygotic twin pregnancies are described as dichorionic and diamniotic.

Monozygotic twinning (identical)

Monozygotic twins (30% of twins) are derived from the splitting of a single embryo and the configuration of placentation depends on the age of the embryo when the split occurred (see Fig. 29.2). Division that occurs at or before the eight-cell stage (3 days post-fertilization) will occur before the outer chorion has differentiated and will therefore give rise to two separate embryos that will each proceed to form their own chorion. These twin pregnancies, like dizygotic twins, will therefore be diamniotic and dichorionic. Embryo division at the blastocyst stage (4–8 days post-fertilization) will occur after the chorion has started to differentiate and therefore the fetuses will share an outer chorion (placenta and outer chorionic membrane). These twins will be monochorionic diamniotic, and are the most common form of monozygotic twins. Division of the embryo between 8 and 14 days will result in the inner amniotic cavity and membrane being shared (monochorionic monoamniotic twins). Splitting beyond 14 days following fertilization is extremely rare, giving rise to conjoined twins (Fig. 29.3 and Table 29.1).

In monochorionic twins, the shared placental mass inevitably contains several vascular anastomoses between the two fetal-placental circulations. The very presence of a shared vascular system dictates that the well-being of each

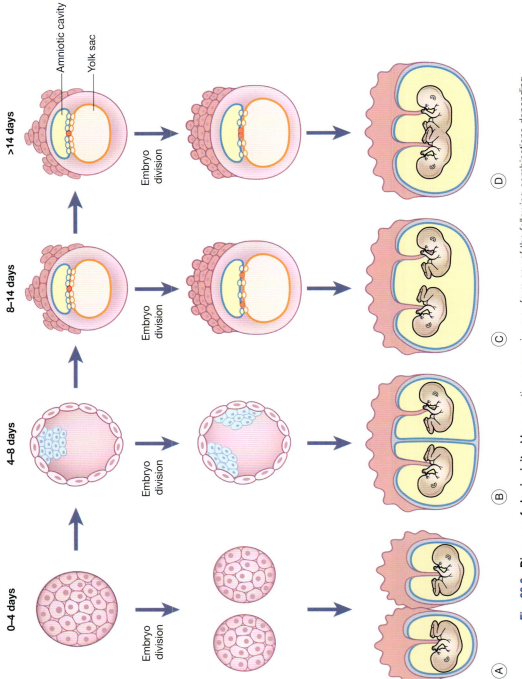

Fig. 29.2 Diagram of chorionicity. Monozygotic pregnancies may form any of the following combinations depending on the timing of embryo division: **(A)** dichorionic diamniotic; **(B)** monochorionic diamniotic; **(C)** monochorionic monoamniotic; **(D)** conjoined twins.

Table 29.1	Chorionicity in monozygous twins		
Timing of embryonic separation after fertilization	**Number of chorions**	**Number of amniotic sacs**	**Percentage of monozygous twins**
<4 days	Dichorionic	Diamniotic	30%
4–8 days	Monochorionic	Diamniotic	66%
8–14 days	Monochorionic	Monoamniotic	3%
>14 days	Monochorionic (conjoined)	Monoamniotic	<1%

Table 29.2	Fetal loss by chorionicity	
	Dichorionic	**Monochorionic**
Fetal loss before 24 weeks	1.8%	12.2%
Fetal loss after 24 weeks	1.6%	2.8%
Delivery before 32 weeks	5.5%	9.2%

The high early fetal mortality in monochorionic pregnancy before 24 weeks is probably largely the result of severe early-onset TTTS (see later).

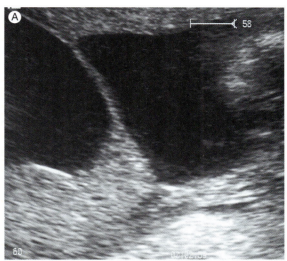

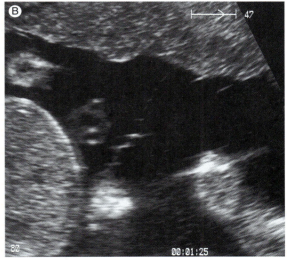

Fig. 29.4 **(A) Dichorionic twins – lambda sign. (B) Monochorionic twins – no lambda sign.** The two amniotic membranes form a 'T' sign as they join the placenta.

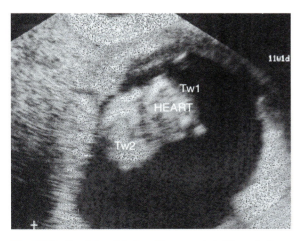

Fig. 29.3 **Conjoined twins.** Diagnosed at 12 weeks' gestation. This is a cross-sectional view through the thoraces of both twins. In view of the shared cardiac structures, management includes the option of termination of pregnancy.

twin is directly dependent on the well-being of the other. The number and nature of these vascular connections places monochorionic twins at risk of specific complications and an increased perinatal loss and morbidity rate.

Chorionicity determination is therefore essential to allow risk stratification (Table 29.2), and has key implications for prenatal diagnosis and antenatal monitoring. It is most easily determined in the first or early second trimester by ultrasound:

- widely separated first-trimester sacs or separate placentae are dichorionic
- those with a 'lambda' or 'twin-peak' sign at the membrane insertion are dichorionic (Fig. 29.4A)
- those with a 'T' sign at the membrane insertion are monochorionic (Fig. 29.4B)

■ different sex fetuses are always dichorionic (and dizygous).

Maternal complications

The incidence of all maternal complications is increased in multiple pregnancy.

Hyperemesis

The increased placental mass, and therefore increased maternal circulating human chorionic gonadotrophin concentration, is associated with an increased incidence and earlier onset of hyperemesis.

Anaemia

There is an increase in the incidence of anaemia associated with multiple pregnancy, which is not completely explained by a haemodilutional effect of the increased plasma volume. The need for iron and folate supplementation should be assessed early in the pregnancy with a full blood count performed at 20–24 weeks' gestation, in addition to the usual antenatal anaemia screen performed at 28 weeks in all pregnancies.

Pre-eclampsia

The incidence of pre-eclampsia in twin pregnancy is three to four times greater than that in singleton pregnancies. It tends to develop earlier and may be more severe. Women carrying a multiple pregnancy should be assessed for any additional risk factor for pre-eclampsia (first pregnancy; age ≥40 years; pregnancy interval of more than 10 years; body mass index of ≥35 kg/m^2 or family history of pre-eclampsia). If one or more additional risk factors exist, the women should be advised to take 75 mg of aspirin daily from 12 weeks until birth as a measure aimed to reduce her overall risk of this complication.

Antepartum haemorrhage

Placenta praevia is more common with multiple gestations because of the larger placental surface. The management of this condition in multiple pregnancy is similar to that of a singleton pregnancy. Placental abruption also appears to be commoner in twin pregnancies.

Thromboembolic disease

Multiple pregnancy is a risk factor for venous thromboembolic disease. This may be due to the adverse effects of the increased size of the pregnant uterus on venous blood flow. Women with multiple pregnancy are also more likely to have other independent risk factors for venous thrombosis such as advanced maternal age, assisted conception, high parity, pre-eclampsia and immobility. Assessment of risk factors for thromboembolic disease should be performed throughout pregnancy. Antenatal thromboprophylaxis may be indicated throughout pregnancy or from 28 weeks' gestation dependent on the number and nature of concurrent risk factors.

Other maternal complications

The mother is also at increased risk of gestational diabetes, general discomfort, varicose veins and dependent oedema, delivery trauma, caesarean section, postpartum haemorrhage, psychological disorders, breastfeeding and parentcraft challenges.

Fetal complications

Chromosomal abnormalities

These are usually confined to one twin (i.e. non-concordant) in dizygotic twins and almost always concordant in monozygotic twins. The maternal age-related risk for carrying at least one fetus with trisomy 21 (Down syndrome) is therefore approximately doubled in dichorionic twin pregnancies (most of which are dizygotic, i.e. the mother carries two individuals each with a risk), but remains unaltered in monochorionic (monozygotic) twins. Maternal serum screening for trisomy 21 performs poorly in twin pregnancy. Nuchal translucency measurement (with or without biochemistry) is a more useful screening test. Analysis of cell-free fetal DNA in the maternal blood (non-invasive prenatal testing) is likely to be the most sensitive and specific screening test for fetal chromosome anomalies, but is not currently freely available within the National Health Service.

If a screening test suggests an increased risk of a chromosome anomaly in any twin, diagnostic testing should be offered. Amniocentesis of each amniotic sac is required in dichorionic pregnancies, and care must be taken to document which sample has come from which sac. Monochorionic (identical twins) only exceptionally have different karyotypes (i.e. rarely there may be post-division loss of some chromosome material in one twin) and sampling of one sac is acceptable unless one has an obvious structural abnormality. Chorionic villous sampling is not usually appropriate for twin pregnancies as it may be difficult to be sure that both placentae have been sampled, particularly if they are lying close together.

Before any screening or invasive diagnostic test is undertaken, the parents should be comprehensively counselled about the psychological difficulties they may face if a risk or diagnosis of an anomaly is confined to a single fetus, and the physical and psychological risks associated with selective termination of one twin.

Structural defects

The incidence of structural fetal abnormality is no different per fetus in a dichorionic pregnancy than from a singleton pregnancy, but it is two- to three-fold greater with monochorionicity. The mother therefore will have a two- to six-fold increased risk of carrying a fetus with a structural abnormality. In monochorionic twins, it is thought that it is the process of embryo division which is inherently teratogenic. Characteristic abnormalities include cardiac defects, neural tube and other central nervous system defects, and gastrointestinal atresia. It is appropriate to offer all those with multiple pregnancies a detailed mid-trimester ultrasound scan. Monochorionic twin pregnancies should be offered an extended ultrasound assessment of fetal heart structure. The abnormalities are usually confined to one twin; for example, if there is a neural tube defect in one twin, the other twin is normal in 85–90% of cases. Selective termination with intracardiac Potassium Chloride (KCl) is possible in dichorionic pregnancies only, and is most safely carried out before 16–20 weeks. The procedure, however, carries a 5% risk of miscarriage of both twins. In monochorionic twins, due to the shared fetoplacental vascular system, specialized cord vessel occlusive techniques may be considered, but carry an increased (10–20%) risk of loss to the other twin due to the invasiveness of this procedure.

Premature birth

Approximately 60% of twin pregnancies result in spontaneous pre-term birth before 37 + 0 weeks' gestation, and approximately 10% deliver before 32 weeks' gestation. Triplet pregnancies typically (75%) result in spontaneous pre-term birth before 35 + 0 weeks' gestation. Twins account for 25% of all premature births, despite accounting for only 3% of births per year. Pre-term delivery is higher in monochorionic compared with dichorionic twins (see Table 29.2). Increased uterine distension, early myometrial contractility and TTTS may be causative factors in premature labour in multiple pregnancy. At present there is no known effective treatment to prevent premature labour. Women should be advised to seek assistance early with any symptoms of suspected pre-term labour so that corticosteroids can be administered to accelerate fetal lung maturation.

Fetal growth restriction

Abdominal palpation is not reliable to monitor fetal growth in multiple pregnancy. Serial ultrasound should be performed to measure fetal abdominal circumferences. Twins typically reflect singleton size charts until 28–30 weeks' gestation and then growth slows. Approximately 30% of twins are small for gestational age by singleton standards and a significant difference in the growth of one twin compared with the other is seen in 12% of pregnancies. This is defined by a discordance in fetal size of 20–25% (the difference in abdominal circumferences divided by the abdominal circumference of the larger twin) and predicts morbidity. Placental dysfunction underlies fetal growth restriction in twin pregnancies, as it does in singleton pregnancies. If diagnosed, growth restriction requires increased surveillance of fetal well-being with umbilical artery Doppler and cardiotocography (CTG)

monitoring, so that delivery can be optimally timed. Monochorionic twins are at increased risk of growth restriction and require a lower threshold for delivery owing to the specific adverse consequences to the co-twin in the event of a single intrauterine death in these twins (see later).

Twins with one fetal death

First-trimester intrauterine death in a twin has not been shown to have adverse consequences for the survivor. This probably also holds true for the early second trimester in dichorionic twins, but loss in the late second or third trimester commonly precipitates labour. The majority of affected pregnancies will deliver both fetuses before 34 weeks' gestation, often within 3 weeks of the loss. Prognosis for a surviving dichorionic fetus is then influenced primarily by its gestation. When a monochorionic twin dies in utero, however, there are additional risks of death (approx. 20%) or cerebral damage (approx. 25%) in the co-twin as a result of the shared fetal-placental circulations. As these are probably related to acute hypotension in the co-twin at the time of the other's death, early delivery of the surviving twin is unlikely to improve its outcome and may compound morbidity if performed at a premature gestation.

Antenatal problems specific to monochorionic twin pregnancies

Twin-to-twin transfusion syndrome

This complicates 10–15% of monochorionic multiple pregnancies and accounts for around 15% of perinatal mortality in twins. In this condition there is a net blood flow from one twin to the other through arterial to venous anastomoses in the shared placenta. The circulation of the recipient becomes hyperdynamic, with the risk of high-output cardiac failure and polyhydramnios. Conversely, the donor develops oliguria and oligohydramnios, and often suffers growth restriction (Figs 29.5). The ultrasound finding of the oligohydramnios-polyhydramnios sequence is the key to establishing an antenatal diagnosis.

Without treatment, TTTS is associated with a >80% pregnancy loss rate. Two interventions have proven useful: serial amniodrainage and laser ablation of the causative placental vascular anastomoses (Fig. 29.6). Evidence has emerged that laser ablation is the most effective intervention (70% survival vs 50% survival with amnioreduction) and therefore is the treatment of choice in all but the mildest form of TTTS. Laser therapy is also associated with a lower rate of significant neurological morbidity in surviving twins compared with amnioreduction (5% vs 15%).

Twin anaemia polycythaemia sequence

In this condition there is a slow low volume transfer of blood from one fetus to the other. This causes one fetus to

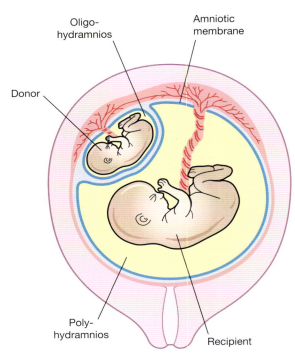

Fig. 29.5 **Monochorionic twins demonstrating TTTS.** (Oligohydramnios-polyhydramnios sequence).

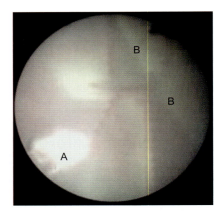

Fig. 29.6 **Fetoscopic laser ablation of vascular anastomoses on the surface of the placenta in the treatment of TTTS.** The laser fibre **(A)** is used to ablate vessels crossing the inter-twin membrane **(B)** from the donor twin as they anastomose with vessels from the recipient twin.

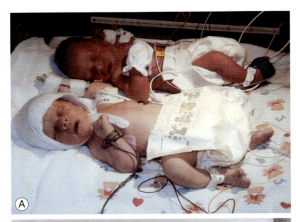

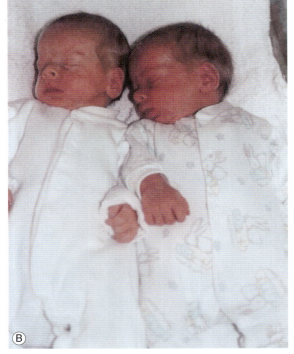

Fig. 29.7 **Twin anaemia polycythaemia sequence.** These monochorionic twins were born at 37 weeks' gestation. Although their weights were almost identical, there was significant difference in haemoglobin concentrations at birth. This is a recently described (chronic) form of fetal-to-fetal transfusion. **(A)** At delivery. **(B)** Post corrective blood transfusion to the anaemic twin (with permission).

become anaemic and the other polycythaemic (Fig. 29.7), without the large haemodynamic fluid shifts seen in TTTS. The liquor volumes are therefore not altered as in TTTS. The anaemic twin may develop hydrops. Intervention is difficult with all potential therapies (intrauterine transfusion, laser therapy and early delivery) having a significant risk of not being effective or of fetal and neonatal morbidity. Screening for the anaemia, which occurs in this condition, can be performed by fetal middle cerebral artery Doppler. In the absence of an ideal therapy, this may only be cost effective following laser therapy for TTTS, where the incidence (up to 13%) is higher than seen in other monochorionic twins (1–2%).

Severe selective intrauterine growth restriction (sIUGR)

If severe sIUGR of one monochorionic twin occurs before viability, selective termination by cord-occlusion techniques may be considered in the interests of the co-twin. sIUGR is associated with an increased risk of in utero demise.

Monoamniotic twins

Twins who occupy a single amniotic sac are at risk of loss due to cord entanglement in utero. Frequent CTG monitoring is required once they reach viability. Delivery is electively planned for 32 weeks' gestation, but indicated earlier if cord compression is suggested by abnormal fetal heart rate patterns on CTG analysis. Delivery should be performed by caesarean section, as the risk of a cord accident is particularly high during labour.

Twin reversed arterial perfusion sequence

If the heart of one monochorionic twin stops, it may continue to be partially perfused by the surviving twin via a large fetal arterial-to-arterial anastomose in the shared placenta. The dead twin undergoes atrophy of its upper body and heart due to the especially poor oxygenation of these tissues, and becomes what has been described as an 'acardiac monster'. The condition is very rare, affecting <1% of monochorionic twins. There is a high incidence of mortality in the normal ('pump') twin due to intrauterine cardiac failure and prematurity. This risk increases with the relative size of the acardiac twin. Cord vessel–occlusive techniques, when performed on large acardiac twins (>50% size of the normal twin), appear to improve survival rates of the normal twin.

Management of pregnancy

Initial visit

It is important to ensure that chorionicity has been established on scan. Ideally this should be performed between 11 and 13 + 6 weeks' gestation, as it becomes increasingly difficult to do so with advancing gestation.

The parents are often excited, and shocked, so initial counselling should be focused and include positive aspects. The parents should be counselled regarding their options for antenatal screening for fetal anomalies and should understand the potential dilemmas that may arise if one normal and one abnormal twin is diagnosed. It should be explained that more frequent antenatal visits will be required to monitor both the maternal and fetal well-being, and that ultrasound will play the key role in fetal assessments. Risk assessment for pre-eclampsia should be undertaken and low-dose aspirin initiated as indicated. The risk of premature delivery, the

optimal timing of delivery in uncomplicated pregnancies and potential modes of delivery should be outlined.

Subsequent visits

Women should be cared for in a dedicated multiple pregnancy clinic by a multidisciplinary team including a specialist obstetrician and midwife. The visits should be timed to coincide with the ultrasound assessments, the schedule of which will depend on chorionicity.

Monochorionic twins:

- every 2 weeks from 16 weeks to survey for TTTS and fetal growth restriction
- detailed structural survey at 18 to 20 weeks' gestation
- detailed fetal cardiac scan at 22 weeks' gestation.

Dichorionic twins:

- detailed structural survey at 18 to 20 weeks' gestation
- every 2–4 weeks from 24 weeks for fetal growth assessment.

The mother should be monitored for complications such as pre-eclampsia and anaemia. Risk assessment for thromboembolic disease should be performed at each visit or emergency admission. Discussions about the risks and management of premature delivery and fetal growth problems are useful at 22–24 weeks' gestation. In uncomplicated pregnancies, discussion around mode of delivery and management of twin labour is useful at 32 weeks' gestation when fetal presentations are unlikely to change. Tailored parentcraft advice or classes should be offered and include dietary, breastfeeding and perinatal mental health advice. Contact details of support groups should be offered.

Management of twin delivery

In uncomplicated twin pregnancies delivery is planned for 37 weeks' gestation in dichorionic twin pregnancies and for 36 weeks' gestation in monochorionic pregnancies. This guidance is based on the increased risk of stillbirth in these populations after these gestations.

Presentations at term are typically:

- cephalic/cephalic (40%)
- cephalic/breech (40%)
- breech/cephalic (10%)
- other, e.g. transverse (10%).

In general, providing the presentation of the first twin is cephalic, the balance of current evidence would suggest that a trial of vaginal birth is appropriate. Significant growth discordance or any other concern of fetal well-being may be a reason to consider caesarean section. If the labour is pre-term (<34 weeks) or if the mother has had a previous caesarean section, many clinicians would also consider delivery by caesarean section.

If labour is induced or spontaneous, the first stage is managed as for singleton pregnancies, and care should be taken to ensure that both twins are being monitored with

CTG, rather than one twin twice. This is best achieved by monitoring twin I with a fetal scalp electrode and twin II with an abdominal transducer.

An experienced obstetrician, an anaesthetist, two paediatricians and two midwives should be present for delivery, and if not already required, a syntocinon infusion should be ready in case uterine activity decreases after delivery of the first twin. After delivery of the first twin, it is often helpful to have someone 'stabilize' the lie of second twin to longitudinal by abdominal palpation while a vaginal examination is performed to assess the station of the presenting part. A portable ultrasound machine is helpful to confirm the lie and presentation of the second twin. The membranes of twin II should not be broken until the presenting part has descended into the pelvis. If twin II lies transversely after the delivery of twin I, external cephalic or breech version is appropriate. If the lie is still transverse, the choice is between performing an internal podalic version (ideally keeping the membranes intact while the obstetrician's hand enters the uterus to identify, grasp and bring down a fetal foot) followed by subsequent breech extraction or performing a caesarean section. The CTG of twin II should be carefully monitored throughout and delivery expedited if suspected fetal distress is observed. This twin has the highest risk of adverse outcome in labour.

A maternal epidural is useful in the management of twin labour, owing to the increased risks of obstetric intervention, particularly assisted delivery of twin II.

Due to the enlarged uterine size, the mother is at risk of atonic postpartum haemorrhage. This should be anticipated. Management of the third stage should be active with the administration of syntocinon or ergometrine. Rapid escalation to a postpartum haemorrhage protocol should follow if indicated by ongoing blood loss. Risk assessment for thromboembolic disease should continue post-delivery.

Triplets and higher multiples

In these cases the perinatal mortality is high, mostly because of the high risk of pre-term labour, and it may be appropriate to discuss reducing the number of fetuses to twins at 12–14 weeks' gestation. With quadruplets or higher order pregnancies, there is likely to be a greater chance of at least one or two survivors if fetal reduction is carried out, despite the miscarriage risk associated with the procedure itself. Reduction of any monochorionic twin pairs will have the greatest positive effect on outcomes. For triplets the situation is less clear. The emotional and ethical problems associated with these decisions are considerable.

Triplets and higher order multiple pregnancies require intensive antenatal care. These pregnancies are best delivered by caesarean section due to the inability to effectively monitor all fetuses in labour and the higher risk of fetal malpresentation.

Key *points*

- It is essential to establish chorionicity by $11 + 0 - 13 + 6$ weeks' gestation in multiple pregnancy to plan and deliver appropriate antenatal care.
- Increasing fetal number and monochorionicity are associated with increased risks of adverse outcomes.
- The shared fetal circulations within a monochorionic placenta can cause specific complications, such as TTTS, but also make the management of other generic twin complications, such as selective fetal growth restriction or anomaly of one twin, more complex.
- Pre-term labour is the commonest cause of neonatal loss and morbidity in multiple pregnancies.

30

Labour and analgesia

Normal labour

Introduction

Labour is a challenging time for mothers and their babies. The success of labour and the ability of the fetus to successfully negotiate a journey through the maternal pelvis depends upon the successful interaction of three variables – the power (contractions), passenger (fetus) and pelvis (bony pelvis and pelvic soft tissues). For women this is often a life-changing event, with the experience that a woman has at this time potentially having both short- and long-term physical and emotional effects. For most women this is a positive, joyous life event, but the challenges faced during labour can potentially result in adverse outcomes for mother and baby. Midwives and obstetricians are intimately involved in the care of women in normal labour, in trying to ensure normality, in recognizing at an early stage when obstetric intervention may be required in the maternal or fetal interest and ensuring that the woman's choices and opinions are respected. The majority of women in the UK will have a normal delivery in pregnancy after 37 weeks' gestation after a healthy uncomplicated pregnancy, with almost two-thirds of women going into labour spontaneously. 40% of these women will be in their first pregnancy. Good communication with women is essential at this time to help them feel supported and in control, with the aim of making birth a positive experience for all concerned.

Evolution and human labour

Labour is defined as the onset of regular uterine activity associated with effacement and dilatation of the cervix and descent of the presenting part through the cervix. The control and timing of delivery is crucial in the survival of any species, and in most, the interval between conception and parturition varies little. This is not the case in human pregnancy, where delivery can occur many weeks before or after the expected date.

Labour in humans is surprisingly hazardous. Evolution ought to have favoured those mothers who deliver without

problems, and yet for those without access to good medical care the lifetime risk of dying from labour and postnatal complications may be as high as 10%

Apes are able to give birth with little problem. Their pelvises are relatively large, the fetal head is relatively small and the fetus is born facing anteriorly. When the Australopithecines adopted an upright posture around 4 million years ago, the pelvic shape became narrower in the anteroposterior plane to allow more efficient weight transfer from the trunk to the femurs. As the fetal head was still relatively small, the Australopithecines were also able to deliver without much problem, although this time the head was in the transverse position.

With further evolution 1.5 million years ago to *Homo erectus* and then *Homo sapiens*, the volume of the brain increased from around 500 mL to 1000–2000 mL. This increased the chance of the head being bigger than the pelvis (cephalopelvic disproportion), and to deliver successfully it became necessary for the head to rotate during delivery. The head entered the pelvic brim in the transverse position as the inlet is widest in the transverse plane, but rotated at the pelvic floor to the anteroposterior plane, which is the widest diameter of the pelvic outlet.

This process requires efficient uterine activity and is aided by 'moulding' of the fetal head. Moulding is possible because the individual skull bones are unfused and can therefore move or even override each other to form the most efficient shape for delivery. The pelvic ligaments, particularly the cartilaginous joint of the symphysis pubis, relax antenatally under the influence of relaxin to maximize the pelvic diameters. Successful delivery also requires the fetus to enter the pelvis in the appropriate position. When these criteria are not met, problems may occur and these are discussed further in Chapter 33. The difficulty with human delivery is related to the balance between our need to run (and therefore have a narrow pelvis) and our need to think (and therefore have a big head).

Primigravid compared with multigravid labour

There is a considerable difference between the labour of a primigravida (a mother having her first labour) and that of a parous woman who has had a previous vaginal delivery (Table 30.1). A successful vaginal delivery first time around usually leads to subsequent deliveries being relatively uneventful. Conversely, a caesarean section or other complications in a first labour can lead to subsequent obstetric problems.

The uterus during pregnancy

The uterus is a thick-walled hollow organ, normally located entirely within the lesser pelvis (Table 30.2) in the non-pregnant state. The smooth muscle fibres interdigitate to form a single functional muscle that increases markedly during pregnancy, mainly by hypertrophy (an increase in size of cells) and to a lesser extent by hyperplasia (an increase in the number of smooth muscle cells).

From early pregnancy onwards the uterus contracts intermittently, and the frequency and amplitude of these contractions increase as labour approaches. These 'Braxton Hicks' contractions are irregular, low frequency and high amplitude in character, and are only occasionally painful. They are thought to begin at a 'pacemaker point' close to the junction of the uterus and the fallopian tube (although this has never been confirmed anatomically) and spread from this point downwards. The intensity of contractions is maximal at the fundus (where the muscle is thickest), intermediate at the mid-zone and least at the lower segment.

The initiation of labour

In humans, despite major advances in molecular biology and the science of reproduction, there is still much that is not known about the physiological processes involved in the initiation of labour. Some of the information, which we have about this process, is derived from animal studies where our understanding is more complete. In some mammals, changing levels of oestrogen and progesterone regulate the timing of onset of labour. In other animals, for example sheep, there is some evidence that the fetal adrenal secretion of corticosteroids is the trigger. In humans, however, the process appears to be more complicated, involving the coordinated inhibition and activation of a variety of factors. Our limited understanding of this process means that any proposed mechanism is hypothetical and open to constant change as our knowledge advances.

There is increasing evidence that human parturition involves activation of inflammatory pathways finally leading to cervical ripening, the onset of uterine activity and membrane rupture. This process appears to be controlled in some way by a complex interaction of various mediators. The onset of labour therefore appears to occur when there is the coordinated 'release' of the uterus and cervix from the inhibitory effects of various pro-pregnancy factors and the simultaneous activation of various pro-labour factors (Box 30.1). How these factors interact and why labour occurs at a specific time (whether pre-term or at term) is unclear and still the subject of much ongoing research.

Table 30.1	The differences between a normal primigravid and multigravid labour
Primigravida	**Multigravida**
Unique psychological experience	
Inefficient uterine action is common, therefore labour is often longer	Uterine action is efficient and the genital tract stretches more easily, therefore labour is usually shorter
The functional capacity of the pelvis is not known – cephalopelvic disproportion is a possibility	Cephalopelvic disproportion is rare. If it occurs, it is usually secondary to some serious problem
Serious injury to the child is relatively more common. The incidence of instrumental delivery is higher	Serious injury to the child is rare. Risk of birth injury is less when the baby is born by propulsion rather than traction
Uterus is virtually immune to rupture	Small risk of uterine rupture, particularly if there is a pre-existing caesarean section scar

Table 30.2	Changes in the uterus and cervix during pregnancy	
	Non-pregnant uterus	**Term uterus**
Weight	50 g	950 g
Length	7.5 cm	30 cm
Depth	2.5 cm	20 cm
Shape	Flattened pear	Ovoid and erect
Position	Anteverted and anteflexed in pelvic cavity	Rotated to right in the abdominal cavity
	Non-pregnant cervix	**Cervix at term**
Length	2.5 cm	2.5 cm
Colour	Pink	Blue and vascular

(Adapted from Harrison JM. The initiation of labour: physiological mechanisms. *Br J Midwifery* 8:281–285, 2000).

Box 30.1

Pro-pregnancy factors and pro-labour factors

Pro-pregnancy factors

- Progesterone
- Nitric oxide
- Catecholamines
- Relaxin

Pro-labour factors

- Oestrogens
- Oxytocin
- Prostaglandins
- Corticotrophin-releasing hormone
- Prostaglandin dehydrogenase
- Inflammatory mediators

Pro-pregnancy factors

Progesterone is derived from the corpus luteum for the first 8 weeks or so of pregnancy and thereafter from the placenta. It has the direct effect of decreasing uterine oxytocin receptor sensitivity and therefore promotes uterine smooth muscle relaxation. Progesterone also seems to have an anti-inflammatory role, and decreases cytokine production and the influx of immune cells into the myometrium and cervix occurring in normal labour. Its role in maintenance of uterine quiescence during pregnancy is illustrated by the fact that the progesterone antagonist mifepristone increases myometrial contractility, and has been successfully used to induce labour. Progesterone withdrawal has been shown in animal studies in sheep and goats to trigger labour. However, human parturition is not associated with a fall in serum progesterone levels, suggesting instead that there may be a 'functional' progesterone withdrawal, perhaps caused by changes in the progesterone receptor. This may lead in turn to a decrease in the transcription of genes which cause uterine relaxation, and an increase in the transcription of genes which increase the sensitivity of the myometrium to uterotonic agents and also cause activation of inflammatory pathways within the cervix and myometrium.

Nitric oxide, a highly reactive free radical, is also a pro-pregnancy factor. Some studies have observed a fall in uterine nitric oxide synthetase activity as pregnancy advances, but these findings are not confirmed in other studies. Nitric oxide may be involved in the process of cervical ripening, which involves remodelling of the extracellular matrix and collagen. Catecholamines act directly on the myometrial cell membrane to alter contractility and beta-sympathomimetics have been used as tocolytics to suppress pre-term labour. The specific roles for catecholamines in physiological terms and the role of the hormone relaxin are unclear, although they may indirectly cause uterine muscle relaxation by stimulating prostacyclin production.

Pro-labour factors

Oxytocin, a nonapeptide from the posterior pituitary, is a potent stimulator of uterine contractility. Circulating levels, however, do not change as term approaches. The rise in oxytocin receptor levels explains the increase in sensitivity of the uterus to circulating levels of oxytocin as pregnancy advances. It is unlikely that the onset of labour in humans is triggered by oxytocin release, but it is clear that oxytocin release during labour increases the frequency and force of uterine contractions.

Changes in oxytocin receptor concentration are mediated in part by activation of the fetal hypothalamic–pituitary axis with release of fetal adrenocorticotrophic hormone. Prostaglandin levels also increase prior to the onset of labour. These are synthesized from arachidonic acid by cyclo-oxygenase (COX), and COX-2 enzyme expression in the fetal membranes has been observed to double by the time labour begins. Prostaglandins promote cervical ripening and stimulate uterine contractility both directly and by upregulation of oxytocin receptors, and there is some evidence that the increased levels may be mediated by maternal corticotrophin-releasing hormone secretion. Inflammatory cells are recruited into the fetal membranes, uterus and cervix at the onset of labour, perhaps as a result of distension of the uterus and/or endocrine hormone signaling from the fetus itself. A number of cytokines are produced (such as interleukin (IL)-8, tumour necrosis factor (TNF)-alpha, IL-6 and IL1B), which in turn set up activation of pro-inflammatory transcription factors. This inflammatory response is thought to contribute to cervical ripening and membrane rupture via an increase in collagenase activity. It may also contribute to an increase in uterine activity by inhibition of progesterone and by activation of contractile genes (COX-2, oxytocin receptor).

The mechanism of normal labour and delivery

(See also Clinical pelvic anatomy, Chapter 1.)

The mechanism of labour involves effacement and then dilatation of the cervix, followed by expulsion of the fetus by uterine contractions. The lower part of the uterus is anchored to the pelvis by the transverse cervical (or cardinal) ligaments, as well as the uterosacral ligaments, allowing the shortening uterine muscle to drive the fetus downwards (Box 30.2).

Cervical ripening

The cervix is composed of a network of collagen fibres embedded in ground substance made of extracellular matrix. During the later stages of pregnancy it softens and begins to efface so that delivery can occur. Prostaglandins increase cervical ripening by inhibiting collagen synthesis and stimulating collagenase activity to break down the collagen. This collagenase activity comes in part, not only from fibroblast cells, but also from an influx of inflammatory cells, supporting the theory that labour is in part like an inflammatory process. Dermatan sulphate (a proteoglycan molecule) is replaced with hyaluronic acid, which is more hydrophilic and the

---

Box 30.2

Summary of the mechanism of the labour

- Head at pelvic brim in left or right occipitolateral position
- Neck flexes so that the presenting diameter is suboccipitobregmatic
- Head descends and engages
- Head reaches the pelvic floor and occiput rotates to occipitoanterior
- Head delivers by extension
- Descent continues and shoulders rotate into the anteroposterior diameter of the pelvis
- Head restitutes (comes into line with the shoulders)
- Anterior shoulder delivered by lateral flexion from downward pressure on the baby's head; posterior shoulder delivered by lateral flexion upwards

water content of the cervix increases. As a result of these changes the concentration of collagen fibres decreases and the cervix becomes softer and ready to dilate. In clinical practice, cervical ripening is assessed using the Bishop score (Table 30.3). The parameters of this score include: cervical length, cervical dilatation, consistency, position and station of the presenting part.

Activation of the myometrium

Contractions in the uterus, like any other smooth muscle, involve Adenosine Triphosphonate (ATP)-dependent binding of myosin to actin. The process involves phosphorylation of the enzyme myosin light chain kinase, which is dependent on calcium and calmodulin for its activity. Hence, calcium-channel blockers and beta agonists inhibit uterine activity by decreasing intracellular free calcium levels, and prosta-glandins and oxytocin increase uterine activity by bringing about an increase in free calcium.

The uterine smooth muscle cells are embedded in a supporting framework of collagen fibres and extracellular matrix. The myometrial fibres communicate with each other by means of gap junctions between cells. These gap junctions facilitate cell signalling and also allow the smooth muscle to act as a syncytium, with contractions spreading from one cell to another. During pregnancy gap junctions are few in number, but as pregnancy advances they increase in concentration and size within the uterus. One of the actions of oestrogen and prostaglandin is to increase gap junction formation, while human chorionic gonadotrophin may decrease their formation.

Descent and delivery of fetus

As the cervix dilates and the uterus contracts, the fetus needs to descend into the pelvis. The widest two points of the fetus are the head in the anteroposterior plane (Fig. 30.1) and the shoulders laterally, from one shoulder tip to the other (bisacromial diameter). The head rotates from a lateral position at the pelvic brim to the anteroposterior position at the outlet (Figs 30.2–30.4). This rotation has the advantage that by the time the head is delivering through the outlet, the shoulders will be entering the inlet in the transverse position, maximizing the chance of successful delivery.

The position of the head as it traverses the canal is described according to the position of the occiput in relation

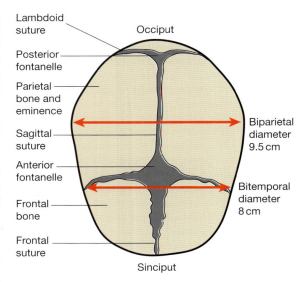

Fig. 30.1 **The fetal skull.** The widest diameter is anteroposterior.

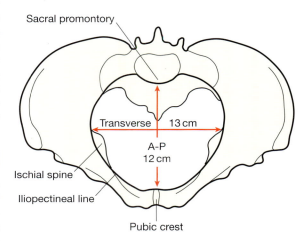

Fig. 30.2 **The maternal pelvic inlet.** The widest diameter is from one side laterally to the other. A-P, anteroposterior.

to the mother's pelvis. The head usually enters the pelvic brim in either the right or the left occipitotransverse position (Fig. 30.5A). The contracting uterus above causes the head to flex so that the smallest diameter is presented for delivery.

As the head descends it reaches the V-shaped pelvic floor at the level of the ischial spines (Fig. 30.5B–D). The shape of the pelvic floor encourages the fundamentally important head rotation. Fig. 30.6 illustrates the tendency for the longest part of the head to fit into the lowest part of the V-shaped gutter, achievable only by a 90° rotation to either the occipitoanterior (OA) or occipitoposterior posi-tion. In most cases the head rotates anteriorly. The conse-quences of posterior rotation are discussed on page 330. The head, now OA, descends beyond the ischial spines

Table 30.3	Bishop score			
Parameter	**0**	**1**	**2**	**3**
Dilatation	<1 cm	1–2 cm	2–4 cm	>4 cm
Length	>4 cm	2–4 cm	1–2 cm	<1 cm
Consistency	Firm	Average	Soft	
Position	Posterior	Mid	Anterior	
Station	−3	−2	−1, 0	+1, +2

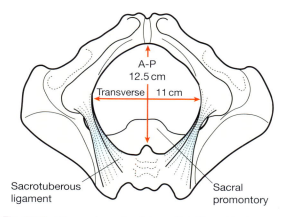

Fig. 30.3 **The maternal pelvic outlet.** The widest diameter is anteroposterior. A-P, anteroposterior.

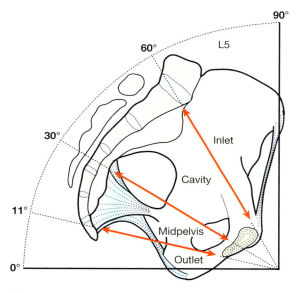

Fig. 30.4 **Lateral view of the pelvis.**

and extends, distending the vulva until it is eventually delivered (Fig. 30.5E & F).

Meanwhile, at the pelvic inlet, the shoulders are now presenting in the transverse position. They too descend to the pelvic floor and rotate to the anteroposterior position in the V of the pelvic floor (Fig. 30.5G). By this time, the head has been completely delivered and it is free to rotate back to the transverse position along with the shoulders. The anterior shoulder can then be delivered by downward traction of the head, so that the lateral traction on the fetal trunk allows the shoulder to be freed from under the pubic arch (see Fig. 30.5G). The posterior shoulder is delivered with upward lateral traction and the rest of the baby usually follows without difficulty (Fig. 30.5H).

The third stage of labour is from delivery of the baby until delivery of the placenta. The uterus contracts, shearing the placenta from the uterine wall, and this separation is often indicated by a small rush of dark blood and a 'lengthening' of the cord. The placenta can then be delivered by gentle cord traction (Fig. 30.5I), but caution is required to avoid uterine inversion.

Diagnosis of labour

The diagnosis of 'labour' is important but often surprisingly difficult. The presence of palpable contractions does not necessarily mean that a woman is in labour, as Braxton Hicks contractions are common antenatally. For labour diagnosis there needs to be *uterine contraction* together with *effacement (thinning) and dilatation of the cervix*.

Effacement has occurred when the entire length of the cervical canal has been 'taken up' into the lower segment of the uterus, a process that begins at the internal os and proceeds downwards to the external os until the cervical tissue becomes continuous with the uterine walls (Fig. 30.7A-C). This is analogous to pulling a polo-necked sweater over your head. It is of note that 'dilatation' refers only to the dilatation of the external os. Again, there is an important difference between primigravid and multigravid labours, as dilatation will not begin in a primigravida until effacement has occurred, whereas both may occur simultaneously in a parous woman (Fig. 30.7).

If there are regular contractions and a fully effaced cervix, the woman can be said to be in labour. If, however, there are contractions with only a partially effaced cervix, further objective evidence must be sought in the form of either a 'show' or spontaneous membrane rupture. A 'show', or bloodstained mucous discharge, has occurred in approximately two-thirds of women by the time of presentation and supports the diagnosis in those with regular contractions. Spontaneous membrane rupture in the presence of regular contractions also confirms the diagnosis.

Rupture of the membranes

Rupture of the fetal membranes is a vital part of normal labour. In 6–12% of labours the membranes will rupture prior to the onset of uterine contractions or cervical dilatation, 'pre-labour rupture of the membranes'. The mother will usually describe the feeling of 'water' leaking vaginally, and if a speculum examination is carried out, a pool of liquor is typically seen in the posterior vaginal fornix. A digital vaginal examination is not routinely indicated, as this increases the risk of introducing infection. If managed conservatively, 60% of mothers will establish in labour spontaneously by 24 h and 90% by 48 h. This conservative management, however, carries a small risk of ascending infection, which may lead to chorioamnionitis. Rarely, chorioamnionitis may progress to rapid overwhelming fetal and maternal sepsis.

Nonetheless, in view of the high chance of spontaneous labour over the first 24 h, a conservative approach may be appropriate. This is provided that the mother is apyrexial, the baby is in cephalic presentation, the liquor is clear and fetal monitoring is normal. In women presenting with rupture of the membranes prior to the onset of labour the risk of serious neonatal infection is 1% compared with 0.5% for women with intact membranes. Induction of labour may be offered after 24 h if there are no signs that labour is becoming established. Women who present with pre-labour rupture of the membranes may also be offered induction of labour on admission, as this may reduce the incidence of neonatal infection with no increase in the rate of caesarean

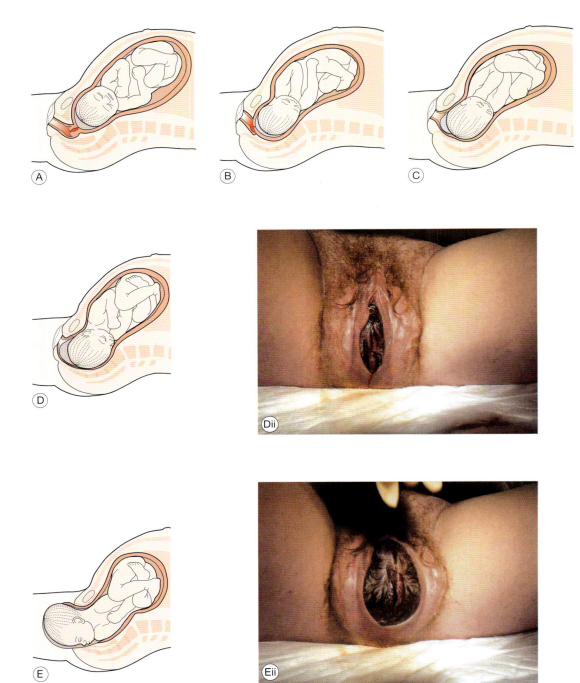

Fig. 30.5   Normal labour; A–I (see text).

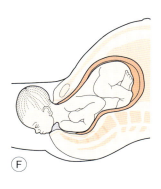
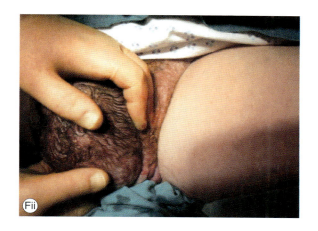
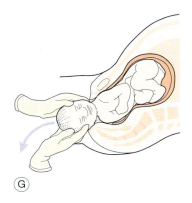
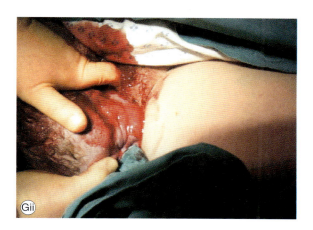
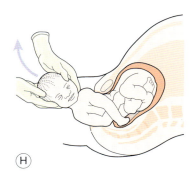
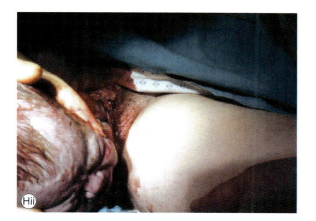

Fig. 30.5, cont'd

continued

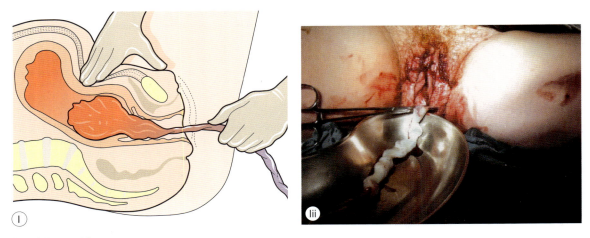

Fig. 30.5, cont'd

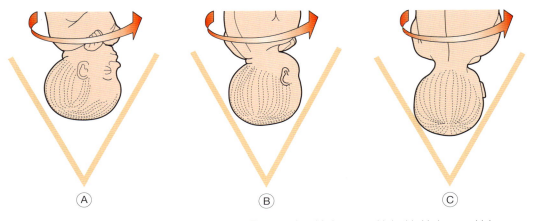

Fig. 30.6 **The head descends onto the pelvic floor.** This runs in a V-shape, and it is this V-shape, which encourages rotation of the fetal head.

	38th week	During first stage of labour	End of first stage of labour
Primigravida	A	B	
Multiparous	A	B	C

Fig. 30.7 **Cervical dilatation – primigravida versus multigravida.** Note that in a multigravida the cervix may dilate before effacement is complete.

delivery. Women with pre-labour rupture of membranes should be counselled about their options, and they and their partners should be involved in the decision-making process. In those managed conservatively, women should be made aware of signs and symptoms of infection and advised to attend hospital if there is any change in the colour or smell of their discharge or any decrease in fetal movements. If there is clinical suspicion of chorioamnionitis, with pyrexia or passage of meconium (see later), delivery must be expedited. Pain and discharge are late features of intrauterine infection.

Clinical progress in labour

Labour is divided into three stages of unequal length (Table 30.4). There is no 'normal' time for the length of labour. However, the mean length of established labour (i.e. from 4 cm dilated, with regular painful contractions) is 8 h for primigravid women but can be up to 18 h. The mean length for second and subsequent labours is 5.5 h but can be up to 12 h. Even after a labour of 40 h the chance of a vaginal delivery is still around 50%. Fetal distress (hypoxia) is only partly related to the length of labour. The highest incidence of caesarean section for distress is in the first hour of labour, probably related to babies already compromised antenatally with some pre-existing problem. Even after 24 h, however, the chance of fetal distress remains low. It is recognized that markedly prolonged labour is associated with subsequent maternal pelvic floor dysfunction and fistulae. There is therefore no 'optimal' length of labour, and each mother should be assessed on an individual basis with her views

being taken into account when making decisions about ongoing management.

First stage

The onset of labour is often gradual, with changes occurring in the cervix and myometrium during pregnancy in preparation for this process. The first stage of labour is timed from the onset of regular uterine activity associated with progressive effacement and dilatation of the cervix. The first stage is complete when the cervix becomes fully dilated (10 cm). Progress in the first stage of labour is measured in terms of dilatation of the cervix and descent of the fetal head.

There are two phases of the first stage. The latent phase describes the time interval between the onset of labour and the completion of effacement. The cervix will be 3–4 cm dilated at the end of this stage. The length of the latent phase is particularly variable, especially for women having their first pregnancy. For some women this stage of labour can be prolonged and potentially unsettling due to the uncertainty associated with the length of time it will take. Women should be supported at this time and encouraged to mobilize if possible. Simple analgesia can be advised and some women may choose to use breathing exercises, massage and immersion in water to help with pain relief. Often women can remain at home in the latent phase and they should be informed that there is no reason to restrict eating and drinking at this time.

The active phase describes the time interval between the end of the latent phase and full dilatation (10 cm). When a woman presents in labour, a risk assessment will be performed to identify whether it is appropriate for her to continue with midwifery-led care. Initial assessment will include a review of her past obstetric history to identify potential complications and this may prompt referral to an obstetric led rather than a midwifery led unit. Baseline recordings of her pulse, blood pressure, temperature and urinalysis should be made along with an assessment of the length, strength and frequency of contractions. Women should be asked if their membranes have ruptured and colour and amount of amniotic fluid lost. Note should also be made of any discharge or bleeding and whether the fetal movements are normal. A vaginal examination is often performed to confirm whether active labour has commenced. An examination is performed to assess fundal height, lie, presentation and engagement of the presenting part. An assessment of the contractions is made by the midwife by palpation of the woman's abdomen and auscultation of the fetal heart is performed with either a handheld Doppler device or a Pinard stethoscope. Some hospitals will perform a cardiotocography (CTG) on low-risk women at first presentation in labour. This is controversial, as the benefit of CTG monitoring in low-risk women has not been proven. However, some women may request a CTG on admission and their wishes should be respected following a discussion about the possible limitations of its use.

Table 30.4	The three stages of labour	
	Stage	**Phases**
First stage	From the onset of labour until the cervix is fully dilated; further subdivided into two phases	(a) Latent – onset of contractions until the cervix is fully effaced and 3–4 cm dilated
		(b) Active – cervical dilatation
Second stage	From full cervical dilatation until the head has delivered. It also has two phases	(a) Propulsive – from full dilatation until head has descended onto the pelvic floor
		(b) Expulsive – from the time the mother has an irresistible desire to bear down and push until the baby is delivered
Third stage	From delivery of the baby until expulsion of the placenta and membranes	

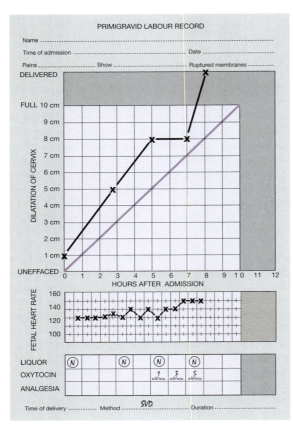

Fig. 30.8 **Partogram suitable for recording a primigravid labour.**

Table 30.5	Vaginal examinations
Findings on vaginal examination	**Details**
Presence or absence of meconium	Meconium staining might suggest fetal distress
Dilatation of the cervix	In centimetres from 0 to 10 cm
Station of the presenting part	In centimetres above or below the ischial spines
Position of the head	With reference to the occiput if cephalic, or sacrum if breech. A note should be made of whether the head is flexed or deflexed
Presence of caput and/or moulding	If excessive, might suggest obstructed labour

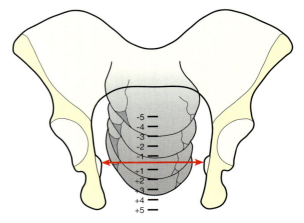

Fig. 30.9 **Descent of the head is described relative to the ischial spines.**

During labour, information about maternal observations (blood pressure, temperature, pulse), fetal heart rate, progressive cervical dilation, descent of the presenting part in fifths palpable, the strength and frequency of contractions and the colour of the amniotic fluid draining are plotted on the partogram. This should be commenced when a woman is established in labour (Fig. 30.8). It forms a graphic record of clinical findings and any relevant events. The purpose is to help early recognition of abnormal labour, to ensure appropriate transfer of care where indicated and to aid continuity of care.

Although there is no research on the ideal frequency of vaginal examinations in labour, the World Health Organization recommends that 4-h vaginal examinations are adequate. These should ideally be performed by the same professional to minimize interobserver variation (Table 30.5). Vaginal examinations should not be regarded as routine; they are unpleasant, may be painful and are associated with a risk of infection even when performed in a 'sterile' manner. The average rate of cervical dilatation in primigravidae is around 1 cm/h, although it is accepted that ½ cm/h can be normal.

Descent of the fetal head is measured in labour by abdominal examination, when the amount of the fetal head palpable above the pelvic brim (in fifths) is documented on the partogram. If only two-fifths or less of the fetal head is palpable abdominally, then the head is determined to be 'engaged' (Fig. 30.9).

On vaginal examination, the 'station' of the fetal head with respect to the ischial spines is recorded. Sometimes it can be difficult to ascertain this accurately, as increasing caput succedaneum (see later) can make the head seem artificially lower in the pelvis on vaginal examination. The ischial spines are designated station zero. When the head is above the spines, it is said to be at −1, −2, −3 or −4 cm. If the head is below the spines, the notation is +1, +2, +3 or +4 cm. If the head is at the level of the ischial spines, it must be engaged.

It is important to note that the 'position' of the head on vaginal examination (VE) is with reference to the occiput, for example occipitoanterior (OA), right occipitotransverse (ROT) or left occipitoposterior (LOP).

'Caput' (succedaneum) is oedema of the scalp owing to pressure of the head against the rim of the cervix and is classified somewhat arbitrarily as '+', '++' or '+++'. 'Moulding' describes the change in head shape, which occurs during labour, made possible by movement of the individual scalp bones. It is arbitrarily termed '+' if the bones are opposed, '++' if they overlap but can be reduced by digital pressure and '+++' if they overlap but cannot be reduced.

Uterine activity is routinely monitored in labour by palpation; measuring length, strength and frequency of contractions. Uterine activity over a 10-min period is plotted on the partogram. Women often report increasing, regular uterine activity at the onset of labour.

In the first stage an assessment of the fetal heart rate is made every 15 min by intermittent auscultation. If any abnormalities are detected by this method, CTG monitoring is advised in the first instance. For some women this may mean transfer to hospital from home or a low-risk midwifery-led setting.

Passage of meconium in itself is not concerning. A healthy term baby will often pass meconium during labour and under these circumstances it will be thin and green/brown in colour. However, passage of thick meconium, which is often more greenish in colour (pea soup), can be a sign of fetal hypoxia or acidosis.

Second stage

This begins when the cervix is fully dilated and ends with delivery of the baby. In a similar way to the first stage of labour, the duration of the second stage of labour is different for nulliparous and parous women. It is generally recommended that for nulliparous women, birth would be expected to take place within 3 h of the start of the active second stage of labour. For parous women, birth would be expected to take place within 2 h of the start of the active second stage of labour in most women. Progress is measured in terms of descent and rotation of the fetal head on vaginal examination. There are two distinct phases:

1. the propulsive/passive phase. This is from full dilatation until the head reaches the pelvic floor. During this time, the head is relatively high in the pelvis, the position is typically occipitotransverse, the lower vagina is not stretched and the mother has no or little urge to push. In many respects it is a natural extension of the first stage of labour
2. the expulsive/active phase. This begins when the fetal head reaches the pelvic floor, the head becomes visible and the mother usually has a strong involuntary desire to push.

With pushing the head usually delivers. Normally it does so in the OA position. After delivery it restitutes, returning to an occipitolateral position by rotating with the shoulders as they descend into the pelvis. The birth attendant then applies lateral traction to the head, moving it in the direction of the mother's back to allow the birth of the anterior fetal shoulder (see earlier). At this point, an oxytocic is injected intramuscularly into the mother's thigh to encourage a prolonged uterine contraction and minimize the chance of postpartum haemorrhage. The head is then lifted anteriorly to allow delivery of the posterior shoulder, after which the rest of the baby is delivered with lateral flexion of the fetal body.

The umbilical cord is clamped and cut. If the baby does not require resuscitation, cord clamping should be delayed and the baby may be placed on the mother's abdomen and skin-to-skin contact encouraged. If this is not the woman's preference, the baby should be wrapped in a warm towel and handed to the parents.

Third stage

This is the time from delivery of the baby to delivery of the placenta and membranes. The third stage of labour can be managed physiologically or actively. Active management of the third stage of labour has been shown to decrease the risk of postpartum haemorrhage and the need for blood transfusion. It involves the use of an oxytocic (as mentioned earlier), deferred clamping and cutting of the cord, and gentle controlled cord traction using the 'Brandt-Andrews' method after separation of the placenta has been diagnosed (see Fig. 30.5I). Placental separation is recognized by apparent lengthening of the cord and a gush of dark blood per vaginam. The operator exerts traction on the cord while the other hand maintains pressure upwards on the fundus. The main risk of cord traction is uterine inversion and the fundus is continually 'guarded' to prevent this (see p. 334). Once the placenta passes the vulva it may be gently twisted to allow the membranes to peel off completely and the uterine fundus is rubbed up to ensure that the uterus is well contracted. Some women may choose to have a physiological third stage of labour; this involves no routine use of uterotonic drugs, no clamping of the cord until pulsation has ceased and delivery of the placenta by maternal effort only. The third stage is prolonged if it is not completed within 30 min after delivery of the baby with active management and within 60 min of delivery of the baby with physiological management.

The labia, vagina and perineum are inspected for tears and sutured if bleeding. Finally, the placenta is examined to ensure it is complete.

The normal blood loss at delivery is about 300 mL. The routine use of an oxytocic following delivery of the anterior shoulder reduces the risk of postpartum haemorrhage by about 60%.

Episiotomies and perineal tears

Episiotomy should not routinely be performed at the time of a normal vaginal delivery, as there is no clear evidence that this reduces the incidence of third- or fourth-degree tears. Midline episiotomy in particular does not protect the perineum or sphincters during childbirth and may impair anal continence. If an episiotomy is to be performed, a right (or less commonly left) posterolateral episiotomy is preferred (Fig. 30.10).

Restricting the use of episiotomy to specific fetal and maternal indications leads to lower rates of posterior perineal trauma, less need for suturing and fewer long-term complications. A spontaneous tear may be less painful than an episiotomy and may also heal better.

Possible indications for an episiotomy are as follows:

- a rigid perineum which is preventing delivery
- if it is judged that a large tear is imminent
- most instrumental deliveries (forceps or ventouse)
- suspected fetal compromise
- shoulder dystocia (to permit access to the birth canal).

Prior to an episiotomy, local anaesthetic is injected into the subcutaneous tissues of the perineum and vagina (unless there is an effective regional block). A right mediolateral cut

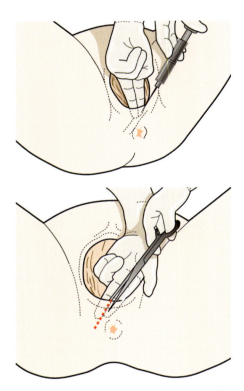

Fig. 30.10 **If required, an episiotomy is usually carried out after infiltration of the perineum with local anaesthesia.**

is made and pressure on the fetal head is maintained so that the delivery is slow and the head remains flexed, minimizing the possibility of the incision extending. The cut should begin at the vaginal fourchette and be at angle of between 45° and 60° to the vertical axis.

Spontaneous tears are categorized into four degrees (Table 30.6). An episiotomy is an iatrogenic second-degree tear. Anterior perineal trauma is classified as any injury to the labia, anterior vagina, urethra or clitoris, and is described as such.

Repair of episiotomies and perineal tears

Before performing repair of a perineal tear or episiotomy, it is important to ensure that the woman has been offered analgesia and that she is in a comfortable position so that the genital area can be adequately examined. Good lighting is essential and the examination should be done gently and with sensitivity. A rectal examination should be performed as part of the procedure to ensure that there is no damage to the anal sphincter or to the perineal muscles.

Repair should be with a rapidly absorbable synthetic material (Dexon or Vicryl Rapide), using a continuous subcuticular (non-locking) technique to minimize short- and long-term problems (Fig. 30.11). These newer materials result in less short-term pain and less analgesic requirements than do older materials, such as catgut and non-absorbable sutures. Good perineal hygiene after delivery is likely to aid

Table 30.6	Classification of spontaneous perineal tears
	Tear involves
First degree	Injury to the vaginal epithelium and vulval skin only
Second degree	Injury to the perineal muscles, but not the anal sphincter
Third degree	Injury to the perineum involving the anal sphincter complex
Fourth degree	Injury to the perineum involving the anal sphincter complex and anal/rectal mucosa

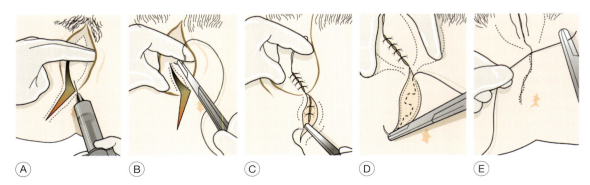

(A)　(B)　(C)　(D)　(E)

Fig. 30.11 **Repair of a perineal tear or episiotomy (see text).**

healing, and the use of ice packs and analgesia may be useful to alleviate discomfort. The use of rectal non-steroidal analgesia may be helpful provided there is no contraindication to its use.

Repair of episiotomy and first- or second-degree tears

The perineum is infiltrated with local anaesthetic (Fig. 30.11A) (unless an epidural is in place or there has been a pudendal block or perineal infiltration prior to delivery). The apex of the vaginal incision or tear is identified and the first suture placed just above this level (Fig. 30.11B) (care is needed because the rectum is just posterior to the vaginal wall).

The use of a loose, continuous non-locking method for vaginal mucosa and perineal muscles and a continuous subcuticular technique for perineal skin is recommended (Fig. 30.11C–E).

Repair of third- or fourth-degree tears

This should be by an experienced clinician, in theatre, with good analgesia, good light, the appropriate instruments and an assistant. The anal mucosa (if involved) is repaired using interrupted dissolving sutures, with the knot of each suture placed in the anal canal. The internal anal sphincter is then identified and its ends approximated and sutured with a monofilament suture such as polydioxanone. Next, the ends of the external anal sphincter are identified and either approximated or overlapped, again with the monofilament suture. The rest is as described earlier for first- and second-degree tears. Antibiotics, laxatives and fibre are important to allow healing.

Analgesia in labour

Although there is an acceptance, to a degree, that labour is a painful experience, we must guard against the inevitability that labour *should* be painful. Mothers, especially primigravidae, find it difficult to conceptualize the amount of pain they may experience or their ability to cope with it until they are in established labour. Mothers may choose to suffer some pain, but the extent to which the mother should experience pain should ideally be agreed, mainly by the mother but in consultation with a midwife and/or obstetrician and/or anaesthetist.

The pain of labour can be severe. It is a complex mix of physiological, psychological and emotional factors and can be difficult to treat. Many different forms of analgesia have been suggested and each has varying efficacies, risk profiles and potential complications.

Pain is unpleasant for the mother, although there is often some amnesia, which can positively influence its perception in retrospect. It is also recognized that the childbirth experience is influenced by maternal expectations and preparation, and by the severity of pain in labour.

Factors influencing pain

The severity of labour pain can vary, depending on obstetric, psychological and emotional factors.

Pain scores have been shown to be higher in primigravid women than in multiparous women, especially if they have not had any antenatal preparation. Reports have also shown that primigravid women generally experience more sensory pain during early labour compared with multiparous women, who experience more intense pain much later in labour, as a result of rapid descent of the fetus.

Long labours are perceived as being more painful. Labour is also reported to be more painful with fetal malposition and, in particular, a woman whose baby is occipitoposterior may experience continuous backache and a prolonged labour.

Physiology of labour pain

There are two components to the pain of labour: visceral (relating to an organ, i.e. the uterus) and somatic (relating to other tissues).

Visceral labour pain occurs during the first stage of childbirth and is due to progressive mechanical dilatation of the cervix, distension of the lower uterine segment and contraction of the uterine muscles. Labour pain may also be as result of the myometrial and cervical ischaemia that occurs during contractions. Severity of this pain mirrors the duration and intensity of contractions. Visceral pain is transmitted by small unmyelinated 'C' fibres, which travel with sympathetic fibres and pass through the uterine, cervical and hypogastric nerve plexuses into the main sympathetic chain. The pain fibres from the sympathetic chain then enter the white rami communicantes associated with the T10 to L1 spinal nerves and pass via their posterior nerve roots to synapse in the dorsal horn of the spinal cord. Chemical mediators involved in this pain transmission include bradykinin, leukotrienes, prostaglandins, serotonin, substance P and lactic acid. This pain is dull in character and is sensitive to opioid drugs.

Somatic labour pain occurs during the late first stage and the second stage of labour, and is due to stretching and distension of the pelvic floor, perineum and vagina. It occurs as a result of descent of the fetus, and during this stage of labour, the uterus contracts more intensely in a rhythmic and regular manner. Somatic pain is transmitted by fine, myelinated, rapidly transmitting 'A delta' fibres. Transmission occurs via the pudendal nerves and perineal branches of the posterior cutaneous nerve of the thigh to S2 to S4 nerve roots. Somatic fibres from the cutaneous branches of the ilioinguinal and genitofemoral nerves also carry afferent fibres to L1 and, to some degree, L2.

All resulting nerve impulses (visceral and somatic) pass to dorsal horn cells and finally to the brain via the spinothalamic tract. Direct pressure of the fetus on the lumbosacral plexus also results in neuropathic pain during labour.

Psychology of labour pain

Maternal control makes labour a more positive experience. Attitudes to pain and pain relief in labour depend on personal aspirations, expectations, cultural factors, learned behaviours, peer group influences, desirability of the pregnancy, previous experiences of pain, pre-existing anxiety or depression, and preparation, education and communication.

Methods of pain relief

Non-pharmacological methods

Maternal support

Psychological support is extremely valuable and allows pharmacological intervention to be minimized. With continuous 1:1 support in labour; mothers need less analgesia, are more likely to have a vaginal delivery and are more satisfied with their labour. The supporting person does not need to be the mother's partner or a midwife, and indeed it may be more useful if they are not part of the mother's social network at all.

Environment

It is recommended that music of the mother's choice be played in labour, that light diet be offered, as long as the labour is uncomplicated, and that the mother is encouraged to be mobile, to walk and to try to achieve comfortable positions; it is recognized that pain is increased by being flat on the back. Positions such as squatting, all fours, or a birthing chair or birthing ball may reduce the need for pharmacological pain relief.

Birthing pools

The use of warm baths and birthing pools (Fig. 30.12) has been shown to reduce pain and the need for regional

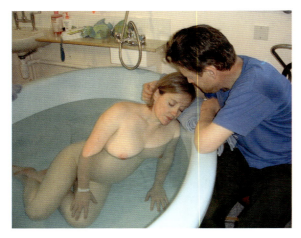

Fig. 30.12   A birthing pool. The environment for labour and delivery is important in reducing the need for pharmacological intervention (with permission).

analgesia. These should not be used within 2 h of the administration of opioids or if the mother is drowsy.

Education

Maternal education has some effect in engendering calm and making expectations realistic; this thereby improves control and reduces pain and distress in labour.

Breathing and relaxation techniques, the playing of music, massage, acupuncture, acupressure and hypnosis are used by many women, but have limited evidence to support their effectiveness. There is no evidence that transcutaneous electrical nerve stimulation (TENS) has any benefit.

Pharmacological methods

Inhaled analgesics

Entonox (a 50:50 mixture of oxygen and nitrous oxide) is commonly used by labouring mothers. Despite its widespread use, studies have shown that it is not a potent analgesic in labour; reassuringly, however, there is moderate evidence for its safety. Any pain relief it offers is limited, and it can lead to nausea, vomiting, drowsiness and light-headedness.

The anaesthetic gases isoflurane, desflurane and sevoflurane can be used safely at sub-anaesthetic concentrations with or without nitrous oxide to improve analgesic efficacy during labour. Although studies have shown that sevoflurane is superior to Entonox in providing pain relief, these gases are not widely available for use in the labour setting.

Systemic opioid analgesia

Systemic opioids have a limited effect, irrespective of the drug, the route or the method of administration. There is some limited evidence that intramuscular diamorphine gives more effective analgesia than other opioids, and it may have fewer side-effects. There is the potential for maternal nausea, vomiting and drowsiness, and short-term respiratory depression and drowsiness in the neonate. Opiates should be avoided if delivery is thought to be likely to occur within 4 h of administration. Antiemetics should be administered when parenteral opioids are used. Women should be aware that the use of opioids during labour may interfere with breastfeeding and bonding after delivery.

Opioids can be given as a subcutaneous or continuous intravenous infusion, which is controlled by the patient (patient-controlled analgesia [PCA]) rather than as intramuscular injections. Remifentanil is often used under these circumstances as it is short acting and women can control dose administration to coincide with contractions.

Pudendal analgesia

The pudendal nerve, derived from the second, third and fourth sacral nerve roots, supplies the vulva and perineum. It crosses the sacrospinous ligament behind the ischial spine along with the pudendal artery (Fig. 30.13), and local infiltration at this point may provide useful perineal analgesia for a low-outlet forceps or ventouse delivery. A pudendal needle

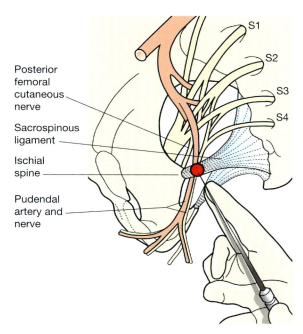

Fig. 30.13 The pudendal nerve runs behind the sacrospinous ligament.

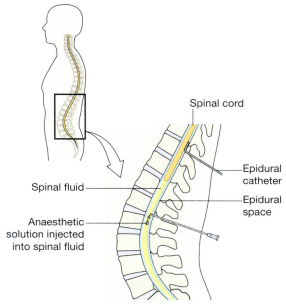

Fig. 30.14 Schematic diagram of the meninges.

is inserted through the sacrospinous ligament, and after aspirating to ensure that the injection is not intravascular, a local anaesthetic is injected behind the ligament on that side. The injection is repeated on the other side and it is usual to infiltrate the perineum directly at the same time.

Regional analgesia

This refers to the delivery of analgesic drugs into the intrathecal (subarachnoid) space or into the epidural space (Fig. 30.14). In obstetric anaesthesia, the introduction of a drug to the intrathecal space tends to be known as 'a spinal' and the introduction of drug to the epidural space, as 'an epidural'.

In general, epidurals are used for analgesia in labour, and spinals as a form of anaesthesia for caesarean section and other operative procedures (Table 30.7). The use of regional techniques for anaesthesia has resulted in a reduction in the use of general anaesthesia for caesarean section and other operative procedures. This in turn has had an impact on maternal morbidity and mortality from anaesthetic causes.

Epidural analgesia for labour

There is good evidence that epidurals provide more effective pain relief than parenteral opioids. The main indication for epidural analgesia is maternal request, but there may be obstetric indications, e.g. in twin delivery to allow manipulation of the second twin if necessary. Continuous electronic fetal monitoring is recommended. Epidurals do not cause a prolonged first stage, do not lead to an increased rate of caesarean section and are not associated with long-term

Table 30.7	Differences between epidural and spinal analgesia	
Epidural		**Spinal**
Extradural catheter placement		Subarachnoid injection
Cannula allows top-up for prolonged use		One-off injection lasting 2–4 h
Analgesic effect may be patchy		Dense and relatively reliable anaesthetic blockade

backache. However, they have been associated with a prolonged second stage and a higher rate of instrumental delivery, but this may be less of an issue with some lower dose regimens. The addition of opioid to the epidural solution allows less local anaesthetic use and therefore greater mobility. Epidural analgesia should be continued until after the third stage and for perineal repair if necessary.

Where labour proceeds to a trial of assisted delivery or caesarean section, or if complications requiring operative intervention are encountered, the epidural can be topped up or a spinal can be used instead.

Side-effects of epidurals (Table 30.8) can arise from the mechanical nature of the technique or from the drugs themselves. Neurological complications from mechanical insertion are rare, but inadvertent dural puncture may occur and ongoing CSF leakage following this can lead to a 'spinal headache'. This leakage can be sealed using a technique known as a 'blood patch'. Side-effects from the local anaesthetic and opioid are hypotension, urinary retention, pyrexia, pruritus, maternal respiratory depression and neonatal respiratory depression. The hypotension results

Table 30.8	Complications of regional analgesia
Complication	**Details**
Dural puncture headache	Occurs due to CSF leak from subarachnoid space. Headache when sitting upright and relieved when lying flat. Blood patch may be necessary to treat.
Hypotension	Fall in blood pressure due to blockage of sympathetic tone to peripheral blood vessels resulting in vasodilatation.
Local anaesthetic toxicity	Systemic toxicity occurs when local anaesthetic is injected into blood vessel. Affects central nervous system and cardiovascular systems, ultimately progressing to cardiovascular collapse and death.
Accidental total spinal block	Occurs with accidental injection of epidural doses of local anaesthetic into the subarachnoid space. Implies anaesthesia has spread to brainstem resulting in loss of consciousness, respiratory arrest and profound hypotension. Treatment involves intubation, ventilation and circulatory support.
Neurological complications	Peripheral nerve injury can occur secondary to direct needle trauma, intraneural injection of local anaesthetic, compression from haematoma or abscess formation, stretch injury or nerve ischemia. Majority of injuries are transient. 95% resolve in 4–6 weeks and 99% resolve in 1 year.
Effects on labour	Epidural analgesia increases assisted vaginal delivery rates unless second stage is actively managed.
Bladder dysfunction	Loss of sensation can predispose to bladder overdistension. This can lead to long-term voiding dysfunction. Bladder care in labour is important and catheterization should be performed in women having difficulty voiding.

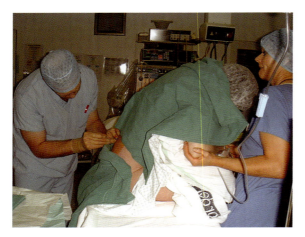

Fig. 30.15 Spinal anaesthesia provides a dense block, which is particularly useful for caesarean section and some instrumental deliveries.

from sympathetic blockade and peripheral vasodilation, and should be managed by lying the patient in the left lateral position, giving oxygen and treating with either intravenous fluids or vasopressors.

Spinal anaesthesia

Spinals can be used primarily for analgesia, but are more commonly used for anaesthesia before caesarean section, instrumental delivery or the surgical management of postpartum complications, such as a retained placenta or the repair of third- and fourth-degree tears (Fig. 30.15). In obstetric anaesthesia, spinals are invariably carried out as a single shot, which provides a dense block for 2–4 h. As with epidurals, the addition of an opioid allows some sparing of the local anaesthetic volume (and therefore dose), which in turn allows some sparing of the side-effects of sympathetic block.

Complications of spinal anaesthesia can again be considered as related to the procedure and related to the drugs. The mechanical complications are similar to those of the epidural. Hypotension also often occurs and is managed as described earlier. A high block (which blocks fibres above T4), however, can lead to bradycardia, which in turn compounds any hypotension. A total spinal is a rare complication in which local anaesthetic affects the brain directly and leads to unconsciousness.

Combined spinal–epidural (CSE) is a technique whereby the epidural space is accessed using an epidural needle and then a spinal needle is passed down the epidural needle and advanced to the intrathecal space. 'Spinal doses' of drugs are then given down the spinal needle and this needle is removed and an epidural catheter introduced down the epidural needle to the epidural space. The epidural catheter can then be 'topped-up' as necessary. CSE is used when rapid-onset analgesia is needed, but the procedure may be prolonged, such that epidural top-ups may be needed too, or when the patient's condition cannot risk the potential sympathetic block, which might occur with a full spinal (cardiac disease) or a high motor block (respiratory disease); a smaller dose spinal can then be used, with the facility to top this up epidurally.

General anaesthesia

General anaesthesia in pregnancy carries more risk than in the non-pregnant patient. As there is reduced gastro-oesophageal tone, increased intra-abdominal mass and reduced gastric emptying, regurgitation of gastric contents and aspiration of these to the lungs is more likely. In addition, as the gastric contents are more acidic in pregnancy, any aspiration is more likely to lead to pneumonitis. Difficult and failed intubation is more likely than in non-pregnant patients because of pregnancy-related obesity. Regional anaesthesia is therefore to be preferred if possible.

Key *points*

- The correct diagnosis of 'labour' is central to good management.
- Labour is considered in three stages: the first from the onset of labour until the cervix is fully dilated, the second from then until delivery of the baby and the third from that point until delivery of the placenta and membranes.
- Compared with a multigravida, the labour of a primigravida is likely to be longer and more likely to result in both instrumental delivery and neonatal injury.
- The choice of analgesia used should be a balanced, well-informed decision, based upon maternal choice following discussion about the efficacy, risks and side-effects of the analgesic methods available.
- Non-pharmacological options include psychological support from a birthing partner, a positive attitude from professionals, remaining mobile and finding comfortable positions, the use of warm baths and birthing pools, and other techniques of the mother's choice.
- Entonox is not a potent analgesic but there is moderate evidence for its efficacy. Systemic opioid analgesia also has limited effect.
- There is good evidence for the analgesic benefits of epidural analgesia compared with systemic opioids. A 'low-dose' local anaesthetic and opioid mixture may be optimal.

31

Monitoring of the fetus in labour

Introduction

The purpose of monitoring the fetus in labour is to identify those who might be at increased risk of death or hypoxic injury, so that delivery can be expedited and harm prevented. Fetal monitoring involves fetal heart rate (FHR) assessment, either by intermittent auscultation or by continuous electronic measurement (cardiotocography, CTG: 'cardio' meaning heart, 'toco' meaning labour). Intermittent auscultation of the fetal heart is appropriate for monitoring fetal condition in labours at 'low risk' of fetal hypoxia, with electronic fetal monitoring being advised in labours at increased risk ('high risk') of hypoxia, or if concern is raised by preceding intermittent auscltation. A 'normal' CTG is good at identifying the non-hypoxic fetus, but the converse is not true regarding an 'abnormal' CTG; there is a high false positive rate and many fetuses suspected to be hypoxic are not. As a consequence, the use of the CTG increases the rate of obstetric intervention in return for little or no neonatal benefit.

The term 'fetal distress' is widely used to describe a clinical scenario where there is concern regarding fetal well-being; unfortunately, the term lacks a precise definition and its use is not encouraged. A standardized categorization of the CTG enables a more meaningful way of communicating the magnitude of concern. Analysis of the electrocardiogram (ECG) waveform in association with the CTG can improve its predictive ability for hypoxia.

Fetal physiology

Fetal oxygenation depends on a number of factors.

Maternal blood supply to the placenta

During a contraction the intramural vessels supplying the placenta are constricted by the smooth muscle fibres of the uterus. Providing the contractions are not too long or too frequent, the placental blood supply has time to recover before the next contraction begins. In hyperstimulation, when the uterus is contracting too frequently, placental oxygenation may be impaired. In other circumstances there may be placental hypoperfusion, for example following the distal sympathetic blockade and associated hypotension, which can occur with spinal or epidural anaesthesia.

Functional capacity of the placenta

A small placenta is less capable of adequate oxygen transfer than a larger placenta. In this condition, the fetus may already be growth restricted prior to the onset of labour and therefore more susceptible to a hypoxic stress. In cases of placental abruption, the resulting partial placental separation leaves a reduced surface area for vascular communication and is therefore less efficient at oxygen exchange.

Fetal circulation

The fetus responds to hypoxia with peripheral vasoconstriction and redistribution of the blood to the heart and the brain. Prolonged vasoconstriction may lead to damage in other organs manifest in the neonatal period, such as the gastrointestinal tract (resulting in necrotizing enterocolitis and kidneys (renal failure). Regardless of the protective effect of such redistribution, in the absence of intervention, prolonged or severe hypoxia and acidosis results in hypoxic brain damage or death.

Persistent or severe hypoxia leads to anaerobic metabolism and acidosis. The acid–base balance within the fetal circulation is a reflection of the degree of oxygenation, and this forms the basis of intrapartum fetal blood sampling (FBS).

Risk assessment

FHR monitoring is recommended to all labouring women. The use of continuous electronic monitoring in 'low-risk' labours may increase the rate of intervention for little or no demonstrable neonatal benefit. It is important to consider which labours are increased risk of hypoxia (so-called 'high-risk' labours) and which are 'low risk'. Some of these factors are outlined in Box 31.1

Meconium staining of the amniotic fluid

Meconium (fetal stool) staining of the amniotic fluid is present in 15% of all deliveries at term and in about 40% at 42 weeks. The mechanism may be stimulation of the vagus (parasympathetic) nerves in utero, causing the fetal bowel to contract and the anal sphincter to relax. This often happens for no particular reason, but it also may occur as a response to fetal hypoxia. While often not of clinical significance, the presence of meconium staining increases the likelihood that there is underlying fetal hypoxia. A 'normal' CTG provides reassurance, but an 'abnormal' CTG is more likely to truly represent fetal hypoxia in the presence of meconium staining.

Meconium staining may give rise to the 'meconium aspiration syndrome'. This is a form of neonatal pneumonitis. Clinical features range from mild neonatal tachypnoea to severe respiratory compromise. The incidence is probably unrelated to the presence or absence of fetal hypoxia, but the syndrome is more likely to be severe if there is associated hypoxia or acidosis; it is also more severe when the meconium is thick.

Meconium can be graded as follows:

Grade 1: good volume of liquor stained lightly with meconium

Grade 2: reasonable volume of liquor with heavy suspension of meconium

Grade 3: thick undiluted meconium of 'pea soup' consistency.

The grading of meconium is subjective and correlates relatively poorly with fetal condition and neonatal outcome, but generally,

---

Box 31.1

Pregnancies at increased risk ('high risk') of fetal hypoxia and acidosis in labour

Fetal factors

- Fetal growth restriction or small for gestational age (see p. 270)

Placental factors

- Hypertension (see p. 253)
- Antepartum haemorrhage (see p. 237)

Obstetric factors

- Precipitate labour (see p. 307)
- Pre-term labour (see p. 263)
- Prolonged labour (see p. 308)
- Induced labours or those augmented with Syntocinon (see p. 305)
- Mothers with epidurals
- Mothers with a previous caesarean section
- Meconium (fetal stool) stained amniotic fluid (see later)

---

the higher the grade the more likely it is to be associated with metabolic acidosis and the meconium aspiration syndrome. It is appropriate to consider continuous electronic FHR recording if meconium staining is identified.

Fetal heart rate recording

Intermittent monitoring (intermittent auscultation)

Assessment of the FHR can be used to provide some information about fetal well-being. In 'low-risk' labours, it is recommended to auscultate the fetal heart every 15 min before and after a contraction during the first stage of labour, and every 5 min between contractions in the second stage of labour. A baseline tachycardia or bradycardia and the presence of decelerations are indications for further evaluation with continuous CTG monitoring. The heart can be auscultated using either a manual Pinard stethoscope or an electronic Doppler detector.

Continuous monitoring (cardiotocography)

A CTG provides a continuous printed or electronic record of the FHR and uterine contractions. The contractions are registered by a pressure monitor supported on the mother's abdomen by an elastic belt, and the FHR is measured using either:

- an abdominal ultrasonic transmitter–receiver Doppler probe, which detects fetal cardiac movements and hence the heart rate

or

- a clip, known as a fetal scalp electrode (FSE), which is attached to the baby's scalp and detects the R–R wave of the fetal ECG. It is usually used if the external abdominal monitoring is technically unsatisfactory.

Analysis of the CTG is undertaken in a systematic fashion, whereby each of the three features are categorized as 'reassuring', 'nonreassuring' or 'abnormal' (Table 31.1). Such an analysis is subsequently distilled in order to provide an

---

Table 31.1	Categorization of the individual features of the intrapartum CTG		
Feature	**Reassuring**	**Nonreassuring**	**Abnormal**
Baseline FHR (bpm)	110–160	100–109 or 161–180	<100 or >180
Variability	5–25	<5 for 30 to 50 min	<5 for >50 min
Decelerations	None or early. Variable with no concerning features for <90 min	Variable with no concerning features for >90 min OR Variable with concerning features in up to 50% of contractions for 30 min OR Late in >50% of contractions for 30 min	Variable with concerning features in >50% contractions for 30 min OR Late decelerations for >30 min OR Acute bradycardia lasting 3 min or more

Note that the presence of accelerations makes acidosis unlikely but the absence of accelerations in the intrapartum period does not in itself indicate hypoxia or acidosis
(Adapted from National Institute for Health and Care Excellence [NICE] 2014).

overall categorization of the CTG as 'normal', 'suspicious' or 'pathological' (Table 31.2).

The baseline FHR is normally between 110 and 160 beats per minute (bpm). This rate represents a balance between the sympathetic and parasympathetic systems. Sustained tachycardia may be associated with prematurity, and the rate slows physiologically with advancing gestation. Tachycardia may also be associated with fetal acidosis (probably as a response to increased sympathetic stimulation) or maternal pyrexia (fetal temperature closely reflects maternal temperature). Fetal cardiac tachydysrhythmias are rare but can cause extremely high heart rates.

Baseline bradycardia is associated with severe fetal acidosis (e.g. following placental abruption, uterine rupture or cord prolapse), but it is more commonly found in the presence of maternal hypotension, typically following epidural analgesia. Fetal congenital heart block is rare, but can occur especially in association with maternal systemic lupus erythematosus. Baseline variability is the fluctuations in the FHR and is due to the balance between the parasympathetic and the sympathetic nervous systems. Since the nervous system of the fetus develops as pregnancy advances, the baseline variability is relatively reduced at earlier gestations. Baseline variability is described as normal, reduced or absent, and it gives a relatively good indication of fetal oxygenation. Normal variability is 5–25 bpm; the commonest reason for loss of baseline variability is the 'sleep' phase of the fetal behavioural cycle, which may last up to 50 min. Loss of variability is also associated with prematurity, fetal acidosis and some drugs administered to the mother (e.g. opiates or benzodiazepines).

Accelerations of the FHR are a sign of a healthy fetus (accelerations indicate the fetus is moving), but their absence in labour is not unusual. Prior to labour there should be at least two accelerations per 15 min, each with an amplitude >15 bpm and lasting for at least 15 seconds.

The presence of decelerations increases the likelihood of fetal hypoxia. Accurate categorization of decelerations is important, but there is often a difference of opinion between clinicians regarding the classification of decelerations; most decelerations in labour are 'variable' in nature (Fig. 31.1). Decelerations represent a reduction in FHR from baseline of at least 15 bpm and last for more than 15 seconds. Early decelerations occur with contractions; the trough of the deceleration coincides with the peak of the contraction. Early decelerations reflect increased vagal tone (intracranial pressure rises during a contraction) and are probably

physiological. As the name suggests, 'variable' decelerations vary in both timing and shape. Variable decelerations probably represent cord compression (particularly in oligohydramnios). Variable decelerations are sometimes sub-categorized into 'typical' and 'atypical' ('atypical' indicates the presence of 'concerning features'). A small increase in FHR at the beginning and end of a variable deceleration (shouldering) suggests that the fetus is coping physiologically with the

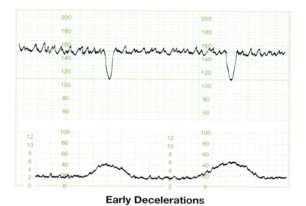

Early Decelerations

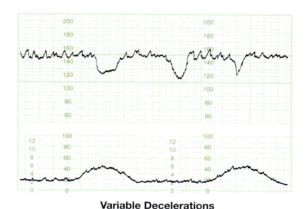

Variable Decelerations

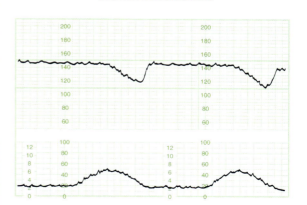

Late Decelerations

Fig. 31.1 Characteristic appearances of CTG decelerations.

Table 31.2	Categorization of the CTG in labour
Normal	**All features reassuring**
Suspicious	One nonreassuring and two reassuring features
Pathological	One abnormal feature or two nonreassuring features

(Adapted from NICE 2014)

hypoxic stress of the intermittent compressions; absence of 'shouldering' is a concerning feature. Other concerning features include duration of deceleration >60 seconds and a biphasic (W) shape. Variable decelerations may resolve if the mother's position is changed. Late decelerations occur more than 15 seconds after the contraction, where the trough of the deceleration typically falls outwith the duration of the contraction. Late decelerations suggest reduced placental perfusion and hypoxia during that period. The recommended actions following categorization of the CTG are summarized in Table 31.3. It is crucial to explain to women in labour your findings and proposed actions.

Fetal electrocardiogram

Analysis of the fetal ECG in labour can improve the specificity (i.e. reduce the number of false positives) of the CTG. A FSE is required to obtain the ECG, the signal from which is a reflection of the electrical activity in the myocardium.

Myocardial hypoxia leads to changes in the ECG waveform. Used in conjunction with the CTG, fetal ECG analysis results in fewer babies with severe metabolic acidosis at birth, fewer babies with neonatal encephalopathy, and fewer operative vaginal deliveries. The use of fetal ECG with CTG also reduces the need for FBS. The fetal ECG is used in many but not all maternity units.

Fetal blood sampling

Also known as fetal scalp sampling, this is a diagnostic test for fetal acidosis. The CTG is used as a screening test to detect the fetus who is experiencing hypoxia and acidosis. The CTG is highly sensitive (good at detecting true positives) but very poorly specific (there are many false positives). CTG use leads to an approximately four-fold increase in caesarean section rates for presumed fetal hypoxia, a figure much reduced if FBS is used to identify a normal pH in the false positives.

The principal indication for undertaking a FBS is the presence of a 'pathological' CTG, where knowledge of the fetal pH is likely to influence the management of the pregnancy. FBS is contraindicated where there is a risk of infection transmitted from the mother (e.g. human immunodeficiency virus, hepatitis B, herpes), a fetal bleeding diathesis (e.g. von Willebrand disease) and before 34 weeks' gestation. FBS is not appropriate in the presence of an acute event necessitating immediate delivery, e.g. cord prolapse and placental abruption; consideration of the whole clinical picture is crucial.

Technique of fetal blood sampling

Explanation is given to the mother and her verbal consent to proceed is obtained. The mother is placed in the lithotomy position with 15° lateral tilt, or in the left lateral position.

Immediately prior to undertaking a FBS, the fetal scalp is digitally stimulated; if this prompts an acceleration of the FHR, then the likelihood of fetal acidosis is very low and the indication for a FBS can be reconsidered. An amnioscope appropriate for the dilatation of the cervix is inserted and the scalp is dried with a swab on sponge-holders. The scalp is then sprayed with ethyl chloride to induce hyperaemia and the area is covered with a thin layer of paraffin jelly (so that the blood will form a blob). A blade is used to make a small incision in the scalp and the blob of fetal blood is touched with the capillary tube. Where possible, three samples are taken to ensure consistency of results. The pH of the sample is determined on a near-patient analyser. Serum lactate measurement may be employed as an alternative to determining pH.

Interpretation of results

The scalp blood pH reflects the acid–base status of the fetus at the time of the sample, while the 'base excess' reflects a change over a longer period. Correlation between the CTG and scalp pH is not precise, but as a general rule the greater the number of nonreassuring or pathological features contained in the CTG, the higher the chance of acidosis. It is usual practice to deliver the baby if the pH is 7.20 or below (Table 31.4).

Table 31.3	Actions to be followed when the CTG is categorized as 'suspicious' or 'pathological'	
Category	**Action**
Suspicious	Correct any underlying cause, e.g. maternal hypotension, uterine hyperstimulation
	Adopt one or more conservative measures, e.g. change maternal position, adjust Syntocinon infusion
Pathological	Exclude an acute event, e.g. placental abruption, cord prolapse
	Correct hyperstimulation, i.e. stop Syntocinon, consider tocolysis
	Adopt conservative measures, e.g. change of maternal position, correct maternal hypotension
	Consider FBS or expedite delivery

(Adapted from NICE 2014)

Table 31.4	Categorization of pH results following FBS	
pH		
>7.25	Normal	No action
7.21–7.25	Borderline	Repeat in 30–60 min if not delivered
7.20 or below	Abnormal	Instrumental vaginal delivery or caesarean section

Fetal monitoring scenarios (Figs 31.2–31.9)

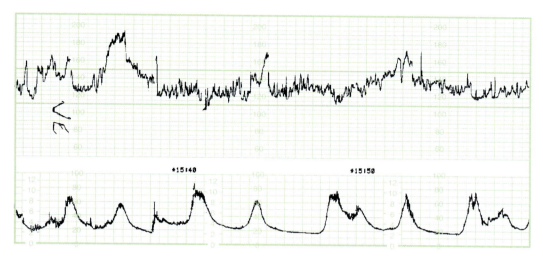

Fig. 31.2   A 29-year-old para 2, with a history of two previous normal deliveries admitted in labour at term. The cervix was 3 cm dilated on vaginal examination) and fully effaced, but there was thick meconium staining. The CTG was reassuring with a baseline of 130 bpm, good baseline variability and presence of accelerations. She was given diamorphine for pain relief.

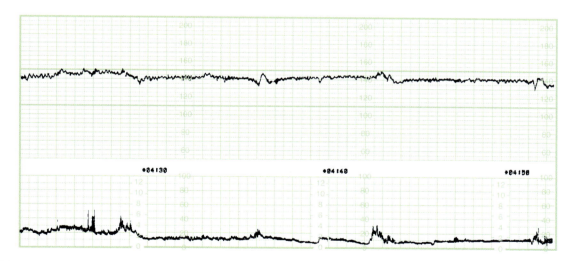

Fig. 31.3   After a further 2 h, baseline variability was reduced. Although there were no decelerations, it was recognized that meconium staining increases the risk of fetal hypoxia and FBS was performed. The pH was 7.31 (normal) and she went on to have a normal delivery 3 h later.

Fig. 31.4 A 40-year-old primigravida was admitted after spontaneous rupture of membranes at term. The amniotic fluid was clear and she was having mild contractions every 8 min. The CTG baseline was 130–140 bpm with normal variability but there were variable decelerations. These are not uncommon after membrane rupture, as amniotic fluid cushions the cord and cord compression is less likely. The decelerations resolved with change of maternal position, but she required a caesarean section for failure to progress beyond 8 cm.

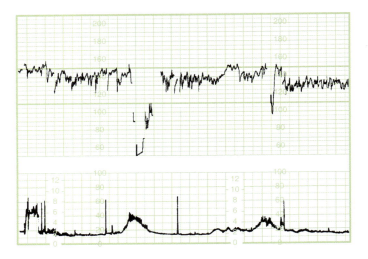

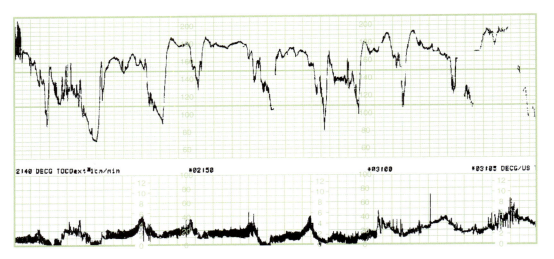

Fig. 31.5 A 27-year-old primigravida was induced at 40 weeks + 12 days, as she was 'post-dates'. After prostaglandin gel was administered vaginally, the cervix was suitable for membrane rupture and the induction was continued with a Syntocinon infusion. This CTG was seen at 6 cm dilatation and it shows a baseline around 180 bpm (tachycardia) with reduced variability and atypical decelerations; the CTG was 'pathological'. FBS revealed a pH of 7.28, but on repetition 30 min later, the pH was 7.19. By this time, the cervix was fully dilated and the baby was delivered by ventouse extraction. The baby was born in good condition.

Long-term prognosis following delivery

There are two key issues to be considered here:

1. whether a particular infant, born with apparent compromise, will later turn out to be neurologically normal, i.e. prospective prediction
2. whether an infant, later discovered to be affected by cerebral abnormality, sustained its injury prior to the onset of labour or as the result of some intrapartum insult, i.e. retrospective evaluation.

Before considering these two overlapping issues, it should be noted that the term 'birth asphyxia' is best avoided unless there is evidence of a pale baby with no tone and not breathing, with evidence of metabolic acidosis on cord arterial blood.

Prospective prediction

The actual length of time and degree of hypoxia required to produce cerebral palsy in a previously healthy fetus are unknown, but there are specific mechanisms which protect the fetus for considerably longer than an adult with similar blood gas concentrations. Nonetheless, hypoxia, whether of antenatal or intrapartum origin, can cause cerebral injury, and attempts have been made to correlate status at delivery

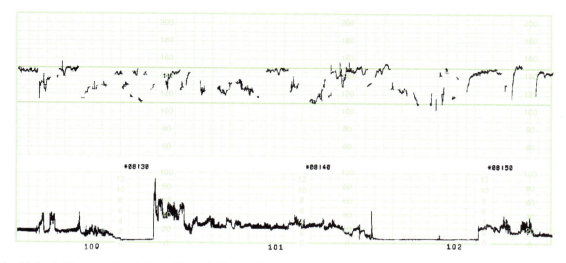

Fig. 31.6 **A 19-year-old primigravida weighing 105 kg was admitted in early labour.** The CTG shows poor pick-up from the abdominal Doppler probe, and after the membranes were ruptured, a scalp clip was applied. The subsequent CTG was reassuring and she had a normal delivery.

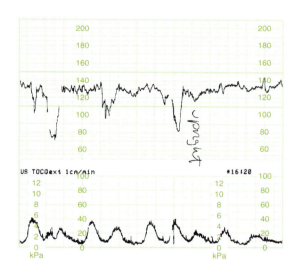

Fig. 31.7 **A 26-year-old primigravida was induced at 33 weeks for worsening pre-eclampsia.** The fetus was small for gestational age, but the amniotic fluid volume was normal on ultrasound and the antenatal CTG was normal. Eight hours after vaginal administration of prostaglandin gel, with the cervix still closed, there were three variable decelerations. While the reassuring baseline FHR and baseline variability might have warranted more conservative management in a normally grown, term fetus in labour, the underlying risk factors for fetal hypoxia were sufficient to warrant delivery by caesarean section. The baby, weighing 1.6 kg, had Apgar scores of 9 and 10 at 1 and 5 min, respectively, and made uneventful progress. It is crucial to consider the whole clinical picture when interpreting the CTG.

with long-term neurological outcome. CTG abnormalities, Apgar scores, neonatal behaviour and neonatal brain imaging have all been evaluated.

The CTG and Apgar scores are of very limited value in assessing long-term prognosis. There is a high incidence of 'abnormal' CTGs in what are later shown to be normal infants. The same is true for Apgar scores, which are intended as a guide to the need for resuscitation rather than a reflection of the degree of hypoxic injury. Low Apgar scores do not indicate the cause of the baby's poor condition, and are a reflection of its immediate status.

Abnormal neonatal behaviour, referred to as 'neonatal encephalopathy', is considerably more useful. This is a clinically defined syndrome of disturbed neurological function occurring during the first week after birth; characterized by

difficulty with initiating and maintaining respiration, depression of tone and reflexes, altered level of consciousness and seizures. There are three grades:

1. hyperalert and jittery with reduced tone and dilated pupils. This usually resolves within 24 h without long-term sequelae
2. lethargic, with seizures and a weak suck. There is an approximately 20% chance of severe sequelae
3. flaccid, no suck, no Moro reflex and prolonged seizures. The chance of severe sequelae is approximately 70–80%.

The prognosis is generally good if the baby does not develop Grade 3 neonatal encephalopathy or if Grade 2 neonatal encephalopathy lasts less than 5 days.

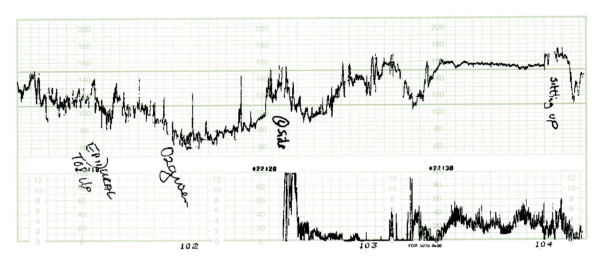

Fig. 31.8 **A 34-year-old primigravida in spontaneous labour at term had an epidural sited when 4 cm dilated.** After epidural top-up there was a fetal bradycardia, which evolved into a tachycardia before returning to normal. It is recognized that the maternal hypotension associated with regional anaesthesia leads to placental hypoperfusion and fetal bradycardia. The bradycardia usually resolves spontaneously or following maternal fluid volume expansion.

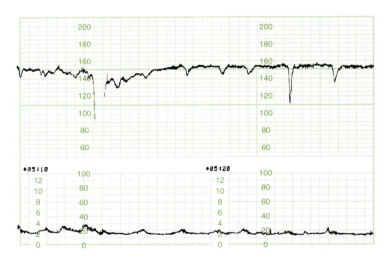

Fig. 31.9 **A primigravida at term who was admitted from home in spontaneous labour at 8 cm dilatation.** The CTG has reduced variability and there are shallow late decelerations. A fetal blood sample showed a pH of 7.09 and an emergency caesarean section was performed. The baby had Apgar scores of 3 at 1 min and 7 at 5 min, and weighed 2.23 kg. The baby's subsequent progress was normal. Although seemingly 'low risk', this pregnancy was affected by undiagnosed fetal growth restriction.

Radiological assessment is also of value in assessing long-term neurological function. The prognosis is good if a computed tomography or magnetic resonance imaging scan appears normal but is not as good if there is evidence of cerebral damage. At term, partial but prolonged hypoxia (as indicated by repeated decelerations with loss of variability over a prolonged period) may give rise to motor cortical atrophy and quadriplegia; if the hypoxia is sudden and profound (as with a prolonged bradycardia), it is more likely to result in injury to the thalamus, giving rise to an athetoid or dyskinetic type of cerebral palsy.

Early cerebral oedema suggests a recent event, as oedema usually appears within 6–12 h of an insult and clears by 4 days afterwards. Further clinical evaluation may be available from an electroencephalograph (EEG). The incidence of death or handicap is low if the EEG is normal. Often, however, despite these measures, the prognosis cannot be defined with accuracy and only long-term follow-up will reveal the true clinical picture.

Retrospective evaluation

Cerebral palsy, which is characterized by non-progressive abnormal control of movement or posture, is usually not diagnosed until months or years after birth, and it is often at this point that questions are asked about whether the cause lay in some difficulty with the delivery. In many instances, it is impossible to say whether the cerebral insult was antenatal in origin (usually of an unspecified nature) or whether it occurred in labour, but this apparently academic point has two important implications. First, if most cases of cerebral palsy are antenatal in origin, then intrapartum monitoring and subsequent intervention will have little impact upon eventual outcomes. Second, there may be medicolegal ramifications. If a cerebral insult is found to have occurred as the result of negligence during labour, a substantial sum of money will be paid in compensation.

Epidemiological studies suggest that in about 90% of cases, the cerebral injury is antenatal in origin, and that in the remaining 10%, the problems may have been the result of intrapartum difficulties. In particular, there is a strong association between cerebral palsy and prematurity, fetal growth restriction, intrauterine infection, fetal coagulation disorders, antepartum haemorrhage and chromosomal or congenital anomalies.

There are sometimes conflicting views about the criteria required to implicate intrapartum events as the cause of cerebral palsy. One set of views is expressed in Box 31.2.

The large majority of neurological pathologies causing cerebral palsy occur as a result of multifactorial and mostly unpreventable reasons during either fetal development or the neonatal period. This, however, is not an excuse for substandard intrapartum care and every effort should be made to identify and act upon identifiable causes of potential cerebral injury.

Box 31.2

Criteria often used to define an acute intrapartum hypoxic event as the cause of later cerebral injury

- Evidence is required of a metabolic acidosis in an intrapartum fetal blood sample, umbilical arterial cord or in very early neonatal blood. Metabolic acidaemia at birth is, however, comparatively common (2% of all births), and the vast majority of these infants do not develop cerebral palsy. An appropriate cut-off point that correlates with a risk of neurological deficit may be a pH of <7.00 and a base deficit of >16 mmol/L
- There should be early onset of severe or moderate neonatal encephalopathy
- Cerebral palsy should be of the spastic quadriplegic or dyskinetic type. Spastic quadriplegia, and less commonly, dyskinetic cerebral palsy are the only subtypes of cerebral palsy associated with hypoxic intrapartum events at term

---

Key *points*

- The purpose of monitoring the fetus in labour is to identify those who might be at risk of hypoxic injury, so that delivery can then be expedited prior to irreversible harm. This monitoring involves FHR assessment, either with intermittent auscultation or by continuous electronic measurement (CTG).
- FBS is used to reduce the incidence of false positive diagnosis of fetal acidosis.
- Interpretation of a CTG has to take account of the whole clinical situation rather than the CTG in isolation.
- Meconium (fetal stool) staining of the liquor increases the chance that there is underlying fetal hypoxia.
- The fetal ECG, when used in combination with the CTG, leads to fewer acidotic babies with fewer operative deliveries.
- Cerebral palsy is usually the result of antenatal factors rather than intrapartum hypoxia and acidosis.

32 Induction of labour

Introduction

Induction of labour is one of the most common obstetric interventions, occurring in approximately 20% of pregnancies in the UK. It is indicated when the risks of continuing the pregnancy are felt to be greater than the risks of delivery, and is more commonly carried out in the interests of the fetus than the mother. The decision is often difficult, particularly at pre-term gestations, and many factors, including the availability of neonatal facilities, must be considered. There needs to be a careful discussion about the risks and benefits with the mother, especially as the process may have an impact on the woman's experience of labour.

It should be noted that 'induction' is different from 'augmentation'. Induction refers to the process of starting labour and can only be applied to someone who is not already labouring. Augmentation describes the process of accelerating labour which is already underway.

Indication

The most common indication for induction is prolonged pregnancy. For 5–10% of women their pregnancies continue beyond 42 weeks. The chance of perinatal death increases as the pregnancy continues, rising from 1 : 1000 at 37 weeks to 6 : 1000 at 43 weeks. Although absolute numbers are small, it is not unreasonable to advocate induction of otherwise uncomplicated pregnancies at 41 + 0 to 42 + 0 weeks. The risk of stillbirth also increases with maternal age, with a rate of 0.75/1000 for mothers <35 years compared with around 2.5/1000 in women aged ≥40 years. Women >40 years may therefore be offered induction at 40 weeks rather than waiting to >41 weeks. There are many other indications for induction (see below).

Potential indications for induction

- Maternal diabetes, including gestational diabetes
- Twin pregnancy
- Pre-labour rupture of membranes
- Fetal growth restriction and suspected fetal compromise
- Hypertensive disorders of pregnancy including pre-eclampsia
- Deteriorating maternal medical conditions (e.g. cardiac or renal disease)
- Maternal request

Contraindications

Induction is contraindicated in situations where a vaginal delivery is contraindicated, such as placenta praevia or transverse lie. Real caution is required in those who have had a previous caesarean section or uterine surgery, as induction carries an increased risk of uterine scar rupture compared to the risk associated with spontaneous labour. Many clinicians would therefore consider a previous caesarean to be a contraindication to induction unless the cervix was very favourable, and awaiting spontaneous labour or carrying out an elective caesarean may be a safer option. There is also an increased risk of hyperstimulation with induction in those who have had a previous history of precipitate labour.

Methods

Before induction, gestation should again be confirmed, presentation checked and any contraindications excluded. Many induction methods are available including mechanical (Foley catheter insertion or amniotomy) and pharmacological (oxytocins and prostaglandins). Deciding on the most appropriate technique depends on the cervix, as assessed by the Bishop scoring system (Table 32.1 and Box 32.1):

- if the score is ≤6, the cervix should be 'ripened' with prostaglandins (e.g. gel or pessary)
- if >6, either prostaglandins or artificial rupture of the membranes (ARM) ± Syntocinon may be considered.

The pharmacological preparations all cause uterine contractions and have the potential to reduce uterine blood flow and compromise the fetus, therefore cardiotocography (CTG) monitoring is indicated.

Table 32.1	Bishop scoring system for cervical assessment		
Score	**0**	**1**	**2**
Cervical dilatation (cm)	<1	1–2	3–4
Length of cervix (cm)	>2	1–2	<1
Station of presenting part (cm)	Spines –3	Spines –2	Spines –1
Consistency	Firm	Medium	Soft
Position	Posterior	Central	Anterior

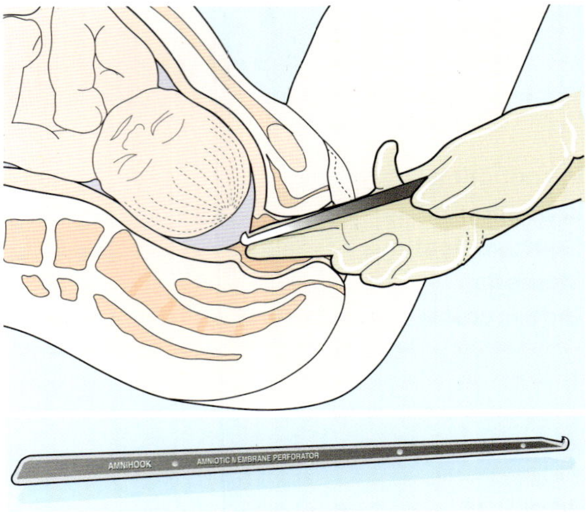

Box 32.1

Overview of induction

- Confirm that the indications are appropriate and that there are no contraindications
- Cervix unfavourable (Bishop score ≤6) → 'ripen' with a vaginal prostaglandin preparation
- Cervix favourable (Bishop score >6) → ARM ± Syntocinon

Fig. 32.1   ARM can be used to induce or augment labour. (Redrawn from Greer IA, Cameron IT, Magowan BA, et al. *Problem-based obstetrics and gynaecology*, Edinburgh: Churchill Livingstone; 2003.)

Unfavourable cervix

Prostaglandins

As discussed on page 304, prostaglandins promote cervical ripening and stimulate uterine contractility. They have been administered via the oral, parenteral and vaginal routes, as well as directly through the cervix and infused into the extra-amniotic space. The main side-effect is gastro-intestinal upset with nausea, vomiting and diarrhoea, which may occur in up to 50% of instances depending on the route of administration. Vaginal preparations have the fewest side-effects.

Prostaglandin E_2 (PGE_2) is used in clinical practice. A gel or tablet is inserted into the posterior fornix and if there is no uterine activity the cervix is reassessed after 6 h. If the Bishop score is <7, further prostaglandin is given and the cervix reassessed 6 h later. Further doses may be given or the patient left for 12–18 h (e.g. overnight). If at any stage the Bishop score is >6, an ARM may be performed, reassessment made in a further 2 h and Syntocinon started if there is no change. Prostaglandins should not be given if there is regular uterine activity, to minimize the risk of hyperstimulation. Misoprostol (a methyl ester of prosta-glandin E_1) can also be used either orally or vaginally but carries a higher incidence of hyperstimulation than PGE_2 preparations.

Sustained-release preparations containing PGE_2 are also available as a polymer-based vaginal insert with retrieval thread. The preparation is placed in the posterior fornix for 24 h and then removed. This technique has the advantage that the insert can be removed if hyperstimulation develops, and there is evidence that it is associated with a reduced likelihood of operative vaginal delivery compared with other prostaglandin formulations.

Favourable cervix

If the cervix is favourable, the choice is between:

- prostaglandins
- ARM
- ARM and Syntocinon.

It remains unclear which of these methods is superior, but there is some evidence that maternal satisfaction and likeli-hood of achieving vaginal delivery within 24 h is greater with prostaglandins. The requirement for analgesia and rates of postpartum haemorrhage may also be lower in this group.

Artificial rupture of the membranes

ARM (or 'amniotomy') may be used for induction in those with a sufficiently favourable cervix and is also used for augmentation. It probably works by a combination of uterine decompression and local prostaglandin release. Another advantage is that it allows assessment of the colour of the liquor (see 'Meconium staining of the amniotic fluid' section, p. 293). Although ARM is effective in the case of a favourable cervix, it is associated with a more frequent need for oxytocin augmentation compared with vaginal prostaglandins.

Before ARM, a vaginal examination is performed. The fetal head should be well applied to the cervix to minimize the risk of cord prolapse. With asepsis, the tips of the index and middle fingers of one hand should be placed through the cervix onto the membranes (Fig. 32.1). The amniotomy hook should be allowed to slide along the groove between these fingers (hook pointing towards the fingers) until reaching the cervix. The point is then turned upwards, breaking the membrane sac. Liquor is usually seen, but may be absent in oligohydramnios or with a well-engaged head. Cord prolapse should be excluded before removing the fingers, then the fetal heart should be rechecked. Absent liquor following ARM should be treated in the same way as meconium staining by carefully monitoring fetal well-being.

Syntocinon

Syntocinon contains a synthetic form of oxytocin, a naturally occurring hormone usually produced by the pituitary gland in labour, which stimulates uterine contractions. This may be used for induction after ARM with a favourable cervix, or for augmentation of a slow, non-obstructed labour. It should only be started after membrane rupture, and continuous CTG monitoring is mandatory. The dose should be titrated against the contractions, aiming for not more than three to four contractions every 10 min. Using Syntocinon is less effective than vaginal prostaglandin (in terms of achieving vaginal delivery within 24 h) and is more likely to be associated with epidural analgesia.

In contrast to the effects of ARM alone for augmentation, early ARM and oxytocin reduces the duration of the first stage of labour by about 90 min and confers a trend to a reduction in rates of caesarean section, but has no effect on maternal satisfaction or neonatal outcome.

Other methods of induction

Membrane sweep

This involves performing a vaginal examination and inserting a finger through the internal cervical os to separate the membranes from the uterine wall, thus releasing endogenous prostaglandins (Fig. 32.2) (often uncomfortable for the mother). Carrying out one sweep after 40 weeks' gestation doubles the incidence of spontaneous labour over controls, especially in those with low Bishop scores. The risk of infection is considered minimal.

Anti-progesterones

Mifepristone, a progesterone antagonist, has been studied in early pregnancy and shown to increase uterine activity, leading to cervical softening. Research into its use as an induction agent later in pregnancy has shown promising results, but it is not yet in clinical use because of fetal safety concerns.

Mechanical methods of induction

Several mechanical induction methods are available including laminaria tents, intracervical insertion of Foley catheters and other balloon devices inserted through the cervix. Increasing evidence suggests that these are as effective as

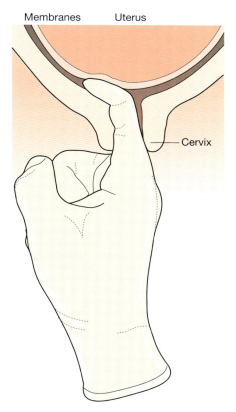

Fig. 32.2 A 'membrane sweep' may increase the incidence of spontaneous labour.

prostaglandins for achieving vaginal delivery within 24 h (with the possible exception of multiparous women), and are associated with similar rates of caesarean section. Mechanical methods confer lower rates of hyperstimulation compared with vaginal prostaglandins. Compared with oxytocin induction alone, caesarean section rates appear to be lower with mechanical methods.

Complications

Induction risks are largely related to the use of 'oxytocics', preparations that are used to stimulate uterine activity. The most concerning side-effect is uterine hyperstimulation, carrying the risk of fetal compromise. Hyperstimulation occurs in 1–5% of prostaglandin-induced labours and is defined as >5 contractions in 10 min for >20 min associated with fetal heart rate abnormalities (detected on CTG monitoring). It necessitates removal of the prostaglandin (if possible), consideration of tocolysis and potentially emergency delivery if the fetal heart changes do not normalize. Induction may also be associated with increased obstetric intervention (including operative vaginal delivery rates), but recent large population studies suggest no increase in caesarean section rates if induction is performed at 41 weeks.

Unsuccessful induction

Despite the aforementioned techniques, induction is sometimes unsuccessful. The plan then depends on the reason for the induction. If it was for some significant fetal or maternal indication, there is probably little choice but to consider caesarean section. If, however, the reason was less pressing (e.g. for post-dates), it may be worth considering a more conservative approach including a repeat induction attempt at a later date. This would depend on an informed discussion with the couple.

33

Malpresentation and slow labour

Introduction

Labour is defined as the onset of regular uterine activity, cervical effacement and dilatation with descent of the presenting part. The length of labour varies among women. First labours on average last 8 h and are unlikely to last over 18 h. Second and subsequent labours last on average 5 h and are unlikely to last over 12 h. In order to determine if labour is progressing adequately it is important to assess cervical dilatation and rate of change, uterine activity and station, and position of the presenting part. The parity of the woman should always be considered for reasons outlined above. National clinical guidelines advise offering vaginal examination every 4 h in addition to abdominal palpation and assessment of vaginal loss.

Abdominal palpation should aim to define the lie, presentation and position of the fetus. The *lie* refers to the long axis of the fetus in relation to the long axis of the uterus. Usually the fetus is longitudinal, but occasionally it may be transverse or oblique. The *presentation* is that part of the fetus that is at the pelvic brim, in other words, the part of the fetus presenting to the pelvic inlet. Normal presentation is the vertex of the fetal head and the word 'malpresentation' describes any non-vertex presentation. This may be of the face, brow, breech, or some other part of the body if the lie is oblique or transverse.

The *position* of the fetus refers to the way in which the presenting part is positioned in relation to the maternal pelvis. Strictly speaking, this refers to any presenting part, but here it will be considered in relation to those fetuses presenting head first (cephalic). As discussed in Chapter 30, the head is usually occipitotransverse at the pelvic brim and rotates to occipitoanterior (OA) at the pelvic floor. 'Malposition' is when the head, coming vertex first, does not rotate to OA, presenting instead as persistent occipitotransverse or occipitoposterior (OP). Vaginal examination should be performed to assess cervical dilatation and effacement in addition to station and position of the fetal head.

The strength, duration and frequency of uterine activity should be evaluated regularly throughout labour, and alongside abdominal and vaginal examination, will assess progress in labour. Uterine overactivity presents as rapid, painful contractions often associated with fetal distress. This can happen spontaneously but is more commonly associated with the use of oxytocics. Inadequate uterine activity is often associated with absent or slow cervical dilatation. Slow labour may result from inadequate uterine activity, cephalopelvic disproportion (CPD) or, more commonly, a combination of the two.

CPD refers to how well the fetal head fits through the pelvis and may occur if the fetal head is too big or the pelvis too small. It is subdivided into 'true' CPD if the head is in the correct position and 'relative' CPD if the obstruction is caused by malposition.

Precipitate labour

Precipitate labour has been defined as expulsion of the fetus (a combined first stage and second stage of labour duration) within less than 2–3 h of the onset of contractions and may result from uterine overactivity.

Excessive uterine activity is commonly termed uterine tachysystole or hyperstimulation. It is defined as more than five uterine contractions per 10 min in at least two consecutive intervals. There may be signs of fetal distress on the cardiotocograph due to interference with the placental blood supply.

Spontaneous hypercontractility, excessive uterine activity not resulting from the administration of medications, is rare. Spontaneous uterine hypercontractility may be associated with placental abruption (see p. 238).

Uterine hyperstimulation occurs much more commonly, however, and by definition is caused by the use of oxytocics. Both oxytocin and prostaglandins may be implicated. The choice of dosage regimens for each represents a compromise between efficacy and the risk of hyperstimulation. The appropriate dose of oxytocin remains controversial, but there is good evidence for starting at a low dose, around 0.5–4 mU/min, and increasing incrementally to 12 mU/min. The dose should be increased no more frequently than every 30 min until there are 4–5 contractions in 10 min. While the licensed maximum dose is currently 20 mU/min, some clinicians support the use of regimens up to 32 or even 40 mU/min.

With prostaglandins, hyperstimulation is also a significant risk but is less likely if their administration is intravaginal rather than oral, intracervical or directly extra-amniotic.

Precipitate labour resulting from either spontaneous hypercontractility or uterine hyperstimulation may lead to fetal distress. Normal labour with sufficient physiological relaxation time allows the oxygenation level of an uncompromised baby to be restored between contractions. However, strong contractions and a shortened relaxation time does not allow the blood supply to the placenta to return to baseline levels before the next contraction, which can result in fetal acidosis (Fig. 33.1). Precipitate labour

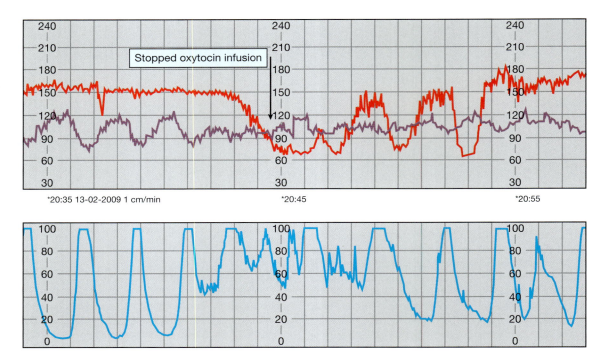

Fig. 33.1 **Cardiotocograph trace in precipitate labour.** There is hyperstimulation secondary to Syntocinon administration. When the Syntocinon is stopped, the contractions become less frequent and the CTG improves.

may also predispose to uterine rupture in parous women, particularly if there is a pre-existing caesarean section scar.

Management of precipitate labour is largely dependent on the fetal condition. If an oxytocin infusion is running, it should be stopped and the woman turned to the left lateral position. A tocolytic agent (a drug to relax the uterine muscle, e.g. a bolus of subcutaneous terbutaline or Glyceryl Trinitrate (GTN) sublingual spray) may be administered. If severe fetal distress is apparent it may be necessary to deliver the baby either instrumentally or by caesarean section, depending on the dilatation of the cervix. If a caesarean section is arranged, it is worth carrying out a vaginal examination prior to starting the operation, as the cervix may dilate rapidly during the time taken in the transfer to theatre, especially in a parous woman.

Precipitate labour is associated with complications for the mother, including: cervical and perineal tears, retained placenta, postpartum haemorrhage and the need for a blood transfusion.

As mentioned earlier, it is important to remember that frequent uterine contractions are also a feature of placental abruption. Contractions with a frequency of more than one every 2 min are highly suggestive of this problem and these frequent contractions may increase the distress of a fetus already compromised by partial placental separation. The diagnosis of placental abruption is even more likely if there is associated lower abdominal pain, backache or vaginal bleeding. As a general rule, tocolytic drugs should not be used to manage the uterine hypercontractility associated with

placental abruption, as uterine relaxation may exacerbate the bleeding and precipitate further placental separation.

Slow labour

Slow progress in labour is usually diagnosed by assessing the rate of cervical dilatation. As discussed on pages 284 and 310, progress can be monitored on a partogram, and alert lines can be used to identify women who are progressing slowly. Early identification and correction of abnormal labour makes it more likely that the mother will achieve a vaginal delivery. The definition of slow labour is controversial; traditional obstetric practice suggested that any nulliparous woman with a rate of cervical dilatation less than 1 cm/h required treatment for slow progress. More recently, a rate of cervical dilatation of <0.5 cm/h has been adopted as the threshold. National clinical guidance suggests a diagnosis of delay in labour should be made when there is dilatation of less than 2 cm in 4 h.

Slow labour is associated with:

- eventual fetal 'distress' and risk of fetal hypoxic injury
- an increased risk of intrauterine infection leading to fetal and maternal morbidity
- maternal anxiety and longer term 'psychological' scarring
- a loss of confidence in those providing maternity care.

These in turn are associated with a greater chance of the mother being delivered by caesarean section or requiring an instrument delivery. The causes of slow labour are summarized in Table 33.1 and the outcome in Table 33.2.

Prolonged latent phase

Chapter 30 describes how the first stage of labour is divided into two parts: the latent phase (from the onset of contractions until the cervix is fully effaced) and the active phase (when the cervix begins to dilate). The normal duration of the latent phase of labour in primigravidae ranges from 1.7 h up to 15.0 h. The latent phase is most likely to be prolonged in those whose cervix is unfavourable, and a prolonged latent phase is therefore much more common in primigravidae (Fig. 33.2).

There is rarely any serious cause for a prolonged latent phase. CPD is usually evident at more advanced stages of cervical dilatation. With a prolonged latent phase, the mother often becomes weary, exhausted and demoralized from what can sometimes be discomfort over a number of days. A prolonged latent phase of labour is associated with more obstetric intervention (e.g. delivery by caesarean section) and poor fetal outcomes (e.g. admission to the neonatal unit). Within reason, it is important to resist the temptation to actively intervene by artificially rupturing the membranes or administering oxytocics, at least until the cervix is 2 or 3 cm dilated and fully effaced with a well-applied presenting part. These measures may actually increase the risk of further obstetric intervention in what might, with patience, have been an uneventful labour. Reassurance, encouragement and appropriate analgesia over this time are extremely important.

Prolonged active phase and secondary arrest

The active phase may be prolonged because of inadequate uterine activity or CPD (Fig. 33.3).

Inadequate uterine activity

The uterus may be hypoactive or incoordinate. A hypoactive uterus is one with low resting tone and only weakly propagated contractions. There is often a longer interval between contractions and the contractions are not particularly painful.

Incoordinate uterine activity may occur because of inadequate 'fundal dominance'. Normal uterine contraction begins at a pacemaker point close to the junction of the

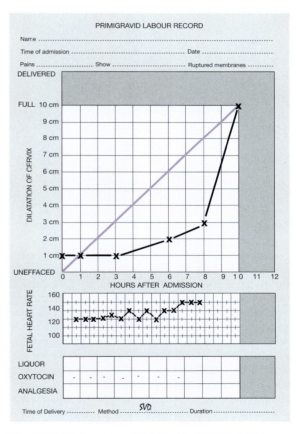

Fig. 33.2 Partogram with prolonged latent phase.

Table 33.1	Clinical classification of slow labour
Clinical features	**Caused by**
Prolonged latent phase	Idiopathic

Prolonged active phase and secondary arrest	Inadequate uterine activity:
	  hypoactive
	  incoordinate
	Obstruction (CPD):
	• true CPD (head too big or pelvis too small)
	• relative CPD (malposition of the head increases the diameter of the presenting part)

Table 33.2	Outcome of delivery based on pattern of labour (%)			
	Cases	**Spontaneous vertex delivery**	**Instrumental delivery**	**Caesarean section**
Normal pattern	65–70	80	18	2
Prolonged latent phase	2–5	75	10	15
Prolonged active phase	20–30	55	30	15
Secondary arrest	5–10	40	35	25

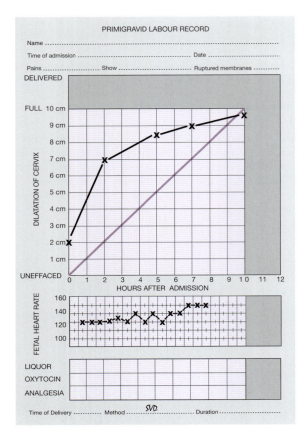

Fig. 33.3 **Partogram with prolonged active phase.**

uterus and the fallopian tube. It spreads from this point downwards, with its intensity maximal at the fundus (where the muscle is thickest), intermediate at the mid-zone and least at the lower segment. Uterine contractions can be described in terms of baseline tone, amplitude, frequency and duration. With incoordinate uterine activity, the intensity profile appears to be reversed, with the maximal intensity in the lower segment (where the muscle is thinnest) and weakest at the fundus. This is much less efficient. The resting tone is increased throughout and the threshold for pain is therefore reached earlier in the contraction. Incoordinate uterine activity is common, especially in women in their first labour. Contractions may be incoordinate in terms of frequency or duration/strength, or a combination of both.

Inadequate uterine activity has no specific cause. It may simply be a developmental feature of the uterine muscle and there is evidence that many will resolve spontaneously given sufficient time. There is also some evidence that inadequate uterine activity is associated with CPD. This is because cervical dilatation itself may improve uterine activity, but it is less likely to occur if the presenting part is pressing less firmly on the cervix.

If progress is satisfactory, there is no need to consider treatment of incoordinate uterine activity. Most will respond well to oxytocics, usually given by a stepwise intravenous

oxytocin infusion, as described earlier. As labour is likely to be prolonged, care should be taken to make sure that the mother does not become dehydrated or ketotic, as this will further exacerbate the uterine problem.

Cephalopelvic disproportion

This may occur because of the following:

1. the baby's head is presenting in the optimal way but is too large relative to the pelvis ('true' CPD). It is diagnosed only if the head does not become engaged despite adequate uterine activity. It is not possible to predict CPD antenatally, and even using the strictest antenatal criteria, many of those considered to be at risk by clinical pelvic assessment will go on to have a vaginal delivery. More complicated attempts to predict CPD using ultrasound measurements of the fetal head together with X-ray or computed tomography pelvimetry measurements have also proved to be unreliable and only lead to unnecessary surgical intervention. Short maternal stature or small shoe size are not predictive of CPD. The only true test is labour itself
2. there is a malpresentation or malposition of the baby's head so that a wider part of the head is being presented to the pelvis. This is 'relative' CPD. It may occur with deflexed malpresentations (particularly of the brow and face, p. 314), but the most common cause of relative CPD occurs when the head rotates to the OP (p. 317) rather than the OA position. The first stage and second stage progress more slowly, and although spontaneous delivery is quite possible with the head coming out 'face to pubis', secondary arrest is not uncommon
3. there is some form of pelvic abnormality. Major abnormalities are uncommon, particularly in affluent societies, and are usually associated with disease, injury or severe nutritional problems. The obstetric classification is based on the shape of the pelvic brim, as it is the pelvic inlet, which seems to be the major determinant of successful delivery (Fig. 33.4).

Pelves with normal shape and bone development

The round 'gynaecoid' pelvis is the commonest, and as would be teleologically predicted by the theory of natural selection, it is obstetrically ideal. The long oval 'anthropoid' pelvis is also relatively common but is associated with OP presentation.

Pelves with abnormal shape and bone development

Defects of nutrition and environment
Minor

The flat-brimmed 'platypelloid' pelvis and the triangular 'android' pelvis are considered to be minor variations

Normal shape and bone development

Round gynecoid pelvis (A)

Long oval anthropoid pelvis (B)

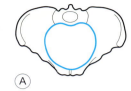
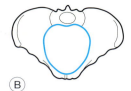

Abnormal shape and bone development

Defects of nutrition and environment

Minor

Flat-brimmed platypelloid pelvis (C)

Triangular android pelvis (D)

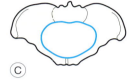
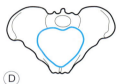

Major

Rickets (E)

Osteomalacia (F)

Disease or injury

Spinal - kyphosis or scoliosis (G)
Pelvic - tumours, fractures
Limbs - childhood polio or a congenitally
        dislocated hip

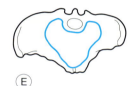
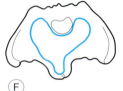

Congenital

Naegele pelvis and (H)
Robert pelvis

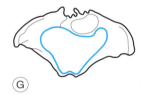
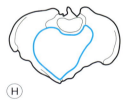

Fig. 33.4   Classification of pelvic shapes.

associated with adverse nutrition in infancy and childhood. The flat-brimmed pelvis is found relatively more commonly in African women and the triangular pelvis in those from southern Europe.

Major

Rickets is caused by prolonged vitamin D deficiency in early life, leading to poorly mineralized bones containing large areas of soft uncalcified osteoid. Weight bearing produces bony deformities by pushing the sacral promontory forward and pivoting the sacrum backwards. The result is a marked reduction in the anteroposterior measurement of the pelvic brim, with possible further mid-cavity narrowing in severe cases as the acetabula are also forced inwards. Low vitamin D concentrations are present in a large proportion of the UK population. It is therefore recommended that women who are pregnant or breastfeeding should have vitamin D supplementation (10 μg a day). Higher risk populations

including women with increased skin pigmentation, obesity or immobility are advised to take at least 1000 units per day.

Disease or injury

Abnormal pressure on the pelvis from kyphosis or scoliosis gradually moulds the pelvis into funnelled or asymmetric shapes. Asymmetrical weight bearing from polio or a congenitally dislocated hip may also mould the pelvis to less favourable proportions. Pelvic fractures may leave the pelvis asymmetrical, and excessive bone formation at the fracture site may further narrow the passage.

Congenital malformations

Congenital absence of one or both sacral masses (Naegele pelvis and Robert pelvis, respectively) results in direct fusion of the sacrum to the ilium and marked narrowing.

Management of slow labour

When progress is slow or when there is secondary arrest, it is important to distinguish whether the cause is inadequate uterine activity or CPD.

The strength of contractions is difficult to assess reliably and cannot be done from a cardiotocograph recording. Direct intrauterine pressure monitoring using a pressure catheter is essentially only a research tool and is rarely, if ever, used in clinical practice. Some idea of the strength can be gained through maternal observation and abdominal palpation of contractions. The examining hand is placed between the umbilicus and the uterine fundus, and the duration and frequency of the uterine contractions is assessed over a 10-min period. With an experienced observer, this can provide useful clinical information. In the presence of CPD there will be caput (a diffuse swelling of the scalp) and moulding (an alteration in the relation of the fetal cranial bones), and malposition or malpresentation may be identified by careful vaginal examination. If delay in labour is suspected or confirmed, amniotomy should be offered with a view to repeat examination in 2 h to ensure adequate progress in labour.

In practice, the clinical decision is whether or not to start an oxytocin infusion. The main risks of starting oxytocin are of:

- hyperstimulation of the uterus and subsequent fetal distress
- rupture of the uterus (this applies almost exclusively to multiparous mothers and is more likely in those with a previous caesarean section scar).

In primigravidae with slow progress or secondary arrest who do not have a prohibitive malpresentation (e.g. brow presentation) it is reasonable to start oxytocin. This is not appropriate if there is suspected fetal distress and should only be after the membranes have been ruptured or have ruptured spontaneously. The aim is to titrate the infusion to the point where the contractions are coming at a frequency of 4–5 every 10 min. Vaginal examinations should be repeated every 3–4 h after the infusion is started to ensure adequate progress. If progress is still inadequate (cervical dilatation has increased by less than 2 cm in 4 h), then operative delivery will be required.

In parous women, the decision is more difficult, mainly because of the risk of uterine rupture (p. 334). Rupture can occur suddenly and leads to expulsion of the fetus into the peritoneal cavity. In this situation, fetal hypoxia and death is not uncommon. If the mother has had a previous vaginal delivery, true CPD is extremely unlikely, but if the only previous delivery was an elective caesarean section (e.g. for breech presentation), there is no guide to the likelihood of true obstruction. Syntocinon should therefore only be used with caution and only in those women thought to have inadequate uterine activity with no evidence of obstruction. Vaginal examinations should again be repeated every 3–4 h to ensure adequate progress, with a lower threshold for caesarean section in those thought to have some degree of CPD.

Malpresentation

As described earlier, 'malpresentation' is a term used to describe any non-vertex presentation. Over 95% of fetuses are in cephalic presentation at term. Malpresentations include face presentation, brow presentation and breech presentation. When the fetus has a cephalic presentation, the presenting diameter is dependent on the degree of flexion or extension of the fetal head – deflexed and brow presentations offer a wide diameter to the pelvic inlet (Table 33.3 and Fig. 33.5).

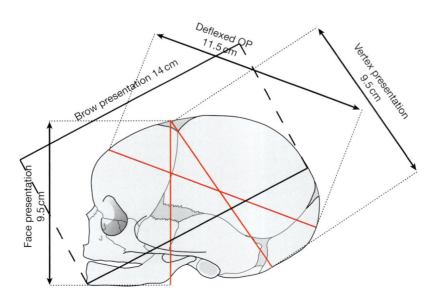

Fig. 33.5 **The presenting diameter is dependent on the degree of flexion or extension of the fetal head.**

Table 33.3	Presenting diameters of the fetal head	
Presentation	**Presenting diameter**	
Vertex	Suboccipitobregmatic	9.5 cm
Deflexed OP	Occipitofrontal	11.5 cm
Brow	Mentovertical	14 cm
Face	Submentobregmatic	9.5 cm

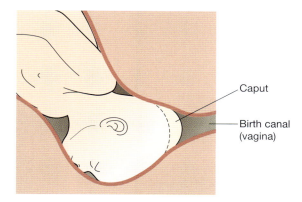

Caput

Birth canal (vagina)

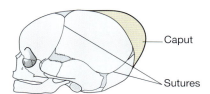

Caput

Sutures

Fig. 33.6 **'Moulding' refers to the change in shape of the fetal skull during labour as it 'moulds' to the birth canal. Caput refers to oedema of the presenting part of the scalp.**

As the fetal skull is made up of individual bony plates (the occipital, sphenoid, temporal and ethmoid bones), which are joined by cartilaginous sutures (the frontal, sagittal, lambdoid and coronal sutures), it has the potential to be 'moulded' during labour. This allows the head to fit the birth canal more closely (Fig. 33.6). Moulding should be distinguished from caput succedaneum, which refers to oedema of the presenting part of the scalp. Both moulding and caput can occur in any cephalic presentation, but are more likely to occur in malpresentation. The presence or absence of moulding and caput should be documented during each vaginal examination in labour; excessive moulding and caput are suggestive of an obstructed labour due to CPD.

Face presentation

This occurs in about 1:500 births and occurs when the fetal head extends right back (hyperextended so that the occiput touches the fetal back) (Fig. 33.7A). It is associated with prematurity, tumours of the fetal neck, loops of cord around the fetal neck, fetal macrosomia and anencephaly. Face presentation is usually only recognized after the onset of labour, and if the face is swollen (Fig. 33.7B) it is easy to confuse this presentation with that of a breech. The position of the face is described with reference to the chin, using the prefix 'mento'. The presenting diameter is submento-bregmatic (9.5 cm) (see Fig. 33.5).

The face usually enters the pelvis with the chin in the transverse position (mentotransverse) and 90% rotated to mentoanterior so that the head is born with flexion (Fig. 33.7C). If mentoposterior, the extending head presents an increasingly wider diameter to the pelvis, leading to worsening relative CPD and impacted obstruction (Fig. 33.7D). A caesarean section is usually required.

Brow presentation

This occurs in only approximately 1:700 and 1:1500 births, and is the least favourable for delivery (Fig. 33.8). The presenting diameter is mentovertical, measuring 14 cm. The supraorbital ridges and the bridge of the nose will be palpable on vaginal examination. The head may flex to become a vertex presentation or extend to a face presentation in early labour. If the brow presentation persists, a caesarean section will be required.

Breech presentation

Breech presentation describes a fetus presenting bottom first. The incidence is around 40% at 20 weeks, 25% at 32 weeks and only 3–4% at term. The chance of a breech presentation turning spontaneously after 38 weeks is <4%. Breech presentation is associated with multiple pregnancy, bicornuate uterus, fibroids, placenta praevia, polyhydramnios and oligohydramnios. It may also rarely be associated with fetal anomaly, particularly neural tube defects, neuromuscular disorders and autosomal trisomies. At term, 65% of breech presentations are frank (extended), with the remainder being flexed or footling (Fig. 33.9). Footling breech carries a 5–20% risk of cord prolapse (p. 325).

Mode of delivery

There has been extensive debate about the safest route of delivery – whether it should be vaginal or by caesarean section. The risks of vaginal delivery are small, but include intracranial injury, widespread bruising, damage to internal organs, spinal cord transection, umbilical cord prolapse and hypoxia following obstruction of the after-coming head. The risks of caesarean section are largely maternal and related to surgical morbidity and mortality. Planned caesarean section is associated with less perinatal mortality and less serious neonatal morbidity than planned vaginal birth at term. The risks of serious maternal complications are much the same, partly because planned vaginal delivery often ends with an intrapartum caesarean section and such caesarean sections carry greater risks than planned elective sections. The

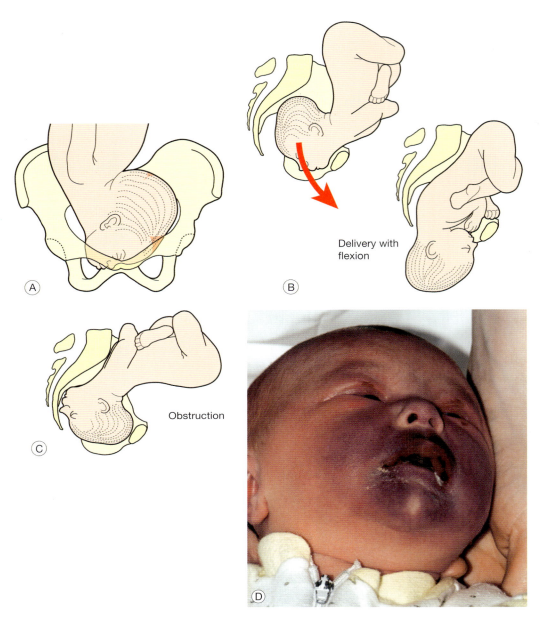

Fig. 33.7   Face presentation. (A) The head enters the pelvic brim in the transverse position. **(B)** Most rotate to the mentoanterior position and deliver without problems. **(C)** Those that rotate to mentoposterior will obstruct. **(D)** Face presentation is often associated with oedema and bruising. This baby recovered without problems.

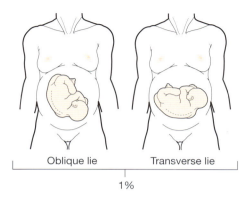

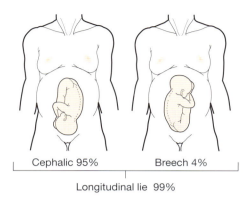

Cephalic 95%   Breech 4%   Oblique lie   Transverse lie

Longitudinal lie 99%   1%

Fig. 33.8 **Fetal lie at term.**

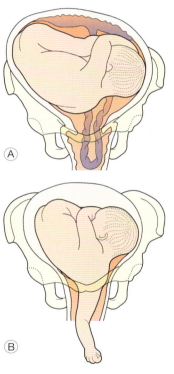

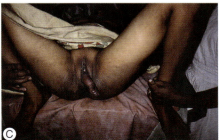

Fig. 33.9 **Transverse lie is associated with (A) cord prolapse, (B) and (C) arm prolapse.**

problem of delivery can be removed if it is possible to turn the baby prior to the onset of labour. This process is called external cephalic version (ECV).

External cephalic version

All women with a breech presentation at term should be offered ECV unless there is an absolute contraindication (outlined in Box 33.1). It is good practice to offer ECV from 36 weeks in nulliparous women and from 37 weeks in multiparous women. The success rate is approximately 50%.

Procedure

A cardiotocograph and ultrasound scan should be performed. Some obstetricians like the patient to be fasted and prepared for theatre, and although this is usually not necessary, it is reasonable to have access to theatre close at hand. ECV is most likely to be successful in parous women when the presenting part is free, the liquor volume is normal, the head is easy to palpate and the uterus feels soft. A flexed breech is more likely to turn than an extended (frank) breech.

Ask the mother to lie flat with a 30° lateral tilt. The use of tocolysis, such as a betamimetic drug, to soften the uterus is associated with an increased success rate. Applying scanning gel to the abdomen allows easier manipulation and permits scanning during the procedure if required. The breech is disengaged if necessary, with the scan probe or hands, and then attempts are made to rotate in the direction in which the baby is facing (i.e. forward roll). The fetal heart should be checked throughout the procedure. If a forward roll is unsuccessful, a backward somersault can be tried. If the procedure is only partially successful (i.e. the fetus is converted to a transverse lie), the fetus should be returned to breech rather than leave it transverse. A CTG should be performed after the procedure is completed. Women who are D negative should undergo testing for fetomaternal haemorrhage and anti-D should be offered.

Caesarean section for breech presentation

The aforementioned evidence considers term pregnancies only. Caesarean section for breech at term carries a small increase in immediate complications in comparison to vaginal birth. The decision to perform a caesarean section has important implications for future pregnancies, such as the risks of opting for vaginal birth after caesarean section, increased risk of complications in future caesarean sections and the risk of an abnormally invasive placenta.

Pre-term breech

For those in pre-term labour with breech presentation, the mode of delivery should be individualized. The decision should be based on stage of labour, type of breech, fetal well-being and the availability of a skilled clinician in vaginal breech delivery.

Vaginal delivery for breech presentation

Women should be assessed and counselled in the antenatal period regarding the risks associated with vaginal breech birth. A higher risk planned vaginal breech birth is expected in the following circumstances: hyperextended neck on ultrasound, high/low estimated fetal weight, footling presentation and evidence of fetal compromise. If a woman presents with an unplanned vaginal breech labour the management plan will depend on the stage of labour and the availability of clinical expertise. Induction of labour is not usually recommended.

The first stage is managed with caution. The role of epidural analgesia is particularly controversial – its use may facilitate manipulation of the fetus, but its presence may inhibit the desire to push, which is particularly important in breech delivery. Augmentation of slow progress should only be considered in the event of inadequate uterine activity in the presence of an epidural. There is no contraindication to a fetal 'scalp' electrode being applied to the breech, providing care is taken to avoid genital injury. A semirecumbent position in an 'all fours' position has been recommended.

At full dilatation, the mother can be encouraged to push. The temptation to pull must be resisted. Ideally, the baby should be left alone to deliver itself ('hands off'), taking care to ensure the back remains uppermost when advancing. If there is undue delay, or there are concerns about fetal well-being (e.g. movements stopping, baby becoming floppy, no response to stimuli), assisted delivery can be used to encourage a more rapid delivery. The techniques of 'hands off' and 'assisted breech' are illustrated in Figs 33.10 and 33.11. Breech extraction may be considered when delivering the second twin (p. 318).

One of the key risks of breech delivery is that pulling may lead the head to extend and therefore become stuck at the pelvic brim. *The importance of maternal effort at this stage, rather than traction from below, cannot be overemphasized – it allows the head to flex and minimizes the risk of it becoming stuck at the pelvic brim.*

Should the head of a pre-term breech become entrapped behind an incompletely dilated cervix, it should first be flexed as far as is possible to narrow the presenting diameter. Failing this, the options are then to incise the cervix at the 4 and 8 o'clock positions (risking massive, potentially fatal maternal haemorrhage) or to push the fetus back up and perform a caesarean section (a very difficult manoeuvre). Because such interventions are hazardous to the mother, it may be preferable to await spontaneous delivery.

All babies presenting by the breech should be examined for developmental dysplasia of the hip and Klumpke paralysis.

Transverse lie and oblique lie

These are uncommon, occurring in less than 1% of deliveries at term (Fig. 33.12). Usually there is no specific cause, but abnormal lie is more common in multiparous women, multiple pregnancies, pre-term labour and polyhydramnios. It may also be associated with placenta praevia, congenital abnormalities of the uterus, lower uterine fibroids and other pelvic masses such as an ovarian cyst.

If transverse lie is identified antenatally, a scan should be undertaken to exclude placenta praevia, polyhydramnios, lower uterine fibroids and a pathologically enlarged fetal head. ECV is usually possible (see earlier), and the mother should be reviewed a few days later to ensure that the lie is still cephalic. She should be advised to come to hospital if there is any suspicion of early labour, as it may still be possible to carry out an ECV at that stage, providing the membranes are still intact. She should also be advised to go to the hospital immediately if there is any suspicion of membrane rupture, as there is a risk of cord prolapse or prolapse of a limb (Fig. 33.13A–C). In view of the small risk of cord prolapse, some clinicians advise that women with a transverse lie or unstable lie (see later) are admitted to hospital from 38 weeks to await birth or until a longitudinal lie is maintained (see Table 46.1).

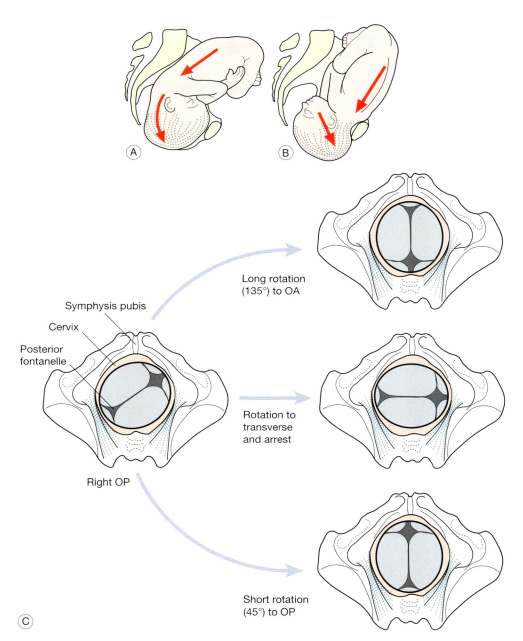

Fig. 33.10 OP position (A) compared with an OA position (B). (C) Occiput rotation.

The knees can be flexed to
deliver the legs

Once the legs are delivered,
it is important to wait for the
body to advance further,
before holding the bony
pelvis firmly as shown

Rotation allows one arm to
be freed, flexed and brought
down....

....while rotation the other
way allows the other arm to
be similarily delivered

After delivery of the other arm,
flexion of the baby's head is
again encouraged by allowing
the breech to hang down....

....and the head is delivered
as for the 'hands off' vaginal
breech delivery

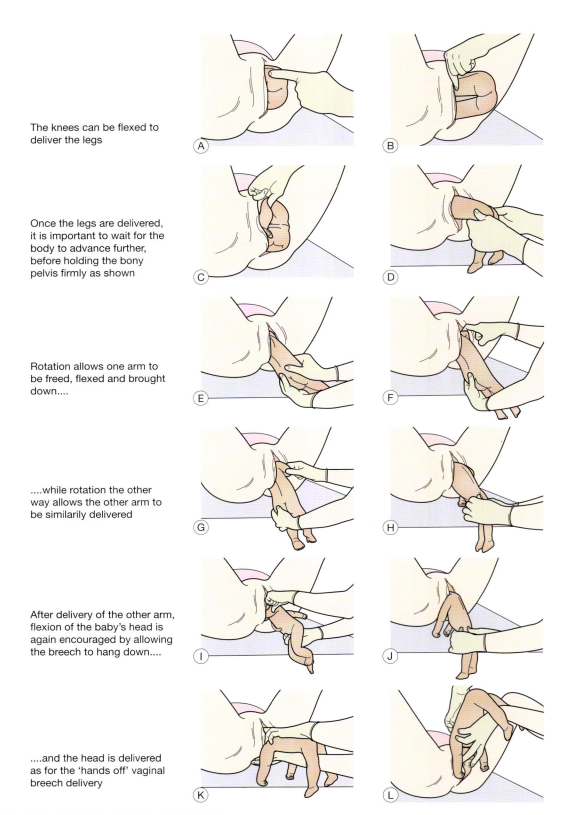

Fig. 33.11 **Assisted vaginal breech delivery.**

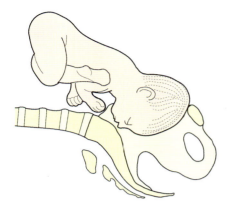

Fig. 33.12   Brow presentation.

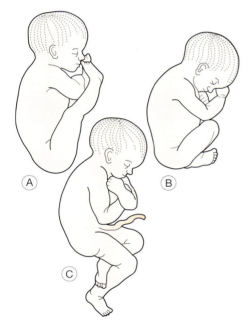

Fig. 33.13   Breech presentation. Those presenting by the breech may be **(A)** extended (or frank); **(B)** flexed; or **(C)** footling.

If the lie is transverse in established labour, particularly after membrane rupture, a caesarean section will usually be required. These caesarean sections can be technically very difficult, and a vertical uterine incision may be necessary to allow adequate access for delivery.

Unstable lie

An unstable lie is one that varies from examination to examination. The options are:

■ manage conservatively, with repeated ECVs as required, and await the spontaneous onset of labour.

Should the membranes rupture with the fetus in a non-cephalic presentation there may be a risk of cord prolapse, and as described earlier, inpatient management is considered appropriate by some

■ arrange to turn the baby to cephalic presentation and then induce labour. This is sometimes referred to as a 'stabilizing induction'. The disadvantage is that the induction itself is not without risks, and the lie may become unstable again even after the membranes have been ruptured

■ carry out a caesarean section.

Malposition

Normally the head engages at the pelvic brim in the occipitotransverse position, flexing as it descends into the pelvic cavity and rotating to OA at the level of the ischial spines. The head then extends as it descends, distending the vulva until it is delivered. In about 10% of pregnancies, the fetal head enters the pelvis in a more OP position than transverse or anterior, either by chance or in association with an unfavourably shaped pelvis, particularly the long oval 'anthropoid' pelvis. The baby is then in a direct occipitoposterior position or with the occiput to the right or left of the midline, referred to as right or left occipitoposterior.

There are then three main possibilities (Fig. 33.14C):

■ the occiput will rotate anteriorly (through approximately 135°) to OA, and then (usually) deliver normally (65%)

■ it will partially rotate to occipitotransverse and not deliver (20%)

■ it will rotate more posteriorly to OP (15%).

Those that remain OP have greater difficulty negotiating the birth canal and are less likely to deliver spontaneously. The normal mechanism of delivery involves extension of the head to OA, but extension is not possible in the OP position and a wider diameter is presented to the outlet (occipitofrontal 11.5 cm) (Table 45.1 and Fig. 33.14A,B). With malposition the first and second stages of labour are usually longer, partly because of the greater presenting diameter (relative CPD), and partly because the head is less well applied to the cervix and therefore less able to facilitate its dilatation. Back pain in labour appears to be more common with OP position. The mother is more likely to request an epidural, is more likely to experience secondary arrest due to relative CPD, and is more likely to require augmentation with Syntocinon.

If the cervix does not reach full dilatation despite Syntocinon, a caesarean section will be required. If full dilatation is reached, it is quite possible for a baby to deliver in the OP position (with the head coming out 'face to pubis') but, not uncommonly, manual rotation, rotational ventouse or Kielland rotational forceps delivery will be required (p. 340). Third- and fourth-degree perineal tears are more likely to occur when a baby delivers in an OP position.

As the breech descends with pushing, it rotates to the anteroposterior and advances over the perineum. It then rotates with the back uppermost. Any movement of the back posteriorly should be corrected.

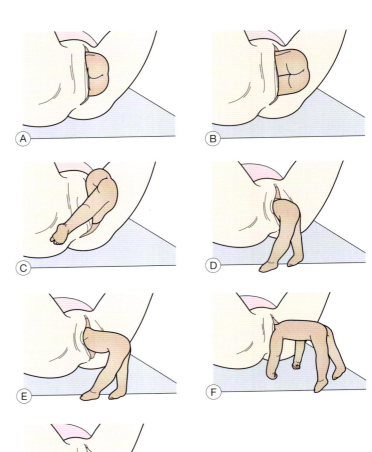

The legs will free themselves as the baby advances, and will hang down

With pushing, the arms will deliver

The breech should be allowed to hang in order for the head to flex, waiting for the nape of the neck to become visible

After delivery of the other arm, flexion of the baby's head is encouraged by placing the second and third fingers of the lower hand over the malar bones on the face, pulling them towards you....

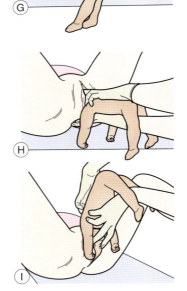

....while the second and third fingers of the other hand are used to push the occiput (back) of the head away from you. With maximum flexion, the head can then be delivered. An episiotomy can be used if necessary

Fig. 33.14 'Hands off' vaginal breech delivery.

34

Obstetric emergencies

Introduction

One woman dies every minute of every day worldwide from a complication of pregnancy. In developed countries, maternal death is uncommon, but evidence from the UK Confidential Enquiry into Maternal Deaths found substandard care in around two-thirds of cases. This is partly a result of the fact that most obstetric emergencies are rare and often unfold with such rapidity that junior medical staff can find themselves facing potentially catastrophic conditions that they may never have seen before, let alone have ever managed.

This chapter will examine the obstetric emergencies listed below:

- amniotic fluid embolism
- prolapsed umbilical cord
- retained placenta
- shoulder dystocia
- uterine inversion
- uterine rupture.

See also haemorrhage (Chapter 25), eclampsia (Chapter 27) and pulmonary embolism (pp. 212–213).

Principles of management

Anticipation and preparation are essential – and they may lead to prevention. For example, if the mother has a history of postpartum haemorrhage, anticipation with intravenous (IV) access, blood sent for group and save in early labour and active management of the third stage may make an important difference to the outcome should the problem recur. If there are risk factors for shoulder dystocia, such as a presumed large fetus in a mother with diabetes and a long first stage of labour, it is important to ensure that an experienced midwife is allocated to care for her and that senior medical staff are present on the labour ward at the time of delivery.

In addition, as life-threatening emergencies are relatively rare, it is important that there should be regular 'fire drills' of obstetric emergencies to ensure that all staff are fully prepared, that equipment is fully functional and that supporting systems (portering, laboratory, etc.) are prepared.

It should also be remembered that emergencies can arise anywhere in the unit, not just in the labour ward. There is now clear evidence of the benefits of formal team training and use of simulation in rare obstetric emergencies. This applies to both technical aspects of delivery and non-technical (team working) aspects of care.

The principles outlined in Box 34.1 can be adapted for initial resuscitation in all obstetric emergencies, which involve maternal compromise. Remember that there are often two lives at stake, and in most emergencies minutes or even seconds count. Remember too, however, that panicking is never helpful. A good principle to remember is that the fetus rarely needs to be resuscitated directly – 'resuscitate the mother and you will resuscitate the fetus'. It should be noted that an obstetric emergency can cause profound lifelong psychological problems for both the mother and her partner. This can manifest itself as postnatal depression, post-traumatic stress syndrome and a real fear of becoming pregnant again. Counselling and debriefing after such experiences should be encouraged both while the woman is in hospital and some weeks later.

Resuscitation

Resuscitation should have a strong focus on the airway, breathing and circulation (ABC) of basic life support, as noted in Box 34.1. The first priority is always the mother, aiming for maternal resuscitation and then (and only then) to consider the welfare of the baby. Resuscitation in pregnancy has some differences from that in a non-pregnant person, as outlined below, but it is still essential to approach the problem by using ABC and then consider possible causes. The 4 Hs and 4 Ts listed in Box 34.2 are helpful.

The key resuscitation differences are that:

- the aorta and vena cava are compressed by the gravid uterus, impeding venous return and reducing cardiac output; there is an increased risk of aspiration of stomach contents resulting from relaxation of the oesophageal–gastric junction (progesterone effect) and the pressure of the uterus
- difficult intubation is more common in the pregnant than in the non-pregnant patient (1:300 vs 1:3000) – short neck and laryngeal oedema

Box 34.1

On identification of an emergency

1. Call for help. Emergency bleep the obstetrical emergency team. This should include a senior obstetrician and anaesthetist, the theatre team, a person skilled in neonatal resuscitation, the midwifery sister, a porter and the junior medical staff.
2. Ensure you have checked the environment is safe for you and apply *ABC* if appropriate:
   - *airway*: place patient head down, maintain airway patency, give correct dose of oxygen (O_2) (15 L/min) via facemask, attach pulse oximeter
   - *breathing*: assess, monitor respiratory rate, ventilate if indicated
   - *circulation*: insert two grey/brown IV cannulae, take full set of bloods (Full Blood Count [FBC] coagulation, cross-match 6 units of blood, urea and electrolytes, and liver function tests). In all cases of severe haemorrhage, give 2 litres [L] of warmed isotonic crystalloid stat.
   - left lateral tilt.
3. Check maternal observations as appropriate, e.g. pulse, blood pressure (BP), O_2 saturation monitoring and bladder catheter for urinary output measurement.
4. *At this point, see the appropriate management guidelines for the particular emergency (e.g. 4 Hs and 4 Ts, Box 34.2).*
5. Consider an ECG, blood glucose measurements, central venous monitoring and an arterial line.
6. Use a compression cuff and warmer to give fluids if rapid administration is indicated.
7. Remember to document fully (ideally allocating a team member to be the scribe) in the notes, including all observations, procedures and actions with date, timings, a signature and a printed name.
8. Remember the mother's partner. Although some partners might wish to wait outside, others may prefer to stay in the room.

Box 34.2

Causes of collapse

4 Hs
- Hypoxia
- Hypovolaemia
- Hypo- and hyper-kalaemia
- Hypothermia

4 Ts
- Thromboembolism
- Toxic (including local anaesthesia)
- Tamponade
- Tension pneumothorax
  Also consider:
- Eclampsia (including magnesium toxicity)
- Amniotic fluid embolus

- chemical pneumonitis is more likely than in the non-pregnant state, owing to the decreased pH of the stomach contents and the increased chance of inhaling the contents because of the changes outlined previously.

It is therefore important in the early stages of resuscitation to:
- tilt the patient to the left by 15–30° (reduces aortocaval compression and increases potential cardiac output by 25%)

- apply cricoid pressure and intubate early, to avoid aspiration of gastric contents and to facilitate oxygenation
- involve a senior obstetrician and anaesthetist immediately or as early as possible (to facilitate intubation and early caesarean section where and when appropriate).

In cases of cardiorespiratory arrest, the revised Resuscitation UK guidelines (2015) should be followed. These have moved the emphasis for basic life support towards a single compression-ventilation ratio of 30:2. If the mother is not delivered, left lateral tilt can be achieved using firm support under the right hip (an assistant can be asked to kneel and use their knees to support the patient in left lateral tilt).

After about 20–22 weeks, it is essential to perform a caesarean section early if resuscitation is unsuccessful (at this gestation, the fundus of the uterus will be at or above the level of the umbilicus). The decision for perimortem caesarean section should be made by 4 min if there is no response to active resuscitation, and the delivery by 5 min (the '4-minute rule'). An anaesthetic is not required in order to proceed. This is primarily to save the life of the mother and forms part of the resuscitation technique. It makes cardiopulmonary resuscitation (CPR) more efficient by:
- increasing venous return
- improving ease of ventilation
- allowing CPR to be carried out in the supine position
- reducing oxygen requirement after delivery.

Amniotic fluid embolism

Epidemiology

This is one of the most catastrophic conditions that can occur in pregnancy. It is rare, with an incidence somewhere between 1.25/100000 and 12.5/100000. As a precise diagnosis can be difficult, it is also difficult to establish an accurate mortality rate, but it is probably around 20–40%.

Aetiology

The exact pathophysiology remains unclear. It was believed that some breakdown occurred in the physiological barrier separating the mother and fetus, allowing a bolus of amniotic fluid to enter the maternal circulation. This bolus moved to the pulmonary circulation and produced massive perfusion failure, bronchospasm and shock. More recently, it has been suggested that the underlying mechanism may be an anaphylactoid reaction to fetal antigens entering the maternal circulation, and individual variations in sensitivity to these antigens are reflected by the severity of the resulting clinical picture.

Risk factors

Amniotic fluid embolism can occur at any time in pregnancy, but it most commonly occurs in labour (70%), after vaginal delivery (11%) and following caesarean section (19%). The following risk factors have been identified:

- multiparity
- placental abruption
- intrauterine death
- induction of labour
- precipitate labour
- multiple pregnancy
- suction termination of pregnancy
- medical termination of pregnancy
- abdominal trauma
- external cephalic version
- amniocentesis.

Clinical features

The clinical picture usually develops almost instantaneously and the diagnosis must be considered in all collapsed obstetric patients. The mother may demonstrate some or all of the signs and symptoms listed in Box 34.3, but classically a woman in late stages of labour or immediately postpartum starts to gasp for air, starts fitting and may have a cardiac arrest. There is often profound disseminated intravascular coagulation (DIC) with massive haemorrhage, coma and death. There are inevitably signs of fetal compromise if it happens prior to delivery.

Diagnosis

The definitive diagnosis is usually at autopsy and is made by confirming the presence of fetal squames in the pulmonary vasculature. It is also possible to confirm the diagnosis in a surviving patient, again by finding fetal squames in washings from the bronchus or in a sample of blood from the right ventricle. In the acute situation, as there is no single clinical or laboratory finding, that can diagnose or exclude amniotic fluid embolism, the diagnosis is made clinically by exclusion.

Box 34.3

Symptoms and signs of amniotic fluid embolus

Symptoms

- Chills
- Shivering
- Sweating
- Anxiety
- Coughing

Signs

- Cyanosis
- Hypotension
- Bronchospasm
- Tachypnoea
- Tachycardia
- Arrhythmias
- Myocardial infarction
- Seizures
- Disseminated intravascular coagulopathy

Management

This is primarily supportive and should be aggressive. There is, however, no evidence that any specific type of intervention significantly improves maternal prognosis. Initial therapy is aimed at supporting cardiac output and management of DIC. If the woman is undelivered, an immediate caesarean section may be appropriate, providing the mother can be stabilized.

A chest X-ray will often show pulmonary oedema and an increase in right atrial and right ventricular size. The electrocardiogram (ECG) demonstrates right ventricular strain and there is a metabolic acidosis (reduction of partial pressures of oxygen and carbon dioxide [pO_2 and pCO_2].

In addition to the initial management of an obstetric emergency (Box 34.1), therapy may include:

- aggressive fluid replacement
- maintenance of cardiac output with a dopamine infusion
- treatment of anaphylaxis with adrenaline (epinephrine), salbutamol, aminophylline and hydrocortisone
- treatment of DIC with fresh frozen plasma and cryoprecipitate
- treatment of haemorrhage after delivery with Syntocinon, ergometrine, carboprost (Haemabate) or misoprostol, and uterine massage
- early transfer to an intensive care unit (ITU) for central monitoring, respiratory support and other therapy, as appropriate.

Prognosis

The outcome for the baby is very poor, with a perinatal mortality rate of approximately 60% and most survivors usually suffering neurological impairment. Maternal outcome in mothers who have suffered a cardiac arrest is complicated by the fact that many are left with serious neurological impairment.

Prolapsed umbilical cord

Definition

'Cord presentation' is defined as the presence of the cord between the presenting part and the membranes prior to membrane rupture. 'Prolapsed umbilical cord' refers to the same situation after membrane rupture where the cord descends through the cervix. The cord can remain alongside the presenting part (occult prolapse) or can pass the presenting part (overt prolapse), and it will be visible or palpable in the vagina (Figs 34.1 and 34.2). Cord prolapse is a true obstetric emergency requiring immediate action.

Epidemiology

The incidence is related to presentation (Table 34.1). Any obstetric condition that precludes a close fit between the fetus and the pelvic inlet makes a cord prolapse more likely,

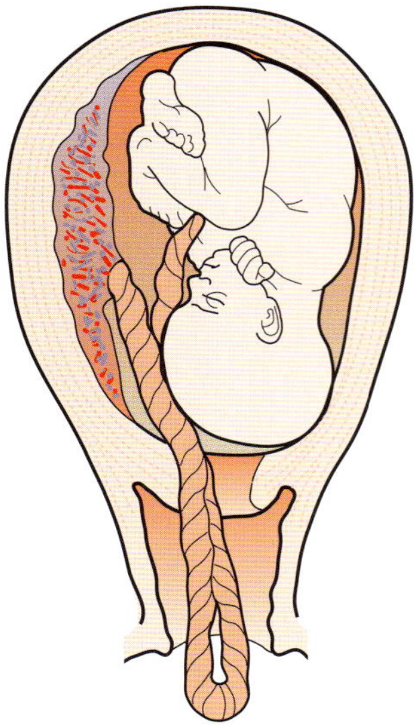

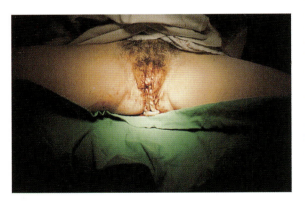

Fig. 34.1 Umbilical cord prolapsing through incompletely dilated cervix. This is due partially to a high presenting part.

Fig. 34.2 The umbilical cord is visible at the introitus. This fetus requires immediate delivery. (Reprinted from Rymer J. Picture tests obstetrics and gynaecology, Fig. 155, p. 78, 1995, by permission of the publisher Churchill Livingstone.)

Table 34.1	Incidence of cord prolapse in relation to presentation
Presentation	**Incidence**
Vertex	0.4%
Frank breech	0.5%
Flexed breech	4–6%
Footling breech	15–18%

particularly breech presentation, malposition, pre-term gestation, polyhydramnios, fetal growth restriction and placenta praevia. Other predisposing factors include a long umbilical cord, artificial rupture of the membranes and being a second twin.

Clinical features/investigation

There are two main insults to the cord, both of which may lead to cessation of fetal blood flow and fetal death. First, there is direct cord compression by the fetal body against the maternal pelvis, and second, there is likely to be cord spasm from exposure to the cool external atmosphere or excessive handling of the cord.

Cardiotocography (CTG) usually indicates fetal compromise in the form of deep variable decelerations or a single prolonged deceleration (Fig. 34.3).

In some instances, the cord is clearly visible protruding through the vagina ('overt' cord prolapse), but it may be found at a vaginal examination carried out in response to some CTG abnormality ('occult' cord prolapse). It is important to routinely exclude cord prolapse following artificial rupture of the membranes or in the presence of variable decelerations of acute onset (this CTG pattern is associated with benign cord compression as well as cord prolapse).

Management

It is important to act swiftly, providing the maternal condition is stable. If there is an abnormal fetal heart pattern (suspicious or pathological) the baby should be delivered immediately. If the cervix is fully dilated, preparation should be made for delivery by forceps or ventouse; if not, by immediate caesarean section (as soon as safely possible). General anesthesia is often required, but a spinal anaesthetic may be used by an experienced anaesthetist in some circumstances. If the fetal heart pattern is normal and the cervix not fully dilated an urgent caesarean section should be arranged, but the fetal heart pattern should be monitored continuously and delivery expedited if this becomes abnormal.

To protect the cord from occlusion during the transfer to theatre, the woman should be placed in the head-down position and a hand placed in the vagina to lift the presenting part up off the cord and prevent cord compression. An alternative is the knee–chest position (Fig. 34.4). Another reasonable approach is to insert a Foley catheter and fill the maternal bladder with 500 mL fluid. The catheter can be spigotted and this will relieve the pressure on the cord. This may be a useful approach when transporting the woman from a community setting. In this setting, if loops of cord are outside the vagina, a gentle attempt can be made to replace them within the vagina. There is a balance to be achieved between excessive cord handling versus leaving the loops exposed to a cold environment, both of which can lead to significant cord spasm.

A tocolytic (e.g. terbutaline 0.25 mg subcutaneously) should be given to minimize uterine contractions. The bladder should be emptied before starting caesarean section. If there is doubt as to fetal viability, for instance if the cord has prolapsed at home or silently on the antenatal ward, it is important to establish fetal viability before embarking on an unnecessary caesarean section. The absence of cord pulsation does not necessarily indicate fetal death, particularly if

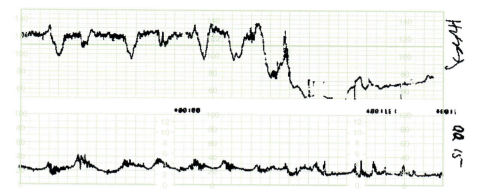

Fig. 34.3 In an occult umbilical cord prolapse the only indication may be CTG abnormalities, which should mandate a vaginal examination.

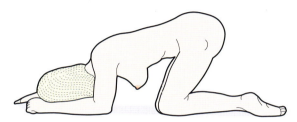

Fig. 34.4   The knee–chest position should be adopted on the way to theatre. Gravity ± an assistant's hand displaces the presenting part away from the umbilical cord.

the prolapse is acute, and the fetal heart itself should be visualized directly by ultrasound. If fetal death has occurred, the mother should be allowed to labour and deliver spontaneously.

Prognosis

Fetal mortality has been reduced over the years with the increasing use of caesarean section and improvement in neonatal intensive care, but it remains around 10%.

Retained placenta

Definition

Retained placenta is defined as failure to deliver the placenta within 30 min of delivery of the baby in active management of the third stage and within 60 min in physiological management of the third stage. Active management involves giving uterotonic drugs (Syntocinon or Syntometrine), deferred clamping and cutting of the cord, and controlled cord traction after signs of separation of the placenta, and has been shown to reduce postpartum haemorrhage by up to 50%. A retained placenta increases the risk of postpartum haemorrhage by a factor of 10 owing to the inability of the uterus to contract down completely. This risk appears to be maximal at 40 min after delivery. Such haemorrhage can be severe and life-threatening, particularly if there has been a partial separation.

Epidemiology

Retained placenta occurs in 2–3% of all vaginal deliveries and is more likely with pre-term gestations; if the baby is delivered before 37 weeks, the incidence increases by a factor of three, and if delivered at 26 weeks, the risk is increased by a factor of 20. It is also more common after a previous caesarean section, and rarely this can be associated with a morbidly adherent placenta.

Pathology

During normal childbirth, 90% of placentas are usually delivered within the first 15 min. Placental delivery is usually preceded by signs of placental separation, i.e. lengthening of the cord, a sudden small gush of dark blood and increased mobility of the uterus. Failure of the placenta to deliver may occur because of an unusually adherent unseparated placenta, or because the placenta has separated successfully but is retained within the uterus by a partially closed cervix. Failure of separation is the much more worrying of these two situations.

An adherent placenta is the result of abnormal placental implantation during the first trimester. Normally, the invading fetal trophoblast cells are arrested by the maternal decidual barrier, probably by the action of a specific form of leucocyte. If this maternal decidual layer is in some way ineffective, the trophoblast cells may invade further than usual and may extend through the myometrium or even as far as the outer serosal layer. The decidual barrier may be rendered ineffective by a number of factors, and is, for example, often thin and scarred following caesarean section. When over-invasion occurs, the placenta becomes abnormally adherent and is referred to as placenta accreta (Box 34.4). *Those with a placenta praevia overlying a previous caesarean section scar are at very high risk of this serious complication.*

Box 34.4

Risk factors for placenta accreta

- Previous caesarean section
- Placenta praevia
- Advanced maternal age
- High parity
- Previous retained placenta
- History of dilatation and curettage or suction termination of pregnancy
- Previous postpartum endometritis

Table 34.2	Classification of abnormal placental attachment	
Type	Incidence	Pathology
Placenta accreta	75–78%	Invades superficially into the myometrium
Placenta increta	17%	Invades deeply into the myometrium
Placenta percreta	5–7%	Invades through the myometrium and penetrates the outer serosal layer of the uterus. It may invade adjacent structures, including bladder and bowel

Morbidly adherent placenta is subdivided into three subgroups: placenta accreta, placenta increta and placenta percreta, depending on the depth of invasion (Table 34.2), though it is often difficult to differentiate these clinically. Both ultrasound assessment (looking for abnormal Doppler blood flow) and magnetic resonance imaging scanning have been used to help diagnose the degree of invasion. However, there is no definitive test which can absolutely exclude this complication prior to delivery. There is loss of the physiological cleavage plane such that the placenta is unable to separate after delivery of the baby, and partial separation or iatrogenic effort at separation may lead to profound haemorrhage.

A particular problem is the increasing prevalence of mothers who have had previous caesarean sections, which in turn increases the incidence of morbidly adherent placenta in subsequent pregnancies. If there is a low anterior placenta in a subsequent pregnancy, there will be a significant risk of placenta accreta and subsequent haemorrhage. If there is a suspicion of abnormal placentation in elective cases, the theatre team must be made aware well in advance. A consultant obstetrician and anaesthetist should be present and cell salvage equipment, cross-matched blood, etc. must be available.

Management

If the patient is bleeding heavily, a retained placenta is an obstetric emergency and treatment must be immediate. Aside from the initial resuscitation measures (discussed earlier) the patient should be transferred to theatre for a manual removal of the placenta.

If there is no bleeding, an initial conservative approach can be adopted. IV access should be established and

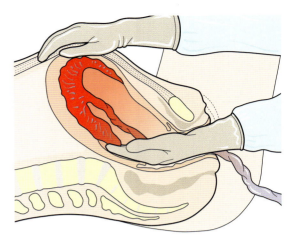

Fig. 34.5 **Manual removal of the placenta.** A cleavage plane is identified with the fingers, which then continue along the plane until the placenta is fully separated from the uterine wall.

cross-match arranged in case bleeding begins, and it is reasonable to wait an hour or so for spontaneous expulsion of the placenta to occur. In the interim, emptying the bladder (e.g. with an indwelling catheter), the use of Syntocinon, and the 'rubbing-up' of a contraction, or breastfeeding, with its resultant physiological release of oxytocin, may help to aid expulsion. If the placenta is still retained after 1 h, the mother should be transferred to theatre for regional or general anaesthesia. Then, under aseptic conditions, a hand is passed into the uterus through the cervix in order to identify the cleavage plane between the placenta and the uterine wall. During the procedure, the uterine fundus is supported through the abdominal wall using the opposite hand. The placenta can then be gently stripped off the uterine wall and delivered (Fig. 34.5). Once it is removed, a contraction should be 'rubbed up' and uterotonics given as required (e.g. a Syntocinon infusion) to reduce the risk of postpartum haemorrhage from an atonic uterus. The procedure must be covered with antibiotics, as there is a significant association between manual removal of the placenta and postpartum endometritis.

If the cleavage plane cannot be found and the placenta is so firmly adherent to the uterine wall as to make removal impossible or dangerous (uterine rupture), the clinical diagnosis is 'placenta accreta'. Subsequent management then depends on the degree of haemorrhage. If there is persistent uncontrollable haemorrhage, a hysterectomy is often required. It may be possible to arrest the haemorrhage using tamponade techniques (using either a balloon or packing within the uterine cavity). If there is no active haemorrhage, conservative management can be considered. With conservative management, when the placenta is left in situ to be absorbed over time, there is a significant incidence of major complications from infection and bleeding, and the patient must be monitored closely for several weeks following discharge. Senior staff must always be involved in management of abnormal placentation when it is suspected or diagnosed.

Sepsis

Sepsis may be defined as an infection, suspected or proven, plus two or more SIRS criteria (Box 34.5). Systemic maternal sepsis remains an important cause of maternal mortality and morbidity in the UK, with the predominant genital organisms being *E. coli*, the group A *Streptococcus* and the group B *Streptococcus*. Early presentation of sepsis (<12 h post-birth) is more likely to be caused by streptococcal infection, particularly group A, and severe continuous pain suggests necrotizing fasciitis. Non-genital infections include pneumonia and influenza. Early recognition and aggressive management of suspected sepsis is important to prevent progression to severe sepsis with multi-organ dysfunction, tissue hypoperfusion and septic shock (Box 34.6).

Full bacteriological and radiological investigation for the source of sepsis is essential, but it should not significantly delay fluid resuscitation and antibiotic therapy. Antibiotics should be given within 60 min of presentation, as this has been shown to reduce mortality by up to 50% – the so-called 'golden hour'. Arterial blood gases, lactate, urea and electrolytes, liver function tests, glucose and clotting are very useful in monitoring the systemic response to sepsis, and this is often best carried out in a high-dependency or intensive care setting.

Box 34.5

Sepsis

Sepsis is an infection, suspected or proven, plus two or more systemic inflammatory response syndrome (SIRS) criteria (see below).

Patients with uncomplicated sepsis need to be observed and monitored to detect early possible organ dysfunction and complications.

Systemic inflammatory response syndrome

This can be triggered by infectious and non-infectious causes such as trauma. It is characterized by any two or more of the following features:

- temperature >38 °C or <36 °C
- tachypnoea >20
- tachycardia >90
- white cell count (WCC) 14
- blood glucose >7.7 mmol/L.

Box 34.6

Severe sepsis

Severe sepsis is defined as sepsis complicated by organ dysfunction.

Criteria for organ dysfunction:

- respiratory: a new or increased O_2 requirement to maintain SpO_2 >90%
- renal: Urine output (UOP) <0.5 mL/kg per h for 2 h or newly raised creatinine (>176 μmol/L)
- hepatic: newly raised bilirubin (>34 μmol/L)
- coagulation: platelets <100, INR >1.5 or APTT >60 seconds
- neurology: altered mental state/Glasgow Coma Scale (GCS).

Criteria for tissue hypoperfusion – organ dysfunction:

- systolic BP <90 or mean arterial pressure (MAP) mean arterial pressure<65 mmHg
- lactate >4 mmol/L.

Shoulder dystocia

Shoulder dystocia is one of the most frightening and threatening obstetric emergencies. There is a need to act quickly in order to prevent serious fetal morbidity and mortality.

Definition

Shoulder dystocia occurs when the fetal anterior shoulder becomes impacted behind the symphysis pubis, preventing delivery. Clinically, it is defined as difficulty delivering the shoulders, requiring obstetric manoeuvres beyond episiotomy and moderate axial traction. Although the incidence overall is around 0.2%, it rises to 0.5% with a fetal weight of over 3.5 kg and 10% with a weight of over 4.5 kg. Shoulder dystocia accounts for 8% of all intrapartum fetal deaths.

Risk factors

Although risk factors have been identified (Box 34.7), they have only very limited predictive value; 50% of shoulder dystocia occurs in normal-sized fetuses and 98% of large fetuses do not have dystocia. It is estimated that 3695 elective caesarean sections would have to be performed in non-diabetic mothers with babies estimated to weigh >4.5 kg in order to avoid one permanent brachial plexus injury.

Clinical features

The baby's head frequently descends slowly and is often delivered as far as the chin and the fetal body is in the pelvis. The head often retracts tightly against the perineum and vulva – this is called the 'turtle sign' and should raise the possibility of an impending shoulder dystocia.

The umbilical cord is trapped and occluded between the fetal trunk and the maternal pelvis, leading to rapid fetal hypoxia and death. The pH drops by an estimated

---

Box 34.7

Risk factors for shoulder dystocia
Antepartum

- Macrosomia
- Past history of dystocia
- Diabetes
- Post-dates
- Obese mother
- High parity
- Male fetus

During first stage of labour

- Prolonged first stage
- Secondary arrest >8 cm
- Mid-cavity arrest

During second stage of labour

- Forceps/ventouse delivery
- Difficulty delivering chin

0.04/min and it therefore takes around 7 min for the pH of a previously uncompromised fetus to fall below pH 7.00. It is estimated that 50% of deaths occur within 5 min.

Neonatal morbidity may result from brachial plexus damage due to excessive downward traction of the head during attempts at delivery. It is possible to damage nerve roots at the level of C5–T1, C5–6 (Erb palsy, Fig. 34.6) or C7–T1 (Klumpke palsy).

While the main concerns for shoulder dystocia relate to the fetus, there may also be maternal complications in the form of genital tract trauma and atonic postpartum haemorrhage. Uterine rupture is rare.

Management

This is an obstetric emergency where seconds count. The aim is to disimpact the anterior shoulder and allow the fetus to be delivered. The mnemonic 'HELPERR' (Advanced Life Support in Obstetrics [ALSO] programme, American Academy of Family Physicians [AAFP], Kansas, USA) is useful to help the clinician through a set of detailed manoeuvres in a calm, logical way. Each manoeuvre is attempted for a maximum of 30 seconds before moving to the next (Fig. 34.7). It is important to avoid excessive traction to reduce the risk of brachial plexus injuries and use the manoeuvers to disimpact the anterior shoulder. Recent simulation evidence suggests that, compared with internal rotation, removal of the posterior arm as the initial internal manoeuvre may be more successful at reducing the degree of brachial plexus stretch and potentially be less traumatic to the fetus. However, in clinical practice practitioners should initially use the manoeuvre they are most familiar with, but be prepared to use other manoeuvres if that is unsuccessful.

If all else fails, there are four 'last resort' measures. These are described here in brief:

1. posterior axillary traction: this manoeuvre involves placing the index fingers of each hand into the posterior fetal axilla, which lies in the sacral curve. A similar technique involves passing a soft catheter between the body and humerus and this allows traction to be applied to the axilla (posterior axillary sling technique)

2. symphysiotomy: the symphyseal joint is split with a scalpel, thereby increasing the pelvic diameters (Fig. 34.8). Both legs must be supported during the process to prevent excessive abduction of the hips

3. one or both clavicles of the fetus may be deliberately fractured to reduce the bisacromial distance

4. the Zavanelli manoeuvre: this involves replacing the head with flexion and rotation, and then delivering by caesarean section. In the largest series to date, out of 59 such procedures, 53 were successful. Generally the fetal outcome is poor, often because this is a manoeuvre of last resort.

Shoulder dystocia remains an extremely serious, unpredictable and relatively rare event. Fetal survival and neurological normality are proportional to the speed of successful resolution.

Uterine inversion

Definition

Uterine inversion is rare, occurring in 1/2000–1/20 000 pregnancies, but as it may quickly lead to maternal death, it is an extremely significant third-stage complication. The uterus may undergo varying degrees of inversion, and in its extreme form, the fundus may pass through the cervix, such that the whole uterus is turned completely inside out. As there is a rich vagal supply to the cervix, the inversion leads to profound vasovagal shock, and this may be exacerbated by massive postpartum haemorrhage secondary to uterine atony.

Pathology

Inversion occurs with active management of the third stage, that is to say it is usually iatrogenic, associated with cord traction before the uterus contracts and placenta separates (Fig. 34.9). It is more likely with a fundal placenta and is found in association with the factors listed in Box 34.8.

Clinical presentation

With complete inversion, the uterus will appear as a bluish-grey mass protruding from the vagina, and in extreme cases there may also be vaginal eversion. The placenta remains attached in about 50% of cases. If the inversion is partial, the only obvious sign may be that of profound shock out of proportion to any blood loss. The diagnosis will require a vaginal examination although an abnormally shaped uterine

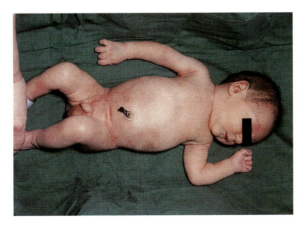

Fig. 34.6 **There is a right-sided Erb palsy following a shoulder dystocia.** The baby was otherwise well. (Reprinted from Rymer J. Picture tests obstetrics and gynaecology, Fig. 168, p. 85, 1995, by permission of the publisher Churchill Livingstone.)

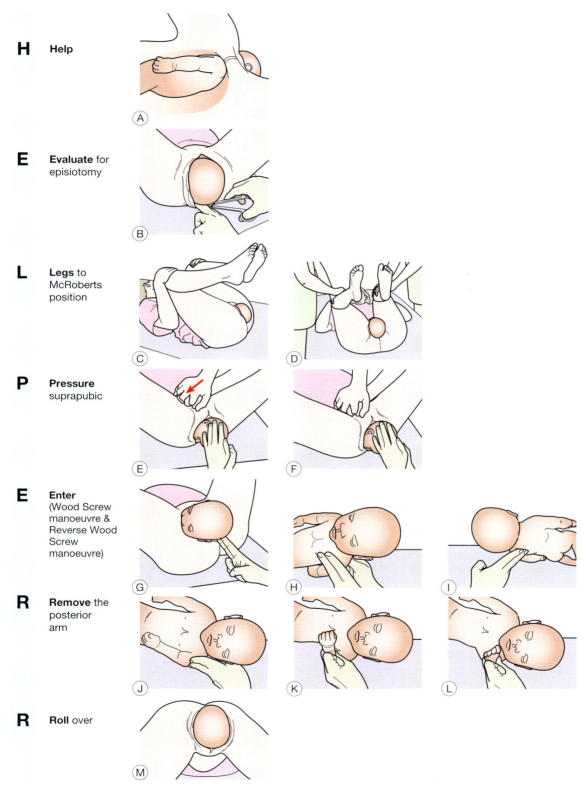

H   Help

E   **Evaluate** for episiotomy

L   **Legs** to McRoberts position

P   **Pressure** suprapubic

E   **Enter** (Wood Screw manoeuvre & Reverse Wood Screw manoeuvre)

R   **Remove** the posterior arm

R   **Roll** over

Fig. 34.7   **Shoulder dystocia.**

continued

H   As with all obstetrics emergencies the first response is to urgently bleep the emergency team. While waiting, use whatever help is available, including the birth partner.

E   This allows room for imminent internal manoeuvres and reduces the frequency of vaginal lacerations.

L   Known as McRoberts manoeuvre. With one midwife to each leg, the mother's legs are flexed hard against her abdomen and at the same slightly abducted outwards. This straightens the sacrum relative to the lumbar vertebrae and rotates the symphysis towards the maternal head, allowing the baby's shoulder to pass under by continuous traction on its head. This manoeuvre is successful in 40–60% of cases.

Attempt delivery for 30 seconds before trying next manoeuvre (applies to each new manoeuvre below)

P   With the legs in the McRoberts position, suprapubic pressure is applied to posterior aspect of the anterior fetal shoulder at an angle of 45° towards the fetal chest in an attempt to rotate the shoulder into the oblique and also to reduce the bisacromial diameter (Rubin I manoeuvre). This is used in conjunction with continuing head traction. If constant suprapubic pressure fails, the assistant can try a rocking movement.

E   There are three basic manoeuvres employed during attempts at internal rotation. The attendant's hand enters the vagina at the 5 and 7 o'clock position, depending where the fetal back is. The middle and index fingers are placed on the posterior aspect of the anterior shoulder and an attempt is made to rotate the shoulder forwards (Rubin II manoeuvre). If this fails, those fingers are kept static and the index and middle finger of the other hand are placed on to the anterior aspect of the posterior shoulder (Wood Screw manoeuvre). Both sets of fingers are again used to attempt rotation. If this fails, the Reverse Wood Screw manoeuvre is attempted. The fingers on the posterior shoulder are withdrawn completely. The fingers on the anterior shoulder slide down the fetal back to lie against the posterior aspect of the posterior shoulder and rotation is attempted again.

R   The hand of the operator is passed into the hollow of the sacrum in front of the fetal chest, the fetal elbow identified, the forearm flexed and then delivered by sweeping it across the fetal chest and face.
Fractures of the humerus are not uncommon with this manoeuvre. It is entirely reasonable to remove the posterior arm before trying any of the 'Enter' rotational manoeuvres (E)

R   It is possible to displace the anterior shoulder during the act of turning the mother over into the all fours position. If not, an attempt can be made to deliver the posterior shoulder first, i.e. the shoulder nearest the ceiling. It is possible to try all the above manoeuvres (except suprapubic pressure) again in this new position.

Fig. 34.7, cont'd

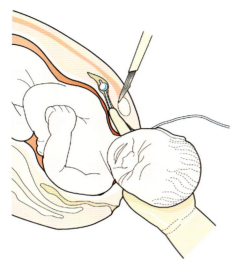

Fig. 34.8 Symphysiotomy. The left forefinger is shown displacing the urethra to the maternal left. A scalpel is positioned above the pubic symphysis and the joint divided anterior to posterior.

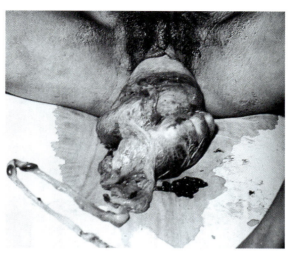

Fig. 34.10 A fatal uterine inversion with the placenta still attached. (Reprinted from Williams Obstetrics, Cunningham FG, Wenstrom KD, Gilstrap LC et al., Fig. 32–25, p. 768, 2001, with permission of The McGraw-Hill Companies.)

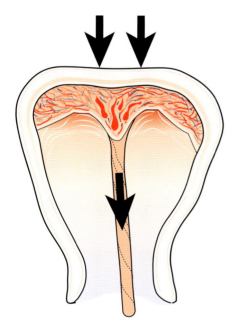

Fig. 34.9 Undue traction on a fundally sited placenta without guarding the uterus may result in uterine inversion.

Box 34.8

Factors associated with uterine inversion
- Previous history
- Fundal placental implantation
- Uterine atony
- Improper management of the third stage
- Abnormally adherent placenta

fundus on abdominal palpation often suggests the diagnosis. Rarely, the presentation is sudden death following neurogenic shock (Fig. 34.10).

Management

Some 90% of patients will have immediate, potentially major life-threatening haemorrhage. In order to minimize vasovagal-induced shock and also haemorrhage, it is imperative to replace the uterus as quickly as is practicable. Immediate resuscitation is required (Box 34.1) and should involve all available obstetric and anaesthetic help. Simultaneous attempts should be made to replace the uterus either within the vagina or possibly back through the cervix if possible. No attempt should be made to separate the placenta, as this may exacerbate the haemorrhage.

One method of reduction is to grasp the uterine fundus with the fingers directed towards the posterior fornix and replace the uterus back into the vagina, pushing the fundus towards the umbilicus and allowing the uterine ligaments to pull the uterus back into position (Fig. 34.11). Alternatively, the centre of the uterus may be indented with three or four fingers and only the centre of the fundus pushed up until it re-inverts. Once re-inversion has occurred, the hand inside the uterus should maintain pressure on the uterine fundus until oxytocics have been given, in order to maintain a contracted uterine state and prevent recurrence.

Should these methods fail, O'Sullivan hydrostatic technique should be employed. This involves passing 2 L of warmed fluid into the vagina using either a ventouse cup or anaesthetic gas tubing. The resulting vaginal distension, especially at the vault, is extremely effective at allowing the uterus to return to the normal position. Up to 5 L of fluid

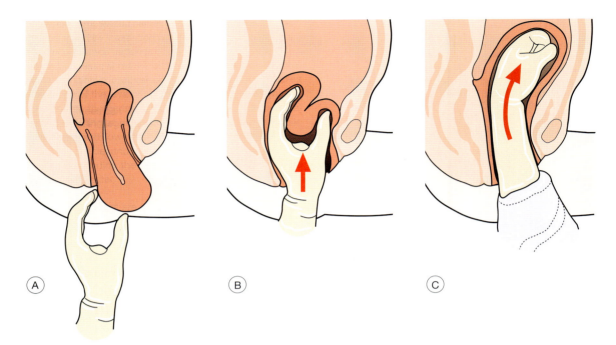

Fig. 34.11 **Replacing an inverted uterus. (A)** Recognition of uterine inversion. **(B)** Replacement of the uterus through the cervix. **(C)** Restitution of the uterus.

may be required to achieve uterine replacement. If successful, the fluid should be allowed to drain and oxytocics given as previously mentioned.

Should all of these attempts fail, a laparotomy is required to aid re-inversion. An incision may be required at the rim of the inversion (Fig. 34.12). Hysterectomy is an option.

Uterine rupture

Loss of the integrity of the wall of the uterus may occur either suddenly or more gradually during the progress of labour. The uterine cavity may communicate directly with the peritoneal cavity (a complete uterine rupture) or be separated from the peritoneal cavity by the visceral peritoneum of the uterus (incomplete uterine rupture or uterine dehiscence).

A complete uterine rupture is a life-threatening emergency often resulting in fetal death, and may lead to maternal death from massive intra-abdominal haemorrhage. Early recourse to caesarean section in 'high risk' parous labours with signs of obstruction is likely to reduce the incidence.

Epidemiology

This obstetric emergency is rare in multiparous women who have had previous vaginal deliveries and virtually unheard of in primigravidae. It does, however, complicate 0.5% of deliveries in those who have had a previous caesarean section, with the rupture occurring at the site of the caesarean section

incision. This risk increases further when oxytocin is used injudiciously and when the number of previous caesarean sections increases. Prostaglandin use is a particular risk and it is assumed that the consequent powerful contractions place a greater strain on the scar. Induction of labour with prostaglandin increases the risk of scar rupture by 14-fold. The risk of rupture is increased yet again if the previous caesarean section was 'classical' rather than 'lower segment' (i.e. midline rather than low transverse uterine incision), and up to a third of pregnancies with classical incisions may be complicated by rupture even several weeks before term. Most obstetricians would offer those with a midline uterine scar an early elective caesarean section. Any woman who has undergone significant uterine surgery (e.g. a myomectomy involving much of the uterine wall) is also at increased risk of uterine rupture and a delivery plan may sometimes require the offer of an elective caesarean section.

Pathology

With complete rupture, the fetus may be extruded into the abdominal cavity. As the rupture can extend laterally into the uterine arteries or broad ligament plexus of veins, there is often severe haemorrhage. Rarely, rupture may occur following direct abdominal trauma, for example a road traffic accident.

In caesarean section scar dehiscence, the fetal membranes remain intact. There is usually minimal bleeding and the rupture does not usually involve the entire scar length.

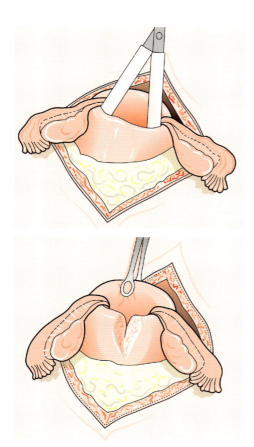

Fig. 34.12 It may be possible to reduce the inversion with division of the involuted rim at laparotomy.

Occasionally, these are found incidentally at caesarean section carried out for other reasons.

Risk factors

There are many risk factors which increase the risk of uterine rupture (Box 34.9), and most of the intrapartum causes are the consequence of increased force being applied to the uterine muscle.

Clinical features

The most common sign of uterine rupture is that of fetal compromise identified by acute onset of significant CTG changes. This occurs in 70% of cases of uterine rupture. Other features include maternal tachycardia, vaginal bleeding (4%), abdominal pain (8%), tenderness and easily palpable fetal parts per abdomen. Occasionally the fetal head is felt to have risen higher on vaginal examination. Dehiscence or rupture may occasionally be identified at a vaginal examination for postpartum haemorrhage. In severe instances, there may be cardiovascular collapse.

Box 34.9

Risk factors associated with uterine rupture

Antepartum rupture (rare)

- Certain congenital malformations of uterus
- External trauma
- Classical caesarean section
- Previous uterine trauma/surgery
- External cephalic version

Intrapartum rupture

- Previous caesarean (especially. induction)
- Previous uterine surgery
- Oxytocin in the multiparous mother
- Precipitate delivery
- Obstructed labour
- Operative vaginal delivery
- Shoulder dystocia
- Breech extraction
- Difficult manual removal of placenta (especially. accreta)

Management

If uterine rupture is suspected, the initial drill of summoning immediate help and resuscitation is followed by an immediate emergency laparotomy to deliver the baby. At the time of laparotomy, it may be possible to repair the defect, especially if this is simple dehiscence of a previous caesarean section scar. If there is massive haemorrhage (more likely if the rupture is complete), or if it does not involve a previous scar, or has led to extension of a scar, an emergency hysterectomy is likely to be required. Most cases of incomplete uterine rupture are not identified at the time of the acute rupture and only become apparent at caesarean section for fetal compromise.

Prognosis

With complete rupture and expulsion of the fetus into the abdominal cavity, the perinatal mortality rate approaches 75%. If untreated, most women would die from haemorrhage and infection.

Key *points*

- Obstetric emergencies are rare and often unfold rapidly. They are often very frightening for all concerned.
- It is extremely important to be prepared to act promptly and to know exactly what to do and when to do it.
- As these emergencies are rare, the labour ward team should participate in regular obstetrical emergency drills training that should include assessment of both technical and non-technical skills (human factor issues).
- Use of mannequins/simulation can facilitate development of appropriate technical skills, team working and communication, improving patient outcomes.

35

Operative delivery

Introduction

The term 'operative delivery' is used to describe both instrumental vaginal delivery (also known as operative vaginal delivery) and caesarean section. Operative deliveries are performed by obstetricians and account for a third or more of all births in most European countries. Caesarean sections can be performed before the onset of labour as either elective or scheduled caesarean sections when planned, or pre-labour emergency caesarean sections when unplanned. All caesarean sections in labour are considered emergency procedures and occur in either the first or second stages of labour, and occasionally after a failed or abandoned attempt at instrumental delivery. Instrumental vaginal delivery using a ventouse (also known as vacuum device) or forceps is only performed in the second stage of labour. It is preferable that instrumental delivery is completed with the first choice of instrument, but in circumstances where the ventouse dislodges close to the perineum, the delivery may be completed with forceps, a situation known as sequential instrumental delivery. The indications for operative delivery can be classified as 'fetal' or 'maternal', with a high degree of overlap.

Instrumental vaginal delivery

The most common indications for instrumental vaginal delivery are suspected fetal compromise (e.g. fetal heart rate abnormalities on cardiotocography) and second-stage delay. Second-stage delay may occur as a result of maternal exhaustion, fetal malposition (occipitoposterior or occipitotransverse) or cephalopelvic disproportion (relative mismatch between the size of the fetus and the birth canal). In practice, the indication for assistance frequently includes both fetal and maternal elements, as a prolonged second stage of labour is often associated with fetal heart rate abnormalities. The criteria in Box 35.1 must be fulfilled before an instrumental vaginal delivery can be safely attempted.

A careful assessment is required prior to instrumental delivery, including abdominal palpation, vaginal examination, assessment of the fetal heart rate, analgesia requirements and the preferences of the labouring woman. There should be no fetal head palpable above the symphysis pubis on abdominal examination (0/5ths), although occasionally one-fifth is palpable in an occipitoposterior position. One of the most difficult parts of assessment is being completely certain of the fetal head position prior to applying the forceps or ventouse. A systematic vaginal examination should determine the orientation of both the anterior and posterior fontanelles, as the most common mistake is diagnosing an occipitoanterior position when in fact it is occipitoposterior. If there is a suspicion from palpation of the sutures that the fetal head is occipitotransverse, it may be helpful to feel for an ear anteriorly under the symphysis pubis. The station of the fetal head should be determined relative to the ischial spines of the mother and the degree of flexion (ideally well flexed with the fetal chin on its chest), caput (scalp swelling) and moulding (overlap of fetal skull bones), and the dimensions of the pelvis should be assessed.

Where uncertainty exists regarding the position of the fetal head, some obstetricians use transabdominal ultrasound to confirm; others will seek a second opinion or re-examine the patient in an operating theatre with good anaesthesia. Incorrect assessment of the fetal head position or the station of the presenting part results in a higher incidence of failed instrumental delivery and morbidity for the mother and baby. An abdominal ultrasound scan can confirm the fetal head position prior to instrumental delivery.

Instrumental vaginal delivery requires a multidisciplinary approach to maximize the likelihood of success and minimize maternal and fetal trauma. In addition to the attending midwife, a practitioner experienced in neonatal resuscitation should be present and the anaesthetist should be frequently involved in the provision of adequate analgesia. Umbilical artery and vein acid–base status should be routinely recorded immediately after delivery.

Complications

Complications include failure with the chosen instrument resulting in either caesarean section or use of sequential instruments. Fetal-neonatal complications include low Apgar scores, fetal acidosis (on cord blood testing), cerebral trauma, cerebral haemorrhage and brachial plexus injury or fractures if shoulder dystocia occurs. Maternal complications include perineal tearing that may involve obstetric anal sphincter injury (third- or fourth-degree tears), postpartum haemorrhage, perineal infection, urinary or bowel incontinence, dyspareunia, or subsequent fear of childbirth). In carefully chosen cases completed by experienced obstetricians the incidence of complications is low. The morbidity associated with instrumental vaginal delivery should be compared with the morbidity associated with a caesarean section in the

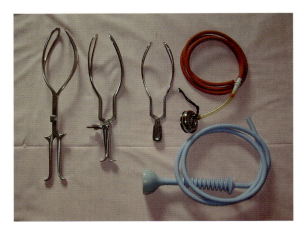

Fig. 35.1   Selected types of forceps and ventouse cups. The forceps, from left to right, are Kielland, Haig Ferguson and Wrigley. The orange tubing is attached to an O'Neill occipitoanterior metal cup, and the blue ventouse is a silastic cup.

second stage of labour, which is a potentially complex procedure associated with maternal and perinatal complications.

Forceps delivery

There are three main types of obstetric forceps (Fig. 35.1):

1. low-cavity outlet forceps (e.g. Wrigley), which are short and light and are used when the head is on the perineum
2. mid-cavity forceps (e.g. Haig Ferguson, Neville-Barnes, Simpson), for use where direct traction is required when the sagittal suture is in the anteroposterior plane (preferably occipitoanterior)
3. Kielland forceps for rotational delivery to an occipitoanterior position from occipitoposterior or occipitotransverse. The reduced pelvic curve of the forceps allows rotation about the axis of the handle.

Low- or mid-cavity non-rotational forceps

The procedure is explained to the mother and her verbal consent to proceed is obtained. The mother is placed in the lithotomy position with her bottom just over the edge of the bed (the bottom half of the bed often lifts away). Using an aseptic technique, the perineum is cleaned and draped, the bladder emptied, and the vaginal examination findings rechecked. A pudendal block and perineal infiltration (local anaesthesia) are inserted if required or the epidural is tested to ensure it is effective. The forceps are assembled discreetly in front of the perineum before application, care being taken to ensure that the pelvic curve of each blade will be sitting over the malar aspect of the baby's head, convex towards the baby's cheeks. Traction is applied in conjunction with the uterine contractions and maternal effort, encouraged by the attending midwife. The rest of the technique is shown in Fig. 35.2.

Rotational forceps

These forceps, known as Kielland forceps (Fig. 35.3), lack the pelvic curve of non-rotational forceps and can be applied directly to the baby's head, if occipitoposterior, to allow gentle rotation to occipitoanterior. After rotation, delivery is as for the mid-cavity forceps. If the baby's head is occipitotransverse, the blades may be applied directly or the anterior blade applied posteriorly before being 'wandered' past the baby's face to the anterior position (Fig. 35.4). These forceps require considerable skill and may be associated with greater maternal injury than rotational ventouse or manual rotation, hence they should only be used by experienced obstetricians.

'Manual rotation' of the head followed by direct traction forceps is an alternative approach to rotational forceps. It is usual to use the right hand for left occipitotransverse or left occipitoposterior (LOT/LOP) positions (Fig. 35.5) and the left hand for right occipitotransverse or right occipitoposterior (ROT/ROP) positions. The fingertips are applied to the lambdoid suture and the fetal head is gently rotated or dragged with a pronation movement. Some operators prefer to rotate during a contraction to minimize the risk of disengaging the head up out of the pelvis. If rotation is successful, it may be necessary to stabilize the new position with one hand while applying non-rotational forceps with the other to prevent the fetal head rotating back again. Delivery with forceps is then completed in the usual way.

Ventouse

Whether to use ventouse or forceps remains an area of debate, but depends to a large degree on the operator's experience and preference. Ventouse has the theoretical advantage that less pelvic space is required – with forceps the diameter of the presenting part includes both the fetal head and the width of the forceps, whereas with the ventouse it is only the diameter of the head that needs to be delivered. The disadvantage is that the mother needs to push well, which may be a limiting factor with maternal fatigue or with dense regional analgesia.

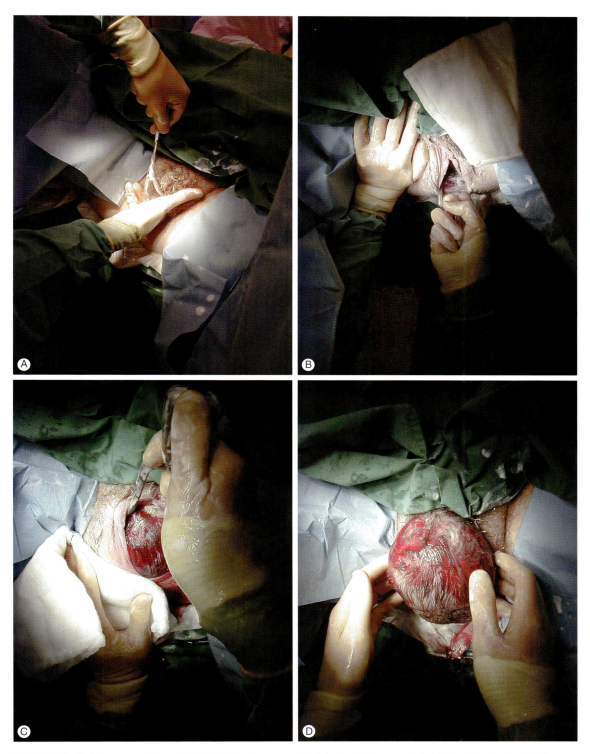

Fig. 35.2 Outlet forceps delivery with Wrigley forceps. The handle in the operator's left hand is inserted to the mother's left side by placing the right hand into the vagina to prevent injury and slipping the blade between the hand and baby's head between contractions **(A)**. Opposite hands are used to insert the right blade, and the blades are locked into position by lowering the handles and allowing articulation to occur gently. Traction is applied by pulling initially downwards at an angle of ~60° – maternal pelvis to obstetrician's pelvis if the obstetrician is sitting **(B)** – with the direction of traction becoming horizontal and then upwards as the baby's head advances over the perineum **(C)**. It is usual to perform an episiotomy as the vulva stretches, but occasionally, as here, this may not be necessary, especially in a parous woman. The forceps are removed after delivery of the baby's head and the remainder of the baby delivered as normal **(D)**.

The use of ventouse compared with forceps is associated with an increased risk of failure, more neonatal cephalhaematomas and retinal haemorrhages, and more low Apgar scores at 5 min, but with less anaesthesia requirements and less maternal perineal or vaginal trauma. No differences in morbidity between ventouse and forceps deliveries were found in the one randomized trial that followed up mothers and children for 5 years.

The use of a soft silastic cup rather than a metal vacuum extractor cup is associated with more failures but fewer neonatal scalp injuries. Silastic cups are therefore often used for occipitoanterior deliveries and a metal occipitoposterior cup or disposable 'Kiwi' cup for transverse and posterior malpositions. Disposable cups (rotational and non-rotational) produce a vacuum using a hand-powered pump and are suitable for single use. The same criteria for safe use apply to ventouse delivery as to forceps (Box 35.1).

The cup should be placed in the midline overlying, or just anterior to, the posterior fontanelle in order to encourage flexion of the head. Failure to correctly position the cup over the 'flexion point' is the commonest reason for ventouse failure. Suction is applied, care being taken to ensure that the vaginal skin is not included under the cup.

Fig. 35.3 **Kielland forceps for rotational delivery.**

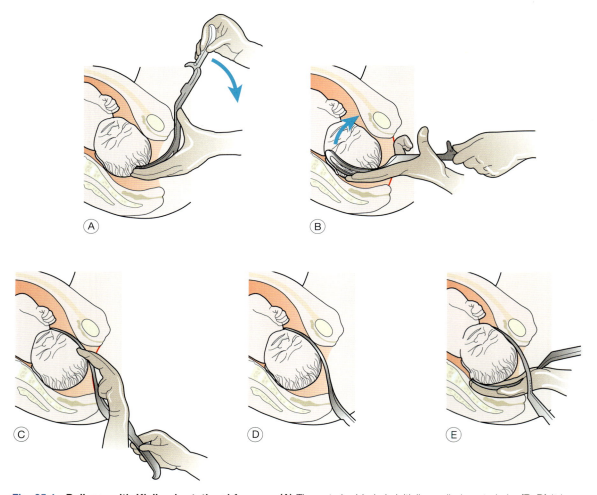

Fig. 35.4 **Delivery with Kielland rotational forceps. (A)** The anterior blade is initially applied posteriorly. **(B–D)** It is then 'wandered' to the anterior position across the baby's face. **(E)** The posterior blade can then be applied and the baby's head rotated to the occipitoanterior position.

Caesarean section

Caesarean section may be:

- pre-labour – this can be elective (planned or scheduled), for example with asymptomatic placenta praevia, severe fetal growth restriction, pre-eclampsia, breech presentation, maternal request or as an emergency (e.g. following a placental abruption)
- in labour (i.e. emergency), usually for the reasons listed under 'forceps' but the cervix is not fully dilated or the mother is fully dilated but unsuitable for instrumental vaginal delivery.

Maternal mortality is higher for emergency caesarean section than for elective; there is also greater morbidity from haemorrhage, infection and thromboembolic disease. Deaths from thromboembolism have been dramatically reduced by the widespread use of appropriate thromboprophylaxis (low-molecular-weight heparin, early mobilization, hydration).

Lower uterine segment caesarean section is by far the most commonly used technique and has a lower rate of subsequent uterine rupture, together with better healing and fewer postoperative complications. A 'classical' caesarean section (vertical uterine incision involving the upper segment of the uterus) will provide better access for a transverse lie, with a vascular anterior placenta praevia, very pre-term fetuses (particularly after spontaneous rupture of the membranes), or where the lower uterine segment is involved with fibroids. Following a vertical uterine incision, the risk of uterine scar rupture in subsequent pregnancies is much greater than with a transverse incision and women are advised not to deliver vaginally following a classical caesarean section.

Preparation for caesarean section includes obtaining maternal consent, intravenous access, group and save (cross-match where increased blood loss is anticipated), sodium citrate ± ranitidine (to reduce the incidence of aspiration of stomach contents into the lungs – Mendelson syndrome), appropriate thromboprophylaxis, antibiotic prophylaxis, anaesthesia (spinal, epidural or general) and bladder catheterization. The details of the operation are outlined in Fig. 35.7.

Complications

Complications of caesarean section include infection (wound, urinary, uterine), postpartum haemorrhage, and less commonly, thromboembolism, and bowel or bladder injury. For the fetus, there is an increased risk of transient tachypnea of the newborn and transfer to the neonatal unit, although this is more likely with pre-labour procedures and at earlier gestational ages. Following a caesarean section there are consequences for any subsequent deliveries.

Subsequent births

In general, women with a previous caesarean section for a non-recurrent indication, e.g. breech, fetal distress or relative

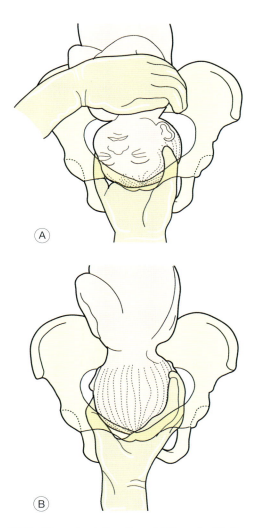

Fig. 35.5 Manual rotation from LOP, as in (A), to direct occipitoanterior (DOA) position, as in (B), using the right hand.

Traction is also applied in the axis of the pelvis as for forceps, but delivery is much more likely to be successful if traction is timed with contractions and maternal effort (Fig. 35.6). The risk of significant fetal injury is increased with the duration of application and with suboptimal positioning.

Although it has been suggested that ventouse should not be used at gestations of less than 36 weeks because of the risk of cephalhaematoma and intracranial haemorrhage, a case–control study suggests that this restriction may be unnecessary. Nonetheless, caution is still required. There is minimal risk of fetal haemorrhage if the extractor is applied after fetal blood sampling or application of a fetal scalp electrode. The ventouse is contraindicated with a face presentation or if there is a possibility of a fetal bleeding disorder.

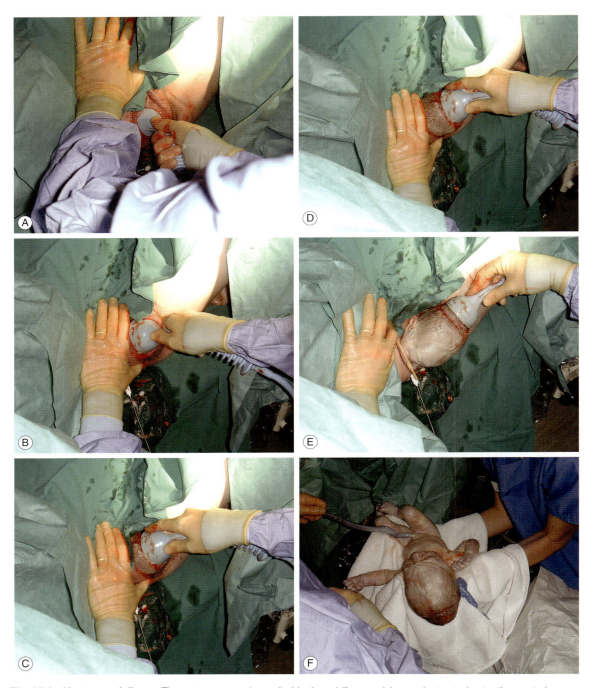

Fig. 35.6 **Ventouse delivery.** The ventouse cup is applied in the midline overlying, or just anterior to, the posterior fontanelle, care being taken to ensure that the vaginal skin is not included under the cup. Traction is then applied to coincide with maternal effort.

cephalopelvic disproportion secondary to fetal malposition (usually occipitoposterior position), should be offered a vaginal birth after caesarean section (VBAC), but elective repeat caesarean section (ERCS) should also be considered. Women with a previous caesarean section are counselled by a senior obstetrician, ideally at the first antenatal visit and again at about 36 weeks' gestation when a care plan can be finalized. Women who attempt VBAC have a vaginal delivery rate of approximately 60–70%. The risk of uterine rupture with attempted VBAC of spontaneous onset is

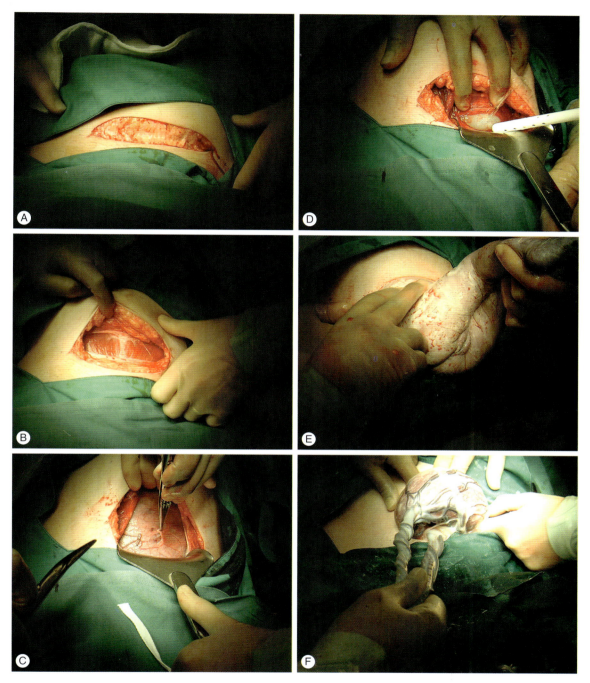

Fig. 35.7 **Delivery by caesarean section.** The table should be tilted 15° to the left side (to reduce aortocaval compression and hypotension) and a lower abdominal transverse incision made, cutting through the fat **(A)** and the rectus sheath **(B)** to open the peritoneum. The bladder is freed **(C)** and pushed down, and a transverse lower segment incision is made in the uterus **(D)**. If the presentation is cephalic, the head is then encouraged through the incision with firm fundal pressure from the assistant. Wrigley forceps are occasionally required. If the baby is presenting by the breech (as here), traction is applied to the baby's pelvis by placing a finger behind each flexed hip to deliver the bottom first **(E)**. If the lie is transverse, a leg should be identified and pulled through the uterine incision to help deliver the baby (i.e. internal podalic version). After delivery, Syntocinon is given intravenously and after uterine contraction, the placenta is delivered **(F)**.

continued

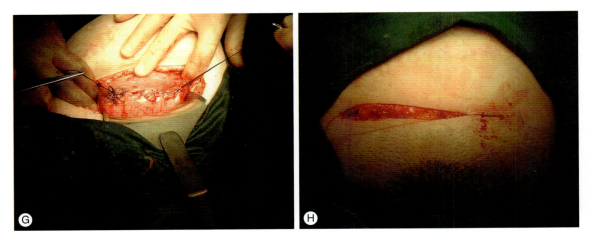

Fig. 30.7, cont'd   Haemostasis is obtained with clamps and a check is made to ensure that the uterus is empty and that there are no ovarian cysts. The incision is closed usually with two layers of dissolving suture to the uterus **(G)**, one layer to the rectus sheath and one layer to the skin **(H)**.

estimated to be approximately 1 in 200–500, being higher if the labour is induced or contractions are stimulated with an oxytocin infusion.

Caesarean section on maternal request

Women who have had a previous difficult delivery or adverse outcome irrespective of the mode of delivery may request an elective caesarean section for a subsequent birth. This may be influenced by both psychological and physical complications. Although in most cases a more straightforward vaginal delivery can reasonably be anticipated next time around, careful consideration of the advantages and disadvantages of an elective delivery is required. Some women request an elective caesarean section for a first birth, where there is no obstetric indication; the advantages and disadvantages need careful consideration before an informed decision can be reached.

> **Key points**
>
> - Operative delivery includes instrumental vaginal delivery by either forceps or ventouse, and caesarean section either pre-labour or during the first or second stages of labour.
> - Operative delivery accounts for a third or more of all births in most European countries.
> - The indications for operative delivery may be fetal or maternal or a combination of both.
> - Forceps may be low-cavity (outlet), mid-cavity or rotational (Kielland), and should only be used when eligibility criteria have been met.
> - The use of ventouse compared with forceps is associated with less maternal perineal trauma but more neonatal trauma and more instrumental delivery failures.
> - Maternal morbidity is higher for emergency than for elective caesarean section.
> - Counselling following a caesarean section needs to address the risks and benefits of VBAC versus ERCS.
> - Operative delivery can result in physical and psychological complications that should be addressed when planning subsequent births.

Stillbirth and neonatal mortality

Introduction

The death of a baby before, or soon after, birth has devastating and long-lasting effects on the families left behind. The loss affects the parents, their families, friends and communities, as well as the staff involved in the baby's care. In this chapter we will explore some of the causes of stillbirths and neonatal deaths in the UK and worldwide, along with their clinical management and strategies for prevention.

There are many different definitions of stillbirth and neonatal death in various countries. The following terms are used in the UK:

- **stillbirth** – a baby delivered with no signs of life that is known to have died after 24 completed weeks of pregnancy. (A baby known to have died before 24 weeks, even if they are delivered after 24 weeks, is classed as a miscarriage or late fetal loss.)
- **antepartum stillbirth** – death before the onset of labour
- **intrapartum stillbirth** – death during labour
- **neonatal death** – a baby that dies in the first 28 days of life
- **early neonatal death** – a baby that dies within the first 7 days
- **late neonatal death** – a baby that dies between 7 and 28 days
- **perinatal mortality rate** – the number of stillbirths and early neonatal deaths per 1000 total births.

International statistics produced by the World Health Organization (WHO) define stillbirths as deaths after 28 weeks or weighing ≥1000 g (as it is not always possible to accurately assess gestation).

Incidence

The stillbirth rate in the UK is around 4.5/1000 live births, and the neonatal death rate is approximately 1.7/1000. The global stillbirth rate is much higher at approximately 18/1000, although it may be as high as 50/1000 in the most under-resourced settings (see Chapter 42 online). The UK stillbirth rate fell during the second half of the 20th century (Fig. 36.1), mainly because of improved general health, better nutrition and wider education, along with improvements in antenatal care. There has been a more gradual fall the

21st century. In affluent countries, a large proportion of neonatal deaths are associated with prematurity (due to either spontaneous or iatrogenic pre-term delivery) and the overall rate of survival varies with the gestation at delivery and the underlying cause.

Stillbirth causes and associations

It is not always possible to identify a specific cause for an individual stillbirth; in almost 50% of stillbirths in the UK the cause is unknown. There are many possible causes of fetal death (Table 36.1) and several classification systems exist which attempt to place stillbirths into descriptive categories. It is important to realize that the presence of a condition does not necessarily mean that it is the cause of death.

Advanced maternal age and maternal obesity are two of the most common associations with stillbirth. Other factors include social deprivation, smoking, non-white ethnicity and domestic violence. The exact aetiology underlying these associations is unclear, but reducing healthcare inequalities is an important way in which stillbirth rates may be reduced.

Management

Diagnosis

In women who experience a stillbirth, approximately half report reduced fetal movements in the days preceding the diagnosis. Other presentations include bleeding or abdominal pain, but for some it is an unexpected finding at a routine antenatal visit or ultrasound.

When fetal death is suspected an ultrasound scan should be performed as soon as possible by an experienced sonographer. A second opinion is recommended if practically possible. As well as the absence of fetal heart activity, other ultrasound features include:

- Spalding sign – overlapping of the fetal skull bones
- hydrops.

It is important that the diagnosis of fetal death is communicated in a sensitive but clear fashion, for example, 'I am extremely sorry but your baby has very sadly died'. If a woman is on her own, offer to call her partner or another person to support her. The initial reaction to the diagnosis differs between couples and no matter the circumstances it is important to allow the family to express their feelings

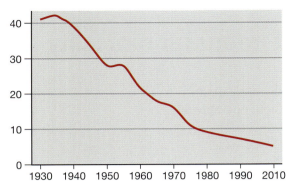

Fig. 36.1 **Stillbirth rates (per 1000 total births) in England and Wales by decade.**

Table 36.1	Causes of fetal death
Fetal	Lethal congenital abnormality Fetal growth restriction Infection Anaemia of fetal origin (e.g. alpha thalassaemia) Fetomaternal haemorrhage Twin-to-twin transfusion syndrome Cord obstruction
Maternal	Metabolic disturbance, e.g. diabetic ketoacidosis Reduced oxygen states, e.g. pulmonary hypertension or cystic fibrosis Antibody production, e.g. rhesus disease Diabetes
Placental mediated ('insufficiency')	Placental abruption Pre-eclampsia Maternal renal disease Antiphospholipid syndromes Thrombophilia Smoking Cocaine use
Structural	Uterine abnormality Uterine rupture Placenta praevia Vasa praevia
Intrapartum	Asphyxia Trauma

freely, which may include anger towards medical or midwifery staff. As long as there are no immediate concerns for the safety of the mother, then allowing the family time alone together to come to terms with the situation may be appropriate.

Immediate management

The first medical priority has to be assessment for underlying acute conditions that might threaten the mother's well-being, such as infection, pre-eclampsia, haemorrhage or disseminated intravascular coagulation (DIC). This should include physical examination, measurement of the blood pressure and urinalysis along with laboratory testing. It is important to test for blood clotting abnormalities, as DIC can be triggered when the fetus has been dead for a while (30% risk after 4 weeks). A Kleihauer test should also be obtained urgently to identify a large fetomaternal haemorrhage, and this can guide the administration of anti-D immunoglobulin in mothers who are rhesus negative.

Delivery

Most women undergo vaginal birth, usually through induction of labour, but all the clinical features should be taken into account when coming to a joint decision about the timing and mode of delivery. Some women express a strong desire for caesarean birth. Such requests should be considered respectfully, but with the advantages and disadvantages being carefully discussed and explored. Whatever is chosen, some women wish to spend some time at home before any intervention – a time to gather thoughts and to make practical arrangements. The mother should be advised that it is not uncommon to feel spurious fetal movement.

Many maternity units have special delivery rooms for women with an intrauterine death, which are more comfortably furnished but are designed such that the safety of the mother is not compromised by lack of immediate access to emergency equipment. Experienced midwifery care is vital along with full access to analgesia as required. An epidural should be available if there are no contraindications, such as infection or DIC.

Psychological care

After delivery, it is important that women and their families are able to spend as much time as they wish with their baby, providing this is their wish. Many parents will choose to name their child. If there is any doubt about the sex of the baby, this can often be resolved within 2 days using quantitative fluorescence polymerase chain reaction. Parents should be offered the opportunity to have photographs of the baby, handprints, footprints and a lock of the baby's hair. Some will wish to leave a toy, family photographs or a letter in the coffin to be with the baby. There may also be particular cultural practices that should be respected, including the need for specific funeral requirements.

Suppression of lactation is of psychological importance to some women following a stillbirth. Up to one-third of women who choose simple methods, such as ice packs, experience severe breast pain. Dopamine agonists are useful but cannot be used in women with hypertension.

Once a couple is ready to be discharged home it is important that the community teams, especially the midwives and the GP, are aware of the events. The community team will continue to support the parents and families through the bereavement process. There are sometimes specialist bereavement teams in hospitals who should also be involved. In addition, support groups, such as those run by the stillbirth and neonatal death charity (Sands), can be particularly helpful.

Investigations

Tests that seek to identify the reason behind the death should be recommended for all parents. These aim to provide an explanation for the death and also inform the planning of any future pregnancies. It is important to recognize that just because an abnormality is found, it is not necessarily the cause of the death and results should be interpreted in light of the clinical findings. These investigations include maternal, fetal and placental tests, and are summarized in Tables 36.2 and 36.3.

Post-mortem

Post-mortem examination of the baby includes determining the weight and length, external examination with clinical photography, skeletal radiography and placental histopathology in addition to conventional autopsy of the baby and placenta. There is the option of a more limited autopsy, excluding certain organs, at the parents' request.

Autopsy can provide key information that is not gained in any other way, but the procedure poses great emotional difficulties for some parents. A simple explanation of the nature of autopsy and its benefits should be offered to all

Table 36.2 Maternal investigations

Test	Reason(s) for test	Additional comments
Haematology and biochemistry (including C-reactive protein and bile salts)	Pre-eclampsia/haemolysis, elevated liver enzymes and low platelets Multi-organ failure in sepsis or haemorrhage Obstetric cholestasis	Platelet count to test for occult DIC (repeat twice weekly if conservative management chosen by mother)
Coagulation studies	DIC	Not a test for the cause of fetal death Sepsis, abruption and pre-eclampsia increase probability of DIC
Kleihauer test	Lethal fetomaternal haemorrhage Decide level of anti-Rh(D) required	Kleihauer should be recommended for all women, not just Rh(D) negative Test should be taken at diagnosis, as red cells clear quickly from maternal circulation
Bacteriology (blood cultures, vaginal and cervical swabs)	Suspected maternal bacterial infection including *Listeria monocytogenes* and *Chlamydia* spp.	Indicated in the presence of maternal pyrexia, infective symptoms or offensive liquor
Serology (parvovirus B19, rubella, cytomegalovirus (CMV), herpes simplex, *Toxoplasma gondii*)	Occult maternal-fetal infection	Stored serum from booking tests can provide baseline serology
Random blood glucose, glycosylated haemoglobin, thyroid function	Occult maternal endocrine disease	Women with gestational diabetes return to normal glucose tolerance within a few hours after an intrauterine fetal death has occurred
Anti-red cell antibody	Immune haemolytic disease Maternal Thrombophilia	Indicated if fetal hydrops present
Thrombophilia screen		Indicated if evidence of fetal growth restriction or placental disease
Parental bloods for karyotype	Parental balanced translocation	Indicated if aneuploidy in fetus or failed fetal testing

Table 36.3 Fetal and placental investigations

Test	Reason(s) for test	Additional comments
Fetal and placental microbiology	Fetal infections	Swabs from maternal and fetal surfaces of the placenta, swab from surface of fetus
Fetal and placental tissues for karyotype (and possible single gene testing)	Aneuploidy Genetic sexing Single gene disorders	Absolutely contraindicated if parents do not wish this (written consent essential)
Post-mortem examination - External - Autopsy - Microscopy - X-ray - Should always include placenta and cord		Absolutely contraindicated if parents do not wish (written consent essential) - External examination should include weight and length measurements - Perinatal pathologist or neonatologist can examine for dysmorphic features if parents do not want a full post-mortem

parents, together with a leaflet and an assurance that the baby will be handled in a dignified manner. However, attempts at persuasion must be avoided. Full parental consent is required for any post-mortem. Even if post-mortem of the baby is declined, the placenta should be sent for examination in all circumstances, as it can provide vital clues as to the cause of death in a significant proportion of cases.

Legal issues

All stillbirths need to be certified by a doctor or midwife and the parents must register the stillbirth within 42 days (21 days in Scotland). Most hospitals will have a bereavement support officer who can advise on the proceedings. Babies born before 24 weeks will not have a death certificate, but the parents can, of course, still arrange a funeral if they wish. Mothers who have delivered a stillborn baby (after 24 weeks) are entitled to normal maternity benefits. There is no requirement to inform the coroner or the procurator fiscal of a stillbirth unless there is suspicion of criminal intent.

Follow-up and next pregnancy

A meeting to discuss the events surrounding their loss and to explain the results of any investigations should be arranged at a time to suit the parents. This is usually around 6–8 weeks after delivery. Returning to the hospital can be extremely distressing for the parents. They should be given the opportunity to recall events and ask any questions they wish. It is important to offer apologies if there have been failures in care and these should be addressed honestly and openly. Ideally, a letter summarizing the discussion should be sent to the parents and their GP.

There is no clear evidence on when couples should plan to conceive again, and this is a personal choice for the individual couple. It is important that the parents are emotionally and physically ready for another pregnancy. Medical care in the next pregnancy will be guided by the nature and cause of the previous loss, but also by the needs and wishes of the mother. In the absence of a specific cause for the previous loss, it is impossible to monitor for specific problems and this brings inevitable uncertainty for the woman. More frequent antenatal visits, particularly with regular growth scans (even if the previous baby was not growth restricted), can provide reassurance and support. Women are often keen to be induced and it is reasonable to view the request sympathetically.

Learning from adverse events

It is an ethical and statutory duty of all healthcare organizations to learn from adverse events. Maternity and neonatal care has a long history of self-reflection, as exemplified by the various national confidential enquiries into maternal and perinatal deaths over the last 60 years. Risk management organizations in the UK require that all perinatal deaths are incident reported and locally investigated to identify lessons that can be learned to improve care. Most maternity units hold regular perinatal mortality meetings for case discussions. These are intended for all healthcare professionals involved in perinatal care, including perinatal pathologists, and they allow a multidisciplinary approach to the case review. In addition to striving for an accurate diagnosis, the team also seeks to define ways in which such a death might be prevented in the future. It is essential that such discussions involve a 'blame-free' approach in order that constructive lessons can be learned. It is also important to recognize that stillbirths are frequently unavoidable, and that neither the healthcare professionals involved, nor the parents themselves, could have foreseen anything.

The perinatal mortality rate has been seen as a broad indicator of the quality of maternity and neonatal services, often adjusted to exclude deaths related to lethal congenital malformations that cannot be avoided. Since 1993 the UK has had a national confidential enquiry into perinatal deaths, most recently this is run by MBRRACE-UK (Mothers and Babies: Reducing Risk through Audits and Confidential Enquiries across the UK). The reports aim to highlight areas of clinical care that could be improved upon in order to reduce poor perinatal outcomes.

Neonatal death

The causes of neonatal death in the most recent MBRRACE-UK report are outlined in Table 36.4. Although only about 8% of babies are born pre-term in the UK, prematurity is associated with very high rates of perinatal deaths, the majority of which occur during the early neonatal period. Most pre-term births relate to spontaneous labour, which itself might be precipitated by bleeding or infection. However, a significant minority of pre-term deliveries are initiated by obstetricians because of serious maternal conditions (e.g. haemorrhage, pre-eclampsia) or fetal disease (e.g. growth restriction, malformation, isoimmunisation or twin-to-twin transfusion syndrome). The direct causes of death among babies born pre-term are varied, but for the majority it is the result of sepsis and/or respiratory

Table 36.4	Causes of neonatal death in the UK, MBRRACE-UK 2014	
Causes of neonatal death in the UK 2014		**Percentage**
Complications after birth		31%
Congenital anomalies		28%
Very premature		13%
Infection		7%
Complications pre-labour		5%
Intrapartum complications		5%
Unknown		5%
Not reported		4%
Placental		2%

failure secondary to respiratory distress syndrome (hyaline membrane disease).

Preventing pre-term birth and its consequences

Interventions to prevent pre-term birth have been a goal for maternity specialists for many years, but with little actual progress. The causes of spontaneous pre-term labour are multifactorial and the rates appear to be rising in the UK. One lifestyle change recommendation to prevent pre-term birth is smoking cessation. Medical interventions, including cervical cerclage (a stitch to keep the cervix closed) and tocolysis (drugs to stop uterine contractions), generate either only small benefits or, more likely, none at all.

In contrast to attempts to prevent pre-term birth, advances in perinatal care have improved the survival rates and quality of survival for many premature infants. Antenatal interventions administered to women at imminent risk of pre-term delivery that improve outcomes include maternal corticosteroids (reduces the incidence of neonatal lung complications), magnesium infusion (neuroprotection, reduces the incidence of cerebral palsy) and intrapartum antibacterial prophylaxis (reduces the incidence of early-onset sepsis from group B *Streptococcus*). Improved neonatal care includes the development of improved techniques for respiratory support, exogenous surfactant administration and more sophisticated feeding schedules. Survival rates have significantly improved (Table 36.5).

Legal aspects

In contrast to stillbirths, deaths that occur in the neonatal period for which the cause of death is unknown, suspicious or related to suboptimal care, should be reported to Her Majesty's Coroner or the procurator fiscal.

Global perspective

As with maternal mortality, reduction in child mortality was highlighted as one of the Millennium Development Goals of

Table 36.5	Neonatal survival rates in countries with advanced health provision, according to gestation
Gestational age	**Neonatal survival rate (to discharge home)**
22 weeks	1%
24 weeks	36%
26 weeks	75%
28 weeks	92%
32 weeks	98%
36 weeks	99%
Term	99.8%

Data for <28 weeks taken from UK EPICURE 2 study (2012).

2000 (MDG-4, now replaced by the Sustainable Development Goals). From 1990 to 2015, the global under-five mortality rate dropped from 90 to 43 deaths per 1000 live births. Despite population growth in developing regions, the overall number of deaths of children under the age of five declined from 12.7 million to 5.9 million. However, 45% (2.6 million) of these deaths are in the neonatal period and this proportion is rising. There are fewer stillbirths worldwide, but nevertheless, 2.1 million babies are stillborn every year. With the 2 million who die in the first week of life, and the further 0.6 million who die before they are 4 weeks old, that means 4.7 million perinatal deaths occurred in 2015.

Causes of death

Determining why babies die in developing countries is difficult because most deaths occur at home and families are often reluctant to seek outside help for a variety of cultural, logistical and economic reasons. Ninety-eight percent of stillbirths occur in low-income countries, with about half of these occurring in labour (compared with <10% in the UK). Globally, the main causes of neonatal death are estimated to be complications of pre-term birth (30%), severe infections (25%), birth asphyxia and trauma (23%), and congenital malformations (7%) (WHO statistics 2008). Up to two-thirds of these deaths can be prevented with known health measures during birth and the first week of life.

Congenital anomalies

This category includes neural tube defects, severe hypothyroidism and congenital rubella syndrome, all of which can be reduced with low-cost interventions; respectively, folic acid, iodinated salt and rubella immunization.

Intrapartum care

Fifty percent of stillbirths in low-income countries occur during labour. Intrapartum events are implicated in a significant proportion of neonatal deaths and can have a significant impact on survivors in terms of cerebral palsy and long-term disability. Birth attendants must be skilled enough to be able to manage normal deliveries avoiding unnecessary interventions, and diagnose and manage or refer women with complications when possible. Approximately 36 million women give birth each year without the help of a trained attendant.

Prematurity

Although pre-term birth is less important proportionately than in affluent countries, globally there are 15 million every year and the figure is rising. It has been estimated that 75% of neonatal deaths related to prematurity could be prevented with simple measures such as antenatal steroids.

Infections

Every year an estimated 30 million newborns acquire a neonatal infection, and 1–2 million of these babies die. The

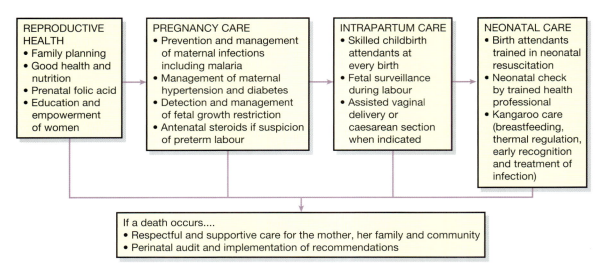

Fig. 36.2 **Prevention and response to perinatal death.** (Adapted from *The Lancet* 'Ending Preventable stillbirths', an executive summary for *The Lancet*'s series, January 2016.)

most common of these infections are early neonatal septicaemia, later neonatal pneumonia, diarrhoea and neonatal tetanus, which together account for around 30% of neonatal deaths. Exclusive breastfeeding helps to prevent many infections in the first month of life. Simple hygiene measures and a clean water supply are also important components in the prevention of infection.

Neonatal tetanus prevention programmes have been a particular success: tetanus has been eliminated in over 100 countries through immunizing mothers with tetanus toxoid, ensuring hygienic delivery practices and maintaining clean care of the umbilical cord stump. Success is not complete, however, with a substantial minority of pregnant women in developing countries still not being fully immunized.

Conclusions

The death of a baby before or shortly after birth is a personal tragedy which is lived out on a global scale. While there are many differences between countries in terms of the size and nature of the problem, there are many common lessons on prevention and care for affected families that can be shared across borders (see Fig 36.2). Improving maternal health and education, preventing pre-term birth, improving hygiene and ensuring skilled birth attendants are challenges that face us all.

Key *points*

- The loss of a baby before or after birth is profoundly distressing for parents, family and friends.
- Most stillbirths are unexpected and almost half of all UK stillbirths are unexplained.
- Some causes of stillbirth can be a serious threat to maternal well-being.
- Investigations seek to explain the death and help plan future pregnancies.
- In developed countries, the large majority of neonatal deaths are associated with pre-term birth.
- Perinatal interventions for prematurity have resulted in better survival rates in recent years.
- Worldwide, infection and birth injury are more common causes of neonatal death.

Physiology

The fetus needs the umbilical cord and placenta for respiration. Within the first minute of life the newborn infant has to adapt to breathing air. Various stimuli, such as hypoxia, cold air and physical contact, will encourage respiratory effort. Most newborn 'resuscitation' is assisting this normal transition process. The 'healthy' fetus will tolerate brief periods of hypoxia (part of the normal birthing process) well. Pathological processes, such as chronic placental insufficiency, acute cord obstruction and infection, add stress to the system and interfere with this normal transition of the infant's ability to cope. Being aware of antecedent events or concerns can help predict which babies might need assistance after delivery.

Physiology of acute hypoxia

Significant hypoxia can occur in utero, or during or after delivery. This hypoxia will stimulate respiratory effort. If the baby fails to start breathing, the baby's oxygen concentration falls further, the baby loses consciousness and enters 'primary apnoea'. The heart rate initially rises then rapidly falls to around half the normal fetal heart rate (~60 beats per minute). Heart rate changes are driven by vagal stimulation and then anaerobic respiration.

After 5–10 min of primary apnoea, spinal centres, which are normally suppressed by higher centres, begin to cause shuddering of the baby's body at a rate of approximately 12/min (agonal gasps). Once this gasping stops, the baby enters 'secondary' (or 'terminal') apnoea. Anaerobic metabolism continues and lactic acidosis causes a further drop in the blood pH. The heart rate will gradually fall and, without intervention, the outcome will be death. The only way to tell whether a non-breathing newborn infant is in primary or secondary apnoea is by assessment of its response to resuscitation. In primary apnoea, nearly all infants will start breathing within a few breaths. In secondary apnoea, the baby will usually gasp for some time before starting regular respiration. In reality, however, both are initially managed in the same way. Circulation does not fail until late in the process and very few infants, therefore, require circulatory support as part of resuscitation. It is this awareness of the normal response to hypoxia in the infant that guides the newborn resuscitation algorithm order, which places a heavy emphasis on airway and breathing support.

Practical aspects of neonatal resuscitation

Before the baby arrives

Team briefing and preparation before the baby arrives can help communication and readiness for the likely scenario. Before the baby arrives think about the following things:
- What are the concerns? (e.g. Gestation? Meconium? Fetal monitoring? Suspected or known anomalies? Risk factors for infection?)
- Can we deal with those concerns? Do we need help?
- Do we have the right equipment and is it working? (e.g. hat, dry towels, heat source, masks, self inflating bag or T-piece resuscitator, suction, resuscitation trolley)
- Are all team members aware of their role?
- If things do not go according to plan A, what is plan B and C?

By outlining the concerns or the expected situation and allocating roles the team can work more efficiently. Clear communication is a key part of working well in a resuscitation team, and that process starts before the baby is born.

Dry, wrap, keep the baby warm and assess

Start a timer on the Resuscitaire or note the time. Dry the baby and then wrap in a warm, dry towel. A naked, wet baby can still become hypothermic despite a warm room, especially if there is a draught. A cold baby has increased oxygen consumption and is more likely to become hypoglycaemic and acidotic. Babies also have a large surface area-to-weight ratio and heat can therefore be lost very quickly. Most of the heat loss is by evaporation, and outcome is therefore improved by drying (Fig. 37.1).

Use this 30–60 second period of drying and stimulating to assess the baby. Assessment consists of: tone, colour, breathing and heart rate.

Apgar score

The Apgar score was proposed as a tool for evaluating a baby's condition at birth and is recorded at 1 and 5 min

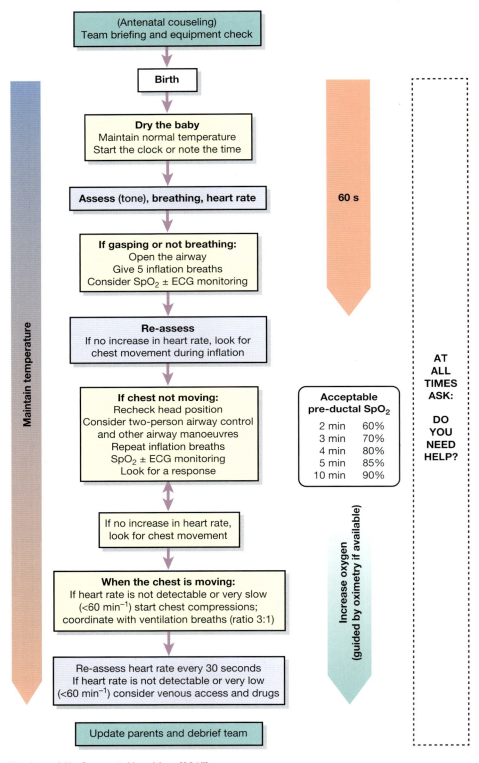

Fig. 37.1   Newborn Life Support Algorithm (2015).

(Table 37.1). Acute clinical assessment will categorize the baby into one of the following three colour groups:

- pink – regular respirations, heart rate fast (>100 bpm). These are healthy babies and they should be kept warm and given to their mothers
- blue – irregular or inadequate respirations, heart rate slow (<100 bpm). If gentle stimulation does not induce effective breathing, the airway should be opened. If the baby responds, no further resuscitation is needed. If not, progress to lung inflation
- blue/white – apnoeic, heart rate slow (<60 bpm). Whether an apnoeic baby is in primary or secondary apnoea, the initial management is the same before.

Airway

Before a baby can breathe the airway needs to be open. The baby's head should be in the neutral position. The normally prominent occiput of a newborn may cause flexion and pharyngeal collapse. A folded towel placed under the neck and shoulders may help to maintain the airway in a neutral position, but take care not to overextend the neck (Fig. 37.2). A jaw thrust may be needed to bring the tongue forward and open the airway, especially if the baby is floppy.

Meconium-stained liquor is relatively common. Fortunately, meconium aspiration is a rare event and often occurs in utero before delivery. If the baby is active, no specific action (other than drying and wrapping the baby) is needed.

Table 37.1	The Apgar scoring system		
Feature	**Score**		
	0	**1**	**2**
Colour	White	Blue	Pink
Tone	None	Poor	Good
Heart rate	<60 bpm	60–100 bpm	>100 bpm
Respiration	None	Gasping	Vigorous
Response to simulation	None	Minimal	Vigorous

(Reproduced with permission from the International Anesthesia Research Society, from: Apgar V. Current researches in anesthesia & analgesia 32(4); 1953. Permission conveyed through Copyright Clearance Center, Inc).

If the baby is not active, inspect the oropharynx with a laryngoscope and aspirate any particulate meconium seen using a soft catheter under direct vision of the vocal cords. Prolonged attempts to suction through the vocal cords should be avoided. The priority should be mask ventilation, especially if bradycardia is ongoing.

Breathing

If the baby is gasping or not breathing, immediately commence artificial ventilation. The first five breaths should be inflation breaths, preferably using air. These breaths are designed to inflate lungs that are fluid filled/collapsed. These should be 2–3 second sustained breaths using a bag valve mask. If available (and staff are trained), a T-piece resuscitator can provide a set peak inspiratory pressure, usually 30 cm H_2O in a term infant, and a positive end expiratory pressure, normally 5 cm H_2O. Use a transparent, soft, reformable mask big enough to cover the nose and mouth of the baby with the baby's mouth open (Fig. 37.3).

The best indication of adequate aeration of the lungs is improvement in the heart rate (if this has been low) or visible chest wall movement; auscultation is less reliable for this assessment. If regular spontaneous breathing has not established after adequate chest inflation, then ventilation breaths should continue at a rate of 30–40 ventilations/min. Ventilation breaths should have a shorter inspiratory phase than inflation breaths. Continue to reassess that the airway is clear and that the chest is rising/falling. If there is no increase in heart rate there are two main explanations. First, and most likely, is inadequate or ineffective aeration of lungs. Second, the baby requires more resuscitation than just aeration of lungs.

Review points to consider if there has been inadequate aeration of the lungs:

- Is the baby in the neutral position? (the most common reason for inadequate ventilation)
- Is the mask the correct size? Is there a good seal around the mask?
- Do you need to perform a jaw thrust? Do you need to use a two-person technique?
- Is there something obstructing the airway, and can you safely remove it?
- Would an airway adjunct like a Guedel airway help?

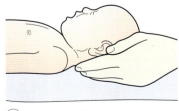 (A) Too flexed

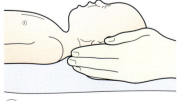 (B) Neutral (correct position)

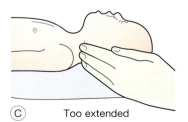 (C) Too extended

Fig. 37.2 Head position.

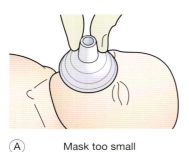
(A) Mask too small

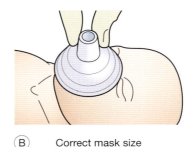
(B) Correct mask size

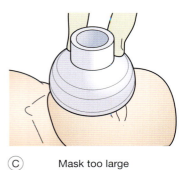
(C) Mask too large

Fig. 37.3 **Mask positioning.**

A Guedel airway should be inserted under direct vision with a laryngoscope as shown in Fig. 37.4. Using a laryngoscope in this way helps prevent trauma. It helps to keep the relatively large infant tongue out of the way as the airway adjunct is inserted. The correct size of airway adjunct should reach from the middle of the chin to the angle of the jaw.

Circulation

Very few infants will require more than aeration of the lungs. The purpose of cardiac compression is to move a small amount of oxygenated blood to the coronary arteries in order to initiate cardiac recovery. There is therefore no point in cardiac compression before the lungs have been inflated.

If the heart rate is not detectable or remains slow (<60 bpm) once the lungs are inflated, chest compressions should be started. The most efficient way of doing this in the neonate is to encircle the chest with both hands so that the fingers lie behind the baby and the thumbs are opposed on the sternum just below the inter-nipple line (Fig. 37.5). Compress the chest to one-third of its depth and perform three compressions for each breath. Compressions are ineffective unless interposed breaths are of good quality and inflate the chest. Asynchronous compressions and breaths will not allow adequate ventilation. Even if the baby is intubated, breaths and compressions should remain synchronous with three chest compressions then one breath. The most common reason for failure of the heart rate to respond, once again, is failure to achieve lung inflation. Once the heart rate is above 60 bpm and rising, cardiac compression can be discontinued.

Drugs

If, after adequate lung inflation and cardiac compressions, the heart rate has not responded, drug therapy should be considered. Airway and breathing must be reassessed as adequate before proceeding to drug therapy. The quickest way to establish reliable vascular access is via an umbilical venous line (or if not possible then an intraosseous needle). Drugs to be considered include:

- adrenaline
- 10% glucose
- sodium bicarbonate.

Using a wall chart/table of predicted weights and the volume to be administered is safer than trying to do drug calculations in a stressful environment.

Adrenaline can also be administered via a tracheal tube, however, absorption is unclear..

Very occasionally, hypovolaemia may be present because of known or suspected blood loss (e.g. antepartum haemorrhage, placenta praevia or vasa praevia). Volume expansion with 0.9% sodium chloride (rather than albumin) may be appropriate. Some units will have rapid access to O negative blood and this may also be appropriate where there is clear blood loss. Occasionally, a baby who has been effectively resuscitated and is pink, with a heart rate over 100 bpm, may not breathe because of the effects of maternal opiates. If respiratory depressant effects are suspected, the baby could be given naloxone intramuscularly. Appropriate airway and ventilation measures are still required, as the effect of naloxone will only last a short time.

Monitoring in neonatal resuscitation

Feeling the base of the umbilical cord for pulsation is not always reliable because absent pulsation does not necessarily mean absent cardiac output. Heart rate can be better assessed by feeling apex beat or listening with a stethoscope, though even this is not infallible. Pulse oximetry provides information on pulse and saturations and can guide requirements for additional oxygen. It is important to be aware that there is a normal transition with oxygen saturation from around 60% at birth to >90% at around 10 minutes of age. The saturations probe should be applied to the (dried) right hand/wrist of the baby to give a pre-ductal measurement.

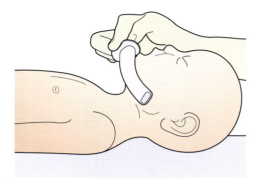

(A) Correct size of Guedel airway

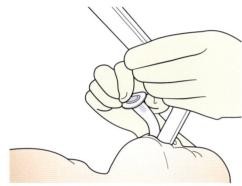

(B) Insertion with a laryngoscope

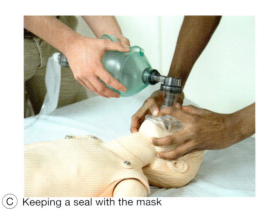

(C) Keeping a seal with the mask

Fig. 37.4 Maintaining the airway. (A) Correct use of Guedel airway. (B) Insertion with a laryngoscope. (C) Two-person technique.

If there is reasonable cardiac output, pulse oximetry will also reliably indicate the heart rate.

Electrocardiogram monitoring can provide a rapid and very accurate examination of the newborn heart rate. In order to be effective, however, there has to be good contact with the skin, i.e. a dry baby.

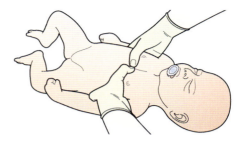

Fig. 37.5 Two-hand technique for cardiac compressions.

Temperature control is also an important part of all newborn stabilization. Hypothermia in pre-term babies increases mortality. Avoiding hyperthermia, especially in term babies with hypoxic-ischaemic injury, is just as critical. Many resuscitation stations will have skin temperature sensor probes or attachments; these can provide automated regulation of heating to maintain the infant's temperature at 36.5–37.5°C.

Pre-term babies

The more pre-term a baby is, the less likely it is to establish adequate respirations. Pre-term babies (especially those <32 weeks) are also likely to be deficient in surfactant. The effort required to breathe is greater and yet the muscles are less developed. One must anticipate that babies born before 32 weeks may need help to establish prompt aeration and ventilation. The paediatric or neonatal team should be called prior to delivery when possible.

Pre-term babies are more likely to become cold (higher surface area:mass ratio) and more likely to be hypoglycaemic (fewer glycogen stores). The temperature of very pre-term babies can be maintained if they are immediately placed in a plastic bag (without drying) under a radiant heater, leaving the face exposed and covering the head with a hat. The delivery room temperature should be maintained above 26°C.

Discontinuation of resuscitation

The outcome for a baby born with no detectable heartbeat that remains undetectable after 10 minutes of effective resuscitated is likely to be poor. The decision to discontinue resuscitation should be taken by a senior member of the team, ideally a consultant.

Debrief and parental communication

It is important to keep parents up to date and explain what is happening. Time for the baby away from the mother should be minimized where possible. It is important to explain to the parents what has happened, potentially why, and what will need to be done (if anything further). A record of events and discussions should be made as soon as possible. Debrief and discussion with team members is just as important. Most infants will do well with minimal need for resuscitation, so in the rare/unexpected circumstances where more intensive efforts are required it can be stressful. Having a formal debrief can alleviate staff concerns and allow for support. By understanding and reflecting on practice we may yield positive changes, improving outcomes for the future.

Practical gynaecology and obstetrics

Introduction

The aim of this chapter is to give a guide on the principles of what to do at a very practical level in a number of common clinical scenarios that you may face when on call. Some of the clinical scenarios are already covered elsewhere in the book, and will be cross referenced, but we make no apology for repetition – looking at a scenario from different angles is always useful in understanding it better. It is also very important to consider *why* something is being done. The 'why' is often overlooked, but it is particularly important when clinical presentations are atypical and when 'out of the box' thinking is therefore required.

The exact management pathway will vary depending on a number of issues:

- How much responsibility you are given and the level of support available. Remember that your seniors are likely to want to be kept informed of what is going on, more than in some other clinical areas
- Who has the primary responsibility for pregnant patients with medical problems?
- Who performs the ultrasound in your unit?
- The skills, equipment, attitudes and culture of staff and patients in your unit.

Some clinical practice varies between hospitals, usually because there is no robust evidence behind quite a few of the things we do, but exploring the reason for these differences can be really interesting and offer a deeper understanding of both the clinical condition and of the systems in which you are working.

Common pitfalls

- Ignoring midwives. Many of them have a huge wealth of experience. Listen very carefully if a midwife tells you they have a hunch there is a problem.

- Interpreting investigations, including cardiotocography (CTG), without seeing the patient. It is very easy to make wrong assumptions.
- Not carrying out pregnancy tests in anyone of reproductive age, i.e. anyone not pre-pubertal or postmenopausal. The answer to the question, 'Could you be pregnant?' is usually, *but not always*, answered honestly.
- Beware of obstetric patients with medical or surgical problems as it is sometimes unclear who is in charge. There is a particular tendency to under-investigate, especially with medically unwell patients who are being managed on a medical ward, as many non-obstetric doctors are nervous of dealing with pregnancy. Ideally, see the patient yourself and speak to the other doctor directly to make sure that you are both clear on the plan.
- Three months into an obstetrics and gynaecology (O&G) job is a risky time. At the start, you will ask lots of questions (you know that you do not know), but by 3–4 months you feel comfortable, relaxed and feel that you understand the job well. You are, however, still relatively inexperienced and you do not know what you do not know! Continue to question.

The 'lows' can be very low, but the highs can be even higher. Enjoy your time in this fascinating speciality – it is a privilege to witness birth, and to share in the joy, and occasional profound sadness, at this most momentous time in our lives.

Lower abdominal pain in gynaecology

Female patients with lower abdominal pain may be referred to either surgery or gynaecology. If the patient has a history and signs consistent with appendicitis (onset over some days, pyrexia, vomiting, possible peritonism) then it is sensible for the patient to be seen first by the surgeons rather than gynaecology. This may vary depending on who does ultrasound scanning and the site of the specialties relative to where the patient is at the time. A collaborative approach, good dialogue and common sense will ensure the best outcome for the patient.

- History must include onset, duration, location, urine symptoms, bleeding, menstrual history, parity and a gynaecological history, including future fertility wishes.
- Examination requires a thorough abdominal examination to locate tenderness or masses, a speculum (to visualize the cervix for discharge or cancer), a bimanual pelvic examination for cervical excitation (blood, or free fluid [inflammation]) and a swab for chlamydia and gonorrhoea.
- A pregnancy test is mandatory, as is a urine dip for signs of urinary tract infection (UTI). Often a full blood count (FBC) and C-reactive protein (CRP) can be helpful for signs of inflammation. (A CRP may sometimes be raised with a normal white cell count [WCC] in acute appendicitis. Inflammatory markers may be raised in an ovarian torsion, but often only subtly or not at all initially.)

Adnexal torsion

An important non-pregnancy-related cause of unilateral adnexal pain is adnexal torsion. This causes severe adnexal pain, not necessarily of sudden onset, often with vomiting and sometimes pyrexia. Treatment is to detort the ovary laparoscopically if possible, though sometimes a unilateral oophorectomy will be required. If the woman is postmenopausal then it is reasonable to offer a bilateral salpingo-oophorectomy.

Ultrasound can aid diagnosis. An ovary with a large ovarian cyst, particularly one that appears dermoid in nature, is more likely to tort. Depending on equipment and skills, colour Doppler may be performed: flow in the ovary suggests torsion is less likely. Do not ask a sonographer to confirm or exclude adnexal torsion but request a comment on likelihood.

Suspected adnexal torsion is a gynaecological emergency, not in the way of a ruptured ectopic pregnancy, but the more quickly a patient is operated on the more likely it is that the ovary will be saved. Diagnosis and prompt intervention can be a challenge due to recognition, surgical skill, access to operating theatre and access to ultrasound.

Liaising and explaining the urgency of this case with general surgical colleagues, theatre staff and anaesthetic colleagues will ensure that all cases awaiting theatre are prioritized appropriately. This is best done face to face where possible.

Sometimes, after 12–18 hours, the pain reduces substantially. This may be because a torted ovary is now necrotic.

Bleeding in early pregnancy

Bleeding in the first or early second trimester is a common cause for presentation. The bleeding may vary from 'spotting' to very heavy vaginal loss.

Causes

Common

- Bleed in continuing pregnancy
- Miscarriage
- Incomplete termination of pregnancy (TOP)
- Ectopic pregnancy

Uncommon but important

- Molar pregnancy
- Cervical pathology, including cancer

Assessment

Adapt to the situation: if stable, a more structured history and examination can be taken, but if not then the patient needs to be stabilized urgently. Take an airway, breathing and circulation (ABC) approach initially. Remember part of 'C' may involve removing products of conception (POC) or operating for ruptured ectopic pregnancy. If a woman is extremely unstable from a suspected ruptured ectopic pregnancy then do not delay getting her to the operating theatre while attempting stabilize ('turning on the tap' is important but do not delay 'sealing the plughole').

History

- Volume of blood
- Previous bleeding in this pregnancy.
- Pain
- Pregnancy history (previous ectopic increases the chance of ectopic this time).
- Previous abdominal surgery (can increase the chance of ectopic pregnancy and make surgery now more technically challenging).
- Fertility (future plans are particularly relevant in a suspected ectopic pregnancy and may guide the procedure, particularly if there is only one tube remaining).
- Cervical smear screening history and any previous post-coital bleeding.

Examination

- Brief general cardiovascular assessment (pulse, blood pressure [BP], capillary refill), check that all is stable.
- Abdominal examination: check for tenderness (increased chance of ectopic pregnancy).
- Speculum examination (assess volume of blood, confirm if it is coming from within the cervix, confirm if POC are present within the cervical os and inspect the cervix for cervical pathology).
- Digital vaginal examination (VE) (again, check the cervix for pathology and whether the os is open) and gentle bimanual examination (assess size of uterus hence likely gestation and presence of adnexal tenderness for possible ectopic pregnancy).

Treatment

- Intravenous (IV) access and fluid resuscitation is required if unstable. FBC, group and save (or cross-match if heavy blood loss) and coagulation screen (if heavy blood loss). Heavy blood loss may need blood products.
- If this is an incomplete miscarriage and there are POC in the cervical os these can be removed carefully using Rampley sponge-holding forceps or similar through a speculum (Fig. 38.1). This is an important skill to learn as it can stop pain in many instances and slow the bleeding quickly. Take the Rampley forceps, keeping the tips sterile, and gently insert just into the cervical os and try to grasp POC. Pull with the aim of removing big pieces whole, rather than piecemeal, where possible.
- Ideally, this should be done on stirrups with good lighting. If you are having to go to casualty or other wards then it might be worth preparing an emergency gynaecology bag of equipment. You may need to trade-off between doing the procedure there, and hence potentially have the woman out of pain quicker, but possibly causing more pain while doing a longer procedure without optimal positioning, or transferring her to somewhere with better equipment. If you are inexperienced it is usually best to try to find the stirrups/good lighting and a Cusco speculum with a ratchet (to free up both your hands).
- A good nurse/chaperone who can support the woman will help you immensely. The woman will often endure the discomfort if there is a good chance that this is definitive management.
- If POC cannot be visualized, but there is a significant amount of bleeding then miscarriage needs to be confirmed by ultrasound in all but critical scenarios.
- Options for treatment with incomplete miscarriage and light bleeding include conservative (await event), medical (misoprostol to speed the delivery of POC) or surgical management of miscarriage (an evacuation of

Empty the uterus

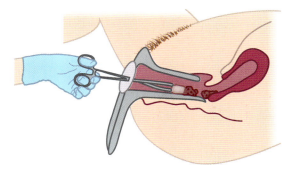

Fig. 38.1 **If there is marked bleeding during a miscarriage, removing tissue from the os can rapidly improve the situation.**

uterus), usually with a suction curettage under general anaesthetic or sedation, or with manual aspiration (surgical management is usually the most appropriate in heavy bleeding).
- In suspected ectopic pregnancy with significant pain or bleeding, surgical management is the treatment of choice, by laparoscopy if possible. Laparotomy is generally most appropriate in very unstable patients. Laparotomy is likely to be a quicker theatre set-up and quicker to access and stop the bleeding in all but the slickest of laparoscopic theatres/teams/operators.

Caveats, tips and pitfalls

- As a ruptured ectopic pregnancy is so risky, you may find yourself relieved to find after a scan that bleeding is due to a miscarriage rather than an ectopic, but remember that the patient may well be devastated. The pregnancy may be wanted or unwanted. You could ask the woman or couple, 'Was it good news or not good news when you found out you were pregnant?' The couple may remember forever the way you discussed this with them.
- The priority of a woman phoning or attending with spotting in early pregnancy may be to get an ultrasound scan quickly to know if her pregnancy is OK. Acknowledging that this is important to her (and not really an entirely unreasonable wish) is likely to be appreciated, even if this is not something that you are able to offer.
- There are suspected ectopic pregnancies that need to go to theatre within an hour, and occasionally those that need to go immediately. Be sure to communicate clearly, assertively and honestly with seniors, theatre staff and anaesthetists how urgent (or not) you feel that the case is.
- If you have the skills to perform, or immediate access to ultrasound, and the woman has no risk factors for cervical cancer and no history of post-coital bleeding pre-pregnancy, then most would consider it reasonable to omit speculum and pelvic examination on first presentation of pain-free spotting, but a speculum is mandatory with repeated episodes of bleeding.
- Ultrasound can be fraught with pitfalls, but these can be mostly avoided if you are sensible. If you have a reasonable degree of scan experience but are not considered 'competent for independent practice' or are unsure in your findings, then be sure to be honest with the patient about your skill level, and ensure the scan is rechecked when next practicably possible. This is particularly important when confirming that a very early pregnancy is intrauterine or confirming a miscarriage. Overconfidence and poor communication with the patient are likely to lead to clinical problems or complaints from your patient. As a junior, diagnosing a very early pregnancy as intrauterine or diagnosing a miscarriage should always be followed

up for confirmation, unless your department has agreed otherwise.

- If you are working in a unit that has much of its scanning done by someone other than the person caring for the patient (be it another doctor, nurse, midwife or a sonographer) you will rely on the wording of the report to determine if this is an intrauterine pregnancy. If you are new to the specialty the descriptions and wording in the report can sometimes be confusing. Be sure to check with a senior staff member or the sonographer if you are unsure whether the report means an intrauterine pregnancy has been confirmed or not. It is also advisable for your own professional development to look at the images yourself, where they are available.
- Spend time if you can in your early pregnancy unit – you will learn a lot.
- It is very important in your interaction with your early pregnancy unit when you are on call, that you are clear on roles and responsibilities. If, for example, you are asked to see a woman with repeated bleeding in early pregnancy with a normal 8-week ultrasound, be sure you are clear whether you, as doctor, are being requested to take over the lead in her care, or whether you are simply being asked do a speculum/pelvic examination to ensure there is no sign of a gynaecological cause (such as cervical cancer). Equally if you ask them to see a patient, be clear on whether, for example, they are taking over her care, or if you are just booking her in for their next available scan slot.
- Managing an incomplete miscarriage is essentially the same as managing an incomplete TOP, but referring to the wrong one to the patient can be extremely upsetting. If it has been a very busy shift in the middle of the night it can be easy to forget which one you are dealing with. Stop and stand outside the room for a few seconds and confirm with the notes and the nurse which case you are about to deal with!
- Except in extremely urgent scenarios, always invest a few minutes in finding out from patients who are going to the operating theatre as an emergency about their fertility situation and plans (as far as is practically and sensitively possible or known). If unexpected events happen this could be invaluable – you cannot ask her while she is asleep!
- Pelvic inflammatory disease (PID) is very uncommon in pregnancy.
- A low BP may be caused by vagal response to POC in the cervical os ('cervical shock'). This can often be accompanied by borderline bradycardia and pain. Hypotension, however, is also a very late sign of severe haemorrhagic shock, so be careful!
- There is a duty of care to provide assistance to a woman with incomplete TOP with significant bleeding/pain, even if you conscientiously object to TOP. It

is courteous to offer help to a colleague who has a greater moral issue with TOP than yourself.

- There are complex regulations about the disposal of POC in some parts of the world. If in doubt keep them to one side in the sluice and seek advice from your gynaecology nurses. Be respectful of POC in front of the patient.

Nausea and vomiting of pregnancy (NVP) and hyperemesis gravidarum (HG)

NVP and HG are common and can be extremely unpleasant. They typically present in the first 11 weeks' gestation, but can continue for many weeks or months. Always rule out other causes. Check urine sample for UTI, take a thorough history (particularly ask about pain, fever, diarrhoea or foreign travel) and examine the abdomen for tenderness.

You may find that your patient, and sometimes their GP, is reluctant to start antiemetics even when clearly indicated. Remember that concerns about the legacy of thalidomide are still deeply ingrained. Most antiemetics have very good safety data and your unit will probably have its own guidelines. Metoclopramide should not be used as first line due to the rare but serious risk of extrapyramidal side-effects, especially in young women.

Aggressive fluid management is the initial cornerstone of treatment and sometimes this, along with IV antiemetics during a few hours' attendance may be sufficient on a first presentation. If the patient is in the late second trimester or beyond you need to check that there is no evidence of pre-eclampsia, and confirm that there is no known cardiac condition where aggressive fluid management could cause pulmonary oedema. Your unit's guidance may have an outpatient treatment plan or admission criteria based on, for instance, urine ketonuria.

Women with hyperemesis are pro-thrombotic: pregnant, dehydrated, and sometimes with reduced mobility. If admitted, they will usually require compression stockings and low-molecular-weight heparin. If hyperemesis is prolonged, start thiamine orally or IV.

Termination of pregnancy

TOP is common and knowledge of the principles, practicalities and procedures is important for everyone, irrespective of their personal views. Your exposure to TOP as a student or junior doctor will vary from limited to a substantial amount depending on the legalities of where you are working, whether it is carried out in the hospital, peripheral clinic, or in the private sector, nurses' roles in the process and if you choose to conscientiously object to TOP. Any healthcare professional can decline to be directly involved, though you should still be aware of the procedures so that you can refer women on to a colleague where appropriate and to understand and manage possible complications if they arise. TOP is rarely seen as a 'glamorous' part of the specialty and therefore, while your senior colleagues crowd around the latest laparoscopic theatre gadget, you may find yourself given surprising autonomy. It can, however, be a very rewarding area to work in, and is often emotionally challenging. Experienced nurses can provide you with a lot of support.

The vast majority of terminations are performed in the first trimester. Termination can theoretically be performed at any gestation by medical or surgical methods. Medical is usually with mifepristone and prostaglandins, normally misoprostol then awaiting delivery. Surgical involves physically removing the pregnancy. Legality, safety, availability of skills, beds and theatre, and local procedural preferences will guide what can be offered. This should be checked before starting the clinic.

Medical termination of pregnancy (MTOP) is most common at all gestations, sometimes as an outpatient. Surgical termination of pregnancy (STOP) involves the use of a suction curette under general anaesthetic. Manual vacuum aspiration (MVA) is generally performed with the patient awake. Both STOP and MVA are usually only carried out in the first trimester, or occasionally after 12–13 weeks. After 22 weeks' gestation, feticide is performed first (as otherwise the fetus may be delivered with signs of life). The upper legal limit for most terminations in England, Wales and Scotland is 24 weeks' gestation. While you may be able to offer a degree of choice to the patient over the mode of termination, be sure to discuss with clinic nurses and seniors before the clinic, or at least before seeing the patient, what modes of TOP are available locally, at what gestation and why, how quickly they can usually be arranged, and if funding is available on the National Health Service (NHS). There is no point offering a woman at 11 weeks + 5 days a surgical TOP if it is only available until 12 weeks and there are no slots available for another week. It is essential to arrange some process afterwards (either follow-up or self-pregnancy test) to ensure that the pregnancy has indeed been terminated.

Women requesting TOP usually tend to arrive by rapid referral from their GP or from a sexual health clinic. The pregnancy is usually dated by ultrasound scan either by the doctor in the clinic or by a sonographer immediately prior to clinic.

Once the woman has had her pregnancy dated, the tasks that need to be performed include the following:

- check personal/contact details, who knows she is here and how she is happy to be contacted (this will make your life or your colleague's life much easier if you have to inform her of a result and only have a home phone number and do not know who else in the house knows that she has been to clinic!)
- establish the O&G history, including previous pregnancies and outcomes, and cervical smear history
- establish contraception history
- establish relevant medical/surgical history
- enquire as to whether the sexual intercourse that led to the conception was consensual and if there are any issues concerning the woman's safety (even if she does not tell you, the fact that you have asked could mean that she discloses later in the procedure)
- ask the reason for the termination (establish if the case meets the criteria of the 1967 Abortion Act) and complete certificate A (which must be done by two doctors)
- confirm that the woman is sure of her decision, and help her talk it through if not
- obtain consent for the procedure and make arrangements (home, ward or theatre)
- prescribe the relevant drugs (mifepristone, misoprostol, analgesia, antiemetics, prophylactic antibiotics and anti-D where needed)
- check FBC and group and save (baseline in case there is significant bleeding, and to check rhesus status for anti-D), and chlamydia/gonorrhoea self-swab
- give contraceptive advice and discuss plans.

Tips/pitfalls

- TOP clinics can provide a good opportunity to develop dating scanning skills, but do not work beyond your skill level. If you are doing the scanning and you are not certain that the pregnancy is intrauterine, request help from a senior practitioner – you need to be absolutely sure the pregnancy is not an ectopic (pain from a ruptured ectopic might be mistaken as pain from the TOP, possibly leading to a hazardous delay in diagnosis).
- Discussing future contraception is a key aspect of both TOP clinic and seeing the patient through the procedure. Read up on contraception and ask clinic staff and/or senior staff what contraception is available. Have the UK Medical Eligibility Criteria (UKMEC) (contraindications to various contraception methods) on your computer screen if the clinic does not have contraception checklists.
- Sometimes a woman will have a friend or partner with her, which can be very helpful for support, but it is important to ensure she is not being coerced by anyone else into having the termination. Most clinics will therefore ask to see her alone at some point, even if only briefly. Check what the local procedure is.
- It is extremely important not to judge, even with non-verbal communication, but equally it is your responsibility to ensure that the woman is clear in her decision. You may therefore sometimes need to have potentially difficult discussions. If in any doubt, it is worth talking it through with the woman again.
- The paperwork for the authorization of abortion and notification following the procedure is straightforward but important. You must have made reasonable efforts to establish that the case meets the criteria of the Abortion Act and it is important to document this

in the case notes. It is good practice for one of the doctors to have directly seen the patient. Whatever you feel about the legislation, actively and knowingly cutting corners here could put both the termination service in your unit and your career at risk.

- Confidentially and information governance is important in all patient care, but TOP is a particularly sensitive area, so be extra careful around these issues – do *not* leave bits of paper with patient details lying around.
- If bleeding and pain is heavier than expected after a MTOP (more common with later gestations) then ensure the woman is stable and check that there are not POC coming from the os (see above). If shock is out of proportion to the volume of bleeding, consider the rare possibility of uterine rupture (rare in first trimester, uncommon but possible later) and check from the scan that this was definitely an intrauterine pregnancy, and could not be a ruptured ectopic.

General principles of antenatal patients seen when on call

There are some principles to be aware of when seeing antenatal patients when on call.

Women with small-for-dates fetuses, previous poor obstetric history, hypertensive disorders, or other issues deemed to make them at higher risk of complications, will usually be seen in an antenatal clinic with senior support. No system is infallible, however, and it is possible that issues can still be picked up incidentally in an on-call setting. You therefore have a degree of responsibility to be aware of, and pick up, any issues concerning the overall pregnancy, even if the only reason you have been asked To see someone is about a rash or a cough. For this reason, it is always prudent to ask if the woman is feeling fetal movements and to briefly check her notes for the symphysis-fundal height (SFH) and BP, and repeat these when you see her (though often the midwife will have this in hand). It is not acceptable to simply put off dealing with significant newly identified or deteriorating antenatal risk factors until the next clinic appointment unless this has been carefully thought through and is deemed reasonable. Do not be falsely reassured by a normal CTG (see below).

Written records usually have a section where it easy to follow trends, such as the SFH growing very little or the BP gradually rising. Be extra careful if the records are stored on a computer system as it is easy to miss a trend on some systems. Do remember that while all healthcare professionals seeing a woman are encouraged to write in her handheld records, she may have forgotten them, or they may not exist, so always ask if she has presented elsewhere.

A key rationale for identifying potential fetal growth restriction (growth slowing down), small for gestational age (SGA) fetuses is to raise the question, 'Is it safer to continue the pregnancy or to deliver the baby?' The same is true of women who experience reduced fetal movements. Although

most go on to have completely normal babies and deliveries, a perception of reduced fetal movements can be a marker for stillbirth. Take it seriously. Each unit should have a guideline on this – read and follow it.

Further investigation and follow-up of SGA, or sometimes delivery, may be indicated. In general, it can help to remember that:

- a normal fetal heart rate on handheld Doppler or Pinard stethoscope only lets you know that the baby is alive at that given moment and is no predictor of well-being
- a normal CTG means that the baby is unlikely to die in the next few hours
- a normal ultrasound scan with fetal size and growth, liquor volume, and umbilical artery Doppler, suggests that, in the absence of unpredictable acute events, there is a very low chance of stillbirth over the coming few weeks.

Hypertensive disorders of pregnancy

The aim of this section is to offer an approach for patients whom you may be asked to see as day attenders with symptoms or signs that could indicate pre-eclampsia. Pre-eclampsia should be considered in all women over 20 weeks' gestation, although in rare cases it can occur earlier, particularly with twins and molar pregnancies. The rationale for identifying pre-eclampsia, as for much of antenatal care, is to guide the decision as to whether, on balance, it is safer for both mother and baby to expedite delivery because stillbirth is slightly commoner in this group.

You will often be asked to see these cases with the results of a 'blood pressure profile' (BP checks usually over 30 min or more), often with urate, urea, creatinine, transaminases, platelets and sometimes a fetal ultrasound scan or CTG. Ask about any symptoms of pre-eclampsia, such as headaches, visual disturbance, epigastric or right hypochondrial pain. You should examine for signs of pre-eclampsia: abdominal examination for SFH, the presence of a fetal heartbeat, hypochondrial tenderness, knee reflexes and check the ankle for clonus. SGA is more common in women with hypertensive disorders of pregnancy and may lower the threshold for further investigation or delivery.

If delivery is advised then a few elements need to be considered: how quickly to do the delivery, whether it is by induction or caesarean section and if there is time to allow antenatal corticosteroids to work to their maximal effect. If the decision is made to continue the pregnancy then you need to consider how frequently and by what methods to monitor the patient, whether admission is required and whether further investigation is needed.

The risk of stillbirth and maternal morbidity or death from pre-eclampsia or eclampsia needs to be balanced against the risks of induction and possible prematurity. It would therefore require severe pre-eclampsia and its potential consequences to recommend delivery at 25 weeks' gestation, whereas most would recommend induction to a woman with even a slightly raised BP if she is beyond 40 weeks' gestation.

Women with hypertension and pre-eclampsia may require antihypertensive therapy to maintain the BP at a reasonable level and thereby minimize the risk of a maternal intracerebral bleed. The antihypertensives can usually be given orally, and are only required intravenously in severe pre-eclampsia or eclampsia. It is essential to be clear that antihypertensive treatment does not 'cure' the underlying condition or improve the outcome for the fetus, and can indeed mask the pre-eclampsia by normalizing the BP.

Never send a woman home with treatment without also considering whether delivery, or steroids, may be indicated – there is a tendency to avoid a decision if you know someone else will be seeing her in two days' time. Always consider the following:

- It is the baby best in or out?
- Are steroids indicated if pre-term delivery is likely?
- How soon should follow-up be, and what should be done at that visit?

Management is usually neither complex nor difficult, but the consequences of getting it wrong can be severe. Normal values and trends are different in pregnancy and despite your best efforts it is easy to subconsciously miss a worrying trend if you are more familiar with looking at non-pregnant results. For these reasons, always discuss these cases with a senior until you have plenty of experience. If your senior is stuck in theatre and everything seems fine you can always send the mother home with a provisional plan and phone them to confirm the plan when you have checked it.

You will learn much more, and it will be far more satisfying for all involved, if you present the case and your proposed management with justification and (politely) ask your senior for their rationale if they have a different management plan from you, rather than just read off results over the phone and wait for an antihypertensive dose and follow-up date in reply. If a woman you have seen returns the next day with an intrauterine fetal death (IUFD), an eclamptic seizure or an abruption, or all three, it does not necessarily mean that you and your senior's management was wrong, but you must be prepared to justify your management plan.

Sepsis in pregnancy

Pregnant women are particularly susceptible to sepsis (see p. 67). You are likely to see women with potential sepsis antenatally, during labour, and postnatally, as well as occasionally in gynaecology.

It is well recognized that covering key initial steps of management quickly and efficiently can be lifesaving. This has resulted in the development of 'Sepsis 6' guidelines in most units in the UK. The aim is to ensure that the basics are done quickly and efficiently, reducing the chance of omission, and helping to identify early those with severe sepsis where critical-care input may be required. The key steps are usually oxygen (if needed), blood cultures, IV broad-spectrum antibiotics, blood tests (including lactate, inflammatory markers and renal function), IV fluids and urine output monitoring. There are also usually triggers to involve more senior input. Midwives will often have extended roles in the tasks they can perform as part of this, aiding efficiency. It is important to familiarize yourself with these protocols in your hospital. Remember particularly that sepsis is not a diagnosis in its own right: you need to think about the source.

While the above developments have undoubtedly been positive, they are not an excuse to switch off to the other possible causes of the signs and symptoms you are seeing. Remember, there may be early sepsis that does not yet meet your unit's criteria, or there may be other causes beyond sepsis that account for the clinical picture (a mildly elevated WCC and tachycardia may tick the boxes for sepsis, but it could also be the presentation of a pulmonary embolus, for example). If you are unsure, by all means give the antibiotics, but start thinking about what else you may need to do. All of this comes back to a good history and examination. The potential harm caused by giving a patient a dose of broad-spectrum antibiotics that may turn out to be unnecessary is generally felt to be outweighed by the gain to getting potentially lifesaving antibiotics administered quickly. By the time the next dose is due preliminary investigation results should be available and there will have been time for events to unfold. Antibiotics can be stopped at this point if infection is felt to be unlikely.

Babies of septic mothers in labour tend to have less favourable outcomes in labour than those with a similar CTG or fetal blood sampling (FBS) and no sepsis. Take this into account during decisions regarding delivery. If labour is not advanced or is progressing slowly, the threshold for caesarean section may be lower. Be sure to remember this when assessing progress and alert seniors to the sepsis if discussing the case.

You will see suspected postnatal sepsis commonly. You need to try and identify the source. Key areas to think about are throat, breasts (mastitis), chest (pneumonia) and uterus (endometritis). Ask about a vaginal discharge and, if present, include a speculum to check for it and send swabs for testing.

Shortness of breath in pregnancy and suspected venous thromboembolism (VTE)

Shortness of breath is a common presentation in pregnancy. It is frequently physiological, but it can be associated with pulmonary embolism (PE). Examine thoroughly and take a detailed history, check inflammatory markers and order a chest X-ray if indicated. Unless you have a specific guideline or validated process in your unit, do not do a D-dimer in pregnant or peripartum women. It is likely to be raised anyway during pregnancy and a negative result is not considered to exclude a deep vein thrombosis (DVT) or PE in pregnancy (the pre-test probability being high).

Signs of DVT (see p. 212) in pregnancy can be subtle, and the consequences of missing it severe. Given the non-invasive nature of a leg Doppler, the threshold for investigating should be very low.

A potential PE, on the other hand, can be a frustrating dilemma as, while signs are sometimes obvious, many present with subtle signs and imaging is often required, even though investigation is frequently normal. The options are a $\dot{Q}$ or $\dot{V}/\dot{Q}$ (ventilation perfusion scan), computerized tomography pulmonary arteriogram (CTPA) or Doppler in both legs. Skills and equipment for these tests (particularly the dye for the $\dot{V}/\dot{Q}$ scan) and their interpretation may not be as easily accessible out of hours or even in working hours. Early conversations with the radiology department about the clinical scenario can therefore be very helpful in these cases. Treatment with low-molecular-weight heparin should be commenced while awaiting investigation, and may reasonably be continued for several days until imaging is complete.

Once a PE has been reasonably excluded, remember that you still do not have a positive diagnosis. It is important to revisit the differential diagnosis and run through this with the team, particularly if the symptoms are still present. Both the medical and obstetric team may need to be involved.

In unwell patients with a suspected PE, summon urgent senior medical, obstetric and anaesthetic assistance and take an ABC approach. If the patient is deemed too unstable to go to CT ask for a portable US (Ultrasound) leg Doppler if it is available. If there is someone present who has any skills in echocardiography the identification of a thrombus within the heart or pulmonary artery can be quick and extremely helpful. Thrombolysis may be appropriate. Rarely, cardiac arrest may occur.

Small vaginal bleed in later pregnancy

It can be a helpful approach to group bleeds in pregnancy into three categories based on gestation:

- first trimester bleeding is common and is unlikely to be life-threatening. Management is as per bleeding in early pregnancy above
- bleeding between 13 and 23 weeks could be due to potential miscarriage (though only approximately 1% of pregnancies miscarry in the second trimester). Here the bleeding is more likely to be heavy and can occasionally be life-threatening
- once the pregnancy has reached 23 weeks it is approaching viability and the well-being (and potential need for further investigation or delivery) of the fetus must be considered in addition to the well-being of the mother.

The cut-off of where to manage these patients varies from unit to unit, so check to make sure you are following your nursing and midwifery colleagues' guidelines.

With bleeding at any stage, it is important to clarify the nature and suspected volume of blood, whether it occurred after sexual intercourse, whether and how often it has happened through (and even before) pregnancy, as well as the cervical smear history. For a small bleed, particularly after 37 weeks, it may simply be 'show', consideration should be given to assessing the cervix, especially if pre-term labour is possible. Continued post-coital bleeding would require a careful clinical assessment of the cervix for any evidence of cervical cancer (uncommon in pregnancy in the UK, but very important). Watery fluid that is blood stained could be a pre-labour rupture of membranes.

Substantial bleeding (>50 mL) is an obvious reason for attendance and an obstetric emergency, but more frequently you will be seeing small bleeds or 'spotting' (usually <5 mL). Most women who have small PV bleeds, particularly spotting, go on to have uncomplicated pregnancies.

The rationale for asking a woman to call the maternity unit is as follows:

- to check through her notes to see if the placenta is low (and that there might be a risk of substantial bleeding from placenta praevia), and to see if anti-D is required
- to confirm all is well with the baby. In the late second or third trimester, a CTG can check for any immediate concerns with fetal well-being
- to check for a cause of bleeding and for any evidence of pre-term labour, pre-term pre-labour rupture of the membranes or abruption.

Tips/pitfalls

Providing the placenta is not low, a speculum examination is important to assess if the os appears closed, whether there is further fresh bleeding coming from the os, if there is cervical ectopy (a benign cause of bleeding), or if there are any appearances to suggest cancer.

A digital VE can add further important information to the examination if the cervix has been difficult to visualize. It is important to remember that a digital VE is a broad term that can involve gently palpating the cervix for dilatation, length and consistency (hence assessing if labour is likely) as is appropriate in this situation. In advanced gestation, a VE is likely to be more vigorous and involve inserting a digit through the os itself, which would be very inappropriate in a pre-term patient unless in labour. There is a theoretical concern by some that this type of VE may result in increased endogenous prostaglandins that may accelerate pre-term labour and reduce time for corticosteroids to work. Some clinicians even have concerns about any type of antenatal digital VE. A pragmatic approach, therefore, is to discuss with a senior colleague before performing digital VE or speculum in pre-term antenatal patients in your early obstetric time.

If the placenta is known to be low or covering the cervical os, a digital VE should generally be avoided (the concern is of causing catastrophic bleeding).

If a placenta is recorded as 'not low' at the 20-week anomaly scan then it cannot 'migrate down' and become a placenta praevia. An anomaly scan is, however, performed by humans and error is possible. If there is clinical concern (e.g. high fetal head despite approaching term, recurrent bleeding), it is best to either check the placental location with ultrasound yourself if you can, review the 20-week scan images if they are accessible or ask for the scan to be repeated.

Women who have bleeding in pregnancy, particularly recurrent, can get frustrated about visits to the hospital, particularly if they have other children to look after at home. The perception (and often reality) is that they come in, are admitted overnight and nothing is done. They then may not see the point in attending and may not call the next time they bleed. Be sure you have an honest conversation with the woman about why she has been asked to come in and the rationale for admission if you feel that admission is warranted.

Differentiating between bleeding and bloody show will seem obvious to experienced midwives and obstetricians, but it is not when you start the job – get someone experienced to have a look with you.

Antenatal vaginal discharge and suspected pre-term pre-labour rupture of membranes

Vaginal discharge is a common antenatal presentation. Common causes include:

- blood
- liquor ± meconium
- urine
- a show
- physiological discharge
- candidiasis.

The cornerstone of management involves checking the history followed by a speculum examination to assess the discharge and take swabs for infection. If blood is seen, then management will be as per Small PV bleed in later pregnancy (see above).

The presence of liquor makes the diagnosis of pre-labour rupture of the membranes (PROM) or pre-term pre-labour rupture of the membranes (PPROM) depending on whether the gestation is before or after 37 weeks (see p. 264). Diagnosis of PPROM is particularly important as it allows preparation for pre-term delivery, including giving prophylactic antibiotics and antenatal corticosteroids if indicated, and induction of labour at an appropriate point. A typical history involves a gush of fluid followed by intermittent fluid leakage. Unless liquor is clearly seen to be leaking without speculum examination, it is best to allow the woman to pass urine and then ask her to lie supine, or in the left lateral position at later gestations, for 30 min unless there are any imminent concerns. This allows for pooling of liquor in the vagina so

that you will be able to identify it. Perform a sterile speculum examination and ask her to cough to see if liquor is present (it is often worth asking for a midwife to look with you if you are inexperienced). If there is no liquor to see then it is important to remember that this is then an *unlikely* PPROM (rather than it being excluded) and explain this to the woman encouraging her to return if there is a further episode. Occasionally further liquor will be lost and it will be later diagnosed as a 'PPROM in hindsight'. Unless this is explained, the woman may later be frustrated about the lack of diagnosis at first presentation, particularly if she develops chorioamnionitis, to which the delayed diagnosis may have contributed. An ultrasound scan for liquor volume can assist the assessment but not make the diagnosis alone. A good history of PPROM, for example, with no liquor on examination yet very little liquor on scan would be strongly suspicious for PPROM. Stress urinary incontinence is common in pregnancy and is a differential diagnosis for the presentation – a smell of urine on the maternity pad would be suggestive of this.

Meconium in the liquor at any gestation is likely to influence the timing of delivery at most gestations, as would a history of group B *Streptococcus* colonization after 34 weeks. Foul smelling liquor, particularly if the history suggests membrane rupture may have occurred some time ago, suggests chorioamnionitis and also strongly favours delivery at most gestations. Antenatal corticosteroids may be contraindicated in significant maternal sepsis for fear of suppressing the immune response. Get senior advice.

Extensive candidiasis can look very like a PPROM. It can also mask a PPROM if the liquor is mixed with watery cheesy discharge. Again, if unsure ask a senior to check.

Admission for induction of labour

Induction of labour is offered when it is thought to be safer for the baby, the mother or both to be delivered, rather than for the pregnancy to continue (p. 308). The exact details of what you do, and what midwives do, will depend on local guidance.

Initial assessment

- Check that a decision has been made for induction, what the indication is and that the gestation and parity are correct.
- Note the degree of urgency and if prioritization is needed.
- Check for capacity issues in the unit and, if it is too busy, consider delaying until quieter.
- Plan any monitoring and management the mother is going to need. If she has pre-eclampsia, how often is a BP check required? Make sure it is clear a CTG should be checked as soon as contractions begin, especially if intrauterine growth restriction (IUGR). The

anaesthetist is likely to want reassurance that the platelets are normal before an epidural can be sited.

- Ensure the woman/couple are briefed on the procedure, i.e. that they understand why the induction is taking place, how long it will take and what will happen after what length of time if labour is not established.
- Check the fetus is cephalic presentation.
- Check for any signs of possible fetal compromise (CTG, clinical growth assessment and any recent ultrasound results) to ensure that there are no signs of compromise. If there are concerns, consider whether induction is advisable at all, and whether additional monitoring will be required.
- Check for absolute or relative contraindications to prostaglandins, such as high parity or previous uterine surgery.
- Perform a cervical assessment ± insert the correct dose of prostaglandins if appropriate (see below)

The principle of the process

The cervix is assessed by VE and scored on a Bishop score (see p. 278). Most policies generally involve a cervical assessment, insertion of Prostaglandins (PGs) if the cervix is unfavourable at set intervals over a period of time, or the use of a slow release preparation, until labour begins. If labour does not begin with prostaglandins, and the cervix has become sufficiently favourable, an amniotomy (or artificial rupture of the membranes [ARM]) can be performed. If labour does not begin within a specified time after ARM, then a Syntocinon infusion should be commenced.

Resist the temptation to ARM too early as the cervix is less likely to dilate, making a caesarean section more likely. The rationale for not continuing to give prostaglandins to a woman who has a favourable cervix is that there is an increased risk of hyperstimulation.

Sometimes after a complete cycle of prostaglandins the cervix is still unfavourable.

At this point it is important to revisit the following before offering further options:

- the indication for the induction (which may mean that the benefits of induction are fewer than continuing, particularly if continuing increases the chance of a caesarean section)
- the urgency of induction
- the woman's views.

Potential options:

- waiting (and possibly going home) for a period of time and then repeating the cycle of prostaglandins
- cancelling the induction and awaiting spontaneous labour
- performing amniotomy on an unfavourable cervix (if the os is open enough to make this possible)
- performing a caesarean section.

Tips/pitfalls

- An ultrasound to check presentation takes seconds and can be a relatively straightforward introduction to learning to scan.
- If you are inexperienced with cervical assessment then aim for the ones where precise estimation is less vital (e.g. the decision has been made for induction earlier that day, or the cervix was previously assessed and found to be very unfavourable). If possible, avoid the ones where getting it right is essential (e.g. those who have completed a full round of prostaglandins, those where PGs may be given in your unit but would be avoided if at all possible – e.g. previous caesarean section, high parity) until you are more experienced.
- Big units may have an 'amniotomy waiting list' for women whose cervixes are favourable and are waiting for capacity on the labour ward. Be sure to liaise closely with the labour ward coordinator and your seniors to ensure this is prioritized appropriately.
- Prostaglandins. Check the label for the one you are giving. They should generally be inserted into the posterior fornix of the vagina and not into the cervix (which would put the woman at increased risk of hyperstimulation).

Labour ward emergencies

General principles

Labour ward emergencies, which despite the name occasionally also occur elsewhere, are truly gripping and have a predominantly positive outcome. Occasionally, however, the outcome is devastating for both the patient and their family. Your role in these emergencies will vary depending on your seniority and who else is around, but even as a medical student it is sometimes possible to make a positive contribution. The main details of these emergencies and how to handle them are covered in Chapter 34, so the purpose here is to suggest a practical approach to selected events.

There is sometimes a mismatch between what is trained for and what is needed. You may, for example, not be able to attend a course on advanced management of obstetric emergencies until later on in your training, yet you may be the most experienced obstetrician on site. You may not be offered any training in obstetric emergencies as 'just an F2 (Foundation year 2 doctor)' but could find yourself on call one night with one registrar and two emergencies happening at once. It therefore helps to think, 'If X happened would I know how to manage it?' Never accept a 'you are too junior to be worrying about this' response and do not underestimate how important the skills you bring from dealing with emergencies outside the obstetric setting can be. Equally, however, remember how capable some experienced midwives can be in dealing with obstetric emergencies and do not be afraid to ask them for help.

A first principle of emergencies is to take measures to actively avoid them happening at all possible. Your role as a junior may be to politely but clearly alert your seniors and colleagues to any potential risk that may have been overlooked, for instance, 'Are we aware that this woman we are about to induce has had three previous caesarean sections?' Other obvious examples include ensuring active management of the third stage of labour is recommended to every woman, as it substantially reduces the risk of postpartum haemorrhage (PPH), and correct delivery of the placenta by controlled cord traction, supporting the uterus using the non-dominant hand, and pulling with just the right amount of traction to minimize the risk of uterine inversion.

There are plenty of grey area examples, and some senior colleagues may disagree with each other, sometimes passionately. Examples might be with suspected fetal macrosomia, especially in mothers with diabetes, and whether they should be delivered by elective caesarean section to remove the risk of shoulder dystocia or whether it is appropriate to induce or augment someone with a previous caesarean due to the increased risk of uterine rupture. This can put you into a potentially challenging position, especially if you are delivering the news to the couple. The woman may have a obstetric management plan that the on-call team is uncomfortable with, or there may be a handover between teams with differing views. If you ask questions politely your seniors will often be open, while professional, about why they hold a particular view. It is a great learning opportunity to mould the way you will practice in what may well remain grey clinical areas.

A second principle is to be as prepared as possible for emergency scenarios and know how to most effectively manage them. This involves knowing not just the principles of how to manage the emergency, but also knowing where things are, who can do what, and who to call in your unit. On your first day, think about checking how to fully open the doors so that the bed can be taken out to the operating theatre, where the light switches, clock and gloves are, how to raise and lower the bed, and how to pull the bottom off the bed. Find out where the forceps/ventouse trolley is, the defibrillator trolley, the haemostatic PPH balloons, cannulas, fluids and uterotonic drugs are kept. If any of the equipment, particularly the haemostatic PPH balloons, are different from those you are used to then ask to take one to familiarize yourself with it; being familiar with a piece of equipment is probably worth the cost of a wasted piece of disposable equipment. Also find out about the system for emergency calls and what commands are recognized, for example an 'obstetric medical emergency' may call a medical team in addition to the usual obstetric team, whereas a 'major obstetric haemorrhage' may alert the blood bank instead. Check the quickest routes around the department; to the operating theatre, to casualty and to where the perimortem caesarean section knife is. Ensure you have the contact bleeps and phone numbers for your senior and if appropriate their senior in case you cannot get your immediate senior in an emergency. It is best to have the contact numbers and preference (home/mobile/page) yourself if your senior is on call from home, as this allows you or a colleague to call them directly straight away, thus allowing the switchboard operators to get on with alerting all others in an emergency.

When the emergency bleep or buzzer goes, look at the clock and note the time, your concept of time will disappear during the emergency. If it is your bleep, listen carefully to where the emergency is; it is easy to forget with the adrenaline, and head straight there. As you enter a labour ward room turn on the lights, if they are not already on, and put on a pair of non-sterile gloves. If not obvious, then ask what the emergency is. Your actions from here will depend on who is in the room and the nature of the emergency. If you are not leading the emergency then always clarify instructions when you are given them and let the person know when you have done their request. Always speak up clearly if you feel something important has been missed, even if it appears obvious. For example, a lack of experience in maternity may mean you are the only person in the room to have the perspective to see that the woman having the massive PPH has stopped breathing and is going blue while the entire team are focused on the 'bottom end'. It might feel uncomfortable at the time but it will feel more uncomfortable afterwards if you know you could have contributed to avoiding an adverse incident, but you did not speak up.

If you witness the start of the emergency then you will need to push the emergency buzzer and then call or ask someone else to call the emergency number. There is sometimes a tendency not to call the emergency number if everyone appears to already be there, but there will often be someone you have not thought of – theatres or porters, for example. You may need to call your consultant at home to come in. Try to ask someone experienced, but available, to call, such as a senior midwife. Make the message succinct, for example: 'Sandra, please could you call Mr Smith at home on his mobile and ask him to come in urgently. Advise him that we are going ahead with a category 1 primary caesarean section for suspected abruption in room 3, and I would like him to be in for potential PPH and complications encountered after delivery. Can you let me know when you have done that please? Thanks.' This explains clearly what is going on and what you need, or do not need, from the consultant. It clearly asks them to attend and is short enough for the person that you are asking to make the call to remember. In some cases, for instance where there is more complex information to pass on, it may be best to call your consultant yourself. Be practical – you could do this on speaker phone while scrubbing up or ask someone to hold the phone to your ear while you are scrubbing. For example: 'Mr Smith, it is Bob your junior registrar and it is 4 a.m. I need you to come in please. Jane Evans, the senior registrar, is carrying out a category 1 caesarean section on an obese woman, and I have an ongoing atonic PPH of 1500 mL at a different caesarean section. I am going through the necessary steps, but will need help if unsuccessful.' This immediately orientates the consultant from sleep, tells them why you are calling for help, why you are calling them specifically, and gives a clear request for what you would like them to do – and it takes around 15 seconds.

Be aware that true emergency scenarios can occasionally require acts that would usually be considered wholly unreasonable. You may be effectively asking a scrub nurse to rush through counts and allow corners to be cut on sterility and cleanliness rituals of their theatre, even occasionally allowing people to operate in their outdoor clothes. The anaesthetist may be giving a general anaesthetic to a patient moments after meeting them. You may find yourself performing a forceps delivery on a patient with no analgesia. All of these can have adverse consequences and must therefore be justified with the information you have at the time. Never intentionally oversell the urgency of something to your colleagues. It could be unforgivable in the event of an adverse outcome. Equally, while the theatre team and anaesthetists will all be familiar with the urgency of some situations, such as fetal bradycardia, especially where it can be heard via a monitor, the urgency may need to be clearly explained and communicated in rarer, more unfamiliar, situations. Good communication is key.

If you are junior and have been rotating through casualty and medical jobs and have attended advanced life-support courses then in the event of a maternal collapse or cardiac arrest you will have a distinct strength over others until the anaesthetist arrives. The 'ABC' approach will come naturally and that you will have recently performed CPR in real life is an advantage. It is likely to have been many years since most of those working on the labour ward, with the exception of the anaesthetist, have performed CPR in real life and drills can only ameliorate this to some extent. Do not be afraid to step up in this uncommon obstetric emergency. Remember left lateral displacement of the uterus and commence perimortem section, or alert someone else to, at around 4 min after a witnessed arrest.

Fetal bradycardia and how to manage it

Most fetal bradycardias resolve spontaneously with no obvious precipitating cause, but when it continues urgent delivery is indicated. While the formal definition is of a reduced fetal heart rate for more than 3 min, most midwives would start manoeuvres, such as moving the mother into the left lateral position to reduce sort of aorto venous pressure, after 1 min and then press the emergency buzzer after 2 min.

How much of the following you would do depends again on your seniority, but you would be expected to deal with these situations relatively independently from an early stage in training. Consider bringing the portable scanner with you on your way to the delivery room. On arrival, ensure that the woman is in the left lateral position. Explain that this situation usually resolves, but that if it does not, her baby will need to be delivered urgently and that is why everyone around her is moving fast. Establish the situation briefly from her midwife, particularly if you are not familiar with the patient, in order to establish the likely resilience of the fetus ask yourself: 'How imminent is delivery?', 'Is labour pre-term?', 'Is there suspected fetal growth restriction?' and 'Are any challenges expected if a caesarean section is required?'

A brief assessment might include quickly confirming the fetal heart rate with an ultrasound scan if it is in the room, but this can be challenging, for instance with obese patients or during contractions. Next ask about pain (consider uterine rupture or abruption) and palpate the uterus (checking uterine tone and fetal size). Perform a VE and, if the fetal heart (FH) is still low and the cervix not fully dilated, insert an indwelling catheter to save time in theatre. Pain between contractions, easily palpable fetal parts and high disengaged presenting part in a woman with previous caesarean section are suspicious for uterine rupture (p. 334, transfer immediately to theatre for rapid delivery). A hard uterus with severe pain and, usually, bleeding is suspicious of abruption (again transfer immediately to theatre for rapid delivery). If the cord is palpably prolapsed and not fully dilated, push the head up off the cord, sit on the bed, ask the midwife to throw a blanket over the patient for dignity if one is immediately available and transfer straight to theatre. Swap places with a midwife when you get there so that you can scrub, ensuring they too keep the head off the cord.

If you do not find a cause but the fetal bradycardia has not resolved, transfer to theatre anyway. Many units will discuss having the patient into the operating theatre 10 min or so after the fetal heart rate dropped and the baby delivered by 15 min, but in some situations, it would be desirable to be quicker than this while in others it would not be possible to be this quick. A woman undergoing induction for significant suspected fetal growth restriction at 36 weeks, for example, who has had a concerning CTG for the past 30 min prior to the bradycardia, probably has a compromised fetus already. There is real urgency here and it would be sensible to alert theatre immediately and transfer her as soon as you have examined her, letting the anaesthetist and theatre staff that know that you are concerned and really need to deliver quickly. A parous woman at 40 weeks with a normal size baby and relatively quick labour so far, on the other hand, who is currently at 9 cm dilated and has a normal CTG, may be about to deliver and it would be reasonable to wait a little longer before transfer, though still alerting the team to stand by.

If the bradycardia persists and the woman is fully dilated, the decision is then whether to undertake a forceps or ventouse delivery, or await spontaneous delivery. It is not uncommon to get fetal bradycardias in otherwise straightforward rapid labours and in time you will come to get a feel for these cases: waiting a short time is reasonable, but preparation for delivery can still be arranged as back-up. A Kiwi ventouse may be especially useful in these cases. In cases where there is a clear suspected cause for the fetal bradycardia and particularly when an instrumental delivery may be more challenging, e.g. a primigravida who has been fully dilated for a while, a choice will need to be made as to the quickest way you (or the most senior practitioner on site) can deliver in this scenario. Sometimes this will be by caesarean section, even if fully dilated.

While transferring to the operating theatre, briefly seek verbal consent for the procedure and consent to explain the outcomes to the woman's partner or any family present while she is recovering. Document the verbal consent later

– never delay to obtain written consent. Communicate with the anaesthetist briefly, but politely, the indication and urgency, and whether there has been any suggestion of pre-eclampsia.

As you arrive in the operating theatre, brief the team succinctly on the case, and if no precipitating cause has been found, it is worth rechecking the fetal heart. If it is still bradycardic, alert everyone to continue to category 1 caesarean section. If the fetal heart has returned to baseline, instruct all to just pause for one moment. Here is a situation needing some judgement. Generally, if the fetal heart goes straight down again proceed with a category 1 caesarean section. If it stays normal then the usual course of events would be to proceed to a spinal and category 2 caesarean section, which has a lower risk to the patient of failed airway than general anaesthetic. In some cases, however, when labour has been progressing well, the CTG was otherwise normal and there was no precipitating cause, then returning to the labour ward may be an option, even if it does mean reversing your decision.

Presuming that a general anaesthetic is going ahead, check that the patient is already catheterized and then scrub quickly. Ask for the sponges, holders and prep the patient while the scrub nurse is preparing their trolley and before the anaesthetist intubates. Voices may occasionally be loud, and it is courteous to call for quiet as the anaesthetist is about to intubate. Then, with their say so, quickly drape and commence the procedure.

While fast entry is important, do take care, especially in second or third caesarean sections, and ask yourself if it is really worth substantially increasing a risk of bowel or bladder injury to reduced delivery time by 30 seconds. Always remember to thank the theatre team and stop for a few moments after delivery.

Shoulder dystocia

This is a very important labour ward emergency, and the life of the baby is truly in immediate danger. The manoeuvres are described in Chapter 34. Learn them. Training prior to being the most experienced person on site in a unit is a challenge. It is unlikely that any of the simulation models available to you are of high enough fidelity to give a realistic feel for the internal manoeuvres and it takes a brave senior colleague to sit and supervise while they watch you perform them in real life. The best one can do is to learn the drills well and discuss with experienced midwives and senior colleagues the difficulties of doing them in practice. Many find the McRoberts position, followed by removing the posterior arm, the most effective initial management plan. Always remove the bottom of the bed before performing the internal manoeuvres and, if they are not succeeding, ask an experienced midwife to try: they may well have done this more often than you. As you deliver the baby it is worth saying something out loud like 'baby facing window'. Medicolegally it will be very important to document whether

the left or right shoulder was anterior, and in the heat of the moment, nobody will have any chance of working out right from left and remembering. Something simple like the above will help with accurate documentation at the end.

Impacted fetal head at caesarean section

An impacted 'stuck' fetal head at caesarean section can be very difficult to deliver. It is worth thinking about this situation even if you are only assisting at a caesarean section as senior back-up may be off site. It is well worth any trainee learning how to 'push up' vaginally even if obstetrics is not your career intention.

Impaction most often happens in advanced labour, frequently when the baby is in an occipitoposterior (OP) position. Anticipate the scenario by always performing a VE immediately before scrubbing for every unplanned caesarean section, unless very urgent. If an impacted head is anticipated you can insert a disimpacting balloon (if available), brief the team and call for senior help from off site if needed. Consider having tocolytics available, and brief the midwife to prepare for a potential push up on the fetal head.

A low operating table or standing on a stool for delivery can be of help.

If it is not possible to deliver the head once the uterus is opened, call for senior help, relax your hand briefly and wait for any contractions to stop (your hand will fatigue quickly otherwise). The aim is then to get under the fetal head with your hand, flex it and lift it out. If not successful, then ask for a 'push' from below: the knees of the woman will be flexed to allow access and the midwife or your assistant can then push the baby's head upwards with at least three fingers. An alternative approach is to try to extract the baby by the breech (this can be surprisingly successful); it may be easier with a tocolytic and the patient in a head-down position. If your hand becomes fatigued you could change table sides and try with your non-dominant hand. After delivery, the area close to the incision in the uterus will usually be torn, and repairing this with a fatigued hand can be difficult; senior help may be available by that point.

After an emergency

After any emergency, it is always important to document carefully, debrief the patient and her partner, and complete any incident forms required. When the outcome has not gone well, try to support your colleagues who will usually have done their best, but may not be feeling they have done so. Try not to jump to conclusions or apportion blame – there is often no blame to be apportioned.

If you feel you have made a mistake, do not try to cover it up, but be honest: this is the only way that you and any others involved will learn. Many things may also have been done well, and there may be lessons to be learned from this too. The only real mistake is the one from which we learn nothing.

Questions

Gynaecology Multiple-choice questions (MCQs)

1. Sarah, aged 17, presents to the gynaecology clinic with her mother. She is concerned that, unlike her friends, she has not yet started having periods. Sarah's mother comments that her daughter has always been a 'late developer', and she is the shortest of her friend group. It also becomes clear that Sarah has not yet developed pubic or axillary hair. You notice in her notes that Sarah is under gastroenterology review for monitoring of inflammatory bowel syndrome, which was recently diagnosed. Which method of investigation is likely to provide a diagnosis?
   a. Plasma FSH, LH, oestriol, prolactin, thyroid function tests.
   b. Karyotype.
   c. X-ray for bone age.
   d. Cranial CT or MRI scan.
   e. None, this is likely to be an example of constitutional delay.

2. Lucy is a 16 year-old girl who has been referred to gynaecology by her GP. She describes a one-year history of cyclical lower abdominal pain and bloating. On examination she has appropriate secondary sexual characteristics and her BMI is 17.5. Her mother's menarche occurred at age 13. You realise that Lucy has not started having periods. What is the most likely cause of this woman's primary amenorrhoea?
   a. Hypogonadotrophic hypogonadism.
   b. Kallman's syndrome.
   c. Congenital absence of the uterus.
   d. Androgen insensitivity syndrome.
   e. Imperforate hymen.

3. Beth and James visit the infertility clinic together. They have been trying to conceive for 13 months and have not succeeded. They are both 26 years old, are medically well and are non- smokers. Beth's BMI is 20 and James' is 24. Her hormone profile is reported as normal and the mid-luteal progesterone confirms that she is ovulating. James' sperm analysis is normal. What is the next most appropriate step in managing this couples' subfertility?
   a. Refer for IVF.
   b. Request hysterosalpingogram.
   c. Refer for ICSE.
   d. Prescribe LH/FSH injections.
   e. Reassure and follow up in 6 months.

4. A 32 year-old woman presents to the infertility clinic. She and her partner have been trying to achieve a second pregnancy for 12 months without success. Their first child is now 4 years old, and this was an uncomplicated pregnancy. She did, however, require to go to theatre postpartum for evacuation of retained placental tissue. She describes that her periods have become very spaced out, and she is worried that the evacuation may have damaged her uterus. On investigation, her early follicular hormone profile is as follows:

LH	35
FSH	40
Oest	120
Test	0.83
PRL	325

   What is the most appropriate treatment for this woman with regard to achieving a pregnancy?
   a. Clomifene for 5 days from day 2 of cycle.
   b. Bromocriptine.
   c. IVF.
   d. Consideration of oocyte donation.
   e. Hysteroscopy and IUD insertion for 3 months.

5. Katherine is a 26-year old science graduate. She has suffered from endometriosis for the past 2 years, originally confirmed by diagnostic laparosopy. As she also wished for contraception, she was started on the COCP. This has not, however, fully relieved her symptoms of pelvic pain and dyspareunia. In her continued management, which of the following is not an option for second line treatment?
   a. Medroxyprogesterone acetate.
   b. GnRH analogue.
   c. Laparoscopic diathermy destruction.
   d. Total laparoscopic hysterectomy.
   e. Ulipristal Acetate.

6. Jane presents to her GP to discuss options for contraception. Which of the following details in her history would signify an absolute contraindication to prescribing the oral contraceptive pill?
   a. 38-year-old woman, smoking 10 cigarettes per day.
   b. 26-year-old woman, with a history of ectopic pregnancy.
   c. 20-year-old woman, who has had previous migraine with aura.
   d. 38-year-old woman, breast feeding at 8 weeks postpartum.
   e. 36-year-old woman, BMI 32.

7. Laura presents to A&E with a 2-hour history of vaginal bleeding and lower abdominal pain. She is a 27 year-old primigravida, currently 7 weeks pregnant. On examination her abdomen is soft and non-tender. Abdominal ultrasound shows a 10 mm intrauterine fetal pole. Speculum examination reveals blood in the vagina and the os is poorly visualised. Which of the following classifications of miscarriage does this represent?
   a. Missed miscarriage.
   b. Threatened miscarriage.
   c. Delayed miscarriage.
   d. Septic miscarriage.
   e. Complete miscarriage.

8. A 23-year-old woman presents to the clinic requesting termination of pregnancy. After appropriate counselling, she decides to proceed with a medical abortion in the knowledge that the pregnancy is currently at 8 weeks gestation. Which of the following drug regimens is appropriate for her management?
   a. Mifepristone, and misoprostol at 24–48 hours.
   b. Feticide intervention and mifepristone and misoprostol at 24–48 hours.
   c. Misoprostol, and mifepristone at 24–48 hours.
   d. Levonorgestrel.
   e. Ulipristal acetate.

9. Katie, aged 19, presents to the sexual health clinic concerned about abnormal vaginal discharge. She describes it as 'milky white' in colour, and she has noticed a 'fishy' odour. She reveals that 3 weeks ago she had unprotected sexual intercourse with a one-off partner and is therefore concerned that she may have an STI. On further questioning, she describes no urinary symptoms, skin changes or abdominal pain; she has, however, noticed episodes of post-coital bleeding over the past year. For contraception, Katie has used the COCP for 3 years. Which of the following pathogens is the most likely cause for this discharge?
   a. Candida albicans.
   b. Chlamydia trachomatis.
   c. Gardnerella vaginalis.
   d. Neisseria gonorrhoea.
   e. Group B streptococcus.

10. Jessica, a 25 year-old woman, presents to her GP describing intense vulval itch over the past 7 days. She was prompted to consult after noticing the appearance of multiple small vulval 'blisters' that morning, which woke her from her sleep due to intense pain and discomfort. She has no relevant past medical history, and no previous episodes such as this. She has one regular male partner who she has been in a relationship with for 2 years. Given the likely diagnosis, which of the following treatment regimes is appropriate for Jessica?
    a. Oral aciclovir for 5 days.
    b. Oral azithromycin stat dose.
    c. Topical clotrimazole pessaries.
    d. Oral metronidazole for 5 days.
    e. Oral azithromycin stat dose and IM ceftriaxone stat dose.

11. Lisa is a 34-year old para 3+0 who presents to gynaecology with heavy menstrual bleeding. Her obstetric history is uncomplicated, but since the birth of her youngest child 2 years ago she has had to use both pads and tampons to manage her periods. On one occasion she describes leaking onto her clothes. Abdominal examination reveals an enlarged, non-tender, bulky uterus. Transvaginal ultrasound scan demonstrates 2 submucous masses, homogenous in nature. Speculum examination is normal. In the management of this condition, after which treatment option is future pregnancy absolutely contraindicated?
    a. Hysteroscopic resection.
    b. GnRH analogues.
    c. Endometrial ablation.
    d. Uterine artery embolization.
    e. Myomectomy.

12. Claire, aged 25, presents to A&E with a 1-day history of lower abdominal pain and vaginal bleeding. Her LMP was 6 weeks ago. She describes that the pain comes and goes and is focused in the right iliac fossa. Occasionally she is experiencing a sharp pain in her right shoulder, however, she things she may have slept badly on it last night. The bleeding is 'dark' and 'like a period'. One examination her BP is 110/70, HR 100, she is exquisitely tender in the RIF and is guarding with rebound tenderness. A urine hCG is positive and serum hCG is 5500 IU/ml. However, on transvaginal scan the uterus is empty, with 'free fluid' in the right adnexa. What is the most appropriate definitive management for this patient?
    a. Medical management: methotrexate.
    b. Surgical management: laparoscopic salpingectomy.
    c. Surgical management: laparotomy and salpingectomy.
    d. Surgical management: laparoscopic hysterectomy.
    e. Conservative management: observation.

13. Mrs Roberts presents to her GP wishing to discuss options for hormone replacement therapy. She is 52 and is experiencing frequent and unpleasant vasomotor symptoms. With regard to counselling women on HRT, which of the following statements is false?
    a. HRT is always prescribed as a combination regimen of oestrogen and progestogen.
    b. If given vaginally, HRT is unlikely to help with vaso-motor symptoms.
    c. Oral HRT has a more beneficial impact on lipid profiles that parenteral HRT.
    d. There is an increased risk of venous thromboembolic disease in the first year of HRT.
    e. Liver disease, thromboembolic disease and history of recurrent venous thromboembolism are contraindications to HRT.

14. Mrs Douglas is a 65 year-old para 4, who presents to the gynaecology clinic describing a feeling of something coming down vaginally, which has developed over the last 3 months. Her children were all born vaginally: the first 3 were uncomplicated however during her last labour she suffered a 3rd degree perineal tear. On examination, there is a grade 2 rectocele and 2nd degree descent of the cervix. With regard to the anatomical attachments of the uterus, which of the following structures provides the greatest degree of support?
    a. Round ligaments.
    b. Ovarian ligaments.
    c. Uterosacral ligaments.
    d. Cardinal ligaments.
    e. Broad ligament.

15. Mrs Richards is a 48-year old woman who presents to urogynaecology. For the past year, she has found herself 'running to the toilet' an increasing number of times each day. Her GP asked her to complete a bladder chart, and on reviewing this it is clear that she voids around 12 times each day. On average, she passes 50 ml with each void. Mrs Richards describes a feeling of 'constant urge'. Numerous urine dipstick tests in primary care have shown no evidence of infection. Given the likely diagnosis, which of the following is the first line treatment?
    a. Supervised pelvic floor exercises.
    b. Solifenacin.
    c. Bladder retraining and lifestyle advice.
    d. Intravesicular botulinum toxin.
    e. Surgical colposuspension.

16. June is a 52-year-old shop assistant who presents to gynaecology via an urgent referral from her GP. She is nulliparous and is currently having regular periods with no perimenopausal symptoms. June believes she may have developed irritable bowel syndrome as she has recently developed irregular abdominal pain and is subjectively bloated. She is unsure of the necessity of a gynaecology referral. In the clinic, a transvaginal scan reveals a multiloculated cyst on the left ovary, approximately 4 cm in diameter. Which of the following factors are used to determine the risk of malignancy in this patient group?
    a. Ultrasound score, symptom score, CA 125.
    b. Ultrasound score, CT score, CA125.
    c. Ultrasound score, menopausal status, serum hCG.
    d. Ultrasound score, menopausal status, CA125.
    e. Ultrasound score x CT score x serum hCG.

17. Mrs Baxter is a 75-year-old retired nurse. She is referred urgently to gynaecology with a 1-week history of vaginal bleeding, and she is extremely concerned. She has a history of PCOS, is nulliparous and is not on HRT. Her menopause occurred aged 57 years. Transvaginal scan demonstrates an endometrial thickness of 6 mm. Speculum examination shows some evidence of atrophic vaginitis. What is the next step in Mrs Baxter's management?
    a. Reassure and prescribe topical oestrogen cream.
    b. Perform endometrial pipelle biopsy.
    c. List for total laparoscopic hysterectomy and bilateral salpingoophorectomy.
    d. Request urgent MRI pelvic.
    e. Take blood for serum CA125.

18. Joanne, a 65-year-old schoolteacher is referred to gynaecology with an 8-week history of worsening vulval itch. She is a para 2 with uncomplicated obstetric and gynaecological history. Joanne tells you she has been commenced on Vitamin B12 injections 'for anaemia'. On examination of her vulva the skin appears generally thin, with areas of white discolouration. What is the most likely diagnosis?
    a. Lichen planus.
    b. Psoriasis.
    c. Lichen sclerosus.
    d. Candidal infection.
    e. Contact dermatitis.

19. Alex is a 24-year-old student who receives a referral to colposcopy after the result of her recent smear showed 'severe dyskaryosis'. Which of the following would be least associated with an increased risk of cervical cancer?
    a. Smoking.
    b. HPV serotype 6.
    c. HPV serotype 18.
    d. Prolonged use of the COCP.
    e. HPV serotype 16.

20. Jennifer, aged 28, presents to early pregnancy triage with vaginal bleeding and lower abdominal pain. She is nulliparous and currently 8 weeks pregnant. She also reveals that she has been struggling with morning sickness, much worse than she had expected. Speculum examination shows a closed cervical os, with a small pool of blood in the posterior fornix. On palpation, the uterus feels large. Abdominal ultrasound shows structurally abnormal trophoblastic and fetal tissue. A diagnosis of molar pregnancy is made and Jennifer is listed for surgical evacuation. Given the clinical picture, what is the likely karyotype of this mole?
    a. 46 XY.
    b. 46 XX.
    c. 69 XXY.
    d. 45 XO.
    e. 47 XXY.

Obstetrics Multiple-choice questions (MCQs)

1. Which of the following is neither a relative nor absolute contraindication to induction of labour?
   a. Previous LUSCS.
   b. Bishop's score of 7.
   c. Low-lying placenta.
   d. Previous precipitate labour.
   e. Grand multi-parity.

2. Which of the following is false about syntocinon?
   a. It can be used for augmentation of labour as well as induction.
   b. It is more effective than vaginal PGs in achieving vaginal delivery within 24h.
   c. Continuous CTG monitoring is recommended following syntocinon infusion.
   d. It should be used with caution in a woman with a previous LUSCS.
   e. It reduces the duration of the 1st stage of labour compared to ARM alone.

3. Which of the following is true regarding breech presentation?
   a. Should always be managed with a caesarean section.
   b. Is more likely in singleton pregnancies.
   c. It is associated with placenta praevia.
   d. It is associated with polyhydramnios and not oligohydramnios.
   e. Most are fixed or footling at term, rather than frank (or extended).

4. With regard to the process of ECV (external cephalic version), which of the following is true:
   a. Should be attempted at 34w in nulliparous women.
   b. Can be attempted in the case of placenta praevia.
   c. Should not be attempted if membranes have already ruptured.
   d. Is usually done in the community setting.
   e. Requires CTG, USS and fetal blood sampling before and after.

5. Which of the following is NOT an absolute contraindication to ECV?
   a. Placenta praevia.
   b. Recent antepartum haemorrhage.
   c. Ruptured membranes.
   d. Morbid maternal obesity.
   e. Major uterine anomaly e.g. fibroids.

6. Which of the following is false about occipitoposterior (OP) position?
   a. Back pain is more common with OP position.
   b. The occiput may rotate to OA and deliver normally.
   c. 3rd and 4th degree tears are more common with OP position.
   d. The mother is more likely to request an epidural.
   e. Haig-Ferguson forceps or rotational ventouse can be used to rotate to OA.

7. Which of these is not required for instrumental delivery?
   a. An empty bladder.
   b. Adequate analgesia.
   c. Ruptured membranes.
   d. Head palpable abdominally.
   e. Cervix fully dilated.

8. Which of the following statements are false about obstetric forceps?
   a. Wrigley's forceps can be used for difficult caesarean sections.
   b. Haig-Ferguson's forceps have a locking mechanism.
   c. Kielland's forceps are rotational forceps.
   d. Ventouse is preferable to forceps in very pre-term deliveries.
   e. Wrigley's forceps are low-cavity forceps.

9. In women with pre-eclampsia, which of the following is NOT an indication for admission?
   a. BP > 150/110 mmHg.
   b. BP > 140/90 mmHg with proteinuria +++.
   c. Headaches and visual disturbance.
   d. Reduced fetal movements.
   e. Postural hypotension.

10. Which of the following drugs should NOT be used in the acute management of pre-eclampsia?
    a. Labetalol
    b. Hydralazine
    c. Magnesium sulphate
    d. Nifedipine
    e. Methyldopa.

11. Which of the following is true concerning CTG monitoring?
    a. Early decelerations are pathological and indicate fetal distress.
    b. Shallow late decelerations may be more worrying than deep ones.
    c. Continuous CTG should be routinely performed in primigravid mothers.
    d. CTG has poor sensitivity but good specificity for assessing pathological patterns.
    e. CTG should be performed following a fetal blood sample result of pH = 7.01.

12. Which of the following is not routinely included in the booking visit?
   a. Past psychiatric history.
   b. HIV testing.
   c. Rhesus status.
   d. Chlamydia testing.
   e. Urine sampling for asymptomatic bacteriuria.

13. Which of the following does gestational diabetes NOT increase the risk of? The fetus of a mother who develops gestational diabetes mellitus is not at increased risk of:
   a. Fetal anomalies such as sacral agenesis.
   b. Macrosomia and shoulder dystocia.
   c. Fetal growth restriction.
   d. Pre-eclampsia.
   e. Stillbirth.

14. Which of the following is true concerning medical disorders of pregnancy?
   a. The antiepileptic drug lamotrigine should not be prescribed in pregnancy as it is teratogenic.
   b. Women at high risk of VTE should be given prophylactic unfractionated heparin to reduce the risk of thromboembolism.
   c. Connective tissue diseases such as SLE tend to be less severe during pregnancy because of the dampening down of the immune system.
   d. Gliclazide is preferable to metformin to control diabetes in pregnancy.
   e. Obstetric cholestasis usually presents after 30w gestation.

15. Which of the following statements are true of prenatal diagnosis?
   a. CVS has a higher overall rate of miscarriage than amniocentesis.
   b. Fetuses with Down's Syndrome are likely to have a low β-hCG and a high PAPP-A.
   c. Amniocentesis is usually carried out after 10 weeks gestation.
   d. Karyotyping can accurately diagnose Fragile X syndrome.
   e. High α-FP is diagnostic of spina bidifa.

16. Which of the following is true of Rhesus disease in pregnancy?
   a. Rh+ mothers with Rh- babies are at risk.
   b. The Keilhauer test is used to test for the presence of the Rh antigen.
   c. Polyhydramnios can indicate rhesus isoimmunisation.
   d. Anti-D should be administered at 28 and 32 weeks.
   e. Most of the population are Rh-.

Case-based questions

1. An 18-year-old primigravid woman is attending her booking scan. She has been experiencing intense morning sickness and has some painless PV bleeding. On examination, her uterus is large for dates, and abdominal USS reveals a "snowstorm" appearance. What is the most likely karyotype of the pregnancy tissue?
   a. 69XXX
   b. 45X0
   c. 47XX
   d. 46XX
   e. 47XXY

2. You are an on-call registrar in obstetrics and gynaecology. A 28-year-old primigravid woman with diabetes is at 41+ weeks, and is giving birth in the labour ward. The midwife calls you urgently to the delivery room and tells you that they are "having problems delivering the shoulders". Which of the following is true of the diagnosis and management of the suspected condition?
   a. Restitution of the head is a worrying sign.
   b. 'Turtlenecking' indicates the shoulders are likely to come naturally.
   c. Episiotomy can help to free space for the shoulders to deliver.
   d. Zavanelli's manoeuvre (flexion and abduction of the hips) can resolve over 80% of cases.
   e. None of the above.

3. Thanks to good teamwork between yourself and the midwives, the woman from the previous question delivers a healthy baby boy. After delivery of the placenta 15 min later, however, she continues to trickle blood. The midwife estimates she has lost around 1.5 L during and immediately following delivery. Which of the following courses of action is in the correct order for managing PPH (not including pharmacological options)?
   a. Abdominal massage → examination under anaesthetic → bimanual compression → balloon tamponade → B Lynch suture.
   b. Examination under anaesthetic → abdominal massage → bimanual compression → B Lynch suture → balloon tamponade.
   c. Bimanual compression → abdominal massage → examination under anaesthetic → Balloon tamponade → B Lynch suture.
   d. Balloon tamponade → bimanual compression → abdominal massage → B Lynch suture → examination under anaesthetic.
   e. B Lynch suture → examination under anaesthetic → balloon tamponade → abdominal compression → bimanual compression.

4. A 30-year-old 30+ woman comes in for a growth scan. You measure the abdominal circumference on the scan and find that it is below the 10th centile. What is the next appropriate course of action?
   a. Reassure and see again in 2 weeks.
   b. Arrange induction of labour.
   c. Doppler ultrasound of the umbilical artery.
   d. Perform a CTG.
   e. Arrange an emergency caesarean section.

5. A 26+2 para 2+0 woman presents with regular uterine contractions. On VE the cervix is almost fully effaced. Which of the following measures are not typically used to inhibit pre-term labour and allow time for steroids take effect?
   a. Oxytocin antagonists
   b. Beta-sympathomimetics
   c. Nifedipine
   d. Antibiotics
   e. Cervical cerclage

Answers

Gynaecology MCQ answers

1. B. Karotype. This is likely.

2. E. Imperforate hymen.

3. B. Request hysterosalpingogram.

4. D. This woman has premature ovarian failure, diagnosed by the high LH/FSH, low oestrogen and menstrual symptoms. Her only option for fertility treatment is therefore oocyte donation. Options A to D describe treatment for other causes of subfertility. 'A'= PCOS. 'B'= prolactinoma. 'E'= Asherman's syndrome. The surgical evacuation is a distractor. Many women will have no problems with fertility after these procedures, and women with Asherman's have a normal hormone profile.

5. E. Ulipristal Acetate.

6. C. These contraindications are defined by UKMEC. Other absolute contraindications include: >35 and smoking >15 cigarettes/ day. Breast-feeding until 6 weeks postpartum.

7. B. In complete miscarriage, the uterus would be empty. In a missed miscarriage, which is also referred to as a delayed miscarriage, there would be no symptoms. The woman is stable and therefore unlikely to be septic.

8. A. Feticide intervention is required for late terminations. Mifepristone is always given before misoprostol. Levonorgestrel and ulipristal acetate are used as emergency contraceptives and therefore inappropriate in this context. Levonorgestrel is licenced for use up until 72 hours, and ulipristal until 5 days.

9. C. The student must be able to diagnose this as bacterial vaginosis, despite distractors. The post-coital bleeding in this case is likely to be attributed to a cervical ectopy, in Katie's case due to her use of the COCP. BV is caused by overgrowth of a number of bacteria, mainly Gardnerella vaginalis.

10. A. This is first episode genital herpes infection and therefore 'A' is the most appropriate treatment. 'B' is the treatment for chlamydia infection. 'C' treats candidal infection. 'D' treats BV. 'E' treats gonorrhoea.

11. C. This woman is likely to have fibroids. 'A' to 'E' are all options for the treatment of fibroids, however pregnancy is absolutely contraindicated after endometrial ablation.

12. B. This woman is haemodynamically stable and therefore is suitable for laparoscopic intervention. Her symptoms and ultrasound findings suggest that there is blood in the peritoneal cavity. In a stable patient, depending on scan findings and serum hCG levels, methotrexate is also an option. In a patient who is markedly unstable, for example with a BP of 60/40, laparotomy may be indicted.

13. A. Progestogens are not required in those women who do not have a uterus.

14. D. Cardinal ligaments.

15. C. Mrs Richards likely is suffering from overactive bladder. Answers 'A' and 'E' describe treatment options for stress incontinence. 'B' and 'D' are also treatment options for OAB, however 'C' is first line.

16. D. Risk of malignancy index.

17. B. Perform endometrial pipelle biopsy.

18. C. Lichen sclerosus is associated with other autoimmune conditions such as pernicious anaemia.

19. B. HPV serotypes 16 and 18 are known to be causative in some cervical malignancies. Smoking and prolonged use of the COCP are also recognised as risk factors. HPV 6 is associated with genital warts.

20. C. The presence of a large uterus and intractable morning sickness suggests molar pregnancy. Ultrasound findings of fetal tissue suggest a partial mole rather than a complete molar pregnancy, and this is consistent with a karyotype of 69 XXY. 46 XX is consistent with complete mole. 45 XO is Turner's syndrome and 47 XXY is Kleinfelter's.

Obstetrics MCQ answers

1. B. Bishop's score of 7. This would indicate that the cervix is favourable for induction.

2. B. It is more effective than vaginal PGs in achieving vaginal delivery within 24h. Vaginal PGs are more effective.

3. C. It is associated with placenta praevia. Breech presentations can be delivered vaginally, are more common in multiple pregnancies and are associated with both polyhydramnios (fetus has space to turn around) and oligohydramnios (fetus does not have space to turn back to correction presentation). Most breech presentations are frank at term.

4. C. Should not be attempted if membranes have already ruptured. ECV after membrane rupture is completely contraindicated. In all cases it is an in-patient procedure. Although very safe, it carries the very small risk of antepartum haemorrhage which may require delivery.

5. D. Morbid maternal obesity. Morbid maternal obesity makes ECV difficult, but it is a relative rather than an absolute contraindication.

6. E. Haig-Ferguson forceps or rotational ventouse can be used to rotate to OA.

    Complications such as pain and tears are more common in OP position, and OPs can rotate spontaneously to OA. Haig Ferguson forceps should only be used in OA position. Rotational ventouse or Kielland forceps may be used to rotate to OA.

7. D. Head palpable abdominally. Head palpable abdominally would indicate that the head is not engaged and therefore instrumental delivery would not be appropriate. If required, a caesarean section would need to be performed.

8. D. Ventouse is preferable to forceps in very pre-term deliveries. All are true except 'D'. Ventouse should be avoided in very pre-term deliveries as large haematomas and head deformities are more common.

9. E. Postural hypotension. Pre-eclampsia is associated with high rather than low blood pressure.

10. E. Methyldopa. Methyldopa has a slow onset of action. Caution should be taken in using nifedipine as it interacts with magnesium sulphate.

11. B. Shallow late decelerations may be more worrying than deep ones. Prolonged shallow decelerations can indicate fetal bradycardia which would be an indication for immediate delivery. Early decelerations are considered normal findings. CTGs are not to be routinely performed precisely because of their low specificity – i.e. they can show pathological findings when there is nothing pathological going on. An FBS result of 7.01 is extremely worrying and should prompt immediate delivery.

12. D. Chlamydia testing. Chlamydia testing is only usually performed in selected groups e.g. under 25s. Asymptomatic bacteruria is often forgotten about, but treating this can reduce the risk of pre-term delivery.

13. A. Fetal anomalies such as sacral agenesis. This would be pre-existing diabetes. GDM can be associated with fetal growth restriction as well as macrosomia.

14. E. Obstetric cholestasis usually presents after 30w gestation. Obstetric cholestasis is typically a late complication of labour (mass effect), so 'E' is correct. Sodium valporate, rather than lamotrigine, is teratogenic. SLE is typically more severe during pregnancy, although other auto-immune conditions such as multiple sclerosis tend to be less severe during pregnancy (and may flare up immediately after). Metformin is commonly used to control diabetes in pregnancy.

15. A. CVS has a higher overall rate of miscarriage than amniocentesis. CVS can be carried out an earlier stage than amniocentesis (after 10w compared to after 15w) but does carry a slightly higher risk of miscarriage (1.5–2% compared to 1%), although this may be related to a higher "background pregnancy loss" rate at an earlier gestation. Fragile X is caused by trinucleotide repeats within the FMR1 gene and cannot be seen on karyotyping. α-FP can indicate neural tube defects it is not diagnostic.

16. C. Polyhydramnios can indicate rhesus isoimmunisation. Polyhydramnios results from fetal anaemia caused by immune-mediated destruction of fetal FBCs. The Kielhauer test measures the amount of fetal Hb in the maternal bloodstream and is used to calculate the required dose of Rh anti-D. Anti-D is usually administered prophylactically at 28 and 34 weeks to Rh- mothers with Rh+ fetuses, although most of the population are Rh+.

Case-based answers

1. D. 46XX. 'A' would be a partial mole: a fetus is usually, but not always, present and this is a possible answer, but the complete mole of 'D' is more likely. B is Turner's, C could be Down's, E is Kleinfelter's.

2. E. None of the above. "E" is correct. Failure of restitution and turtle-necking are worrying signs that suggest shoulder dystocia. Episiotomy is NOT used to free space for the shoulders to deliver, but to allow space for a hand to enter and perform manoeuvres; the obstruction in shoulder dystocia is bony and will not be relieved by cutting through soft tissue. The manoeuvre described in "D" is McRoberts. Zavanelli's is used only in extreme cases – the head is pushed back into the uterus so that the fetus can be delivered by caesarean section.

3. C. Bimanual compression → abdominal massage → examination under anaesthetic → Balloon tamponade → B Lynch suture. Abdominal massage is the simplest and least invasive manoeuvre. Bimanual compression is an effective next step, although this is sometimes performed before moving to theatre. Examination under anaesthetic is the next step, to help to determine the cause of the PPH (the four T's: trauma; tone; tissue; thrombin). Balloon tamponade can be used if the PPH is not resolving, and B Lynch is an invasive procedure to be used in extreme cases. Ligation/embolization of the uterine arteries or even hysterectomy may also be considered.

4. C. Doppler ultrasound of the umbilical artery. If the AC is low, it is appropriate to perform a Doppler ultrasound to see the flow through the placenta. This can determine whether there is placental insufficiency. If the end diastolic flow is absent or reserved, this is a worrying sign and requires urgent senior review. At this stage, it is also important to estimate amniotic fluid volume i.e. oligohydramnios or polyhydramnios.

5. D. Antibiotics. Evidence suggests that treating asymptomatic bacteruria can reduce the risk of pre-term labour, and bacterial vaginosis certainly increases the risk. However, antibiotics are not used generally used in the management of pre-term labour itself. A distinction should be made between pre-term labour and PPROM, as antibiotics are used in PPROM to prevent chorioamnionitis.

Index

Page numbers followed by "*f*" indicate figures, "*t*" indicate tables, "*b*" indicate boxes, and "*e*" indicate online content.

G